RESPIRATORY PHYSIOLOGY

Brent Alexander

ALLIED
HEALTH
PRESS

Respiratory Physiology

Author: **Brent Alexander**

Allied Health Press
4164 Lakeshore Road
Burlington ON L7L 1A4
Canada
www.alliedhealthpress.com
Email: orders@arclereducation.com

ISBN: 978-1-77956-809-0

ABOUT THE AUTHOR

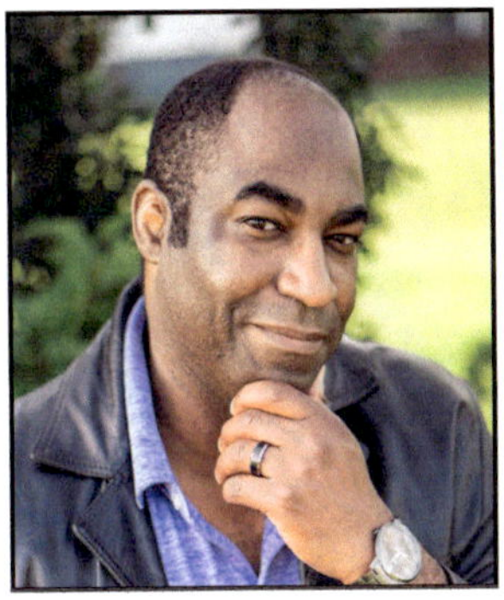

Brent Alexander is a dedicated, senior level, healthcare and life science advisor with over 14 years of medical research and healthcare consulting experience. He is skilled in strategic thinking, data analysis & interpretation, project management, and building relationships. Brent has effectively planned, executed, and evaluated several major medical research projects for organizations such as Suncor Energy Inc., Calgary Flames Hockey Organization, and Own the Podium. Brent has an intrinsic love for science and has expanded on this through gaining academic accolades in maternal/child health and perinatal physiology, as well as in the chronobiological and physiological principles of sleep medicine. Since completing a Masters degree in Medical Science, Brent has previously managed a role as the Clinical Research Coordinator at the Centre for Sleep and Human Performance, a College of Physicians and Surgeons of Alberta, and American Academy of Sleep Medicine accredited sleep centre in Calgary, Alberta. Currently, he holds two positions within Alberta Health Services – _Brent is the Senior Advisor for Public Health, Calgary Zone, providing integration of technology and quality improvement alignment with the clinical operations of immunization and public health programs. He is also a Tissue Specialist with the Southern Alberta Tissue Program where he uses his laboratory experience to expertly assist in the surgical recovery, processing, preservation and distribution of donor tissues that are used for banking, transplantation, and research procedures help improve the quality of life for Albertans. Brent is also an accomplished writer and editor. He has authored and co-authored several abstracts and peer reviewed articles on fever & pregnancy, jet lag & travel fatigue management in elite athletes, and sleep & long-term athletic development (LTAD). In his down time, Brent enjoys staying active through sports and enjoying the outdoors with his wife and son.

Brief Table of Contents

Detailed Table of Contents

CHAPTER 6

Diffusion of Gases in the Lungs 159

CHAPTER 7

Pulmonary Circulation 189

CHAPTER 10

CHAPTER 11

CHAPTER 12

Non-Respiratory Functions of the Lung 343

CHAPTER 13

Respiratory Adjustments in Exercise 375

CHAPTER 14

CHAPTER 15

LIST OF FIGURES

LIST OF TABLES

PREFACE

Respiratory physiology involves how oxygen enters and exits the lungs, how gases diffuse through the alveolar–capillary membrane, and how oxygen and carbon dioxide are transported in the blood between tissues. This is the physical mechanics of breathing, chemical principles governing gas behavior at varying pressures, and the complex way in which the body senses and compensates for changes in the concentrations of oxygen and carbon dioxide. Understanding these processes provides a basic understanding of healthy human function and the basis upon which abnormalities in disease can be interpreted.

In general, respiratory physiology bridges the gap between anatomy, physics, chemistry, and cellular biology to explain how ventilation, gas exchange, and circulation cooperate to achieve homeostasis. The intricate interdependence of lung structure and function allows for efficient oxygen absorption and carbon dioxide expulsion, irrespective of constantly changing demands of different activities and environments. Knowledge of this discipline is not only important for physiologists, but also for clinicians who diagnose and treat lung diseases, biomedical engineers who design ventilators and monitoring devices, and researchers who design new therapies.

Respiratory Physiology offers a broad overview of the fundamental principles governing breathing, gas transport, and ventilation control. The book synthesizes basic concepts with modern discoveries, guiding readers through each significant area in a concise and systematic manner. Emphasizing normal function and common pathological conditions, the book enables one to fully appreciate how the respiratory apparatus adjusts for everyday life, exercise, and through a diseased state.

Chapter 1 provides an overview of the respiratory system, describing its anatomical components—from the nose to the alveoli—and how airway morphology and lung architecture facilitate efficient gas transport. You will learn about structural features such as branching airways, the pleural space, and the chest wall, and how changes in these structures influence lung function.

Chapter 2 discusses the mechanism of breathing. It outlines how pressure gradients are established by muscular contraction and how airflow is determined by compliance and resistance. A detailed discussion is provided for the actions of the diaphragm, intercostal muscles, and accessory muscles, as well as the impact of diseases that alter lung elasticity or airway diameter.

Chapter 3 discusses lung volumes and capacities, introducing the concepts of tidal volume, vital capacity (VC), and residual volume. The chapter discusses how spirometry measures these values and how alterations in volumes and capacities are diagnostic findings in conditions such as restrictive lung disease and obstructive airway diseases.

Chapter 4 addresses alveolar ventilation, the definition of dead space, and demonstrates how air breathed in isn't entirely utilized for gas exchange. Experiments demonstrate the differences between minute ventilation and alveolar ventilation, as well as the benefits of equalizing ventilation to perfusion for optimal gas exchange.

Chapter 5 is a treatment of gas laws and pulmonary pressures, consisting of Boyle's law, Charles's law, Dalton's law of partial pressures, and Henry's law of solubility. The chapter also covers the change in intrapulmonary and intrapleural pressures throughout breathing and how these forces move air and maintain alveolar stability.

Chapter 6 covers diffusion of gases within the lungs and how Fick's law is applied to quantify the transport of oxygen and carbon dioxide through the alveolar–capillary barrier. The diffusion rate is discussed in relation to membrane thickness, surface area, and partial pressure differences, illustrated by means of an analogy to disease and healthy conditions.

Chapter 7 describes pulmonary circulation, including the structure of lung vasculature and the low-pressure, high-compliance nature of the lung vasculature. Regulation of pulmonary vascular resistance, the effects of gravity on blood flow distribution, and mechanisms of hypoxic vasoconstriction to maximize ventilation–perfusion matching are included.

Chapter 8 deals with oxygen transport. After a discussion of oxygen binding to hemoglobin and the oxygen–hemoglobin dissociation curve, the chapter goes on to explain how pH, temperature, and 2,3-bisphosphoglycerate shift the curve. It also calculates oxygen content in arterial and mixed venous blood during various physiological conditions.

Chapter 9 analyzes carbon dioxide transport within the blood and illustrates how CO_2 is transported in solution, as bicarbonate, and protein-bound. Particular attention is devoted to the chloride shift, the role of carbonic anhydrase, and acid–base implications of CO_2 transport within the blood.

Chapter 10 discusses the regulation of breathing. Neural circuits in the brainstem, central and peripheral chemoreceptors, and higher centers for modulation of voluntary and emotional control of respiration are considered. Coordination of chemical and neural messages ensures that ventilation is adjusted according to metabolic needs.

Chapter 11 reviews pulmonary function tests (PFTs), with particular focus on methods such as spirometry, plethysmography, and assessment of diffusing capacity. Interpretation of test results allows clinicians to distinguish between obstructive, restrictive, and mixed patterns of lung impairment.

Chapter 12 explains the non-respiratory functions of the lung, including metabolic processes such as the conversion of angiotensin I to angiotensin II, the removal of circulating mediators, and the filtration of small thrombi. Immunological lung functions for protection against pathogens are also explained.

Chapter 13 examines respiratory adaptation to exercise. The chapter explains how exercise alters ventilation, cardiac output, and blood distribution to meet increased oxygen requirements and CO_2 elimination. Terms like the ventilatory threshold and training adaptations are defined.

Chapter 14 explores comparative respiratory physiology and respiratory development. It traces the development of lung structure and function from fetal development to mature life, comparing respiratory systems across species and how variations in anatomy and control mechanisms reflect diverse ecological and metabolic demands.

Chapter 15 discusses the pathophysiology of common respiratory disorders. Each of the primary disease categories—e.g., asthma, chronic obstructive pulmonary disease (COPD), pulmonary fibrosis, and acute respiratory distress syndrome (ARDS)—is discussed in relation to its underlying physiological disturbance, diagnostic criteria, and broad principles of management.

This book serves as a standard textbook for advanced undergraduate and graduate students of physiology, medicine, respiratory therapy, and related sciences. It is also helpful as a reference for clinicians who wish to solidify their understanding of respiratory function and for researchers who require a solid grasp of fundamental principles. Teachers will find helpful the rational progression of topics for course planning, and clinicians will welcome the explicit descriptions of how physiological principles apply to patient care. Whether as a primary textbook or an ancillary, this work aims to provide readers with the facts they need to understand normal respiratory function, interpret diagnostic data, and appreciate the physiological basis of respiratory disease.

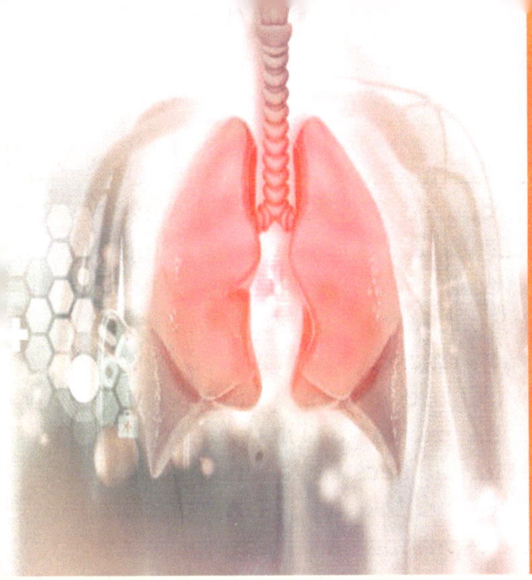

Chapter 1

INTRODUCTION TO RESPIRATORY SYSTEM

Contents

Introduction

The respiratory system is crucial in the body because it plays a vital role in keeping us alive. The primary role of this network is to ensure oxygen enters the blood and carbon dioxide leaves it which is called gas exchange. As well as helping with breathing, the respiratory system is involved in thermoregulation, making sounds, and smelling. The way the lungs, trachea, and diaphragm interact emphasizes the need to know their anatomy and functions. As the respiratory and cardiovascular systems are closely interrelated, any issue in either system can have a significant impact on health and wellness. Therefore, examining how the respiratory system functions and its composition provides a basic understanding necessary to explore its various parts in detail. A detailed examination of the respiratory system reveals numerous essential components that enable its functions. The structural organization includes conducting zones and respiratory zones, which have different functions in breathing. The nasal cavity, pharynx, larynx, trachea, bronchi, and bronchioles are part of the conducting zone, which helps air move to and from the lungs. Alternatively, the respiratory zone consists of the alveoli, where gases are exchanged. Due to this division, it is evident that the respiratory system is complex; to comprehend how airflow and gas exchange function, one must understand these zones. The respiratory epithelium, which contains cilia and mucous, is responsible for filtering and moistening the air going into the lungs, thus defending against infections and allergies. The complexity of the respiratory system is also evident in research on its health and diseases, highlighting the importance of understanding its detailed structure. Besides its basic function, the respiratory system is essential for disease control and management. For instance, understanding the interplay between respiratory and environmental factors can highlight how exposure to pollutants or allergens impacts lung health, leading to conditions such as asthma or chronic obstructive pulmonary disease (COPD). Also, medical research is working to discover the causes of respiratory diseases which helps create new treatments. As detailed in numerous medical sources, covering both the healthy and unhealthy aspects of breathing, it is essential to continue using integrated approaches to educate people and improve public respiratory health. A comprehensive overview of the respiratory system serves not only to enhance our knowledge of its structure and function but also to inform strategies for improving respiratory health and addressing emerging health challenges, ultimately ensuring better outcomes for individuals and communities alike (Bekish et al., 2014; N/A, 2025).

Definition of the Respiratory System

The respiratory system is basically a network of organs that helps the body exchange gases with the air around it. The main task of this system is to give oxygen to the blood and remove the carbon dioxide produced by cells. Oxygen enters the blood and carbon dioxide leaves the blood mostly in the alveoli, which are tiny air sacs in the lungs. The respiratory system also consists of the nasal cavity, trachea, bronchi and lungs and all these parts are necessary for proper ventilation and gas exchange. The respiratory system is crucial for life because it encompasses both its structure and the key functions that support it. The respiratory anatomy includes both conducting and respiratory zones, and these zones are connected but have different roles. The conducting zone contains the nasal passages, pharynx, larynx, trachea, and bronchi, primarily to filter, warm, and moisten the air entering the body, thereby protecting the lungs. The respiratory zone, comprising the respiratory bronchioles, alveolar ducts, and alveoli, is the primary area for gas exchange.

This division highlights that the respiratory system is a complex system, and all its parts must work together to maintain the body's balance. The organization and function of the respiratory system have evolved to allow organisms to handle their metabolic needs in different environments. Studies on the respiratory system continue to improve, highlighting the critical relationship between its structure and its function in the body. To understand the respiratory system's definition, one must know how its elements cooperate to ensure enough gas exchange and support metabolism. Things become more complicated because medical terms are used to describe the system, and some terms previously used by doctors are still questioned by science. For instance, the need for precise terminology underscores the significance of clarity in scientific communication, as terms should accurately represent the anatomy and function of the respiratory system (Al Mehzaa et al., 2019). Consequently, ongoing discourse in medical semantics encourages the refinement of terms to establish a more logical and practical vocabulary that aligns with advancements in respiratory science and clinical practice, thus promoting better integration and understanding across related fields (N/A, 2025) (Figure 1.1).

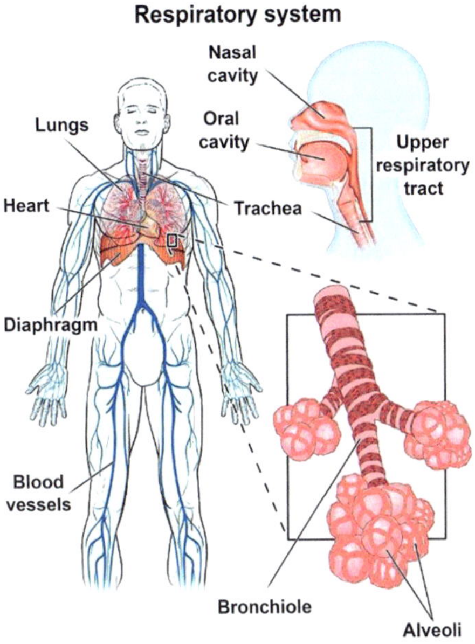

Figure 1.1. Respiratory system.

Source: https://my.clevelandclinic.org/-/scassets/images/org/health/articles/respiratory-system.

Importance of the Respiratory System in Human Physiology

Homeostasis and cellular function are supported by the respiratory system, which helps exchange gases. Oxygen is necessary for aerobic metabolism, the primary process by which energy is generated in human cells. When we inhale, air rich in oxygen reaches the lungs, passes through the alveoli, and enters our bloodstream. Carbon dioxide, which is formed during cellular respiration, is released when we exhale. It is an essential for both making energy and regulating the acidity of blood, which helps maintain the body's acid-base balance. the respiratory system is crucial for maintaining health, as any problems with gas exchange can cause metabolic issues and health complications. The respiratory system also defends the body by shielding it from pathogens and harmful substances in the air. Several parts of the respiratory system and reflexes are involved in cleaning, humidifying, and warming the air as it moves toward the lungs. Particulates and microbes are caught by nasal hairs, and mucus and cilia help move the mucus up so it can be either coughed out or swallowed. It is significant for preventing infections and diseases of the lungs, for example, pneumonia and bronchitis. Also, the immune response is assisted by immune cells in the lung tissues, which respond to pathogens inhaled through the lungs. Thus, the respiratory system is not solely a conduit for air; it is also an active participant in the body's defense mechanisms against disease, thereby reinforcing its importance in human physiology (Bekish et al., 2014, 2017). Additionally, the respiratory system is closely connected to other organ systems, which underscores its significant role in human physiology. While gas exchange is occurring, the cardiovascular and respiratory systems work in collaboration: oxygenated blood is delivered to tissues and organs, and deoxygenated blood is returned to the lungs for reoxygenation. It demonstrates that the respiratory system plays a crucial role in metabolic functions within the body. Additionally, the system responds to both physical activity and emotions by adjusting breathing rates, demonstrating its ability to adapt to various situations. Exercise increases the body's need for oxygen, so breathing rate and depth increase to meet the needs of the body. The interconnectedness of systems emphasizes the respiratory system's immense importance, not just for oxygen delivery but also for overall physiological coordination and harmony (Bekish et al., 2014; Bekish et al., 2017).

1.1. Functions of the Respiratory System

Maintaining homeostasis in the body depends on the many essential roles of the respiratory system. Primarily, it is responsible for gas exchange, facilitating the intake of oxygen (O_2) and the expulsion of carbon dioxide (CO_2). Oxygen enters the blood, and carbon dioxide is released primarily in the alveoli. The respiratory system is also essential for regulating blood pH by working with the bicarbonate buffer system, which controls CO_2 levels. It is essential, since it helps maintain the balance of acids and bases, which affects cellular activity and metabolism. The respiratory system is crucial for maintaining the body's balance and cellular activities due to its role in gas exchange and pH regulation. In addition to gas exchange, the respiratory system supports other vital functions that enhance health and the environment. A good example is olfaction, the sense of smell, which is made possible by receptors in the nasal cavity. This sense is vital for spotting things in the environment that influence our appetite and social life. Additionally, the respiratory system helps regulate body temperature by changing the air temperature before it reaches the lungs. It is necessary to protect the sensitive tissues in the lungs. Additionally, the mucociliary escalator, which utilizes cilia and mucus, aids in removing and expelling foreign particles and pathogens, thereby protecting the immune system and lungs. Thus, these extra roles prove that the respiratory system is not just for gas exchange. The respiratory system stands out in immune defense because it is the first line of defense against harmful pathogens. The bronchus-associated lymphoid tissue (BALT) is a key component of this immune response, as it helps orchestrate the defense against inhaled pathogens, particularly in avian species (Dalamani et al., 2006). Humans have similar defenses because many immune cells, such as macrophages, are found in the respiratory system, working to detect and stop threats. Moreover, the presence of secretory immunoglobulin A (IgA) on mucosal surfaces provides a humoral defense against bacteria and viruses. The way BALT and mucosal immune factors work together strengthens the respiratory system's ability to fight infections, which helps maintain health. By understanding these immune functions, we can gain deeper insights into the respiratory systems comprehensive role in protecting the body from disease (Bekish et al., 2017).

1.1.1. Gas Exchange: Oxygen and Carbon Dioxide

The respiratory system relies on gas exchange, which primarily involves the exchange of oxygen and carbon dioxide between the alveoli in the lungs and the bloodstream. Oxygen, needed for cellular respiration, moves from the alveoli into the capillaries because there is a difference in oxygen levels. This process occurs easily because the alveoli have a large surface area and are very thin. Carbon dioxide, which is a waste product of metabolism, is carried from the blood into the alveoli and then expelled when we breathe out. This process maintains cellular energy and also helps the body regulate its acid-base balance, demonstrating that gas exchange in the respiratory system is crucial. Factors affecting the efficiency of gas exchange are the pressures of the gases and the area where diffusion occurs. Partial pressure gradients cause movement of oxygen and carbon dioxide; oxygen can enter circulation because its partial pressure is higher in the alveoli than in the blood. This same process happens for carbon dioxide (which is more concentrated in the blood than in the alveoli) allowing it to be eliminated. If pneumonia or pulmonary edema disturbed, which leads to poor gas exchange and hypoxia, illustrating the importance of the lungs being in balance to handle oxygen and carbon dioxide effectively in various situations. Both external respiration, which happens in the lungs, and internal respiration, which is the use of oxygen and creation of carbon dioxide at the cellular level, play a role in how gases are exchanged in the body. Additionally, organisms have different respiratory systems that match their ability to live in various environments. Marine mammals have special features that enable them to hold their breath for an extended period and utilize gas efficiently during dives. Understanding these diverse mechanisms broadens our comprehension of physiological variations across species. It underscores the intricate relationship between structural anatomy and functional capacities of the respiratory system in facilitating gas exchange under various conditions, as detailed in comprehensive studies of respiration processes and their underlying principles (Bekish et al., 2014; N/A, 2025) (Figure 1.2).

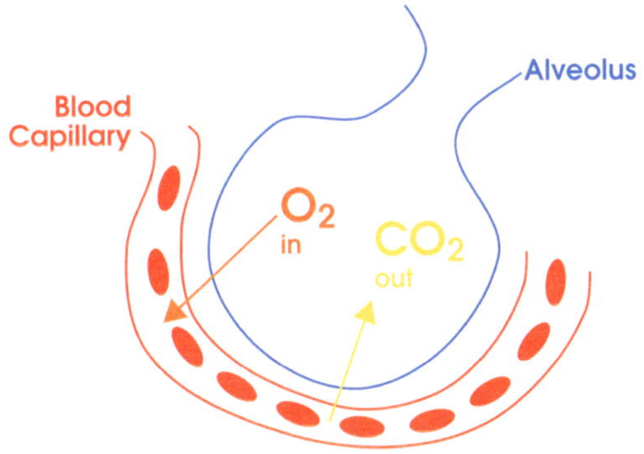

Figure 1.2. Gas exchange in humans. Oxygen and carbon dioxide switch places between a capillary (part of the bloodstream) and an alveolus (an air sac in the lungs).

Source: https://upload.wikimedia.org/wikipedia/commons/thumb/c/c4/Gas_exchange_in_the_aveolus_simple_%28en%29.svg/1024px-Gas_exchange_in_the_aveolus_simple_%28en%29.svg.png.

1.1.2. Regulation of Blood pH

Maintaining the pH of blood is crucial for homeostasis in the human body, and this is primarily controlled by the respiratory system. The blood pH is carefully kept within the range of 7.35 and 7.45, which is necessary for proper enzyme action and metabolism. The respiratory system plays a vital role in this regulation by managing the levels of carbon dioxide (CO_2), a byproduct of cellular respiration. When CO_2 levels increase, it reacts with water in the body to form carbonic acid (H_2CO_3), which can lower blood pH, leading to acidosis. Breathing out CO_2 increases pH, which can lead to alkalosis. The respiratory system's ability to regulate the amount of air it takes in and lets out is crucial for maintaining blood acidity balance and overall bodily equilibrium. The relationship between the respiratory system and the renal system highlights the importance of maintaining blood pH. Although the respiratory system can quickly adjust to CO_2 levels, it is the kidneys that help maintain a balanced pH over a longer period by regulating the movement of bicarbonate and hydrogen ions. The buffering system helps maintain pH balance, along with the changes in breathing. When respiratory function is compromised, such as in chronic obstructive pulmonary disease (COPD), the inability to expel CO_2 leads to respiratory acidosis. Due to these conditions, it is evident that the body utilizes both systems to maintain a blood pH level close to the required level for stability. It demonstrates that human biology is complex and that multiple organ systems are required to maintain balance. Problems with maintaining pH can be very harmful to health, which highlights the respiratory system's role in keeping metabolism balanced. The presence of acidosis or alkalosis can disrupt various cellular activities, including nerve communication and muscle function. A person may show signs of respiratory distress, confusion or muscle changes, so quick action by a doctor is required. to blood pH imbalances. Understanding these mechanisms enables healthcare professionals to develop targeted treatments for conditions associated with blood pH imbalances. In addition, the respiratory system helps manage the pH of blood, which is needed for living healthy. As education in physiology continues to evolve, resources such as laboratory manuals and updated bibliographies serve to enhance our understanding of these intricate biological processes (Beebe et al., 2019; N/A, 2025) (Figure 1.3).

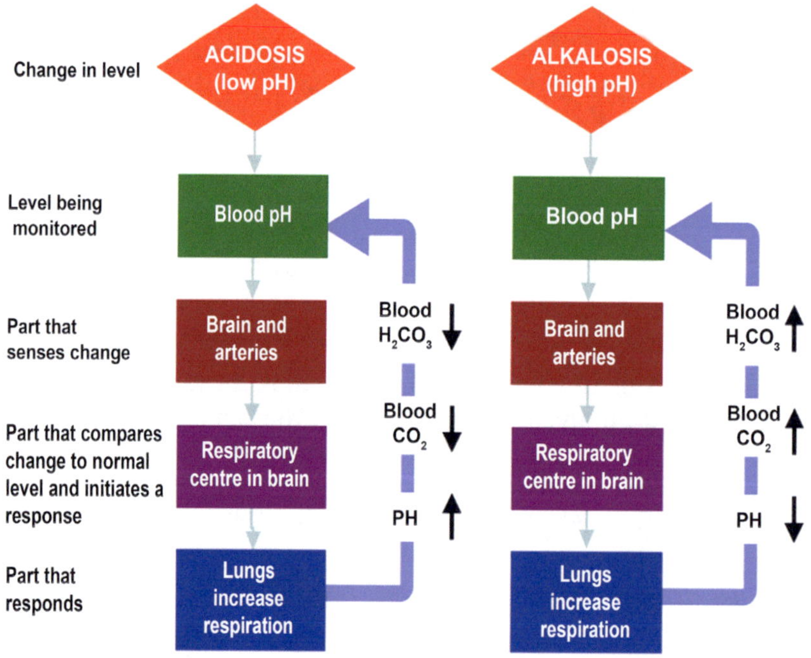

Figure 1.3. Respiratory regulation of blood pH.

Source: https://letstalkscience.ca/sites/default/files/styles/width_800px/public/2021-11/Respiratory-regulation-of-blood-pH.png?itok=Wp77tX9E.

1.1.3. Protection Against Pathogens and Irritants

The respiratory system helps protect the lungs by utilizing various anatomical and physiological mechanisms against environmental hazards. The nasal cavity is important because it filters the air we breathe, and the mucous membranes catch and trap dust, particles, and germs. Ciliated epithelial cells also help by transporting the trapped particles toward the throat, which allows them to be removed with a swallow or a cough. Additionally, immune cells, such as macrophages and lymphocytes, in the respiratory system enable the body to detect and eliminate pathogens before they cause infections quickly. These initial barriers play a key role in keeping the respiratory system healthy and preventing many respiratory diseases, which proves how vital their structure is for protection. In addition to using mechanical filters, the respiratory system employs biochemical methods to prevent pathogens and irritants from causing harm. Mucus secretion works by trapping harmful particles and also including substances like lysozyme and defensins that fight microbes. They are designed to eliminate bacteria and viruses that attempt to enter the respiratory tract. Airborne pollutants can cause oxidative stress which makes it harder for people with asthma or COPD to breathe. Research has established that oxidative stress can lead to significant lung damage, compromising the protective functions of the respiratory system, and emphasizing the necessity of maintaining antioxidant levels to mitigate these effects (Sabuncuo et al., 2022). Therefore, a combination of structural and biochemical defenses is necessary to provide robust protection against airborne pathogens and irritants. Pathological conditions such as cystic fibrosis (CF) illustrate the consequences of compromised protective mechanisms within the respiratory system. The thick mucus in CF patients helps specific pathogens, mainly Pseudomonas aeruginosa, to thrive, which can cause serious harm to the lungs. The interplay among host defenses, altered microbiota, and environmental factors complicates the infection landscape, leading to a cycle of chronic inflammation and lung injury (Anjali et al., 2016). The complexity suggests that single approaches may not be sufficient, so combining different strategies is crucial for effective treatment and care. Knowing how pathogens affect the lungs and how the body responds helps develop new therapies that improve lung function and resistance to infections. So, to keep people safe from pathogens and irritants, research and innovation in respiratory health must continue.

1.2. Structural Anatomy of the Respiratory System

The proper structure of the respiratory system is essential for it to function effectively, exchange gases efficiently, and maintain homeostasis. The system starts at the external nasal passages and ends in the alveoli of the lungs which are responsible for most oxygen and carbon dioxide exchange. The nasal cavity, pharynx, and larynx in the upper respiratory tract clean, heat, and add moisture to the air we inhale. However, the lower respiratory tract consists of the trachea, bronchi, and bronchioles, which ultimately end at the alveolar sacs. Each of these structures is carefully designed to optimize airflow and ensure the respiratory surfaces remain moist, which is essential for effective gas exchange (Bekish et al., 2014). Additionally, the respiratory system becomes increasingly specialized as it progresses from large airways to the tiny alveoli. The trachea is maintained in an open and stable position by C-shaped cartilage rings. When the bronchi reach the lungs, they continue to branch into bronchioles, and these branching bronchioles end in alveoli, which significantly increase the area for gas exchange. Alveolar walls are very thin, consisting of only one layer of epithelial cells and coated with surfactant, which reduces surface tension. This anatomical design ensures that oxygen can diffuse rapidly into the blood while allowing carbon dioxide to exit, highlighting the efficiency of the system (Bekish et al., 2017). The way the respiratory system is organized is both useful and represents changes brought about by evolution to support metabolism. All these segments and structures have evolved to help the lung respond to its environment, enhance breathing, and support various body functions. For example, the extra surface area of the alveoli enables more efficient gas exchange, which helps active organisms maintain their high metabolic rates. Connective tissues give the airways their structure, which keeps them open during breathing, allowing air to move freely. As a whole, the structural anatomy of the respiratory system exemplifies a complex interplay between form and function that underpins the essential processes of respiration and gas exchange, making it a crucial area of study within human physiology (Bekish et al., 2014).

1.2.1. Upper Respiratory Tract Components

The upper respiratory tract facilitates early gas exchange by conditioning, filtering, and humidifying the air we breathe in. The main parts of the respiratory system are the nasal cavity, pharynx, and larynx, and each plays a significant role in breathing. The nasal cavity, which is covered with mucosa and cilia, is the first place where airborne pathogens and particles are stopped. It moistens the air and helps with smelling, which is vital for survival. Because the nasal turbinates are so detailed, they increase the air flow surface area, which helps allow the air to become more efficient before it reaches the lungs. The pharynx, which follows the nasal cavity, allows air and food to move through it, showing the connection between the respiratory and digestive systems. The pharynx is divided into the nasopharynx, oropharynx, and laryngopharynx, which each play essential roles in breathing. The nasopharynx which is behind the nasal cavity, is mainly responsible for air passage and contains the adenoids that help with the immune system. Food and air enter the body through the oropharynx and laryngopharynx, which facilitate swallowing. This multifunctionality is crucial, as it prevents aspiration and directs air efficiently towards the larynx, where vocalization occurs, ultimately linking respiratory function with communication, an ability that has evolved significantly in humans as detailed in recent studies on motor evolution (John, 2008). The larynx, which is the voice box, is essential in the upper respiratory tract for both making sound and guarding the lower airways. The larynx, composed of cartilage, houses the vocal cords and plays a crucial role in producing sounds by vibrating and modulating them. Also, while swallowing, the epiglottis, a component of the larynx, closes over the trachea, stopping food from entering the lungs, which demonstrates how the respiratory and digestive systems work together. The careful orchestration of these functions is vital for maintaining airway patency and ensuring effective communication, highlighting the importance of the upper respiratory components within the broader context of respiratory system performance (Beebe et al., 2019) (Figure 1.4).

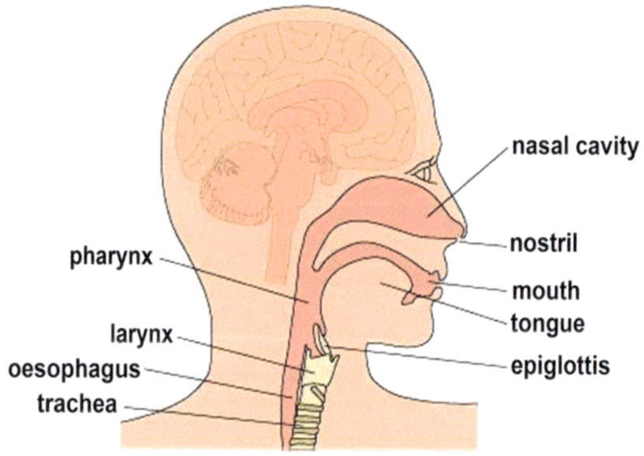

Figure 1.4. Structures of the upper respiratory tract.

Source: https://www.open.edu/openlearn/science-maths-technology/blood-and-the-respiratory-system/content-section-1.1.1.

1.2.2. Lower Respiratory Tract Components

Essential parts of the lower respiratory tract play a significant role in gas exchange and the functioning of the lungs. This part of the respiratory system starts with the trachea, which branches into the primary bronchi and these further branch into secondary and tertiary bronchi in each lung. The complex bronchial tree evenly distributes air to all parts of the lungs, thereby increasing the area for oxygen and carbon dioxide exchange. The airways are supported by smooth muscle and cartilage, which help keep them open and permit them to change size during breathing. It is essential to know the structure of the lower respiratory tract because diseases in this area can seriously affect breathing, which is the primary job of the respiratory system. The alveoli, which are the primary components of gas exchange, are located at the end of the bronchial system. Alveoli are small, balloon-shaped structures arranged in groups, allowing for a large surface area for taking in oxygen and expelling carbon dioxide. The alveolar walls have only one layer of epithelial cells, which helps gases move quickly through them. Thanks to surfactant, a lipoprotein made by type II alveolar cells, the surface tension of the lungs is reduced, and alveoli do not collapse when air is exhaled, which increases the lung's ability to expand. The close relationship between the alveoli and the pulmonary capillaries is crucial; any disturbance can lead to impaired gas exchange and may cause various lung diseases. As highlighted in current research, addressing the challenges posed by lung diseases is imperative given their rising prevalence and the limited therapeutic options available (Cryan et al., 2015). Additionally, understanding how the lower respiratory tract functions is essential to advance treatment and facilitate better patient recovery. Both structural changes and inflammation can be seen in the impact of COPD and asthma on breathing. Recently, tissue engineering has garnered increased attention as a means to repair airway tissues and enhance lung function. Strategies that involve the use of biomaterials and stem cell therapies aim not only to restore structural integrity but also to enhance the functional capacity of the lower respiratory tract (Cryan et al., 2015). Given the significant health burden posed by lower respiratory diseases, it becomes increasingly critical to foster a comprehensive understanding of the underlying anatomy and mechanisms involved to innovate therapeutic approaches that can profoundly influence respiratory health outcomes (Figure 1.5).

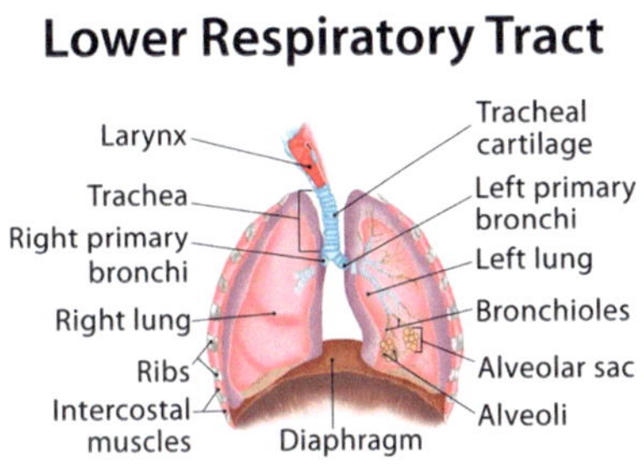

Figure 1.5. Lower respiratory tract.

Source: https://i0.wp.com/student-nurse-life.com/wp-content/uploads/2021/02/Lower-Respiratory-Tract.jpg?resize=750%2C536.

1.2.3. Supporting Structures: Thoracic Cavity and Diaphragm

The lungs and heart are both protected and supported by the thoracic cavity, which is an integral part of the respiratory system. The rib cage, which surrounds this cavity, both protects it and facilitates breathing movement. The rib cage is composed of 12 pairs of ribs, vertebrae, and the sternum, and it helps protect the thoracic organs while also participating in breathing. The lungs are found inside this cavity, and a double-membrane pleura surrounds them to make sure there is a negative pressure, which helps prevent the lungs from collapsing. The way the thoracic cavity is constructed and arranged facilitates effective gas exchange. The way the ribs and spine are constructed allows the thoracic cavity to change in size and pressure, which supports the movement of air through the lungs. The diaphragm, which forms a dome between the thoracic and abdominal cavities, is the primary muscle in the breathing process.

The diaphragm is crucial for breathing because it contracts and flattens during inhalation, creating a vacuum that enables air to move into the lungs. It helps make more space in the thorax and also supports breathing which improves how gas moves in and out of the lungs. During exhalation, the diaphragm relaxes which causes the lungs to shrink and release air. Evidence suggests that the correct placement of the diaphragm enables people to breathe more efficiently in clinical settings. For instance, patient positioning can influence pulmonary aeration and the effective removal of bronchial secretions, highlighting the diaphragm's role beyond mere respiration and underscoring its importance in patient care within the intensive care unit (ICU) context, as suggested in the findings related to optimal patient postures for improved respiratory capacity (Grigoriadis et al., 2009). The movement of the thoracic cavity and diaphragm is better understood by learning about diffusion in the alveoli. The proper transfer of gases is possible only if the supporting structures are strong and work as they should. A mathematical model examining gas diffusion in alveolar regions suggests that variations in the distribution of red blood cells (RBCs) can significantly influence lung-diffusing capacity, highlighting the importance of both anatomical and physiological factors in respiratory health (Kulish et al., 2006). Because the thoracic support structures and diaphragm work in tandem, the entire respiratory system functions effectively. Consequently, any impairment to these structures can lead to compromised respiration, highlighting their critical importance in both health and clinical recovery scenarios (Figure 1.6).

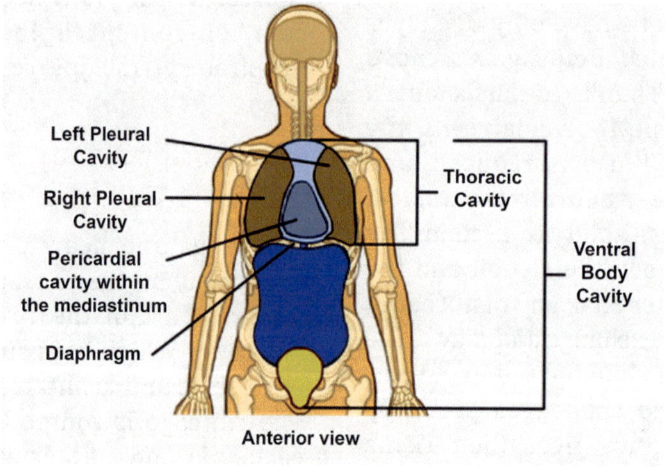

Figure 1.6. The thoracic cavity is the superior cavity in the ventral body cavity.

Source: https://images.my.labster.com/v2/BPS/52977293-f6f5-4177-b41d-6467b5129fb7/BPS_ThoracicCavity.en.x512.png.

1.3. Major Organs of the Respiratory System

Many vital organs in the respiratory system cooperate to help the body exchange gases, which is necessary for life. All the major organs in the respiratory system are the lungs, trachea, bronchi, and diaphragm, each with its own purpose. The lungs, the primary organs of respiration, take in oxygen and remove carbon dioxide from the blood. The trachea carries air to the lungs, which are reached by the air through the bronchi. The system of airways in the bronchi and bronchioles narrows as they branch, which facilitates gas exchange. The arrangement of the airways ensures that air is filtered, warmed, and moistened before reaching the alveoli, where vital gas exchange takes place. In addition to breathing, these organs also protect the body from airborne diseases through their immune defenses. The BALT in birds shows that respiratory organs can both help breathing and provide immunity. It was mentioned that BALT structures are orderly and strengthen as the organism grows, illustrating how the immune system can adapt more effectively with age. Lung interstitial tissues contain tissue macrophages and lymphocytes, which show the key role immune cells play in protecting the lungs and fighting off infections. This dual functionality highlights the importance of a comprehensive understanding of respiratory anatomy and physiology, as disruptions in either aspect can lead to significant health challenges, including increased susceptibility to respiratory diseases (Dalamani et al., 2006). Additionally, understanding the respiratory zones is crucial for comprehending how these organs work in the context of the entire body. People usually separate the respiratory system into conducting and respiratory zones. The conducting zone, which contains the trachea and bronchi, helps move air. The respiratory zone, with the alveoli, is where air is exchanged with oxygen and carbon dioxide. It points out that the respiratory system needs to work well at both moving air and exchanging gases. Many features of the lungs, such as their large surface area and thin walls, are designed for this purpose. As the knowledge of respiratory organs expands, it becomes increasingly apparent how intricately they are connected to overall health, facilitating not only respiration but also playing vital roles in immune defense and homeostasis (Bekish et al., 2014).

1.3.1. Nose and Nasal Cavity

The respiratory system relies on the nose and nasal cavity, which help make breathing effective and filter the first breath of air. Inside the nasal cavity are turbinates, which are bony structures that help filter, humidify, and regulate the temperature of air. The nasal passages heat and moisten the air before it reaches the lungs, which is crucial for the health of the respiratory system and for efficient gas exchange. The mucus membranes in the nose catch pathogens and small particles, which support the immune system. Therefore, the well-being of the nasal structures is crucial for proper breathing and protection against pollutants. The nose and nasal cavity are essential for breathing and also for the sense of smell which is very important for humans. The olfactory epithelium, located in the upper part of the nasal cavity, contains sensory receptors that detect chemicals in the air and also influence our sense of taste and enjoyment of food. It helps people survive by enabling them to recognize dangers, such as rotten food or hazardous substances. Additionally, when we smell something, our emotions are involved, illustrating the connection between the nose and brain activity. The potential for intranasal drug delivery for therapeutic purposes further emphasizes the significance of the nasal cavity in neuroscience, as it enables access to the central nervous system (CNS) without the hurdles presented by systemic administration methods (Erd et al., 2018; Keller et al., 2021). Due to research into intranasal drug administration, scientists have discovered that the nose and nasal cavity can be utilized to deliver drugs directly to the brain. This method has several advantages, including the ability to bypass the blood-brain barrier (BBB), thereby enhancing drug bioavailability and minimizing systemic side effects, while requiring lower doses compared to oral routes. Given that many neurological disorders pose challenges in treatment due to poor drug penetration capabilities, the use of the nasal route is an innovative strategy that capitalizes on the anatomical and physiological features of the nasal cavity (Keller et al., 2021). Studies emphasize the importance of understanding the nasal barrier's structure and function, as well as optimizing formulations for improved drug absorption, which may revolutionize therapeutic approaches for patients with neurodegenerative and psychiatric conditions (Erd et al., 2018). Through this research, further insights into the intricate relationship between the respiratory system and neurological health management are being unraveled (Figure 1.7).

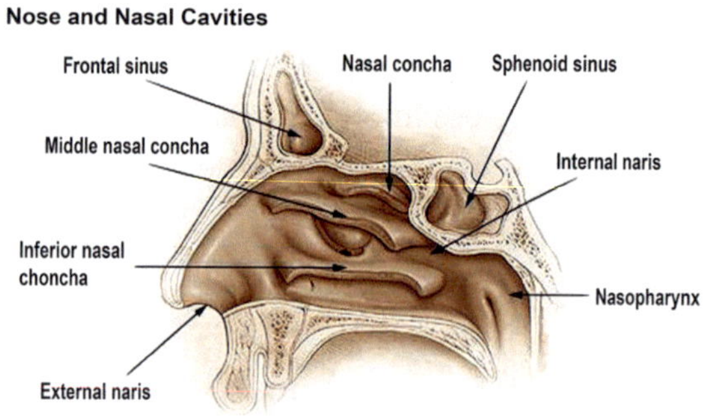

Figure 1.7. Nose and nasal cavity.

Source: https://training.seer.cancer.gov/images/anatomy/respiratory/nose_nasal_cavities.jpg.

1.3.2. Lungs and Alveoli

Gas exchange and maintaining the body's balance depend mainly on the lungs, which are the primary organs of respiration. The lungs, composed of many tissues and alveoli, efficiently allow oxygen to reach the blood and expel carbon dioxide. Due to this design, the surface area is large, which facilitates the body's use of diffusion during breathing. Alveoli, which are tiny air sacs in the lungs, play a key role in gas exchange by connecting the air and blood. The structure of the lungs is designed to function efficiently, featuring a thin epithelial layer that facilitates the easy movement of gases, allowing blood to be quickly oxygenated. It is essential to understand the relationship between the lungs and alveoli to comprehend the primary processes of respiration. Alveoli are connected to many capillaries, which highlights their primary function in gas exchange. A substance called surfactant lines each alveolus, which helps prevent them from collapsing when air is breathed out. remain open and stable, which the surfactant helps to achieve. Also, the immune system defends the alveoli from harmful substances and diseases. The BALT is involved in the immune response in these areas by reacting to various environmental factors, as recent studies have highlighted. Such findings underscore the importance of alveolar health in preventing respiratory diseases, as dysfunction in this system can lead to severe complications and chronic conditions, such as COPD or asthma, which can significantly burden public health (Ak et al., 2021) (Figure 1.8).

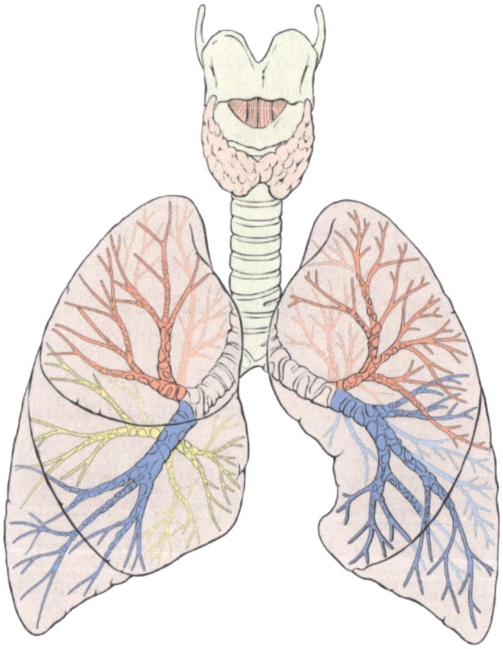

Figure 1.8. Lungs diagram with internal details.

Source: https://upload.wikimedia.org/wikipedia/commons/thumb/a/a1/Lungs_diagram_detailed.svg/800px-Lungs_diagram_detailed.svg.png.

Lung tissue engineering appears to be a promising way to tackle respiratory problems. As chronic lung diseases are becoming more prevalent, finding new ways to treat them is crucial for achieving better patient outcomes. It involves building structures that have the structure and functions of lung tissue. They are designed to enhance healing from airway injuries and provide alternative options to traditional methods and organ transplants. It is crucial for alveoli to be well-engineered for the respiratory system to function correctly. The ongoing exploration of biomaterials and the cellular signaling processes that promote healing holds significant implications for regenerative medicine, as it addresses the urgent need for effective interventions in the treatment of respiratory diseases (Cryan et al., 2015). Such innovative approaches may pave the way for revolutionary therapies that significantly alter the management of lung-related health issues (Figure 1.9).

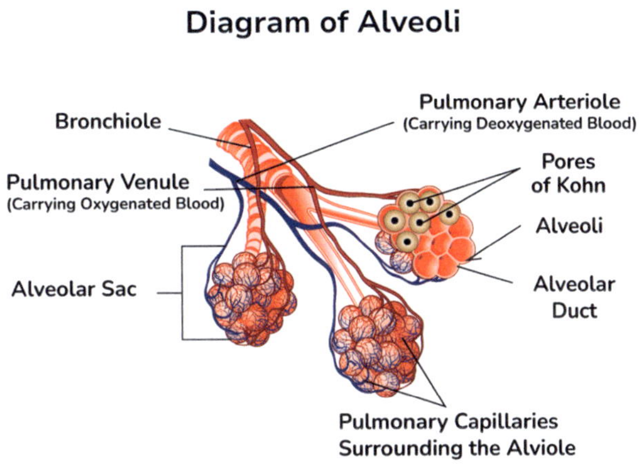

Figure 1.9. Diagram of alveoli.

Source: https://media.geeksforgeeks.org/wp-content/uploads/20240402102643/Diagram-of-Alveoli.png.

1.3.3. Trachea and Bronchi

Air is moved through the respiratory system mainly by the trachea and bronchi. The trachea, also known as the windpipe, is the primary central airway that transports inhaled air from the larynx to the bronchi and directs it to the lungs. The trachea is composed of C-shaped rings of cartilage, which keep it both strong and flexible during breathing. The trachea splits into right and left bronchi, which then branch into bronchioles inside the lungs. This detailed network is vital for air to reach all areas of the lungs, so gas exchange and cell respiration can work well. A clear path for airflow is maintained in the body by the way the trachea and bronchi are built which is necessary for homeostasis. Besides their shape, the trachea and bronchi play important roles in supporting good respiratory health. They primarily help move air, but they also contribute to the process of filtering and humidifying the air we breathe. The inner part of the trachea and bronchi has ciliated epithelial cells and goblet cells that produce mucus, which catches dust, germs, and other small particles. The mucociliary escalator system is lungs, which is essential in improving their function. The smooth muscle around the bronchi helps the airway to narrow or widen, which controls how much air moves through the lungs. In this context, the trachea and bronchi not only serve as conduits but also play an active role in preserving respiratory integrity and function within the respiratory system (Figure 1.10).

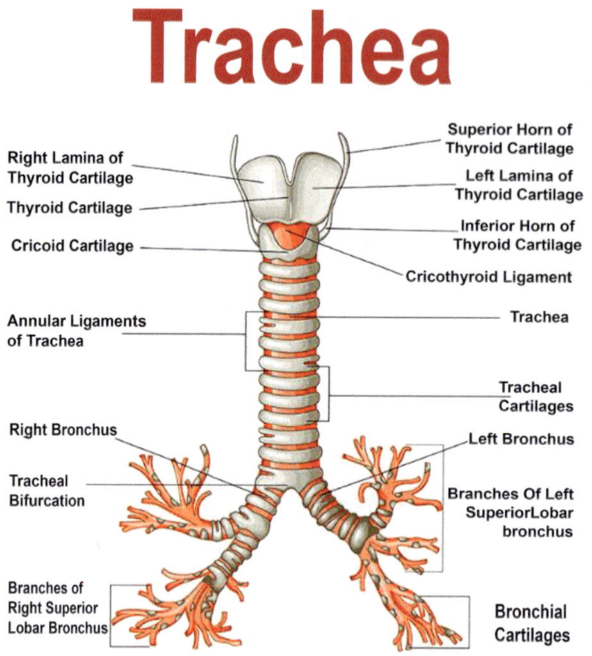

Figure 1.10. Trachea.

Source: https://assets.lybrate.com/imgs/tic/enadp/image-of-the-trachea.jpg.

Advances in respiratory studies have highlighted the need for improved models to investigate the function of the trachea and bronchi. The fact that animal lungs differ from human lungs makes it challenging to apply animal research to humans, so in vitro systems are now more critical. Three-dimensional organoids and organs-on-a-chip are being examined to see if they can replicate the functions and responses of tracheal and bronchial epithelial cells in a controlled way.

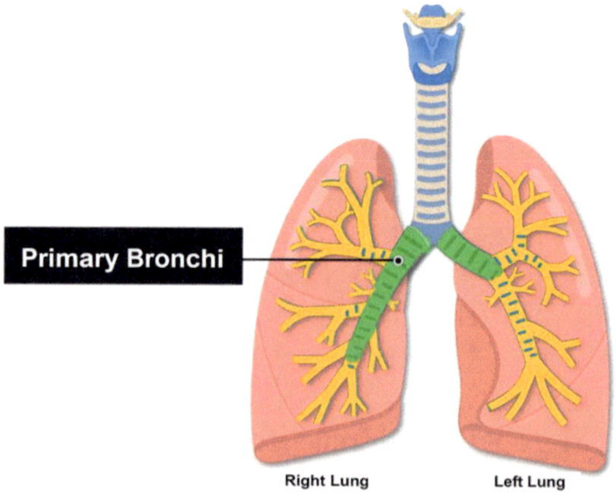

Figure 1.11. Primary bronchi.

Source: https://www.getbodysmart.com/wp-content/uploads/2017/10/Primary-Bronchi-1024x732.png.

They help explain how diseases, regeneration, and pollution affect the lungs. By allowing for the examination of human lung physiology in vitro, such approaches could complement traditional studies and enhance our understanding of respiratory function and disease, ultimately informing therapeutic strategies for respiratory conditions (Gkatzis et al., 2018; Thomas et al., 2018) (Figure 1.11).

1.4. Types of Respiration

The respiratory system is essential for life, as it carries out respiration, which can be broadly categorized into aerobic and anaerobic forms. Energy is produced efficiently in aerobic respiration, a process that occurs when oxygen is present and is utilized by many multicellular organisms. During this process, glucose is oxidized to produce carbon dioxide, water, and adenosine triphosphate (ATP), the energy currency of cells. When cells use aerobic respiration, they can make up to 36 ATP molecules from just one molecule of glucose, which is much more efficient than anaerobic respiration. When there is not enough oxygen, organisms use anaerobic respiration, which breaks down glucose only partially and produces substances like lactic acid or ethanol. Understanding these two types of respiration provides insight into how organisms adapt to their environments, maximizing energy production and survival (Breit et al., 2018). One more critical point about respiration is distinguishing between external and internal respiration. External respiration happens when gases are exchanged between the air and the blood in the lungs. Mostly, oxygen from the air we breathe enters the blood, and carbon dioxide leaves the blood as we breathe out. With internal respiration, oxygen is taken up by cells and used in cellular respiration and carbon dioxide is released as waste. They are essential for keeping homeostasis so that cells can carry out their metabolic activities. The efficiency of both external and internal respiration is crucial for the overall functionality of the respiratory system, as interconnected mechanisms ensure that organisms can thrive despite varying environmental conditions (Natalia et al., 2016). Depending on the metabolic condition, an organism may change the way it breathes. Muscle cells may switch to anaerobic respiration during intense exercise when oxygen is not available enough which causes lactic acid to build up and makes the body feel tired. When there is, and muscles obtain sufficient energy. Because energy production can be flexible, organisms can adapt to varying oxygen levels and energy needs as they evolve. Yeast and similar organisms can utilize either aerobic or anaerobic respiration, depending on whether oxygen is present, demonstrating the flexibility of respiration. As research progresses, the intricate relationships between respiration types and physiological states continue to emerge, emphasizing their roles in health and disease management (Breit et al., 2018).

1.4.1. External Respiration: Gas Exchange in the Lungs

Maintaining homeostasis in the human body depends on external respiration. Here, the lungs help transfer gases, mainly oxygen and carbon dioxide, between the air and the blood through the alveoli. Air from the atmosphere is breathed in and moves to the alveoli, allowing the oxygen-rich air to come into contact with the pulmonary capillaries. Oxygen , and carbon dioxide, which is produced by the body, moves out of the blood and into the alveoli to be exhaled. The gas exchange keeps the cellular respiration going by making sure that oxygen is available and carbon dioxide is removed efficiently, which is anessential for metabolism. The way the lungs are built plays a significant role in determining how effectively external respiration happens. The lungs have millions of small air sacs called alveoli, which are grouped in grape-like groups to allow more gas exchange. The thinness of alveoli walls, which is often only one cell layer, makes it easy for gases to diffuse between the air in the alveoli and the blood in the nearby capillaries. Surfactant, which is present in the alveoli, is necessary because it stops them from collapsing and improves the movement of gases. This structural adaptation, combined with a large surface area, enables the lungs to be highly effective in oxygenating the blood and removing carbon dioxide, thereby providing the basis for efficient external respiration under various physiological conditions (Beebe et al., 2019).

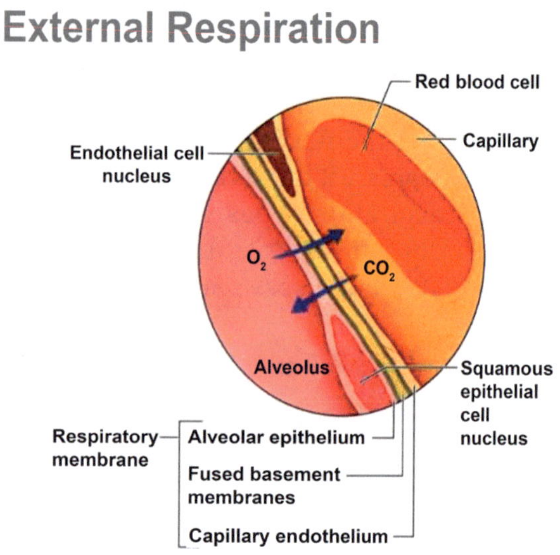

Figure 1.12. External respiration.

Source: https://image2.slideserve.com/5370082/external-respiration-l.jpg.

Additionally, various physiological processes, including ventilation, diffusion, and perfusion, regulate external respiration. Ventilation occurs when air moves in and out of the lungs due to pressure changes caused by the diaphragm and intercostal muscles. In the alveoli, gases diffuse across the respiratory membrane due to pressure differences, allowing oxygen to enter the blood and carbon dioxide to leave. The third dimension, perfusion, refers to the movement of blood through the pulmonary capillaries surrounding the alveoli, which helps oxygenate the blood and remove excess carbon dioxide. Each of these components must function optimally for adequate external respiration, as impairments in any of these areas can lead to decreased gas exchange efficiency, resulting in respiratory distress or failure (Bekish et al., 2017) (Figure 1.12).

1.4.2. Internal Respiration: Gas Exchange at the Cellular Level

Through internal respiration, the body exchanges gases between the blood and its cells. At the cellular level, this type of respiration enables O2 to reach the tissues from the blood and allows CO_2 to move from the cells into the blood. Gases move from regions with a high concentration to areas with a low concentration, which is what drives the process. Oxygen is required in cellular respiration to produce ATP, the energy the cell uses, illustrating the connection between respiration and metabolism. Such an exchange is necessary to keep cells active and to maintain metabolic balance, since cells need oxygen to do aerobic respiration, which is more efficient than anaerobic respiration. Several factors affect how efficiently internal respiration occurs, such as blood flow, the area for diffusion, and the levels of O_2 and CO_2 in the blood and tissues. If someone exercises more, the body uses more oxygen which causes the blood to flow more to the muscles. More blood flow to the lungs enables oxygen to be delivered and carbon dioxide to be eliminated, which helps maintain the body's balance. Moreover, the amount of gas pressure in the blood can influence the rate of diffusion; when oxygen in the alveoli is higher, more oxygen is taken up by the blood, which makes internal respiration work more effectively. This indicates that enhancing various bodily functions facilitates gas exchange and cellular respiration. Additionally, understanding how internal respirations function is crucial because they impact numerous other aspects of health and physiology. For example, conditions that impair circulation, such as cardiovascular diseases (CVDs) or shock, can significantly hinder the efficiency of internal respiration, leading to cellular hypoxia and potential tissue damage. For many medical and health situations, a lack of oxygen can bring about significant problems. Therefore, both clinicians and researchers who aim to address respiratory and cardiovascular health issues should possess a clear understanding of how internal respiration functions and how it is regulated. Future studies may investigate therapeutic interventions that could enhance internal respiration, particularly in pathological states, thereby improving patient outcomes and tissue viability (Bekish et al., 2014, 2017) (Figure 1.13).

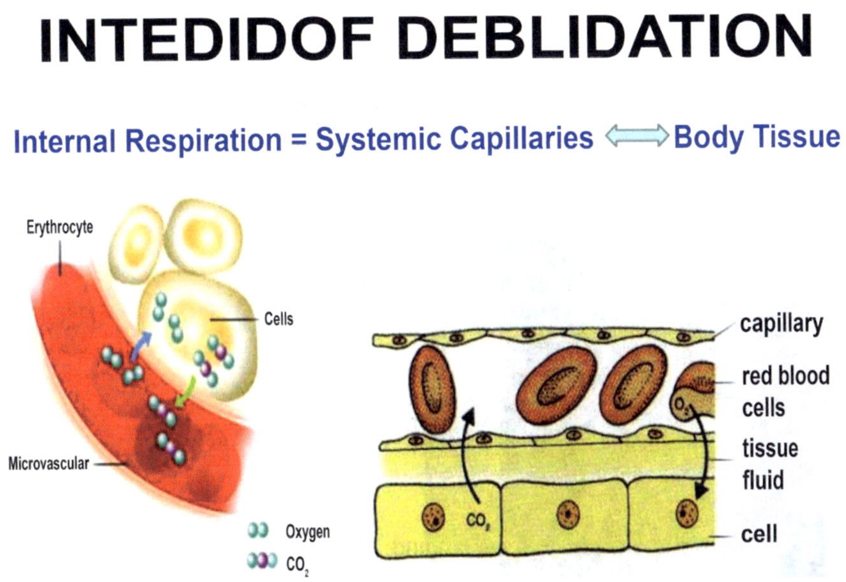

Figure 1.13. Internal respiration.

Source: https://image1.slideserve.com/3321367/internal-respiration-systemic-capillaries-body-tissue-l.jpg.

1.4.3. Cellular Respiration: Energy Production in Cells

Cellular respiration is responsible for making energy available to the cell by changing nutrients into ATP, which is the primary energy molecule. The process consists of three essential parts: glycolysis, the Krebs cycle, and oxidative phosphorylation. In the cytoplasm, glucose is broken down by glycolysis into pyruvate, a process that yields two ATP molecules and two NADH molecules. The subsequent Krebs cycle takes place in the mitochondria, producing additional NADH and flavin adenine dinucleotide (FADH2) while releasing carbon dioxide as a byproduct. Most ATP is created in oxidative phosphorylation when electrons from NADH and FADH2 are transferred through the electron transport chain, which culminates in the reduction of oxygen to water. The way biochemical reactions are coordinated in cellular respiration proves its importance for life. Cellular respiration is facilitated by the respiratory system, which enables the exchange of gases necessary for ATP production. Oxygen is taken in through breathing, enters the lungs, and diffuses into the blood, which then carries it to cells throughout the body. The electron transport chain ends with oxygen, which is crucial for aerobic respiration, as it enables the creation of up to 34 ATP molecules from one molecule of glucose. If there is no oxygen, cells switch to anaerobic respiration, which is less efficient but still allows them to produce ATP by means of fermentation, with lactic acid or ethanol as a result. The respiratory system is needed to supply oxygen to cells and also to get rid of carbon dioxide, which is produced when cells use energy. In addition to producing energy, cellular respiration facilitates various metabolic pathways within cells, thereby supporting the body's metabolic stability. pathways, which demonstrates the flexibility of this metabolic system. The ketogenic diet can, under certain conditions, increase the body's use of fat for energy, causing it to produce ketone bodies. During times when carbohydrates are limited, such as fasting, this alternative energy source is essential, proving that cellular respiration can change with changes in diet. Ultimately, the intricate relationship between cellular respiration and the respiratory system is critical for maintaining energy balance and supporting cellular function across various physiological contexts, reflecting the complex interactions between different biological systems in sustaining life (Max et al., 2021; Zhuet al., 2022) (Figure 1.14).

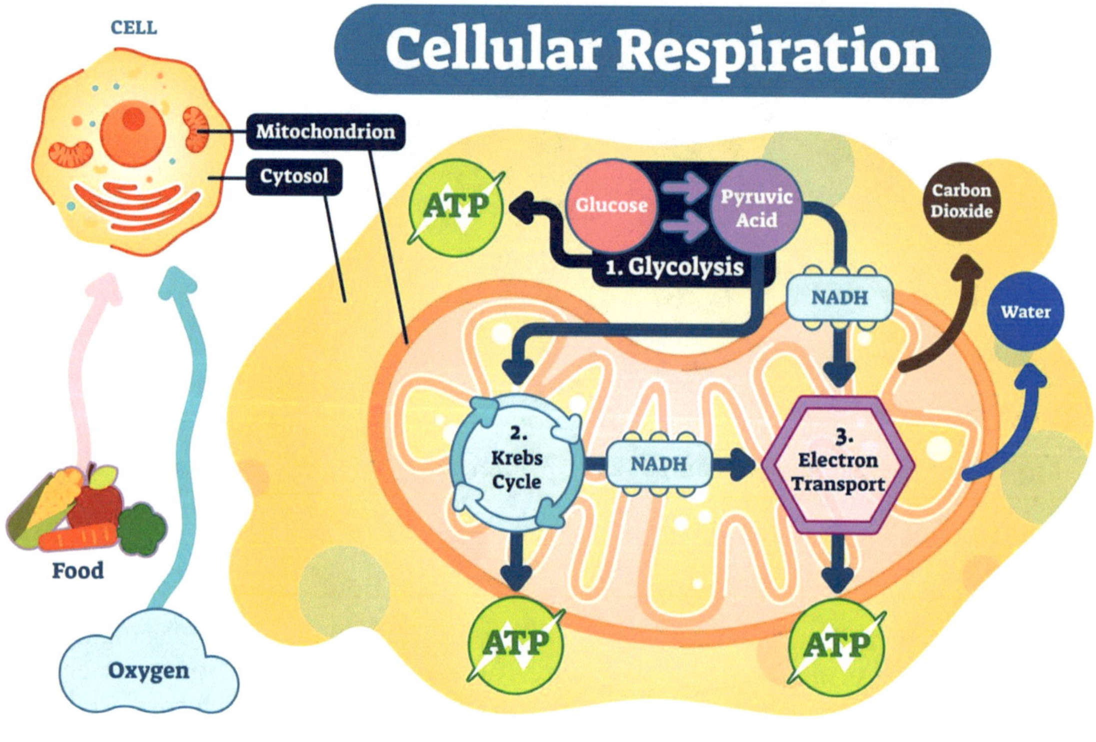

Figure 1.14. Cellular respiration.

Source: https://www.thoughtco.com/thmb/jZkrJoMIeDRpTxSMz_M-C2UJTfE=/1500x1000/filters:no_upscale():max_bytes(150000):strip_icc()/cellular_respiration-8fcc3f1ad3e54a828dabc02146ce4307.jpg.

1.5. Zones of the Respiratory System

The respiratory system is composed of distinct parts that facilitate gas exchange and maintain the health of the respiratory system. The conducting zone, which is mainly the nasal cavity, pharynx, larynx, trachea, bronchi, and bronchioles, allows air to enter the lungs. The region filters, warms up, and humidifies the air, so that only clean and suitable air gets to the alveoli. The intricate structural organization of these pathways, including ciliated epithelium and mucous glands, illustrates the system's capacity to protect against pathogens and particulates, effectively contributing to homeostasis within the respiratory system (Bekish et al., 2014). Unlike the digestive zone, it is in the respiratory zone that oxygen and carbon dioxide are exchanged.

The region contains respiratory bronchioles, alveolar ducts, and many alveoli, which are the most important for gas exchange. The large surface area of the alveoli, together with the thin walls of the pulmonary capillaries, helps oxygen pass into the blood and carbon dioxide leave it. Understanding this zones physiology is crucial for addressing various pathological conditions, such as COPD and pulmonary fibrosis, which can severely impair respiratory function and gas exchange (Bekish et al., 2017). It is also essential to understand how the conducting and respiratory zones interact to see the overall effectiveness of the respiratory system. The transition from conducting airways to respiratory units is an example of how evolution has helped animals breathe effectively. Additionally, distinguishing between these zones helps clinicians develop effective assessment and treatment plans. For example, recognizing the importance of airways in asthma suggests that treatment should target both the lungs and airways. As research continues to expand our understanding of these zones, practical therapeutic approaches will increasingly rely on comprehensive knowledge of respiratory system anatomy and physiology (Bekish et al., 2014).

1.5.1. Conducting Zone: Pathways for Air Movement

The conducting zone helps air move to the lungs, allowing oxygen to be exchanged with the alveoli. In this zone are the nasal cavity, pharynx, larynx, trachea, bronchi, and bronchioles. All the parts are designed to filter, humidify, and warm the air that enters the lungs. The nasal cavity is lined with mucous membranes and cilia, which filter out dirt and germs, allowing cleaner air to reach the lungs. It is crucial to perform this filtration first, as it protects the sensitive tissues in the lungs from harm caused by pollutants and pathogens inhaled from the air. The trachea is a central passage through which air enters the bronchi, which then divide into smaller bronchioles. These structures, which are part of the conducting zone, get smaller as they continue to allow air into the alveoli. At this point, the trachea splits into two primary bronchi, which is essential because it shows how air is optimally distributed in the lungs. Bronchoconstriction and bronchodilation of airways in the lungs are possible because smooth muscle is present in the walls of bronchi and bronchioles. Being able to adjust is essential for the lungs to function effectively in various activities and conditions. The mucociliary escalator is clearly essential for respiratory health during the conducting zone. The movement of cilia and mucus together helps remove debris and harmful microbes from the airways, preventing infection and inflammation. Any interruption in this system may cause respiratory diseases, highlighting the importance of all parts of the conducting zone. A better grasp of these pathways is used to develop strategies that improve breathing and address problems such as asthma and COPD. Thus, by comprehensively examining the conducting zones pathways, we gain valuable insights into the broader context of the respiratory system, which is pivotal for sustaining life through effective gas exchange and homeostasis (Bekish et al., 2014; Beebe et al., 2019) (Figure 1.15).

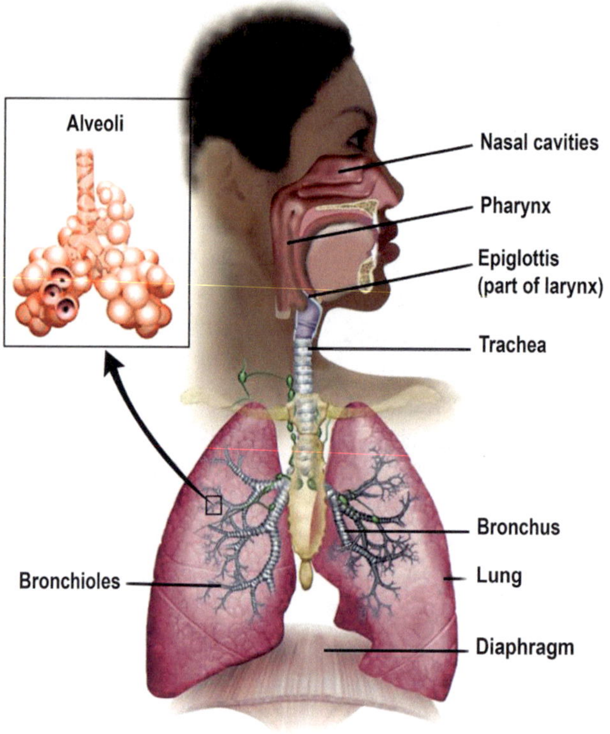

Figure 1.15. Conducting zone.

Source: https://files.mtstatic.com/site_ 7338/55038/0?Expires= 1746681310&Signature= ezobACd7qY28zF1bsZQMbh7Hpf~ HFgKpwy~ ~ymni4ddb5FAsTCcZTJLb2dvdtgInl4QPBU KDGqL30W9qULXyAXN0oAPr8ksPXJoCoIYSAEY7sb NnsWf6jD0Ls5KQRLPf4e6~ERqxw088i-7vrva 4~ZYxLyZJMEsSqRt1~HuwuNk_&Key- Pair-Id=APKAJ5Y 6AV4GI7A555NA.

1.5.2. Respiratory Zone: Sites of Gas Exchange

The respiratory zone in the lungs is necessary for the exchange of oxygen and carbon dioxide between the air and the bloodstream. The main parts in this zone are the alveoli, respiratory bronchioles, and alveolar ducts. There are many tiny alveoli in the lungs, and together they provide the lungs with approximately 70 square meters of surface area. The alveoli have thin, fragile walls, mostly made up of a single layer of epithelial cells, which helps gases move quickly. This way of organizing the lungs helps maintain the substantial differences in oxygen and carbon dioxide levels, which allows oxygen to enter the blood and carbon dioxide to be removed. The alveoli in the respiratory zone are close to many capillaries, which helps gases exchange easily. Since the pulmonary veins are very close to the alveolar walls, oxygen can enter the blood from the air in the lungs and carbon dioxide can leave the blood and enter the air. Differences in partial pressures are what drive this exchange, which helps explain the efficiency of breathing. Alveolar macrophages play a crucial role in maintaining the health of the respiratory zone, as they eliminate foreign particles and pathogens that could impede the exchange of gases. These factors are essential to grasp because they show the many ways respiratory physiology affects our health. Also, the respiratory zones are closely connected to the immune system in the lungs. Because pathogens regularly threaten avian respiratory systems, BALT helps strengthen the immune system which is vital for their well-being. BALT, which is located at the point where the primary and secondary bronchi meet, reaches its full development in birds as they mature, thereby enhancing the immune system's ability to fight respiratory infections. Research indicates that the compartmentalization of immune responses in this tissue may play a pivotal role in how efficiently the lungs respond to different pathogens (Dalamani et al., 2006). This complex interplay between gas exchange and immune defense highlights the respiratory zone's multifaceted importance in maintaining not only respiratory function but also overall health and resilience against disease (Beebe et al., 2019) (Figure 1.16).

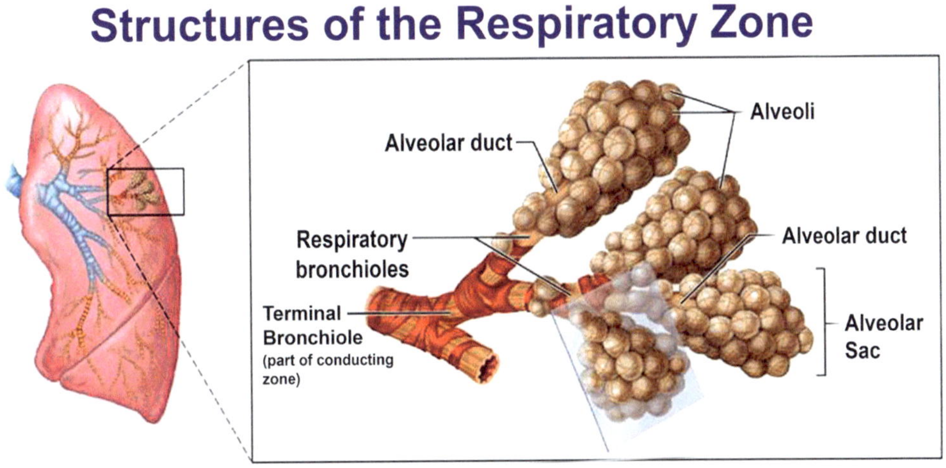

Figure 1.16. Structures of respiratory zone.

Source: https://antranik.org/wp-content/uploads/2024/10/structures-of-respiratory-zone-alveoli-alveolar-duct-alceolar-sac-alveolar-duct-respiratory-bronchioles-terminal-bronchiole.jpg.

1.5.3. Transitional Zone: Areas of Mixed Function

The transitional zone in the respiratory system refers to the parts that carry out functions essential for both moving and refining air. They link the upper and lower respiratory tracts, including the bronchi and bronchioles. The primary purpose of these areas is to ensure that air coming in is warmed, moistened, and cleaned before it reaches the small air sacs in the lungs. Due to this function, the lungs are protected and can work more efficiently to absorb oxygen and eliminate carbon dioxide. Recognizing the importance of these zones underscores the meticulous planning of the respiratory system and highlights the various parts that contribute to its health. In addition to helping with air conditioning, transitional zones play a crucial role in the body's airway defenses. The bronchi and bronchioles are lined with cells that make mucus and cilia, which catch and remove foreign particles, pathogens, and pollutants from the airways. It is essential now, given the increased pollution and rising cases of respiratory diseases. For the airways to remain clear and infections to be avoided, mucus needs to be produced, and the cilia need to move in coordination. As outlined in studies examining the effectiveness of these defense mechanisms, the transitional zones serve as a primary line of defense against airborne threats, thereby contributing to the overall resilience of the respiratory system (Beebe et al., 2019). Besides handling air and defending the body, these zones are also crucial for the physiologic changes needed for exercise and other activities. When we exercise, we use more oxygen, so the bronchi and bronchioles expand to let more air into the alveoli. Neural and hormonal signals facilitate this adjustment, demonstrating that the respiratory system is highly responsive. This flexibility has significant effects, especially in sports and rehabilitation, since it helps guide the way therapists intervene. An appreciation for these complexities reaffirms the necessity of these mixed-function areas in maintaining respiratory efficiency and overall physiological health (Bekish et al., 2014) (Figure 1.17).

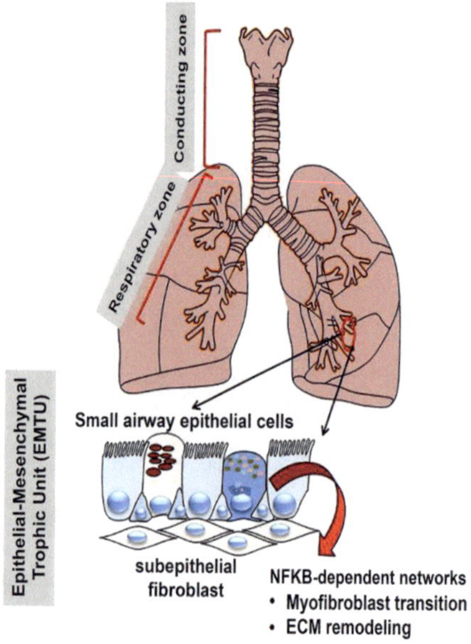

Figure 1.17. Transition zone in airway remodeling.

Source: https://www.researchgate.net/publication/357256227/figure/fig1/AS:11431281251855820@1718383194390/Role-of-the-transition-zone-in-airway-remodeling-Shown-is-a-schematic-view-of-the-human.tif.

SUMMARY

Gas exchange, which is necessary for life, is made possible by the respiratory system, which is a key part of human physiology. Because all parts of its structural anatomy function together, the system is highly efficient at taking in oxygen and expelling carbon dioxide. All the organs involved in breathing, such as the trachea, bronchi, and lungs, are important vital organs since they work together to make breathing both a physical task and an essential part of staying healthy. Besides, understanding the respiratory system's functions reveals its crucial role in various vital processes, including metabolism and acid-base balance, highlighting the multifaceted nature of respiratory physiology. In addition, sorting respiration into external and internal types gives a straightforward way to examine how oxygen is used both in the body as a whole and in individual cells. External respiration is the process of gas exchange in the lungs, and internal respiration is about oxygen entering cells and carbon dioxide leaving them. Due to this division, we can gain a better understanding of airway mechanics and also see how problems in either system may lead to overall health issues. COPD mainly influences external respiration, and this can influence internal respiration, showing how both are linked. Understanding each type of respiration is an essential for understanding how oxygen helps cells, metabolism, and energy production. Lastly, this study of the respiratory system highlights the different zones, including the conducting and respiratory zones, and the functions they perform. The conducting zone, which includes the upper and lower respiratory tracts, is important for removing particles, warming the air, and adding moisture, and the respiratory zone, mainly the alveoli, is where gas exchange happens. Seeing these zones helps explain the changes in the body that support good breathing in different situations. It is essential to use correct and standard descriptions of these zones in medicine, as this helps doctors and other healthcare professionals communicate well. As the literature evolves, it is imperative to ensure terminological coherence to enhance both academic discourse and clinical practice (Bekish et al., 2014; AlMehzaa et al., 2019).

The respiratory system is an important essential for homeostasis in the body because of its functions, how it is built, and the specialized organs it contains. The system primarily facilitates the exchange of gases, allowing oxygen to enter the blood and carbon dioxide to be removed. This key job is made possible by the lungs, trachea, and bronchi, which are built to provide more space for gas exchange. Understanding how the respiratory system is constructed helps us recognize how various diseases can disrupt its functions and compromise health. Research into the mechanisms underpinning respiratory function continues to evolve, further enhancing our comprehension of how these intricate components interact to support life (N/A, 2025). Also, dividing respiration into external and internal forms helps us see when the respiratory system is active during breathing. External respiration deals with the movement of gases between the lungs and the outside, and internal respiration is about the exchange of gases between the blood and tissues. It is essential to know how oxygen is used inside cells and to realize that the body requires more oxygen when we exercise or are sick. Additionally, the separation of zones in the respiratory system, such as the conducting and respiratory zones, illustrates the distinct functions they can perform. These zones differ not only in their structure but also in their specific roles, underscoring the complexity of respiratory physiology (Karolewski et al., 2013). All in all, a detailed look at the respiratory system shows that its different functions, structures and types of respiration are closely connected. All organs and zones in the system play a crucial role in facilitating gas exchange, underscoring the importance of each component in supporting the lungs. By understanding these key points, we not only enhance our understanding of human physiology but also lay a foundation for studying respiratory diseases and their treatments. The continual exploration of this area holds promise for improved therapeutic approaches that could enhance the quality of life for individuals suffering from respiratory diseases, fostering a deeper appreciation for the intricate systems that sustain life (N/A, 2025).

CLOSER LOOK

BLOOD PH

Blood pH, a measure of its acidity or alkalinity, usually is slightly alkaline, ranging from 7.35 to 7.45. This narrow range is crucial for maintaining proper bodily functions, as many biochemical reactions depend on it. The body actively regulates blood pH through various mechanisms to keep it within this optimal range (Figure 1.18).

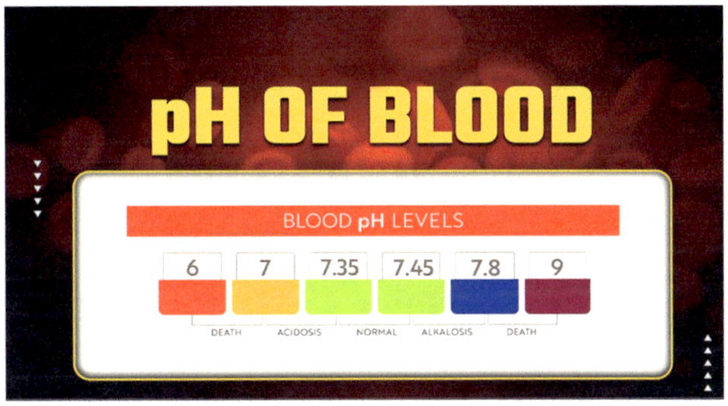

Figure 1.18. pH of blood.

Source: https://static.pw.live/5eb393ee95fab7468a79d189/GLOBAL_CMS_BLOGS/73e56ea7-c69a-4647-9796-d1457dc44e67.jpg.

Key Aspects of Blood pH

- **Normal Range:** 7.35 to 7.45.
- **Slightly Alkaline:** Blood is typically somewhat basic, or alkaline, as it deviates slightly from the neutral pH of 7.0.
- **Importance:** Maintaining this pH is essential for optimal bodily function, as many biochemical reactions are pH-sensitive.
- **Regulation:** The body utilizes a combination of chemical buffers, respiratory adjustments, and kidney function to maintain a stable blood pH.
- **Disorders:** Deviations from the normal pH range, either acidic (pH below 7.35) or alkaline (pH above 7.45), can indicate underlying health problems.

Regulation Mechanisms

- **Chemical Buffers:** The most rapid response to pH changes involves chemical buffers, like the bicarbonate buffer system, which can neutralize acids and bases in the blood.
- **Respiratory Changes:** Breathing rate and depth can be adjusted to influence carbon dioxide levels, which affect blood pH.
- **Kidney Function:** The kidneys excrete excess acids or retain bases in the urine to further regulate blood pH.

Clinical Significance

- **Acidosis:** A blood pH below 7.35 indicates acidosis, which various factors like respiratory or metabolic issues can cause.
- **Alkalosis:** A blood pH above 7.45 indicates alkalosis, also resulting from respiratory or metabolic imbalances.
- **Diagnosis:** Blood gas analysis, which measures pH, carbon dioxide, and bicarbonate levels, is a key tool for diagnosing and monitoring acid-base disorders.

REFERENCES

1. Abdul, N., Sarwani, L., Fatima, A., James, H., Ebrahim, H., Almehzaa, A., & Chakravarty, M. (2019). Exploring use of incorrect terminology used in medical sciences: quest for scientific and academic verity. *Journal of Education and Practice*. https://doi.org/10.7176/jep/10-6-19Beebe, L., Hesse, D., & Massey, A. (2019). *UGA Anatomy and Physiology 2 Lab Manual* (3rd ed.). https://core.ac.uk/download/217306575.pdf (accessed on 31st May 2025).
2. Bekish, V. J., & Zorina, V. V. (2014). *Biology*. https://core.ac.uk/download/80152204.pdf (accessed on 31st May 2025).
3. Bekish, V. J., Logishinets, I. A., & Zorina, V. V. (2017). *Practical Book on Biology*. https://core.ac.uk/download/80152210.pdf (accessed on 31st May 2025).
4. Bhagirath, A. Y., Li, Y., Somayajula, D., Dadashi, M., Badr, S., & Duan, K. (2016). Cystic fibrosis lung environment and Pseudomonas aeruginosa infection. *BMC Pulmonary Medicine, 16*. https://doi.org/10.1186/s12890-016-0339-5 (accessed on 31st May 2025).
5. Breit, S., Kupferberg, A., Rogler, G., & Hasler, G. (2018). Vagus nerve as modulator of the brain–gut axis in psychiatric and inflammatory disorders. *Frontiers in Psychiatry, 9*. https://doi.org/10.3389/fpsyt.2018.00044 (accessed on 31st May 2025).
6. Cryan, S. A., Gilbert, J. L., O'Brien, F., & O'Dea, et al. (2015). *Respiratory Tissue Engineering: Current Status and Opportunities for the Future*. https://core.ac.uk/download/pdf/60777392.pdf (accessed on 31st May 2025).
7. Dalamani, G., Kaspers, B., & Reese, S. (2006). *The Avian Lung-Associated Immune System*. https://core.ac.uk/download/12174987.pdf (accessed on 31st May 2025).
8. Erdő, F., Bors, L. A., Farkas, D. L., Bajza, Á., & Gizurarson, S. (2018). Evaluation of intranasal delivery route of drug administration for brain targeting. *Brain Research Bulletin, 143*, 155–170. https://doi.org/10.1016/j.brainresbull.2018.10.009 (accessed on 31st May 2025).
9. Gkatzis, K., Taghizadeh, S., Huh, D., Stainier, D. Y. R., & Bellusci, S. (2018). Use of three-dimensional organoids and lung-on-a-chip methods to study lung development, regeneration and disease. *European Respiratory Journal, 52*, 1800876. https://doi.org/10.1183/13993003.00876-2018 (accessed on 31st May 2025).
10. Grigoriadis, K., Efstathiou, I., Petrianos, I., Bakalidou, D., Armaganidis, A., & Vasileiadis, G. (2009). *Improvement of Patient's Ventilation by Correcting the Slid Recumbent Position in the ICU. 1*. https://www.semanticscholar.org/paper/d49a9494f68f75fe1b472ed2c19a5382c2fff31e (accessed on 31st May 2025).
11. Karolewski, P., Oleksyn, J., Schnitzer, S. A., & Wyka, et al. (2013). *Phenotypic Correlates of the Lianescent Growth Form: A Review*. https://core.ac.uk/download/237217373.pdf (accessed on 31st May 2025).
12. Keeley, T. P., & Mann, G. E. (2018). Defining physiological normoxia for improved translation of cell physiology to animal models and humans. *Physiological Reviews, 99*, 161–234. https://doi.org/10.1152/physrev.00041.2017 (accessed on 31st May 2025).
13. Keller, L. A., Merkel, O. M., & Popp, A. (2021). Intranasal drug delivery: Opportunities and toxicologic challenges during drug development. *Drug Delivery and Translational Research, 12*, 735–757. https://doi.org/10.1007/s13346-020-00891-5 (accessed on 31st May 2025).

14. Kulish, V., Lage, J. L., & Sourin, A. (2006). Fundamentals of alveolar gas diffusion: Mathematical modeling and visualization. *WIT Transactions on State-of-the-Art in Science and Engineering, 24.* https://www.semanticscholar.org/paper/b899714d0aba93a33ed2a36335f7d5b59134067e (accessed on 31st May 2025).

15. Møller, I. M., Rasmusson, A. G., & Van, A. O. (2021). Plant mitochondria – past, present and future. *The Plant Journal, 108,* 912–959. https://doi.org/10.1111/tpj.15495 (accessed on 31st May 2025).

16. N/A. (2025). *Aerospace Medicine and Biology: A Continuing Bibliography with Indexes, Supplement 128, May 1974.* https://core.ac.uk/download/pdf/42893566.pdf (accessed on 31st May 2025).

17. N/A. (2025). *Aerospace Medicine and Biology: A Continuing Bibliography with Indexes (Supplement 309).* https://core.ac.uk/download/pdf/42832898.pdf (accessed on 31st May 2025).

18. Parlak, A. T. (2021). *Bronchus-Associated Lymphoid Tissue (BALT) Histology and its Role in Various Pathologies.* https://core.ac.uk/download/479934915.pdf (accessed on 31st May 2025).

19. Pérez, H. N., Díaz, S., Garnier, É., Lavorel, S., Poorter, H., Jaureguiberry, P., Bret-Harte, M. S., et al. (2016). Corrigendum to: New handbook for standardized measurement of plant functional traits worldwide. *Australian Journal of Botany, 64,* 715. https://doi.org/10.1071/bt12225_co (accessed on 31st May 2025).

20. Sabuncuoğlu, S., Yalçınkaya, A., Zhou, X., Münch, G., Chang, D., Borrelli, E., Le, N. A., et al. (2022). Importance of oxidative stress and antioxidant system in health and disease. *Biochemistry.* https://doi.org/10.5772/intechopen.100949 (accessed on 31st May 2025).

21. Skoyles, J. R. (2008). Respiratory, postural and spatio-kinetic motor stabilization, internal models, top-down timed motor coordination and expanded cerebello-cerebral circuitry: A review. *Nature Precedings.* https://core.ac.uk/download/pdf/1569872.pdf (accessed on 31st May 2025).

22. Zhu, H., Bi, D., Zhang, Y., Kong, C., Du, J., Wu, X., Wei, Q., et al. (2022). Ketogenic diet for human diseases: The underlying mechanisms and potential for clinical implementations. *Signal Transduction and Targeted Therapy, 7.* https://doi.org/10.1038/s41392-021-00831-w (accessed on 31st May 2025).

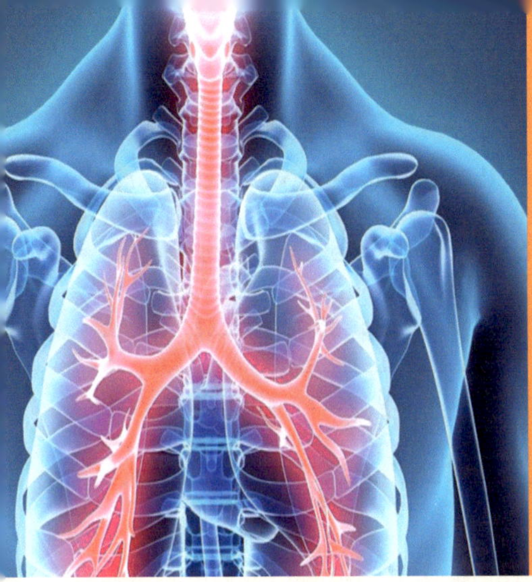

Chapter 2

MECHANICS OF BREATHING

Contents

Introduction

The way breathing functions is an integral part of respiratory physiology, showing the detailed steps that allow gas exchange in the body. Because oxygen is crucial for cellular metabolism, understanding how intrapleural and intra-alveolar pressures impact these functions is essential. When inhaling, the air pressure in the lungs decreases below the air pressure outside, which pulls air into the lungs. The negative pressure is caused by the muscles tightening and the lungs being flexible, illustrating the connection between anatomy and respiratory actions. The lungs to expand and shrink easily because of their elastic properties, which help ventilation work smoothly. Exploring these mechanics helps a person see the many details of respiration and the laws of physics that keep life going, which is helpful in studying what affects breathing. Besides pressure, how the lungs stretch and bend is significant when discussing breathing. Lung compliance refers to the lungs' ability to stretch, and elasticity describes how they return to their original shape after being stretched. Diseases, pressures, or aging can all cause changes in the properties of the respiratory system, which can alter its function. For example, a disease such as pulmonary fibrosis can impair the lungs' ability to function, making it harder to inhale and reducing lung function. Likewise, when elasticity is reduced, expiration becomes less effective, which can cause air to be trapped and result in respiratory distress. According to Negahdar (2012), mechanical changes in lung properties often go unnoticed until they significantly impact lung function. This emphasizes the importance of understanding compliance and elasticity, as they play a crucial role in maintaining respiratory health. Additionally, the muscles of inspiration and expiration facilitate breathing. The diaphragm and intercostal muscles are the primary muscles of inspiration, contracting to expand the thoracic cavity and thereby reduce the pressure inside the lungs. On the other hand, expiration may happen without effort, through the elasticity of the lungs and chest wall, or it can be done by using accessory muscles. For adequate ventilation and oxygenation to happen, the respiratory muscles must work efficiently. In conditions such as cystic fibrosis (CF), as highlighted in Adrian (2012), the increased mucus production can obstruct airflow, making the mechanics of breathing more demanding. When we examine pressures, lung properties, and muscular actions together, we can gain insight into the basic functions of the respiratory system and the challenges in maintaining metabolic balance.

Definition of Breathing Mechanics

Ventilation, or the movement of air in and out of the lungs, depends on the interaction of many physical and physiological forces. Breathing mechanics primarily concerns the interaction between intrapleural pressure, intra-alveolar pressure, and the elasticity of the lungs. Because intrapleural pressure is below atmospheric pressure, it helps the lungs expand when we breathe in. During breathing, the pressure inside the alveoli goes above and below atmospheric pressure, which allows air move in and out of them. The efficiency of gas exchange depends on these pressure changes, which are influenced by the elasticity and compliance of the lungs. Knowing these fundamental ideas is necessary to understand how breathing works and its effects on respiratory health. Respiratory muscles play an active role in facilitating breathing, not just the lungs.

The diaphragm and intercostal muscles primarily help change the size of the chest and create the pressure differences necessary for breathing. When inspired, the diaphragm moves downward, making the thoracic cavity larger, which reduces the pressure inside the lungs and pulls air in. Alternatively, when we are active, the muscles of the abdomen and ribs can contract, which boosts intrapleural pressure and helps us expel air from the lungs. Muscles must work hard enough to beat the resistance from the elastic lungs and the friction in the airways. Efforts to quantify these muscle dynamics and their contributions to ventilation have profound implications for understanding conditions such as asthma or chronic obstructive pulmonary disease (COPD), where breathing mechanics can be significantly disrupted. Surfactant is crucial in breathing because it affects both lung compliance and the effort required to breathe. Surfactant (which is produced by alveolar cells) consists of lipids and proteins and reduces surface tension in the alveoli, allowing them to maintain their shape and prevent collapse during expiration. A decrease in surface tension is vital for good gas exchange and lower effort in breathing, mainly at the end of each breath when pressure in the lungs is lowest. The surfactant system helps open collapsed alveoli, which helps newborns and people with breathing problems by reducing the effects of surface tension. As seen in preterm infants, a lack of adequate surfactant can lead to significant respiratory distress, underscoring the importance of understanding its role in the mechanics of breathing and its therapeutic implications for addressing respiratory failure (Motta, 2012) (Figure 2.1).

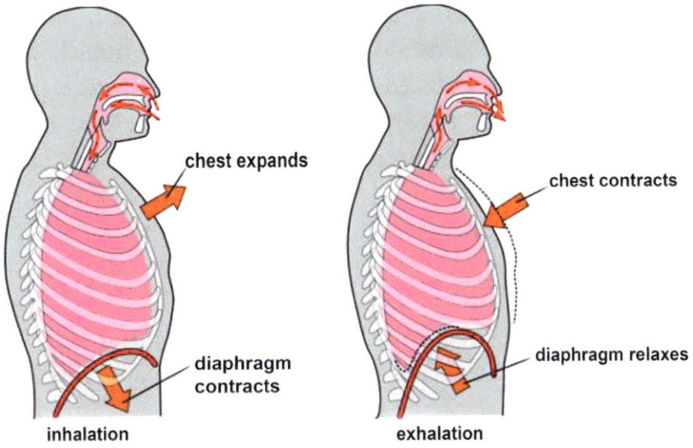

Figure 2.1. Mechanism of breathing.

Source: https://infinitylearn.com/surge/wp-content/uploads/2023/09/Breathing.png.webp.

Importance of Understanding Respiratory Physiology

Knowing respiratory physiology well is essential for understanding how breathing is controlled. The way intrapleural and intra-alveolar pressures change during breathing is significant for lung function. Being aware of how these pressures interact helps healthcare professionals diagnose and treat many lung diseases accurately. An example is pneumothorax, which occurs when there are inappropriate pressure differences, affecting the normal breathing process. Additionally, measuring lung compliance and elasticity provides valuable insights into how breathing functions. When people have less compliance, it may indicate pulmonary fibrosis, which requires treatment. Recognizing these physiological concepts fosters a holistic view of respiratory health. It establishes a foundation for understanding the complex interactions within the respiratory system, thereby emphasizing the importance of this knowledge in clinical practice and research (Knutsen et al., 1976) and discovering how the muscles of inspiration and expiration work improves our understanding of respiratory mechanics. The breathing process mainly depends on the diaphragm and intercostal muscles, and knowing their roles helps explain conditions that affect breathing, such as muscular dystrophies or spinal cord injuries. Examining how these muscles cooperate reveals the complexity of controlling breathing and the adjustments required for exercise and changes in altitude. Understanding how breathing in and breathing out work is essential for both assessing respiratory health and creating rehabilitation plans for patients with lung problems. As respiratory physiology intersects with various medical fields (including pulmonology, critical care, and sports medicine), professionals need to be well-versed in these concepts to promote optimal patient care and improve treatment outcomes (Chatterjee et al., 1997). The role of surfactant in lung function shows why it is vital to understand respiratory physiology in detail. Surfactant reduces the tension at the surface of the alveoli, which prevents atelectasis and improves the lungs' ability to expand. A disruption in surfactant production or function can result in severe conditions, such as neonatal respiratory distress syndrome (RDS), thereby necessitating interventions that target this surfactant system to support lung function and improve oxygenation. In addition, studying the role of surfactants helps explain how fluid exchange across the pulmonary-capillary wall is regulated, which is essential for keeping the respiratory system balanced. Improvements in biomedical research help reveal the details of respiratory physiology, which supports the creation of new treatments for respiratory diseases. Thus, cultivating a thorough understanding of respiratory physiology is essential for fostering innovation and improving patient care within the healthcare sector (Knutsen et al., 1976).

Overview of Key Concepts to be Discussed

To understand respiratory physiology well, one needs to know how breathing works. The relationship between intrapleural and intra-alveolar pressures is significant, since it decides how air enters and leaves the lungs. The pressure inside the pleural cavity, known as intrapleural pressure, is always lower than the atmospheric pressure outside, which helps the lungs expand during inhalation. During inhalation, the pressure inside the alveoli drops below the atmospheric pressure, and it rises above it when we exhale. Because of this relationship, the lungs can ventilate and exchange oxygen efficiently. Therefore, we can now examine other factors, such as lung compliance and elasticity, which will be discussed in more detail later. Lung compliance and elasticity are crucial in understanding how the lungs respond to breathing pressures. Lung compliance refers to the lungs' ability to stretch easily when transpulmonary pressure is altered. Lung elasticity refers to the ability of the lungs to return to their original size after being stretched or filled with air. They significantly affect the effort needed to breathe in and breathe out. Pulmonary fibrosis or emphysema can change these mechanical aspects, which results in higher effort and less effective gas exchange. As this chapter progresses, the implications of compliance and elasticity on respiratory function will be examined, providing insights into their roles in both health and disease (Ltd WKIP). Respiration is made possible by the actions of the diaphragm and intercostal muscles, which control most of the movement. The diaphragm contracts and flattens downward, and the intercostal muscles move the ribs up, which widens the chest cavity and decreases pressure within the alveoli. On the other hand, expiration is usually an automatic process in which the lung tissues recoil and the diaphragm and intercostal muscles relax, allowing air to be pushed out. Also, surfactant, which is secreted by type II alveolar cells, helps decrease the surface tension in the alveoli, allowing the lungs to expand more easily and making breathing less tiring.

2.1. Intrapleural Pressure

Lung expansion and contraction are made possible in breathing by the role of intrapleural pressure. Because of the lungs and chest wall's elasticity, the pressure in the pleural cavity is always lower than atmospheric pressure. The maintenance of this negative intrapleural pressure is crucial during active inspiration, as it creates a pressure gradient that allows air to flow from areas of high pressure (the atmosphere) into areas of low pressure (the alveoli). Since intrapleural pressure and lung volume are closely connected, this variable is significant for breathing, as it regulates airflow and gas exchange at the alveolar membrane. Because of this, understanding intrapleural pressure is important for both medical discussions and clinical assessments of lung function. The connection between intrapleural pressure and lung compliance demonstrates its role in the process of breathing. During the breathing cycle, the pressure within the chest cavity (intrapleural pressure) affects how easily the lungs can expand. When you inhale, the pressure inside the chest drops, causing the alveoli to expand and lowering their pressure, which draws air into them. On the other hand, when we exhale, the systems of compliance are put to the test, because positive pressures in the chest can make it harder to let air out, especially when compliance is low, such as in pulmonary fibrosis. Thus, an understanding of how intrapleural pressure influences lung compliance provides a clearer picture of respiratory mechanics and the various factors that may impede effective breathing (Daphalapurkar et al., 2023). Intrapleural pressure plays a crucial role in determining the way we breathe. All the energy expended on breathing comes from the inhalation and exhalation phases, and these phases are significantly influenced by the intrapleural pressures. If the airways become narrower or the lungs become less elastic, breathing becomes more difficult. Also, when mucus is present in the bronchi, it makes breathing more difficult by raising the resistance to airflow, which forces the respiratory muscles to work harder.

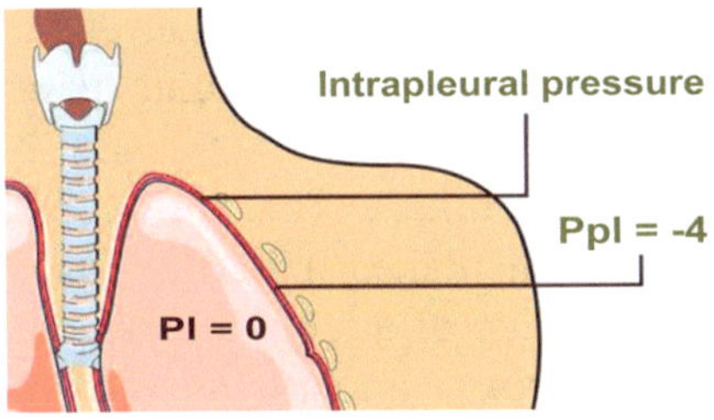

Figure 2.2. Illustration of the intrapleural cavity indicating its pressure.

Source: https://images.my.labster.com/v2/AIR/3a207ba8-34c7-44de-a12b-bb3e6583c42c/AIR_Theory_IntrapleuralCavity.en.x512.png.

Current studies are employing advanced models to investigate the relationship between intrapleural pressure, mucus viscosity, and airflow resistance. These insights are instrumental in understanding not only healthy respiratory mechanics but also the pathology of respiratory diseases, underscoring the complexity and critical nature of intrapleural pressure in respiratory physiology (Ahookhosh et al., 2023) (Figure 2.2).

2.1.1. Definition and Significance of Intrapleural Pressure

The pressure within the pleural cavity (known as intrapleural pressure) plays a crucial role in breathing. The pressure inside the lungs is usually less than atmospheric pressure, which helps the lungs enlarge as air is inhaled. Having negative intra-alveolar pressure is necessary because it draws the lungs outward as the thorax increases in size, causing the lungs to fill with air. The process of air entering the lungs depends on the reduction in intrapleural pressure, which is necessary for the alveoli to expand and fill with air, so it is very important for respiration. Understanding how intrapleural pressure affects lung mechanics is crucial for understanding how the respiratory muscles function properly during breathing in and out. Besides helping the lungs expand, intrapleural pressure plays a role in maintaining the stability of the thoracic cavity. The negative pressure holds the lungs against the chest, preventing them from collapsing as air is exhaled. It is essential for this adhesion to maintain the lungs' proper structure and ventilation. If intrapleural pressure is not normal such as in pneumothorax, the lungs do not work correctly. In some cases, the intense positive pressure can make the lungs collapse which is called atelectasis. Thus, the regulation of intrapleural pressure is essential not only for ensuring effective breathing but also for maintaining pulmonary mechanics and overall respiratory health (Pal et al., 2016). Besides affecting the chest cavity, intrapleural pressure contributes to the body's reactions to different breathing problems. For example, when you exercise intensely, your body requires more oxygen, which necessitates that your lungs work more efficiently. When this happens, the increased intrapleural pressure helps the lungs expand and allows fast air movement. Both the autonomic nervous system (ANS) and respiratory muscles dynamically adjust to maintain a sufficient negative intrapleural pressure, ensuring that it remains adequate for effective gas exchange. Intrapleural pressure is not only involved in the mechanics of breathing but also helps the respiratory system adjust to various situations within the body. Understanding these dynamics is vital for comprehending both normal and compromised respiratory mechanics (Pal et al., 2016).

2.1.2. Factors Affecting Intrapleural Pressure

Intrapleural pressure is influenced by several factors, which interact with the mechanics of breathing during both inhalation and exhalation. At rest, the pressure inside the intrapleural space is lower than the outside pressure, which is needed for the lungs to fill with air. The diaphragm mainly changes the pressure and intercostal muscles contracting when we inhale which widens the chest cavity and increases the size of the intrapleural space. Due to the lowered intrapleural pressure, air can enter the lungs, illustrating the direct relationship between effort and lung function. When expiration begins, these muscles relax, which raises intrapleural pressure and helps expel air from the lungs. It is crucial to understand how these muscles interact to see how gas exchange happens properly in the lungs. In addition to muscles, the flexibility and elasticity of the lungs play a crucial role in controlling intrapleural pressure. The ability of the lungs to expand under pressure is called compliance and it straightaway affects the movement of air into the alveoli. Due to higher compliance, the lungs can expand more, which helps maintain low intrapleural pressures during inhalation. When someone has lung fibrosis or pneumonia, reduced compliance causes their lungs to stiffen, requiring higher pressure inside the chest to ventilate properly. The elasticity of lung tissue, which allows it to return to its original size after being stretched, also helps maintain stable intrapleural pressures during breathing. Studies indicate that the structural integrity and properties of lung tissue influence both compliance and elastance, demonstrating that pathological alterations can significantly impact respiratory mechanics (Daphalapurkar et al., 2023). Surfactant which comes from type II alveolar cells and is made of lipids and proteins, is essential for controlling intrapleural pressures. Surfactant reduces the resistance at the air-liquid interface in the alveoli, which helps the lungs expand more easily when you inhale. This function matters a lot for premature infants, since they often lack surfactant, which makes it harder for them to breathe, and their pressure inside the lungs is unstable. The absence of adequate surfactant also contributes to the collapse of alveoli, increasing the risk of atelectasis and further complicating the respiratory dynamics (Shanny et al., 2016). For this reason, it is essential to understand the relationship between surfactant, lung function and intrapleural pressure to improve respiratory care, mainly for neonates and people with lung disorders. All of these elements together demonstrate the considerable care required to maintain proper respiratory function.

2.1.3. Role in Lung Inflation and Deflation

Lung inflation and deflation are directly connected to how pressures inside the lungs, such as intrapleural and intra-alveolar pressures, are balanced. Inspiration is caused by the diaphragm and intercostal muscles contracting, which results in a vacuum in the thoracic cavity and allows the lungs to expand. Due to this expansion, the pressure inside the alveoli decreases, allowing air to enter the lungs. The elasticity of lung tissue is important, since it helps air move smoothly and the lungs to fill properly. As expiration happens, the muscles relax and the lung tissues stretch back, which produces positive pressure inside the alveoli and forces air out of the lungs. Ventilation and gas exchange in the body are crucial to homeostasis, and this cycle ensures they function efficiently. Surfactant is very important for the process of lung inflation. Because surfactant contains phospholipids produced by type II alveolar cells, it decreases the surface tension in the alveoli, making the lungs more flexible. Because surface tension is reduced, the alveoli can expand more easily when out, and remain open when exhaling. Because of surfactant, neonates can easily adjust from the fluid-filled uterus to breathing air outside the womb. At this critical juncture, the surfactant system must efficiently work to facilitate lung recruitment by reducing surface tension, thereby promoting inflation and ensuring proper gas exchange (Motta, 2012). Because of surfactant, the lungs can continue to breathe normally and avoid problems such as atelectasis that might result from underinflated alveoli. The mechanical function of the respiratory muscles also is crucial for the lungs to effectively fill with air, and later and expel it. When you inhale, the diaphragm contracts, making the thoracic cavity smaller and lowering air pressure, which facilitates airflow into the lungs. During expiration, especially when forced, the abdominal muscles contract and push the diaphragm upward, which allows air to leave the lungs more quickly. The pressures created by muscles have to handle airway friction and the stretch of lung tissue to allow air to move efficiently. Understanding this interplay is further informed by mathematical models that analyze airflow dynamics, highlighting the importance of both muscle strength and lung compliance in determining respiratory efficiency (Giamagas et al., 2018). Collectively, the interplay of pressures, surfactant function, and muscle actions highlights the complex mechanisms governing lung inflation and deflation, which are essential for effective respiratory function (Figure 2.3).

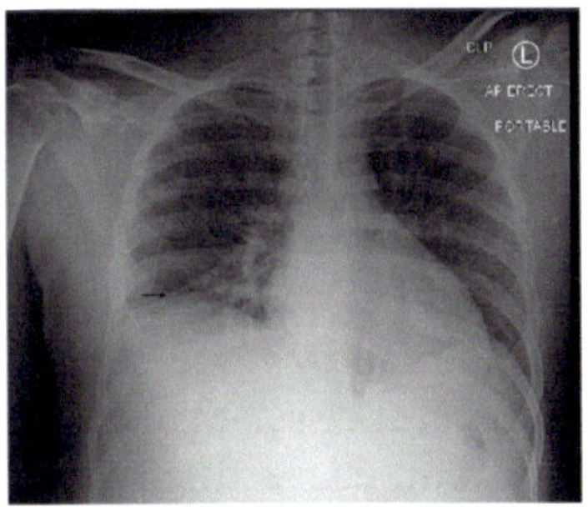

Figure 2.3. Suboptimal lung inflation with bibasilar atelectasis.

Source: https://www.researchgate.net/publication/354937595/figure/fig1/AS:1080241942474879@1634561157833/Suboptimal-lung-inflation-with-bibasilar-atelectasis-identified-by-arrow.jpg.

2.2. Intra-Alveolar Pressure

Alveolar pressure, which is the same as intra-alveolar pressure, is essential for breathing because it helps control the movement of air into and out of the lungs. The pressure here refers to the pressure inside the alveoli, where gas exchange occurs. When we inhale, the diaphragm contracts, which increases the size of the thoracic cavity and lowers the air pressure in the alveoli below the pressure in the air outside. The air moves into the lungs because of the pressure gradient. When the lungs are expiring, the diaphragm relaxes and the thoracic cavity shrinks, which increases the pressure inside the alveoli and forces air out of the lungs. In short, the way pressure changes in the lungs is necessary for proper ventilation and for getting oxygen to the blood and removing carbon dioxide. Several factors influence intra-alveolar pressure, including lung compliance and the presence of surfactant. Lung compliance refers to the lungs' ability to expand more easily; this means that a higher compliance will cause a greater change in lung volume for the exact pressure change. A substance called surfactant which comes from type II alveolar cells, reduces the surface tension inside the alveoli, so they do not collapse and can expand more easily during breathing. Because asthma can alter the structure of the lungs, the relationship between intra-alveolar pressure and lung compliance is crucial. In asthma, for instance, inflammation and bronchoconstriction can hinder airflow, thereby altering normal intra-alveolar pressure dynamics and complicating the breathing process, particularly in severe cases marked by hypercapnic respiratory failure (Eva, 2023). Additionally, factors such as mucus can impact the resistance to airflow and alter the pressure within the alveoli. Mucus buildup in the airways can cause them to narrow, increasing the effort required to breathe and altering the pressure differences. In a study of viscoelastic lung compliance and airflow resistance, it was found that the mechanics of airflow are affected by the physical properties of mucus within the bronchioles (Daphalapurkar et al., 2023). Such a situation is important and critical in diseases where mucus production increases, such as in COPD or CF. Understanding these interactions is crucial for developing effective therapeutic strategies that improve lung function and optimize respiratory mechanics, thereby ensuring that intra-alveolar pressure remains within the physiological range necessary for adequate ventilation (Figure 2.4).

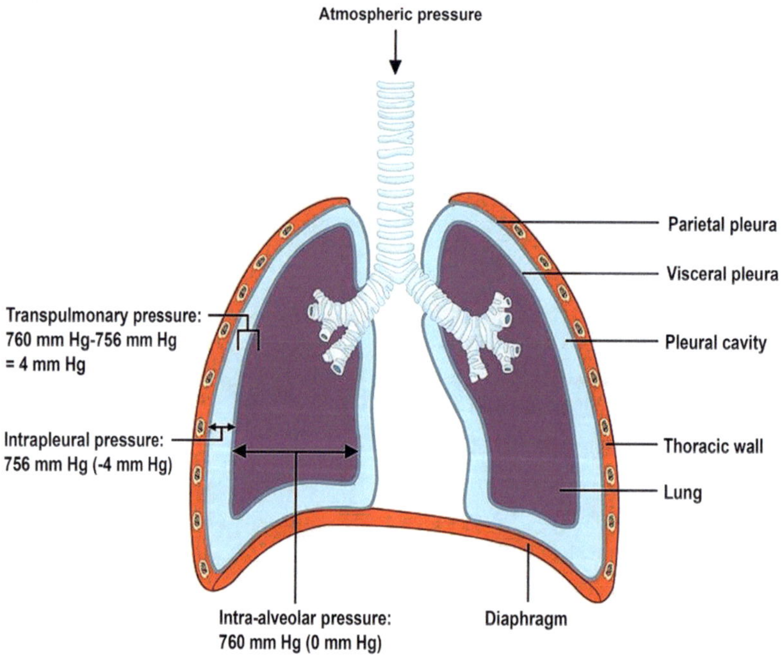

Figure 2.4. Image illustrating transpulmonary, intrapleural and intra-alveolar pressure.

Source: https://upload.wikimedia.org/wikipedia/commons/thumb/2/2c/2315_Intrapulmonary_and_Intrapleural_Pressure.jpg/800px-2315_Intrapulmonary_and_Intrapleural_Pressure.jpg.

2.2.1. Definition and Measurement of Intra-Alveolar Pressure

Alveolar pressure, which is another name for intra-alveolar pressure, is vital in breathing because it shows the pressure inside the alveoli during breathing. Alveolar pressure, which is the pressure of air in the alveoli, helps gas exchange between the lungs and blood. Pressure in the lungs is lower than outside air pressure when you breathe in, allowing air to enter, and higher when you breathe out, pushing the air out. Measuring intra-alveolar pressure accurately is crucial for studying respiratory mechanics, which is typically achieved by using specialized pressure sensors or manometers that provide real-time data on breathing changes. To understand respiratory function and diseases, it is essential to comprehend these dynamics. Besides its measurement, intra-alveolar pressure is closely related to lung compliance and elastic recoil. The mode in which the lungs expand and contract depends on these elements, which also change the pressure in the alveoli. A drop in lung compliance may cause the air pressure in alveoli to rise during inhalation, which makes breathing less effective. In the case of obstructive lung diseases, the ability to control air pressures may be affected, which can cause difficulties with gas exchange. Examining these pressures and their effect on lung mechanics helps explain various respiratory disorders by highlighting the connection between pressure in the alveoli and the amount of air the lungs can hold. Research combining different scales of measurement, as observed in the wide-ranging modeling of lung mechanics, can further refine our understanding of these interactions (Anne-Lauzon et al., 2012). Additionally, intra-alveolar pressure assessment must consider the role of surfactant, a surface-active substance that helps maintain stable pressures within the alveoli. Making surfactants is crucial in preventing the collapse of alveoli when the pressure within them changes during breathing. Lung diseases and injuries can influence the surfactant and the way the lung works, which may result in altered pressures in the air sacs during breathing. The integration of advanced imaging techniques, such as 4-D CT, enables a more nuanced understanding of how both regional and global lung function impacts intra-alveolar pressure dynamics (Negahdar, 2012). Recognizing the multifactorial nature of intra-alveolar pressures informs both clinical assessments and therapeutic approaches for various pulmonary conditions, emphasizing the need for continued research and innovation in respiratory physiology (Figure 2.5).

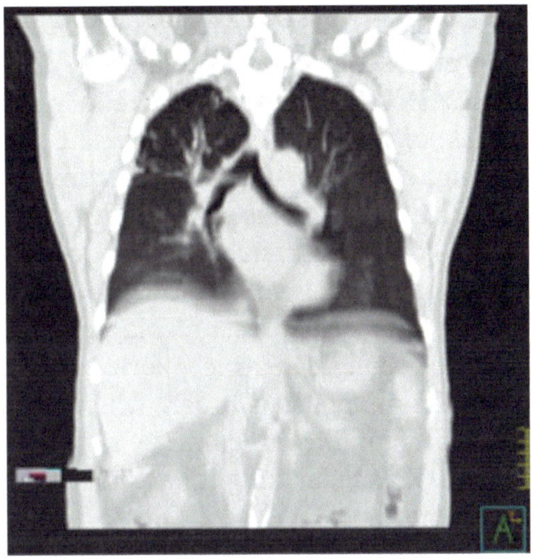

Figure 2.5. Coronal images of the eight breathing phases of the 4D CT (a)–(h) and (i) the slow CT for the patient undergoing audio-visual training.

Source: https://www.researchgate.net/profile/George-Starkschall/publication/8492785/figure/fig9/AS:394411973332996@1471046550115/Coronal-images-of-the-eight-breathing-phases-of-the-4D-CT-a-h-and-i-the-slow-CT-for.png.

2.2.2. Relationship with Atmospheric Pressure

To understand breathing, it is essential to know how atmospheric pressure and lung mechanics are related. Atmospheric pressure, which comes from the weight of air, is very important for both breathing in and breathing out. The diaphragm and intercostal muscles tighten during inhalation, which lowers the pressure inside the chest to a level lower than the outside air pressure. Because the pressure outside is higher, air is drawn into the lungs, demonstrating that atmospheric pressure helps keep breathing possible. When air pressure differs, for example, at high altitudes, the usual ways the lungs work can be affected, which impacts oxygen uptake and lung function. Due to these pressure gradients, it is evident that optimal air conditions are necessary for effective gas exchange and optimal respiratory health. Lung tissues are elastic, which demonstrates the link between atmospheric pressure and respiratory mechanics. Being able to stretch and recoil is called elasticity, and it is very important, crucial for the lungs to function well in ventilation. When atmospheric pressure is low, understanding lung compliance is crucial. Compliance, which is the amount of lung volume change for every change in intrapleural pressure, may be affected negatively by changes in atmospheric conditions. A disease like pulmonary fibrosis, which changes the flexibility of the lungs, may significantly reduce compliance, making it hard for a person to breathe normally.

An enhanced understanding of how lung compliance and external pressure interact can inform clinical approaches for managing patients with respiratory diseases, ensuring that interventions are tailored to maintain optimal lung function amidst changing environmental pressures (Daphalapurkar et al., 2023). Additionally, the role of surfactant in maintaining healthy lung function during changes in air pressure is crucial. Thanks to the surfactant, which is secreted by the alveolar cells, the alveoli can expand easily when air is inhaled. When there is a change in the air pressure around the lungs, surfactant helps maintain alveolar stability and stops them from collapsing, which might cause atelectasis. The level of surficial tension can be adjusted by surfactants, which is essential for preventing instabilities caused by changes in external pressure. Consequently, understanding both atmospheric influences and the biomechanical properties of lung structures, including the role of surfactant, is vital for comprehending the complexities of respiratory mechanics and the work of breathing (Negahdar, 2012).

2.2.3. Impact on Gas Exchange Efficiency

The exchange of gas in the lungs is highly influenced by mechanical factors, particularly the pressures within the pleural and alveolar spaces. They are necessary to keep the lungs inflated and facilitate breathing. Negative intrapleural pressure helps the lungs expand during breathing, and changes in intra-alveolar pressure facilitate effective gas exchange. A decrease in intrapleural pressure, which occurs in some lung diseases, makes the lungs less flexible and reduces the body's ability to exchange gases. Reduced compliance means the lungs do not inflate to their full capacity, which reduces the amount of surface area for diffusion. This interplay between pressures underscores the vital mechanics of breathing, revealing how even slight alterations can disrupt the delicate balance necessary for optimal gas exchange (Falkenström et al., 2010). The elasticity and compliance of the lungs are also very important for efficient gas exchange. Good compliance helps the lungs expand more, which is essential for ventilation. In cases like pulmonary fibrosis, the lungs become stiffer due to reduced elasticity, making it harder to inhale and exhale air. The elasticity of the lungs, derived from their strong structure, enables them to expel air containing carbon dioxide. If the lungs do not empty properly, carbon dioxide is not removed, which can upset the acid-base balance in the blood. Such cases make it clear that how the lungs work directly affects gas exchange and the supply of oxygen to tissues. Exploring these relationships elucidates the importance of maintaining lung mechanics for preserving respiratory efficiency (Falkenström et al., 2010). In any discussion about how efficiently the lungs exchange gases, surfactant in the alveoli plays a crucial role. Surfactants are made up of lipids and proteins and help. It helps reduce the tension at the air-liquid boundary in the alveoli, so the alveoli do not collapse when you breathe out, and the lungs are evenly inflated. Surfactant increases the lungs' ability to stretch and prevents collapse, which helps them exchange more gases with less air. Insufficient surfactant production or function, as seen in conditions like neonatal respiratory distress syndrome (RDS), drastically reduces gas exchange efficiency, resulting in hypoxemia and respiratory failure. The interplay among surfactant dynamics, lung compliance, and mechanical pressures exemplifies the intricate mechanisms that contribute to effective gas exchange, emphasizing the necessity for therapeutic interventions when these systems are compromised (Drasovean et al., 2023).

2.3. Lung Compliance

The mechanism of the lungs' expansion and contraction during breathing depends on their 'compliance', making it a crucial understanding. Lung compliance refers to the extent to which the lungs expand in response to an increase in pressure inside the chest, indicating the elasticity of both the lungs and the chest wall. It takes minimal effort for a highly compliant lung to expand, but a lung with less compliance needs much more effort to expand. Lung compliance may decrease in pulmonary fibrosis or increase in emphysema, which affects how well the lungs function. Furthermore, the effectiveness of the respiratory muscles, especially the diaphragm and intercostal muscles, greatly relies on the lung compliance, as any increase in effort required to achieve ventilation can increase the work of breathing (Cuttano et al., 2013). The function of surfactant in making the lungs more compliant is crucial. Surfactant, a lipoprotein produced by alveolar epithelial cells, decreases the surface tension between air and liquid in the alveoli. Because of this reduction, alveoli remain stable, do not collapse as air is exhaled, and become more flexible. If the level of surfactant is too low, such as in neonatal RDS, the extra surface tension decreases how much the lungs can expand and how well gases are exchanged. Therefore, the respiratory muscles must work harder because they must push against the greater resistance in the airways. The interaction between surfactant, lung compliance, and the mechanics of breathing underscores the intricate physiological balance necessary for adequate respiration, highlighting the importance of understanding these factors in contexts such as mechanical ventilation and treatment of respiratory illnesses (Negahdar, 2012). When treating patients with respiratory distress, assessing lung compliance is very important. When lung compliance is not standard, it may show an underlying disease and can have a significant effect on how treatment is chosen.

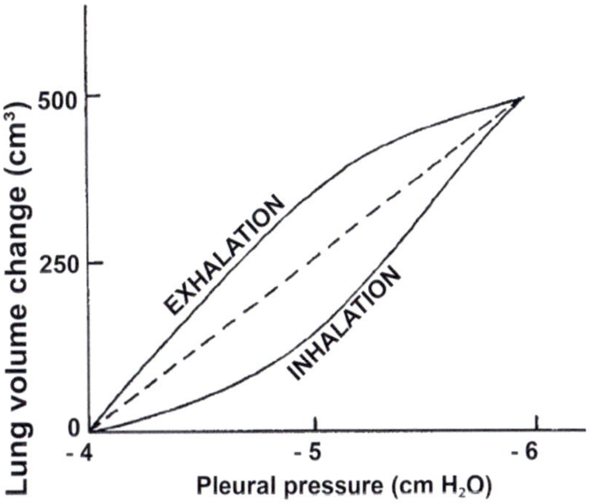

Figure 2.6. Compliance diagram of the two lungs in a normal person.

Source: https://www.researchgate.net/profile/Dulli-Agrawal-2/publication/252275502/figure/fig1/AS:298022601805827@1448065533454/Compliance-diagram-of-the-two-lungs-in-a-normal-person.png.

For example, in people on a ventilator, checking compliance helps establish the correct ventilator settings and enhance gas exchange. Additionally, understanding the relationship between regional lung compliance and overall function can inform therapeutic approaches, such as the application of lung protective strategies in patients with acute respiratory distress syndrome (ARDS). Innovations in imaging techniques, including four-dimensional computed tomography (CT), have further enhanced our ability to assess regional lung mechanics, allowing for a more personalized approach to treatment based on quantifiable metrics of lung compliance (Negahdar, 2012; Cuttano et al., 2013). These advancements emphasize the importance of a detailed understanding of lung compliance within the broader context of respiratory health and disease management (Figure 2.6).

2.3.1. Definition of Lung Compliance and Its Importance

Lung compliance refers to the ability of the lung to stretch in response to changes in pressure, primarily during inhalation. The change in lung volume for every unit increase in pressure is used to define it, which is often expressed as the ratio of volume to pressure across the whole lung surface area. High compliance is a sign that the lungs can open up well, which helps with ventilation, but low compliance usually means the lungs are stiff and hard to open. Due to this characteristic, the efficiency of breathing and the way the lungs function are significantly influenced. A healthy person's lungs are flexible, so the effort needed to breathe is less, and the lungs can ventilate well and keep the blood oxygenated, which supports the metabolism in all parts of the body. Lung compliance matters in both basic breathing and in medical diagnosis and treatment. Pulmonary fibrosis, emphysema, and ARDS are some of the conditions where abnormal lung compliance is often found. As a result, expanding the lungs is more difficult, which makes breathing harder and causes respiratory distress. Evaluating lung compliance in a timely manner helps doctors determine the severity of the patient's condition and choose the most effective treatment, such as mechanical ventilation or medication. In addition, knowing about lung compliance helps healthcare workers understand how external things—like positioning and surfactant—can affect breathing, which supports better choices in emergencies. Lung compliance is closely tied to the effects of surface tension in the alveoli which is essential for surfactants in respiration. The lipoprotein surfactant, produced by type II alveolar cells, reduces the stress on the alveoli and keeps them from collapsing, which significantly improves the flexibility of the lungs. In premature infants, this relationship is significant because they might not have enough surfactant which can cause respiratory problems such as neonatal RDS. Additionally, understanding how surfactant affects lung compliance can inform the development of treatments that enhance breathing. Therefore, maintaining optimal lung compliance is not merely a matter of physiological importance but has profound implications for both individual health and broader public health considerations in managing respiratory diseases and conditions, as noted in previous studies (Knutsen et al., 1976; Hoo et al., 2005).

2.3.2. Factors Influencing Lung Compliance

Lung compliance is essential for breathing, demonstrating how the lungs are able to expand and contract in response to changes in air pressure. The way the lung is built and the presence of surfactant are among the main reasons for lung compliance. The lung parenchyma is viscoelastic, and it is the elastic fibers that enable the lung to stretch and return to its original shape. If elastic fibers are damaged, typically due to pulmonary fibrosis, the lungs become less flexible, making it harder for them to expand during inhalation. Also, when mucus plugs the airways, it makes it harder for air to move in and out of the lungs which affects how well the lungs can function. It is essential to understand these factors to develop effective treatments that enhance lung function, particularly in individuals with diseases that impair lung compliance. Lung compliance is also strongly affected by pulmonary surfactant, which is made and released by type II alveolar cells. The presence of surfactant reduces the tension at the air-liquid interface in the alveoli, which allows them to expand when breathing in and prevents them from collapsing when breathing out. A lack or problem with surfactant, which is common in neonatal RDS, makes breathing more difficult and uses more energy. A change in the makeup of surfactant, as occurs in CF, can lead to increased airway obstruction and mucus production, which further exacerbates the decline in lung compliance. CF is known to cause increased mucus production, which results in bronchiectasis and airway consolidation, making it very hard for air to move through the lungs. Improving the effectiveness of surfactants may help optimize lung compliance in patients, potentially leading to enhanced respiratory function and improved overall health. Besides physical exercise, the way a person is positioned and the environment are important for lung compliance. For example, changing your body position can change the pressure within your chest, which can make it easier or harder to breathe; lying down often takes more effort than standing. Exercise also helps improve lung compliance by building stronger muscles and enhancing respiratory function, which allows air to move more easily and the lungs to recoil more effectively. Pollution and other environmental issues may cause chronic inflammation and harm the lungs, which makes compliance worse. The literature emphasizes that understanding how mucus affects airflow resistance is crucial. A lower viscosity of mucus, correlated with a higher frequency of breath cycles, can facilitate effective lung mechanics and improve compliance, suggesting that therapeutic measures should be aimed at managing mucus properties to enhance respiratory function (Adrian, 2012; Daphalapurkar et al., 2023) (Figure 2.7).

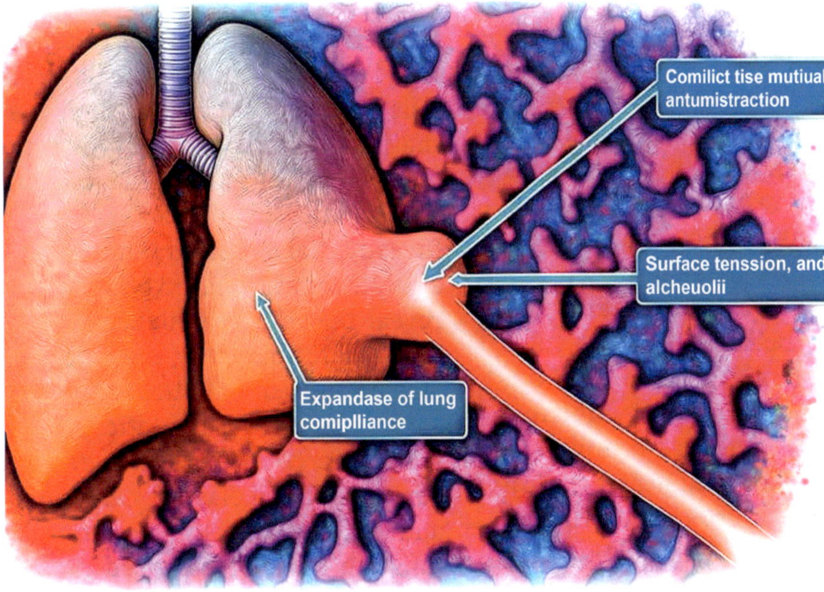

Figure 2.7. Factors influencing lung compliance.

Source: https://esoftskills.com/wp-content/uploads/2024/01/factors_influencing_lung_compliance.jpg.

2.3.3. Clinical Implications of Altered Lung Compliance

A change in lung compliance can have significant effects on patients who have different respiratory conditions. Lung compliance refers to the lungs' ability to expand and contract in response to changes in pressure, which is crucial for effective breathing. When compliance falls, which can happen in pulmonary fibrotic diseases, patients have to work harder to breathe. The lungs have to work harder to bring in the same amount of air, which makes the muscles used for breathing tired. Therefore, healthcare providers regularly use spirometry to assess a patient's lung function and determine the extent to which the disease is affecting them. By understanding the impact of altered compliance on breathing efficiency, clinicians can tailor therapeutic interventions to mitigate respiratory distress, ultimately improving patient outcomes in those with compromised lung function (Knutsen et al., 1976). Surfactant is crucial for maintaining the lungs' flexibility and compliance. Because of the surfactant, the alveoli can expand more easily when we breathe in. If surfactant is missing, such as in premature infants or adults with ARDS, the lungs have very reduced compliance of this, atelectasis and difficulty with gas exchange occur, which changes how patients are treated. For example, surfactant replacement therapy was developed to address these issues, which highlights a change in treatment plans that helps patients comply better. When clinicians understand the mechanisms involved, they can select treatments that enhance lung function. Thus, a comprehensive grasp of compliance dynamics is indispensable for informed clinical decision-making in respiratory care (Hoo et al., 2005). Considering the potential long-term effects of altered lung compliance is crucial for patient care. It has been found through research that infants with respiratory problems or those exposed to difficulties during pregnancy often experience lung function problems as they grow older. They emphasize that early intervention and regular monitoring are crucial. By studying lung compliance, it becomes possible to identify individuals at risk and design targeted interventions to prevent serious lung diseases. If healthcare providers are aware that non-compliance can lead to chronic lung diseases, they can offer patients guidance on lifestyle changes and schedule regular check-ups. These strategies are paramount in improving the quality of life and reducing healthcare costs associated with chronic respiratory diseases, emphasizing the necessity for vigilance in managing altered lung compliance throughout patients' lifespans (Knutsen et al., 1976).

2.4. Lung Elasticity

Lung elasticity is significant for breathing, as it affects how the lungs and the respiratory system function. Because the lung parenchyma is elastic, the lungs can expand when we inhale and contract when we exhale. Usually, the elastic fibers in the lungs help the alveoli go back to their original position after every breath. However, illnesses such as those that cause too much mucus can seriously reduce how elastic the lungs are. Changes in lung mechanics can make breathing more difficult, which may impact how air flows and how gas exchange occurs. Investigations into the rheological properties and structural characteristics of lung tissues reveal that the compliance of the lungs is not solely determined by the elastin and collagen matrix, but is also influenced by external factors, such as mucus accumulation, which can induce resistance (Daphalapurkar et al., 2023). Lung compliance and elasticity are opposite in health and disease. Lung stiffness and the ease of lung inflation must be balanced for the respiratory system to function properly. If airway resistance increases because of a disease, such as in CF, it leads to a loss of lung elasticity. Due to the thick mucus in CF, the small airways become blocked, making the lungs less flexible and increasing the effort required to breathe. As a result, breathing becomes more difficult for the lungs, which have to work harder to supply the body with sufficient oxygen. It is supported by research that clearing mucus well can help reduce some of these problems, which is why interventions for better airway clearance are essential. By minimizing mucus retention, not only is the lung's capacity restored, but the work required for breathing is also diminished, thereby improving overall respiratory function (Adrian, 2012). The interaction between lung elasticity and surfactant helps each other, adding to the complexity of breathing. The surfactant, a lipoprotein complex produced by alveolar type II cells, helps prevent the air in the alveoli from collecting at the surface, thereby preventing them from collapsing during exhalation. It increases the elasticity of the lungs, allowing them to expand more easily with less effort. If surfactant production is interrupted, such as in some neonatal lung diseases, the lungs become very elastic, and this interferes with proper breathing. It is crucial to understand how elasticity, surfactant, and mucus work together to facilitate breathing. Improved insights into these relationships can pave the way for enhanced therapeutic strategies that target not only mucus clearance but also the restoration of ideal lung elasticity and compliance, thereby fundamentally contributing to better management of respiratory ailments (Daphalapurkar et al., 2023).

2.4.1. Definition and Role of Lung Elasticity in Breathing

Lung elasticity is crucial for breathing, as it determines how the lungs expand and contract during each breath. It is mainly the elastic fibers in lung tissue and the surface tension from the fluid in alveoli that make the lungs elastic. Because of this property, the lungs can expand during inhalation and then recoil during exhalation. If a lung is elastic, it can return to its resting size after being inflated, which helps with ventilation and gas exchange. If the lungs are not elastic enough, as in emphysema, the balance between breathing in and out is disrupted, and it becomes harder to breathe, so lung elasticity is essential for healthy breathing. How elastic the lungs are directly affects how easily they can be expanded, which is called lung compliance. When the lungs are elastic, they are more able to fill with air, which is essential for breathing. If the lungs are not elastic enough, compliance decreases, which makes the respiratory muscles work harder to ventilate the lungs properly. Many factors, such as age, environment, and specific health issues, can affect the elasticity and compliance of the lungs over time.

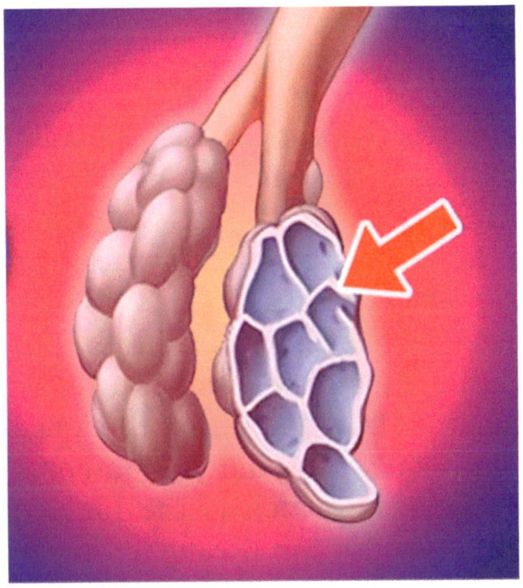

Figure 2.8. Lung elasticity.

Source: https://i.ytimg.com/vi/KYmrI_vYCus/maxresdefault.jpg.

For instance, progressive lung diseases can stiffen the lung tissue or damage the elastic fibers, thereby limiting the lungs' ability to expand effectively during inhalation, ultimately impacting the efficiency of gas exchange within the alveoli (Biga et al., 2019). Understanding these relationships enables doctors to diagnose and effectively treat respiratory problems. Additionally, surfactant is crucial for maintaining the elasticity of the lungs. Alveolar cells make surfactant, which reduces tension at the surface of the alveoli, keeping them from collapsing and supporting lung elasticity during breathing. Because surfactant reduces surface tension, the lungs can expand and contract more effectively, which facilitates efficient gas exchange. A lack of surfactant can cause breathing problems, which are most apparent in neonatal RDS. The balance between lung elasticity and surfactant is vital for the lungs to work correctly. Overall, lung elasticity is integral not just for physical lung mechanics but also for ensuring that ventilation and gas exchange proceed optimally (Biga et al., 2019) (Figure 2.8).

2.4.2. Mechanisms Contributing to Lung Elasticity

Lungs stretch and shrink easily, a trait which helps enable efficiency in breathing. It is primarily due to the presence of collagen and elastin fibers in the lung tissue that gives the lung its elasticity. Due to these fibers, the lungs can expand during inhalation and recoil during exhalation, facilitating the smooth movement of air in and out of the lungs. Lung tissue's viscoelastic quality is important for lung compliance, which is the lung's ability to stretch and let air through, and this can be affected by diseases. The integration of continuum-based numerical modeling has significantly advanced the understanding of these relationships, revealing that changes in the material properties of lung tissue can have a substantial influence on resistance to airflow and overall lung function (Daphalapurkar et al., 2023). Surfactant greatly helps the lungs expand and contract by lowering the tension on the alveoli walls. Because of this mixture of lipids and proteins, a monolayer is created at the air-liquid boundary in alveoli, which helps the alveoli remain stable and prevents them from collapsing when you breathe out. As surfactant reduces surface tension, the small air sacs in the lungs remain open, allowing the lungs to be more flexible, which in turn facilitates gas exchange. In conditions such as CF, where mucus secretion is excessive and affects surfactant function, the interplay between mucus and surfactant can lead to increased work of breathing and compromised lung elasticity (Adrian, 2012). So, keeping the surfactant working properly helps the lung return to its normal position after each breath. Also, the active nature of lung elasticity can be changed by factors outside the body, such as mucus in the airways. The way mucus behaves such as how viscous it is, significantly affects airflow and how the lungs work. According to findings, conditions that lead to increased mucus production, such as bronchiectasis or CF, not only impede bronchial airflow but also disrupt the normal viscoelastic balance of the lungs (Daphalapurkar et al., 2023). Improving the way mucus is cleared from the lungs is crucial for these patients, as it helps the airways function better and reduces the risk of further lung damage. So, the processes involved in lung elasticity are all linked, which explains why both lung parts and external influences are essential for good lung and breathing health.

2.4.3. Effects of Decreased Elasticity on Respiratory Function

The lungs need to be flexible to work properly and the elasticity of lung tissue provides this flexibility. If lung elasticity declines, which is common in emphysema and other respiratory diseases, the way air is brought into the lungs is greatly affected. Reduced elasticity leads to the lungs becoming less compliant, thus making it more difficult for the thoracic cavity to expand properly during inhalation. Consequently, the alveoli receive less air, which makes it harder for gas exchange to happen. Because the lungs must quickly expand and contract during exercise or when breathing quickly, lung elasticity is significant for breathing well. Therefore, when elasticity is reduced, it can make it very difficult for a person to do even simple activities, and this can cause the respiratory muscles to work harder as they try to move air through the stiffened lungs. Besides affecting how the lungs work, reduced elasticity can also impact the overall health of the lungs. The way lung tissues behave viscoelastically is essential for the flow of air into and out of the lungs. If lung tissue loses its elasticity, as in COPD, it can cause airflow to become more difficult, making it easier for mucus to accumulate in the airways. This becomes especially clear in cases of mucus plugging, which adds additional obstacles for airflow during ventilation. Especially, the interaction between airflow resistance and compliance underscores the importance of having effective airway clearance methods. As illustrated in findings on CF, excessive mucus production can lead to bronchiectasis and further diminish lung function, underscoring the need to address both the structural and physiological aspects of lung health to optimize respiratory efficiency (Adrian, 2012). It is clear from examining the broader results of decreased lung elasticity that these changes can significantly impact the way people breathe. If elastic recoil is not working well, more energy is needed to breathe, which puts more strain on the respiratory muscles. Using the accessory muscles of respiration, such as the sternocleidomastoid and scalenes, can cause tiredness and discomfort in those affected. Additionally, the new breathing patterns and increased effort can accelerate the decline of lung function over time. Consequently, developing strategies to improve lung elasticity through targeted therapies, pulmonary rehabilitation (PR), and optimal management of secretions becomes essential for restoring respiratory function and enhancing quality of life (Daphalapurkar et al., 2023). Addressing these factors holistically can help mitigate the adverse effects imposed by decreased lung elasticity on both the mechanical and functional aspects of respiration (Figure 2.9).

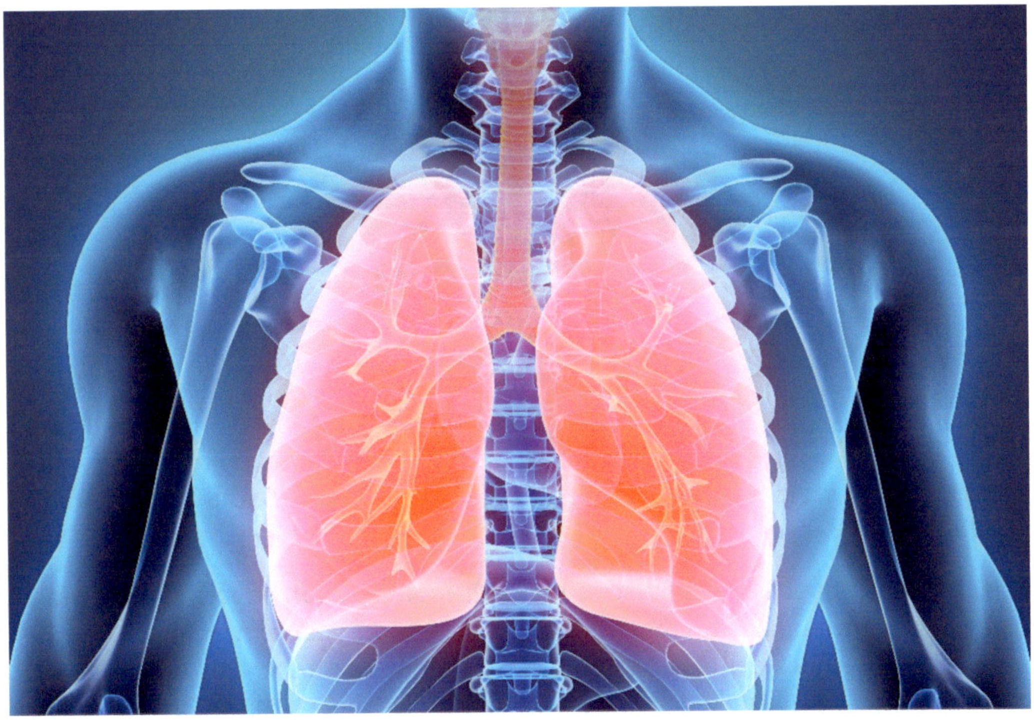

Figure 2.9. Anatomical illustration of the human lungs within the thoracic cavity.

Source: https://images.ctfassets.net/yixw23k2v6vo/gH6gQyKmEr8YfZHhWaiyw/c8830b629ff2791c713a6c29a4db6ded/GettyImages-530196490-3000x2000.jpg.

2.5. Muscles of Inspiration

The muscles of inspiration are necessary for breathing, since they help bring air into the lungs. When you are inspired, the diaphragm, a dome-shaped muscle below the lungs, contracts and flattens which makes the pressure in the thoracic cavity lower. Due to the reduced pressure, air is drawn into the alveoli, where gas exchange occurs. The diaphragm works with extra muscles such as the external intercostals and scalene muscles, to help with breathing. The muscles working together expand the chest and lower the pressure between the lungs and the chest, which allows air move into the lungs more easily. Learning about the biomechanics of these muscles is essential for understanding breathing problems and finding effective ways to treat them. The effectiveness of the muscles of inspiration is closely related to the compliance and elasticity of the lungs. The lung stretches and expands as pressure changes, which is called compliance. It is able to return to its original size after being stretched, a property known as elasticity.

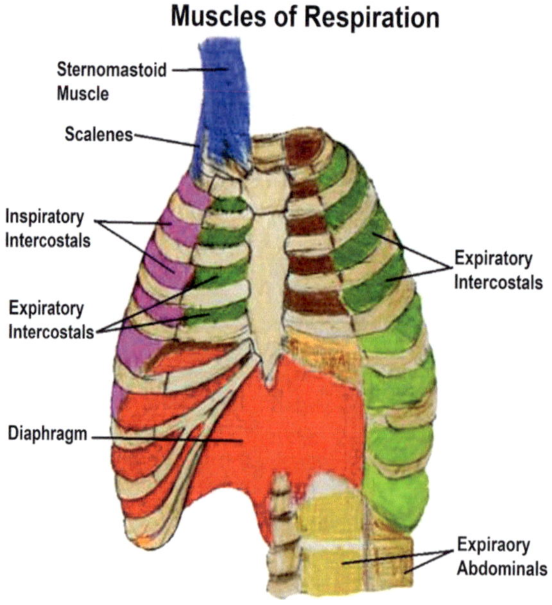

Figure 2.10. Muscles of inspiration.

Source: https://ars.els-cdn.com/content/image/3-s2.0-B9780323900508000017-f01-11-9780323900508.jpg.

Because of these properties, the muscles of inspiration function effectively, allowing the lungs to expand easily when we inhale. On the other hand, lower compliance may suggest problems such as pulmonary fibrosis, where the lungs' structure is altered and this makes breathing harder. Such changes can be quantitatively studied through various models that simulate airflow and compliance, demonstrating a clear connection between muscle function and lung mechanics (Daphalapurkar et al., 2023). Thus, the link between muscles and lung function demonstrates that respiratory physiology is not a simple process. Additionally, surfactant in the lungs is essential for the proper functioning of the muscles that help us breathe and for the mechanics of respiration. Surfactant, which is made by type II alveolar cells, helps lower the tension at the air-liquid interface in the alveoli, so they do not collapse when you breathe out. Surfactant increases lung compliance, enabling the diaphragm and other muscles to function more effectively. If surfactant levels are low, as often occurs in neonatal RDS, it can cause the baby to breathe harder and experience difficulty with oxygenation. This highlights not only the importance of muscular input but also the biochemical environment in which these muscles operate (Chen et al., 2019). A comprehensive understanding of these factors is crucial for developing therapeutic strategies that enhance respiratory function in patients with compromised respiratory function, ultimately highlighting the intricate interplay between muscular mechanics and lung physiology (Figure 2.10).

2.5.1. Primary Muscles Involved in Inspiration

The muscles that are most important for inspiration include the diaphragm and the intercostal muscles which must all work together. The diaphragm, which is a dome-shaped muscle at the bottom of the thoracic cavity, is very important during inhalation. A contraction of the diaphragm causes it to flatten and move downward, which increases the vertical space in the chest cavity. Because of this contraction, the pressure inside the lungs becomes lower than the pressure outside, allowing air to enter the lungs.

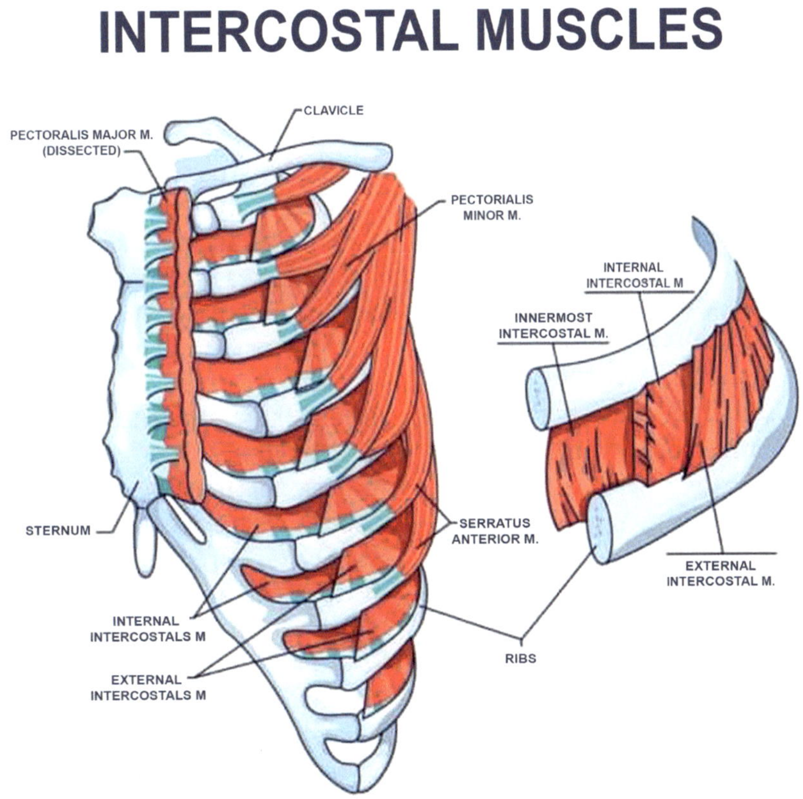

Figure 2.11. Intercostal muscles.

Source: https://centenoschultz.com/wp-content/uploads/Depositphotos_520938088_S-600x600.jpg.

At the same time, the external intercostal muscles (found between the ribs) help lift the rib cage, enlarge the thoracic area, and allow more air to enter. Due to this mechanism, the lungs can properly ventilate and maintain their compliance, which is crucial for efficient gas exchange. If more effort is needed for breathing, such as during exercise or when someone is short of breath, the accessory muscles of respiration become more critical. The scalene and sternocleidomastoid muscles help to raise the first and second ribs, which support breathing in by increasing the size of the thoracic cavity. These accessory muscles are critical in pathological conditions where the primary muscles may be compromised, such as in diseases like idiopathic pulmonary fibrosis (IPF) or during acute respiratory distress. Understanding the functional synergy between these muscle groups is crucial for comprehending the overall mechanics of breathing, particularly in relation to how variations in muscle activation affect intrapulmonary pressure changes and lung compliance, which in turn impact gas exchange efficacy, as noted in studies on pulmonary mechanics (Chen et al., 2019). Fatigue in the muscles is another vital reason that inspiration is affected, mainly when breathing is difficult. Using the inspiratory muscles for an extended period can make them tired, which can reduce their efficiency and affect how well the lungs are ventilated. In babies born prematurely, who often have RDS, using both main and supporting muscles is crucial, as their lungs may not be strong enough to provide the necessary tidal volumes for proper breathing. Here, an understanding of the interplay between mechanical ventilation strategies and the physiological capabilities of these muscles becomes vital to ensure optimal support for the neonatal lung, thus preserving long-term health outcomes (Shanny et al., 2016). As research evolves, exploring these aspects can significantly advance our understanding of respiratory mechanics and the intricate balance between muscle function and pulmonary physiology (Figure 2.11).

2.5.2. Role of Accessory Muscles During Heavy Breathing

Accessory muscles are used more during heavy breathing because the body needs more oxygen. During regular breathing, the diaphragm and intercostal muscles are used; however, in more demanding situations, such as intense exercise or when someone is short of breath, additional muscles are also engaged. The sternocleidomastoid, scalene, and pectoralis minor accessory muscles work to widen the thoracic cavity and increase the lung volume over the usual tidal volume. It helps reduce the pressure inside the chest and the air sacs, which allows more air to be taken in. This demonstrates that the body can adapt by utilizing these muscles, illustrating how muscle function and respiration work together to maintain balance when a person is exerting themselves. Breathing becomes harder when accessory muscles are used because they help change the lung's elasticity and make it harder to breathe in air. If the breathing rate is high, the lung and chest wall's natural elasticity, which helps maintain standard respiratory mechanics, might be affected. Accessory muscles help alleviate this problem by expanding the chest more, resulting in larger lung volumes and improved air exchange. At the same time, being active like this means they have to work harder to breathe, which can cause tiredness and breathing problems if done for a long time. Examining how these muscles are activated helps us understand the overall workings of breathing and their impact on health. In chronic respiratory conditions, such as asthma or COPD, people often need to use accessory muscles to assist with breathing. Due to increased airway resistance, patients must exert extra effort from their accessory muscles to breathe normally. Relying on the ventilator for a long time may show that the lungs are becoming less flexible and compliant, which affects the person's breathing. Using breathing techniques that engage a patient's accessory muscles can be beneficial. Using these techniques improves lung function by increasing tidal volume without placing excessive strain on the primary breathing muscles, which highlights the role of accessory muscles in all respiratory conditions. The study of these dynamics reveals essential considerations in the management of respiratory diseases, emphasizing the integral role of accessory muscles under varying breathing conditions (Figure 2.12).

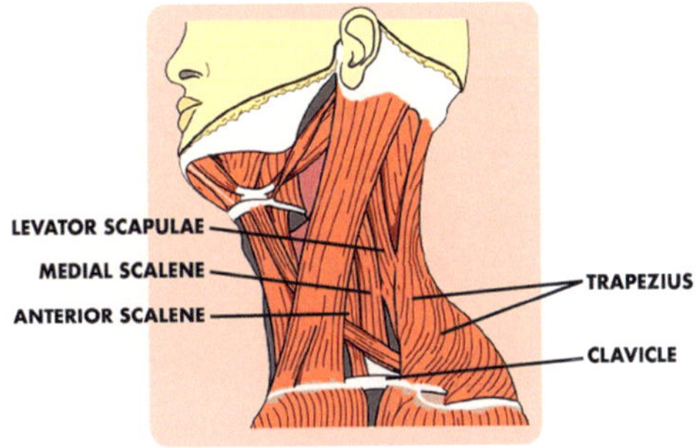

Figure 2.12. Accessory muscles for breathing.

Source: https://rosept.com/sites/default/files/breathing_-_accessory_muscles2x.png.

2.5.3. Neurological Control of Inspiratory Muscles

Most of the breathing process is controlled by nerves that activate the inspiratory muscles, which are crucial to the process of respiration. The medulla oblongata and pons which are part of the brainstem, are responsible for coordinating the breathing rhythms. The ventral respiratory group stimulates the diaphragm and intercostals to contract which allows the lungs to expand. Due to this contraction, the air pressure within the alveoli decreases, allowing air to move into the lungs. Additionally, sensory feedback from peripheral chemoreceptors and mechanoreceptors informs the central nervous system (CNS) of the body's oxygen and carbon dioxide levels, allowing for an adaptive response to varied metabolic demands. The body is able to manage gas exchange effectively due to the intricate connections within the nervous system. When the brain initiates the inspiratory phase, it also regulates the activity of muscles necessary for maintaining proper tidal volume and the mechanics of the lungs. The diaphragm is mainly in charge of breathing in, and it gets its commands from the phrenic nerve, which is then adjusted by signals from the spine and brain. Additionally, accessory muscles such as the scalenes and sternocleidomastoid are used more often when breathing is harder, particularly during exercise or in health problems like asthma. Due to this recruitment, the lungs are able to maintain the optimal level of compliance and elasticity as the body requires.

Being able to respond quickly is an important essential for normal breathing and also for removing carbon dioxide and delivering oxygen, which demonstrates the strong relationship between the brain and the respiratory system. Additionally, understanding how the nervous system controls the muscles used in breathing is crucial for developing new treatments for individuals with respiratory failure or nervous system disorders. To provide the best care, mechanical ventilation requires an understanding of the role of the inspiratory muscles under the influence of nerves, allowing for the selection of the right settings and modes for patient-ventilator synchronization. Assessments of breathing strength and nerve function in the clinic can help choose treatments to support or enhance breathing in patients with respiratory problems. Thus, investigating the neural pathways involved in inspiratory muscle control offers critical insights not just into basic respiratory physiology, but also into developing effective treatment strategies for managing respiratory insufficiency and improving patient outcomes in diverse healthcare settings (Falkenström et al., 2010; Drasovean et al., 2023) (Figure 2.13).

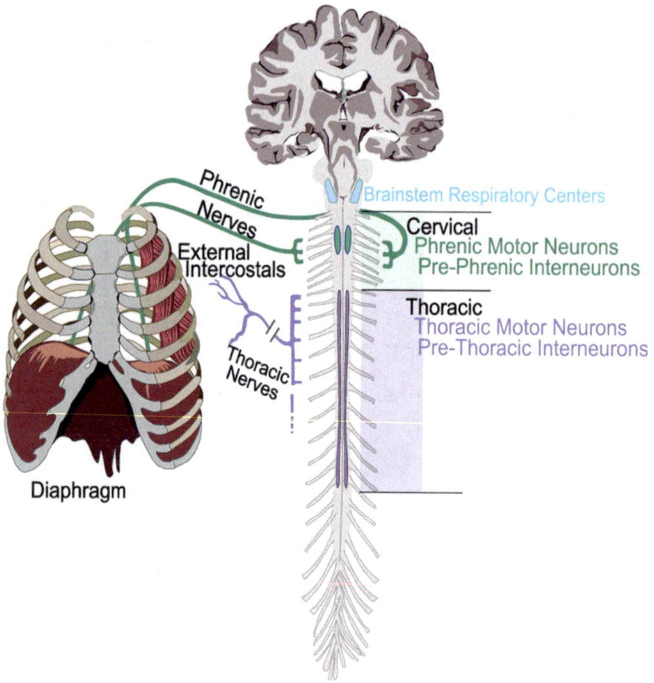

Figure 2.13. Central organization for the neural control of breathing.

Source: https://www.researchgate.net/profile/Ian-Malone/publication/353094269/figure/fig1/AS:1055352057520129@1628626946504/Central-organization-for-the-neural-control-of-breathing-Timing-and-coordination-of.png.

2.6. Muscles of Expiration

The process of expiration depends on a combination of muscles that are very important for breathing. Expiration can be described as either passive or active. The lungs are passively deflated by the natural elasticity of the lungs and the surface tension in the alveoli, which is made possible by pulmonary surfactant. But, when you are active and breathing hard, it is primarily the action of specific muscles that is most important. The primary muscles at work are the internal intercostals and the abdominals, which contract to squeeze the chest cavity and push air out more forcefully. The muscle contraction temporarily raises pressure inside the chest, which increases the pressure inside the alveoli and forces air out of the lungs, showing that good muscle coordination is essential for breathing. The muscles used for expiration become especially important in cases like CF. Due to the thickened mucus, patients often struggle to breathe and must use their breathing muscles more to clear their airways and obtain sufficient oxygen. Alterations in lung compliance and airflow resistance, as noted in research, can hinder effective expiration, leading to a build-up of carbon dioxide and decreased oxygenation (Daphalapurkar et al., 2023). So, it is imperative for the internal intercostals and abdominal muscles to produce enough pressure, both for breathing and to keep the lungs' gases in balance. These dynamics make it clear that people with respiratory diseases often struggle, as the effort required to exhale is significantly greater due to changes in their lungs. Expiratory muscles play a part in breathing that is greater than just helping with exhalation. If lung compliance is altered or elasticity is reduced, as happens in various respiratory diseases, the effort needed to breathe out may increase significantly. Research has shown that conditions resulting in increased mucus viscosity can heighten expiratory resistance, further complicating the breathing process (Adrian, 2012). So, it is crucial for the lungs to be flexible and elastic and for the muscles used in breathing to be strong, to maintain breathing. Moreover, effective airway clearance mechanisms, enhanced by the muscles of expiration, are essential in mitigating long-term lung damage in patients, underscoring the multifaceted functions these muscles serve within the broader context of pulmonary health and disease management (Figure 2.14).

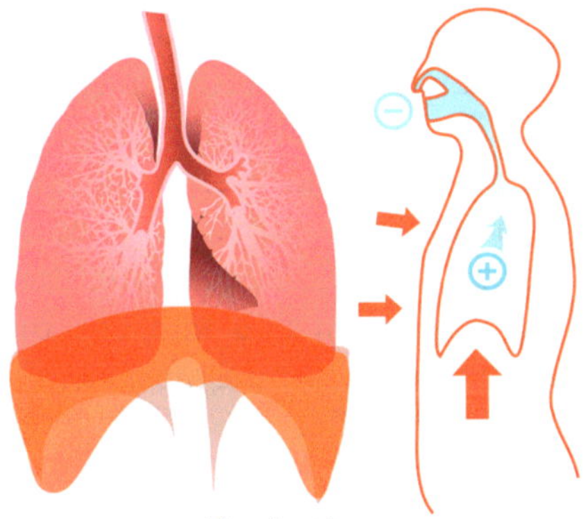

Figure 2.14. Diagram showing expiration.

Source: https://upload.wikimedia.org/wikipedia/commons/thumb/3/33/Expiration_diagram.svg/800px-Expiration_diagram.svg.png.

2.6.1. Primary Muscles Involved in Expiration

The way we breathe out depends closely on the main muscles controlling this part of breathing. Unlike inhaling, which is mainly controlled by the diaphragm and external intercostal muscles, expiration usually occurs without effort when you are resting. The elasticity of the lungs, which is due to their tissue, helps air to move out of the alveoli as intrapleural pressure goes up. However, when someone is forced to exhale, the use of additional muscles becomes crucial. The internal intercostal muscles and others are important since they pull the ribs down in which reduces the size of the thoracic cavity and helps you to exhale. Understanding the distinct actions of these muscle groups enhances our comprehension of respiratory efficiency and overall lung function (Zdeňka et al., 2023). When someone is distressed or has COPD, they rely on accessory muscles much more. Forced expiration is assisted by the abdominal muscles such as the rectus abdominis, transverse abdominis, and obliques, which raise the pressure inside the abdomen. Due to this pressure, the diaphragm moves upward, which helps to reduce thoracic volume and quickly expel air. Using auxiliary muscles is necessary to increase the speed of airflow out of the lungs when breathing hard. Examining these muscles helps us understand that the body can maintain good ventilation in both healthy and diseased states. Accessory muscle activity often signifies inadequate performance of primary muscles, highlighting the importance of muscle efficiency in respiratory health (Joseph et al., 2017). Because breathing out depends on both the lungs and the muscles, respiratory physiology is a complex process. The efficiency of muscle function during expiration depends on the elasticity and compliance of the lungs. Damage to these properties, as in restrictive lung disease, can make it much harder for the expiratory muscles to function properly, resulting in more difficult breathing. Additionally, breathing is influenced by surface tension within the alveoli and the presence of surfactant. Because of surfactant, surface tension is lowered, so the air sacs in the lungs do not collapse, and breathing is easier. Consequently, an integrated view of inspiratory and expiratory muscle function, lung compliance, and the role of surfactant is essential for understanding the overall mechanics of breathing and the compensatory mechanisms that come into play under various health conditions (Zdeňka et al., 2023) (Figure 2.15).

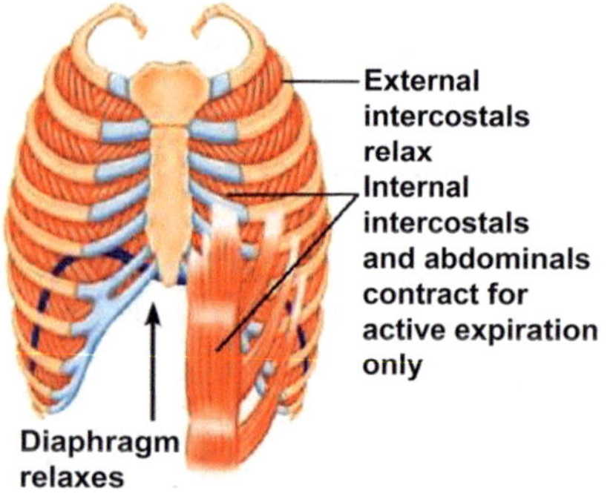

Figure 2.15. Expiration muscles.

Source: https://www.evolvingsciences.com/wpimages/wpf49cf6d1_05_06.jpg.

2.6.2. Role of Passive Vs. Active Expiration

In respiratory mechanics, expiration is a crucial process, and it is divided into passive and active expiration. Quiet breathing causes passive expiration, which occurs naturally as the lungs and chest wall spring back. When the diaphragm and intercostal muscles relax, the lungs shrink, which raises the pressure inside the air sacs and pushes air out. Due to the lung compliance and elasticity of the thoracic cavity, this mechanism is energy-efficient, allowing the body to exchange gases with minimal effort from the muscles. Notably, the dynamics of passive expiration are further influenced by factors such as lung elasticity and intrapleural pressure, which help maintain the fluid dynamics necessary for adequate ventilation. For example, active expiration is used when breathing is stronger, for instance, during exercise or when someone is struggling to breathe. This occurs when additional muscles, such as the abdominal and internal intercostal muscles, are engaged to help expel air more quickly. Active expiration rapidly shrinks the lungs and can have a significant impact on the pressure inside the lungs and chest, which affects how we breathe. During active expiration, the muscles involved in breathing must work harder, which requires more energy due to the increased resistance in the airways. The distinction between the two modes emphasizes how the body adapts to varying physiological demands, ensuring that respiratory efficiency is maintained under differing conditions of activity (Dem et al., 2020). Learning about the interaction between passive and active expiration provides important insights into breathing and its impact on patient care. It is crucial for professionals in anesthesiology and pulmonary medicine to understand these respiratory processes, as they play a vital role in these fields. Noticing when and how these mechanisms are active can help choose the best therapy for patients with weakened respiratory function. By recognizing the role of intrapleural and intra-alveolar pressures, lung compliance, and the influence of respiratory muscles, healthcare providers can better understand the complexities of ventilation and tailor their approaches to improve outcomes in patients undergoing anesthesia or suffering from pulmonary ailments.

2.6.3. Impact of Expiratory Muscle Function on Breathing Efficiency

Expiratory muscles are not given as much attention as inspiratory muscles, but they are crucial for efficient breathing and minimizing the effort required to breathe. Good expiration is possible only when the abdominal and intercostal muscles work together to contract. Being active helps expel air from the lungs, allowing them to be ventilated more fully. When the expiratory muscles are working well, they help keep the intra-alveolar pressure high, which improves the removal of carbon dioxide from the blood, keeping the acid-base balance stable. The link between strong expiratory muscles and better breathing efficiency proves that muscle function is necessary for both regular and intense breathing and failing to use the muscles well can result in less efficient breathing and more energy being used. The breathing difficulties associated with COPD are a prime example of the impact of weakened expiratory muscles. When airways are blocked in COPD, expelling air can be difficult, which leads to air becoming trapped and the lungs expanding too much. Due to changes in lung mechanics, there is increased pressure inside the alveoli and decreased compliance, which makes it harder to breathe and reduces the ability to exchange gases. A patient with weak expiratory muscles may be unable to use accessory muscles, resulting in ineffective breathing patterns. Therefore, breathing becomes less efficient, and the body has to use more energy, leading to greater fatigue and a reduced ability to work out. Rehabilitation exercises targeting the expiratory muscles can enhance the breathing ability of patients with these conditions, thereby improving their overall respiratory function and quality of life. Additionally, the relationship between how the expiratory muscles function and how the lungs expand and contract should be considered when evaluating breathing efficiency. Because of the surfactant, the tension on the surface of the alveoli is reduced, which improves the lungs' ability to expand. However, during forced expiration, coordinated contractions of expiratory muscles can further facilitate the functional residual capacity (FRC) by stabilizing lung volumes and optimizing airflow dynamics. There is a strong relationship between the surfactant and the expiratory muscles, indicating that both are crucial for effective breathing. By strengthening the muscles used for exhaling, it is possible to improve overall lung function, as demonstrated by the use of targeted therapies for various respiratory diseases. Therefore, integrating specific training programs for expiratory muscles in clinical settings may yield significant improvements in breathing efficiency, affirming their vital contribution to respiratory health (Davies et al., 2000; Falkenström et al., 2010) (Figure 2.16).

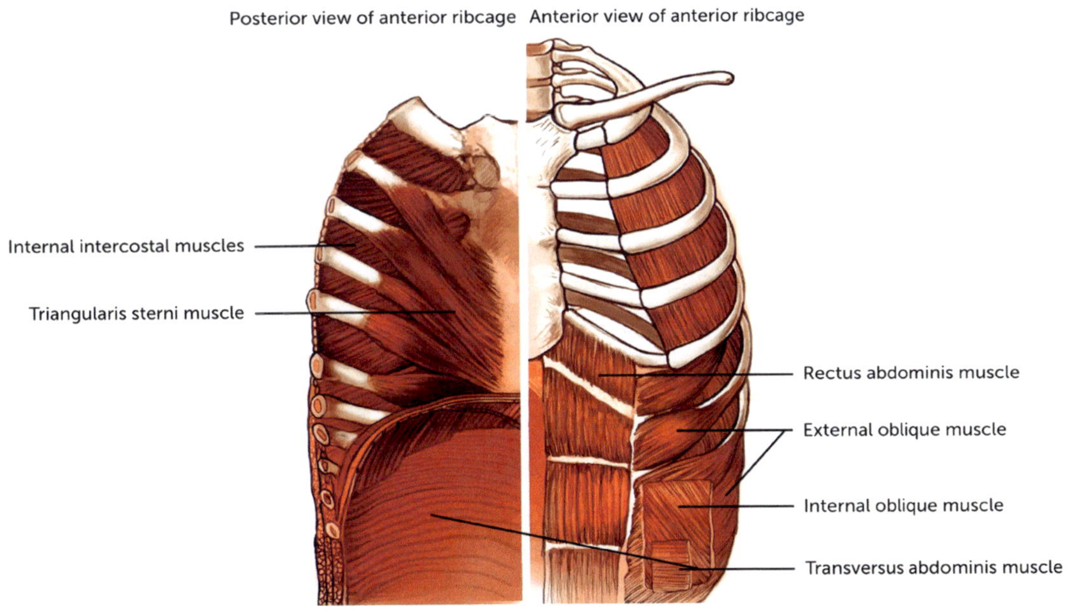

Figure 2.16. The expiratory muscles of the respiratory muscle pump.

Source: https://media.springernature.com/full/springer-static/image/art%3A10.1007%2Fs00134-019-05664-4/MediaObjects/134_2019_5664_Fig1_HTML.png?as=webp.

SUMMARY

Many physiological factors interact to help the lungs exchange gases efficiently. The function of the lungs depends on intrapleural and intra-alveolar pressures, which change to let air be inhaled and exhaled. How the lungs stretch and return to normal is reflected in lung compliance and elasticity, and this affects such interactions. Respiratory function depends on the lungs' ability to adjust to different amounts of air which highlights how important these mechanical properties are. Numerous studies have demonstrated that understanding these concepts is crucial for identifying and addressing health issues that affect breathing. In addition, the muscles involved in breathing in and out play a crucial role in explaining how breathing works. The diaphragm and intercostal muscles are for changing the volume of the thorax, which affects the pressures in the chest that help the lungs expand. At the same time, changes in lung compliance can occur with various diseases, which may necessitate a personalized approach to treating the lungs. Conditions such as CF can cause the mucus in the lungs to change, which affects how easily air can move through the lungs. By combining research, it is clear that specific therapies, such as airway clearance techniques, are effective in managing these conditions. It emphasizes the need to continue studying the detailed mechanisms involved in human respiration. In addition, surfactant plays a key part in lowering surface tension inside the alveoli, which is anessential for the stability and compliance of the lungs. Surfactant improves the stretchiness of the lungs and makes breathing easier, which helps gas exchange. The detailed models of lung mechanics clearly show that surfactant, lung structure, and airflow all play essential roles together. As current research continues to evolve, it is crucial to address how these foundational elements may vary in pathological states, particularly in terms of mucus viscosity and clearance, as noted in studies on CF (Adrian, 2012; Daphalapurkar et al., 2023). Understanding these relationships enables doctors to effectively treat and manage the health of individuals with lung issues.

The way we breathe primarily depends on the interaction between intrapleural and intra-alveolar pressures. When air enters the thoracic cavity, the diaphragm and intercostal muscles tighten, making the pressure inside the chest lower, which helps air enter the lungs. When the lungs expand, the pressure inside them becomes lower, which draws air in and overcomes the elasticity of the lung tissue. When the alveoli are full, the pressure inside them goes above atmospheric pressure, which makes air move out as you breathe out. The relationship between these pressures governs both phases, and understanding them is crucial for insights into normal respiratory function and pathophysiological conditions that might arise due to imbalances or abnormalities in this intricate process, highlighted by mathematical models of lung dynamics that provide deeper insights into airflow patterns during breathing cycles (Giamagas et al., 2018). The compliance and elasticity of the lungs are crucial for effective breathing. When pressure is applied, the lungs expand (compliance) and afterwards, they return to their original state (elasticity). Such physical properties are essential for breathing, and when there are pulmonary diseases, changes in these factors can significantly affect how well a person breathes. An example is that lung compliance decreases in pulmonary fibrosis but increases in emphysema. The surfactant, which is produced by alveolar cells, helps to keep the alveoli stable by decreasing surface tension. This decrease in surface tension increases lung compliance and prevents alveolar collapse. Effective interaction between these factors drives optimal lung mechanics, demonstrating their importance not only in health but also in clinical contexts where respiratory function is compromised (Motta, 2012). Breathing is made efficient by the muscles of inspiration and expiration, which control the mechanical steps of breathing. Inspiration causes the diaphragm and external intercostal muscles to contract, which enlarges the chest and makes it easier to inhale. In a healthy adult, expiration happens mostly by itself, relying on the lungs and chest wall's elasticity. Still, during forced expiration, muscles in the abdomen and between the ribs are used to help expel air. Breathing is the effort needed to resist and overcome the elastic and resistive forces during each mechanical movement. Additionally, when airways encounter resistance, the size of the airways and the volume of air in the lungs significantly influence the rate at which air moves. Understanding the mechanics of these muscular systems and the role of surfactant in optimizing lung function is vital for addressing breathing difficulties, particularly in vulnerable populations such as premature infants (Giamagas et al., 2018).

CLOSER LOOK

ALVEOLAR CELLS

Alveolar cells are the specialized epithelial cells that line the tiny air sacs (alveoli) in the lungs, playing a crucial role in gas exchange and lung function. Two main types of alveolar cells exist: Type I and Type II pneumocytes, with alveolar macrophages also present. Type I cells are thin and squamous, facilitating rapid gas exchange, while Type II cells produce surfactant, a substance that reduces surface tension and prevents the alveoli from collapsing (Figure 2.17).

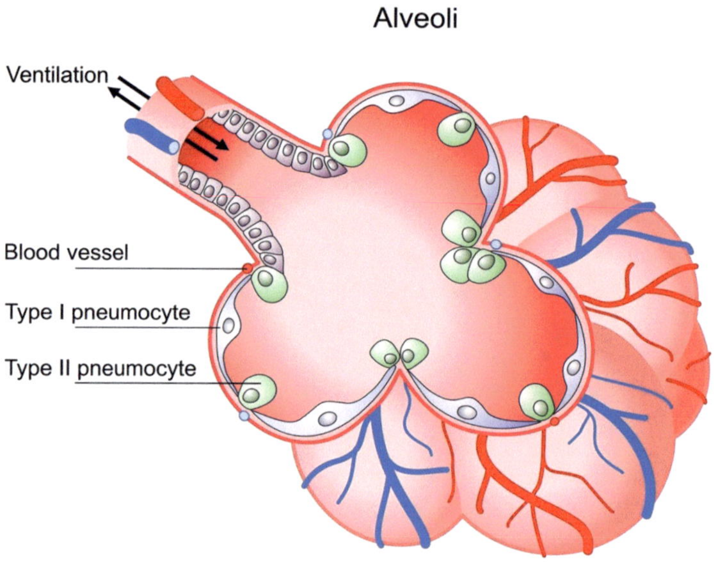

Figure 2.17. Structural anatomy of an alveolar cell.

Source: https://scx2.b-cdn.net/gfx/news/2020/usingalveola.jpg.

Types of Alveolar Cells

- **Type I Pneumocytes:** These thin, squamous cells cover the majority of the alveolar surface (about 95%) and form the air-blood barrier where gas exchange takes place.
- **Type II Pneumocytes:** These cuboidal cells are smaller and fewer in number than Type I cells, but they are crucial for producing and storing surfactant. Surfactant is a complex mixture of phospholipids and proteins that reduces the surface tension at the air-liquid interface within the alveoli, preventing them from collapsing during exhalation.
- **Alveolar Macrophages:** These specialized immune cells reside in the alveoli and play a crucial role in clearing debris and pathogens from the lungs.

Functions of Alveolar Cells

- **Gas Exchange:** Type I cells are responsible for facilitating the rapid diffusion of oxygen into the bloodstream and the removal of carbon dioxide from the bloodstream.
- **Surfactant Production:** Type II cells produce surfactant, which is essential for maintaining alveolar stability and preventing lung damage.
- **Defense:** Alveolar macrophages phagocytose foreign particles and pathogens, protecting the lungs from infection and damage.
- **Repair and Regeneration:** Type II cells can differentiate into Type I cells, enabling the repair of the alveolar epithelium following injury.

REFERENCES

1. Biga, L., Quick, D., Dawson, S., Harwell, A., Hopkins, R., Kaufmann, J., LeMaster, M., et al. (2019). *Anatomy & Physiology*. http://books.google.com/books?id=0fu7zgEACAAJ&dq=definition+and+role+of+lung+elasticity+in+breathing+mechanics+intrapleural+intra-alveolar+pressures+lung+compliance+surfactant+work+of+breathing&hl=&source=gbs_api (accessed on 31st May 2025).
2. Chatterjee, S. (1997). *A Quantitative Estimation of Regulation and Transport Limitations in the Human Cardiopulmonary System*. https://core.ac.uk/download/38901093.pdf (accessed on 31st May 2025).
3. Chen, L., & Zhao, X. (2019). Characterization of air flow and lung function in the pulmonary acinus by fluid-structure interaction in idiopathic interstitial pneumonias. *PLoS ONE, 14*, e0214441. https://doi.org/10.1371/journal.pone.0214441 (accessed on 31st May 2025).
4. Cuttano, A., Scaramuzzo, R. T., Ciantelli, M., Baldoli, L., Bellanti, G., Gentile, S., Cecchi, F., et al. (2013). MEchatronic REspiratory System SImulator for Neonatal Applications (MERESSINA) project: A novel bioengineering goal. *Medical Devices: Evidence and Research*. https://doi.org/10.2147/mder.s45524 (accessed on 31st May 2025).
5. Daphalapurkar, N., Riglin, J., Mohan, A., Harris, J. F., & Bernardin, J. D. (2023). Quasi-dynamic breathing model of the lung incorporating viscoelasticity of the lung tissue. *International Journal for Numerical Methods in Biomedical Engineering, 39*. https://doi.org/10.1002/cnm.3744 (accessed on 31st May 2025).
6. Davies, A. (2000). *Studies of Lung Function*. https://core.ac.uk/download/429712282.pdf (accessed on 31st May 2025).
7. Demırdöven, B. T., & Koca, U. (2020). Mechanical ventilation. *Op Acc J Bio Sci & Res, 2*(2). https://biogenericpublishers.com/pdf/JBGSR.MS.ID.00039.pdf (accessed on 31st May 2025).
8. Drasovean, Y. (2023). *Breathe Easy: RT Student Resource for Mechanical Ventilation*. https://core.ac.uk/download/622362223.pdf (accessed on 31st May 2025).
9. Duke, J. W., Gladstone, I. M., Sheel, A. W., & Lovering, A. T. (2017). Premature birth affects the degree of airway dysanapsis and mechanical ventilatory constraints. *Experimental Physiology, 103*, 261–275. https://doi.org/10.1113/ep086588 (accessed on 31st May 2025).
10. Falkenström, F., Granstrom, F., & Holmqvist, R. (2010). *Mechanical Ventilation*. https://core.ac.uk/download/pdf/35276663.pdf (accessed on 31st May 2025).
11. Giamagas, G., & Monokrousos, N. (2018). *Integrated Computational Simulation of the Mechanics of Breathing*. https://core.ac.uk/download/pdf/159785755.pdf (accessed on 31st May 2025).
12. H, A. (2012). Airways Clearance Techniques in Cystic Fibrosis: Physiology, devices and the future. *InTech eBooks*. https://doi.org/10.5772/30243Ahookhosh, K., Vanoirbeek, J., & Vande, V. G. (2023). Lung function measurements in preclinical research: What has been done and where is it headed? *Frontiers in Physiology, 14*. https://doi.org/10.3389/fphys.2023.1130096 (accessed on 31st May 2025).
13. Hamid, M. S. A. (2000). *Penyediaan Modul Pembelajaran Secara Komputer (Computer Aided Fixed Learning Module–CAFLM)*. https://core.ac.uk/download/288478761.pdf (accessed on 31st May 2025).

14. Hoo, A. F. (2005). *Application and Interpretation of Forced Expiratory Manoeuvres in Infancy.* https://core.ac.uk/download/29141594.pdf (accessed on 31st May 2025).

15. Knutsen, G. L. (1976). *The Influence of Age, Sex and Weight on Respiratory Function in the Sedate Canine.* https://core.ac.uk/download/212846424.pdf (accessed on 31st May 2025).

16. Lauzon, A. M., Bates, J. H. T., Donovan, G. M., Tawhai, M. H., Sneyd, J., & Sanderson, M. J. (2012). A multi-scale approach to airway hyperresponsiveness: From molecule to organ. *Frontiers in Physiology, 3.* https://doi.org/10.3389/fphys.2012.00191 (accessed on 31st May 2025).

17. Lozano, S. M., & Newnam, K. M. (2016). Modalities of mechanical ventilation. *Advances in Neonatal Care, 16*, 99–107. https://doi.org/10.1097/anc.0000000000000272 (accessed on 31st May 2025).

18. Motta, A. (2012). *A New System to Monitor Changes of Lung Mechanics During Resuscitation of Newborns by FOT.* https://www.politesi.polimi.it/bitstream/10589/77825/3/2013_04_Motta.pdf (accessed on 31st May 2025).

19. Navrátilová, Z., Komínková, E., & Petřek, M. (2023). The immune response in the pathophysiology of pulmonary diseases. *Physiology.* https://doi.org/10.5772/intechopen.112587 (accessed on 31st May 2025)

20. Negahdar, M. (2012). *3-D Lung Deformation and Function from Respiratory-Gated 4-D X-ray CT Images: Application to Radiation Treatment Planning.* https://doi.org/10.18297/etd/1048 (accessed on 31st May 2025).

21. Pal, G. K., Pal, P., & Nanda, N. (2016). *Comprehensive Textbook of Medical Physiology – Two Volume Set.* JP Medical Ltd. http://books.google.com/books?id=J2-_DQAAQBAJ&dq=Intrapleural+pressure+definition+significance+mechanics+breathing+lung+compliance+elasticity+muscles+inspiration+expiration+surfactant+work+of+breathing&hl=&source=gbs_api (accessed on 31st May 2025).

22. Sánchez, E. (2023). Acute respiratory failure in exacerbations of bronchial asthma. *IntechOpen eBooks.* https://doi.org/10.5772/intechopen.110278 (accessed on 31st May 2025).

23. Wilson, W. C., & Benumof, J. L. (2025). *Physiology of the Airway.* https://pulmo-ua.com/wp-content/uploads/2021/12/wilson2013.pdf (accessed on 31st May 2025).

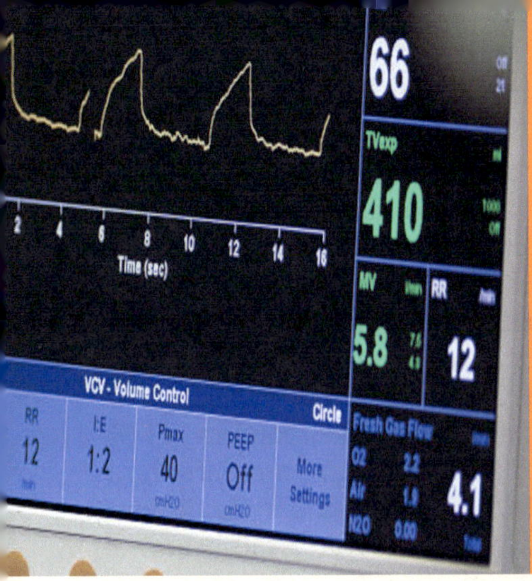

Chapter 3

LUNG VOLUMES AND CAPACITIES

Contents

Introduction

The respiratory system in humans is essential because it helps maintain homeostasis mainly by controlling gas exchange. It is to know lung volumes and capacities to evaluate respiratory health and function, since they help understand how well the lungs are ventilating, diffusing gases, and how much capacity they have. In clinical settings, various techniques are employed to measure these values, enabling healthcare professionals to diagnose and monitor conditions like asthma, chronic obstructive pulmonary disease (COPD), and pulmonary fibrosis. Due to age, sex, body composition, and fitness, breathing patterns and volumes can change, so it is essential to consider these factors to provide accurate assessments and suitable treatments. Research on lung volumes and capacities is related to many metabolic processes. For instance, human breath contains a myriad of endogenous volatile organic compounds (VOCs), reflective of ongoing physiological activities, which can be utilized diagnostically in clinical settings. Understanding the numbers that relate the composition of exhaled air to blood levels improves understanding of how the lungs function. Such research also looks at specific compounds, for example, isoprene, by taking real-time measurements to understand how ventilation, perfusion and metabolic rates are related when someone exercises. Although breath analysis is becoming increasingly popular, we still need to carefully study the main principles that govern lung volumes and capacities. As well as looking at the body's systems that control the lungs, lung volumes are essential for understanding exercise and rehabilitation. Maximal inspiratory and expiratory volumes which are performance indicators, are closely connected to how well someone can exercise and how long they can keep it up. Athletes and patients recovering from breathing illnesses can benefit from these volumes, as they can receive rehabilitation plans to enhance their lung capacity and overall performance. Additionally, incorporating breath analysis, particularly in relation to VOCs, can lead to improved methods for supporting and enhancing lung health and function. Learning about lung volumes and capacities in different ways helps doctors and also aids efforts to improve respiratory health for everyone.

Definition of Lung Volumes and Capacities

Measuring lung volumes and capacities is crucial for understanding how effectively the lungs function and how efficiently they exchange gases. Lung volumes refer to the different amounts of air the lungs can contain during other parts of breathing. These volumes can be classified into several categories: tidal volume (TV), inspiratory reserve volume (IRV), expiratory reserve volume (ERV), and residual volume (RV). Tidal volume is the amount of air breathed in or out during normal breathing, and IRV and ERV are the additional air that can be taken in or breathed out when needed. After a complete exhalation, some air is left in the lungs, which is called residual volume and helps stop the lungs from collapsing. All of these measurements are used to find out lung capacities, which are essential for both clinical tests and understanding lung diseases. It is also necessary to understand lung capacities, which are composed of various lung volumes. The most commonly referenced capacities include vital capacity (VC), functional residual capacity (FRC), and total lung capacity (TLC). VC measures how much air can be exhaled after taking the deepest possible breath, which indicates the health of the lungs and respiratory muscles. Functional residual capacity (FRC) represents the volume of air present in the lungs after passive exhalation, indicating the lungs' ability to maintain optimal oxygen exchange during rest. TLC includes all the lung volumes and shows the maximum air the lungs can hold.

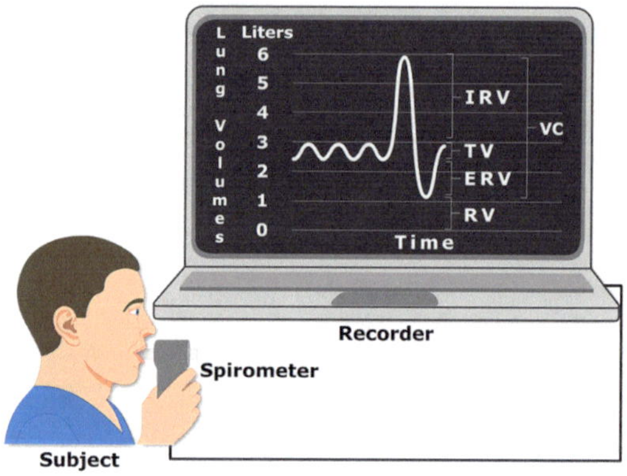

Figure 3.1. Measurement of lung volumes using a spirometer.

Source: https://www.getbodysmart.com/wp-content/uploads/2017/09/Featured-Image-Lung-Volumes-and-Capacities-1.png.

These functions give valuable signs of lung health, which are essential for identifying COPD and other lung diseases in hospitals. New studies show that physical fitness is essential for lung health and how it can be affected by lifestyle. A study found that older individuals who exercise regularly, such as through running, have higher FVC and FEV1 values than those who do not.

The findings indicated that runners had greater lung capacity and function than non-runners and even exceeded population norms in some aspects (Buras et al., 2004). Therefore, exercising regularly can help strengthen the muscles around the lungs and improve breathing, which shows why staying active is essential for the lungs. Emphasizing the interplay between physical fitness and lung capacity can provide valuable insights into preventive health strategies for maintaining optimal lung health throughout life (Figure 3.1).

Importance of Understanding Lung Function

Understanding lung function is crucial for doctors and researchers, as it informs the diagnosis and treatment of various lung diseases. Measuring lung volumes and capacities enables healthcare professionals to assess how well the lungs function and identify any deviations from the norm. For instance, individuals with COPD typically demonstrate reduced forced vital capacity (FVC) and an increased RV, which signals impaired respiratory mechanics. Additionally, with personalized medicine, it is now evident that treatments should be tailored to each patient's specific lung function. A thorough assessment of lung volumes allows practitioners to design better treatment plans that meet the particular needs of each patient which can improve their health and quality of life. Additionally, understanding lung function is crucial for individuals whose environment or genetics predispose them to risk. Studies indicate that high-altitude natives, such as Peruvian women of Quechua descent, exhibit enlarged vital capacities and residual volumes when compared to their sea-level counterparts (Barker et al., 2012). These changes in the body are necessary for people to deal with the lower oxygen at high altitudes. When researchers study what affects lung volumes, they learn about both individual abilities and the adjustments populations make to harsh conditions. Having this knowledge can guide public health efforts to prevent respiratory problems in various communities, which improves the well-being of those groups. Lastly, the implications of lung function knowledge extend into chronic conditions such as multiple sclerosis (MS), highlighting the multifaceted nature of pulmonary health. Research has shown that implementing a Respiratory Muscle Training Program can significantly improve total lung volumes (TLVs) and reduce fatigue among MS patients (Anisha et al., 2018). It points out that strong respiratory health plays a significant role in reducing the effects of chronic disease and that specific interventions can make the lungs more effective. Thus, considering lung volumes and capacities in medical care is essential because it helps treat chronic conditions well and leads to better outcomes and quality of life for patients. To advance both personal and community health, it is essential to understand how the lungs function, highlighting the value of lung function in medicine and healthcare.

3.1. Definitions of Lung Volumes

Lung volumes are essential to understand for checking how the lungs are working and for diagnosing different lung problems. Different air volumes in the lungs are referred to as lung volumes and occur at various points during the breathing cycle. The primary components include TV, ERV, IRV, and RV. The tidal volume is the amount of air we normally breathe in or out, and expiratory and IRVs show how much more air can be expelled or inhaled than this. After a person exhales as much air as possible, some air remains in the lungs, known as residual volume, which helps prevent the alveoli from collapsing and keeps the lungs flexible. Such definitions of lung volumes not only facilitate a clearer understanding of pulmonary mechanics but also serve as a foundation for interpreting various pulmonary function tests (PFTs). It is important to measure and define lung volumes correctly in clinical work to diagnose COPD, asthma, and restrictive lung diseases. If TLC is reduced, this can indicate lung pathology that limits airflow. Conversely, if TLC is increased, it may suggest obstructive diseases where air becomes trapped. Due to these differences, healthcare professionals can design tailored treatment plans for patients. Spirometry and body plethysmography, which are advanced diagnostic methods, depend on having accurate lung volume definitions. These steps, being part of routine clinical care, highlight the importance of knowing lung volumes.

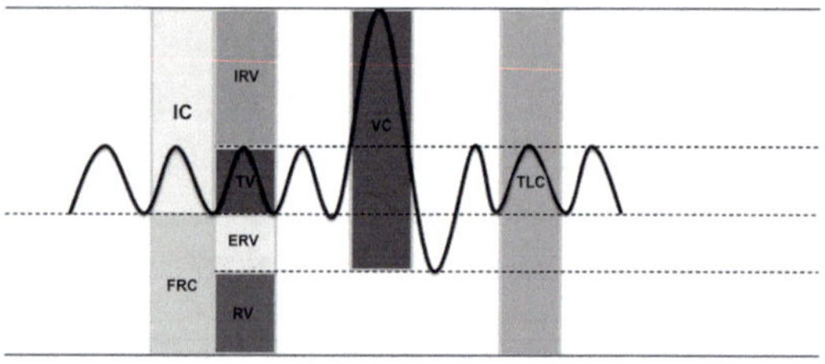

Figure 3.2. Lung volumes. Inspiratory capacity (IC), functional residual capacity (FRC), inspiratory reserve volume (IRV), tidal volume (TV), expiratory reserve volume (ERV), residual volume (RV), vital capacity (VC), total lung capacity (TLC).

Source: https://www.researchgate.net/publication/345028772/figure/fig1/AS:11431281397488630@1745515505040/Lung-volumes-Inspiratory-capacity-IC-functional-residual-capacity-FRC-inspiratory.tif.

Moreover, new research into lung mechanics is continually helping us understand how changes in lung capacity correlate with diseases in the respiratory system. People have begun to focus more on the connection between lung volumes and overall metabolic activity. Several studies have found that the gases released during respiration, including trace gases, can reveal information about how the body metabolizes substances. Exhaled nitric oxide, which is now standardized by task forces, can indicate the extent of inflammation in the lungs and how much the lungs change in size. Because lung function and metabolic markers are related, it is essential to use comprehensive tools in clinical settings. Examining volumetric definitions can, therefore, aid in more accurate diagnosis and treatment of respiratory diseases. Moreover, ongoing studies are examining the impact of breathing patterns and exercise on lung gas exchange dynamics, thus enriching our understanding of the complexities surrounding lung volumes and their clinical relevance (Amann et al., 2010; Alessandri et al., 2018) (Figure 3.2).

3.1.1. Tidal Volume (TV)

The study of lung volumes and capacities depends on understanding TV, which is the amount of air breathed in or out in a typical breath. Usually, an average adult breathes in about 500 milliliters of air per breath and this is a fundamental part of how the lungs work. TV supports the efficient exchange of gases in the alveoli so that the body can meet all its energy needs. When the tidal volume is lower than usual, it may indicate that the lungs are unable to expand properly, which is common in restrictive lung diseases. By regularly assessing tidal volume through PFTs, clinicians gain insight into an individual's respiratory status and can tailor interventions to enhance lung function and overall health (Anisha et al., 2018). In addition, tidal volume plays a significant role in understanding how various conditions affect breathing. Research has indicated that individuals with diseases such as multiple sclerosis (MS) may experience reduced tidal volumes due to the weakness of respiratory muscles, thereby impacting their TLC. A study investigating the influence of a Respiratory Muscle Training Program on patients with MS demonstrated a marked improvement in their lung volumes and capacities after a regimen targeting muscle endurance and strength (Anisha et al., 2018). The results highlight the importance of monitoring tidal volume when assessing lung function, as changes in it can significantly impact a patient's health and daily life. So, having an appropriate tidal volume is necessary for proper breathing and oxygen delivery in any medical setting. Measuring tidal volume is crucial for understanding the health of the lungs and the progression of diseases. For those who practice, spirometry provides valuable information about tidal volume and its impact on respiratory health. With advancements in technology, simple tests can now be performed in various healthcare environments, enabling the detection of pulmonary issues at earlier stages (Swaminathan et al., 1999). Tidal volume is more than a clinical number; it includes several critical life-sustaining processes. As research continues to uncover the complexities of tidal volume, its role in assessing lung capacities will remain central, guiding both the understanding and management of respiratory disorders effectively (Figure 3.3).

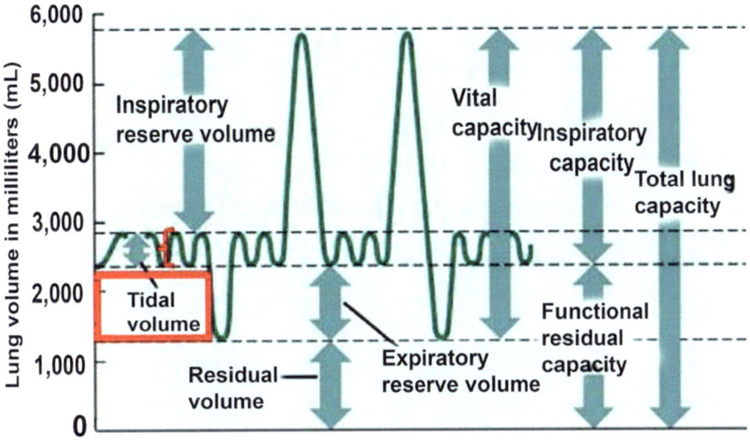

Figure 3.3. Tidal volume.

Source: https://image.slideserve.com/1379611/tidal-volume-tv-l.jpg.

3.1.2. Inspiratory Reserve Volume (IRV)

Respiratory physiology relies on IRV as a crucial component of lung volumes. The IRV is the maximum amount of air a person can take in after a normal breath, and it is essential for checking respiratory capacity and lung function. It matters significantly in medical settings, as changes in IRV may indicate different respiratory problems or inefficiencies. Understanding the dynamics of IRV not only aids in diagnosing conditions like obstructive sleep apnea (OSA) or COPD but also enhances our comprehension of how lifestyle factors, such as obesity and physical inactivity, might impede respiratory health. It demonstrates that checking lung volumes, particularly IRV, is essential to obtain a comprehensive understanding of lung function. Research has demonstrated that body composition has a significant impact on IRV. A review of studies found that obese individuals tend to have a higher IRV than those who are not obese, which suggests that having excess body fat changes how the lungs work. Specifically, the study documented an average IRV of 2.44 ± 0.47 L among obese women, contrasted with 1.87 ± 0.42 L in their non-obese peers (Azevedo et al., 2008). According to the results, obesity might cause the IRV to go up which is essential since the ERV is lower in these individuals. They demonstrate a strong link between body composition and lung capacity, indicating that both factors should be considered in treating and assessing lung diseases. Substances also play an essential role in how IRV works. Studies done recently suggest that taking vitamins, for example, vitamin C, can help boost lung function measurements such as IRV. For instance, research analyzing the effects of ascorbic acid demonstrated increases in IRV among subjects after supplementation, suggesting a protective beneficial role for this vitamin in lung health (Agaba et al., 2005). It highlights the role of biology in breathing, as well as the effects of diet on lung health. By promoting awareness of how lifestyle choices and nutritional interventions can bolster respiratory capacity, practitioners can adopt a more holistic approach to managing lung health, ultimately improving the quality of life for individuals with compromised pulmonary function (Figure 3.4).

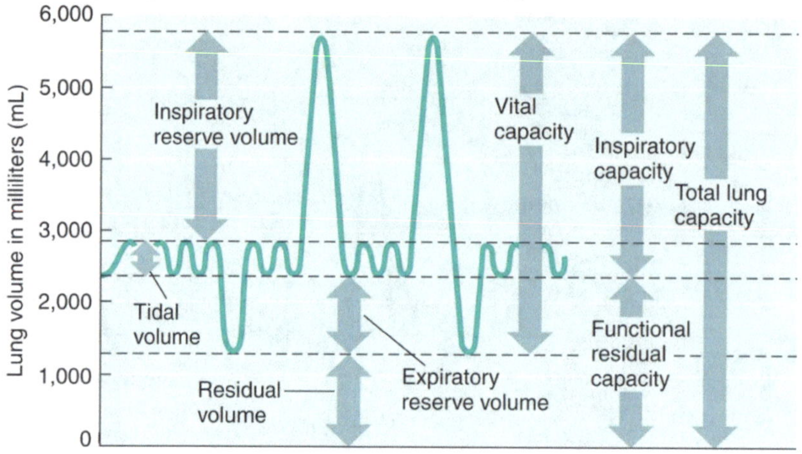

Figure 3.4. Inspiratory reserve volume (IRV).

Source: https://treatcurefast.com/wp-content/uploads/2021/10/slide_1.jpg.

3.1.3. Expiratory Reserve Volume (ERV)

ERV is a key part of lung function, which refers to the extra air you can force out after your normal breath. It is essential for understanding both the mechanics of breathing and the health of the lungs. ERV is crucial for assessing various respiratory disorders, particularly in individuals with restricted lung diseases or obesity. Having a low ERV can cause someone to have less lung capacity, which shows how valuable it is to keep the expiratory function strong. Factors such as age, sex, and body mass index (BMI) can significantly influence ERV measurements, making it necessary to consider these variables during clinical assessments. By looking at these variations, we can discover that a lower ERV may cause more difficulty breathing and make exercising more difficult which can lead to COPD. Moreover, ERV and body composition highlight the strong link between obesity and lung function. According to research, having obesity often results in less effective respiration, due to the mechanical pressure from extra body fat. Because lung volumes are reduced, people need to adjust their inhalation technique, which in turn alters their breathing pattern. The additional weight of fat in the abdomen can stop the diaphragm from moving entirely, which reduces the body's ability to expel air. The presence of visceral fat in a population increases the risk of a reduced ERV, which is a significant issue for public health. Such alterations in lung mechanics are particularly relevant to understanding both the prevalence of OSA and associated cardiovascular risks, as reduced lung capacity further exacerbates these conditions, as discussed by Jun (2020) and Dhairya et al. (2020). Additionally, the use of ERV in hospitals enables doctors to identify and treat various respiratory diseases. Changes in lung volume, such as a decrease in ERV, may suggest a disease and help choose the right treatment. For instance, PFTs that assess ERV alongside FVC and forced expiratory volume (FEV) provide comprehensive insights into lung function status. Assessing ERV can help determine how respiratory health changes over time, mainly when examining reactions to treatment in those with chronic lung diseases. In this context, understanding the implications of ERV not only contributes to patient care but also informs broader health strategies aimed at mitigating the effects of conditions associated with reduced lung capacity, further reinforcing the importance of regular assessments as part of respiratory health management (Figure 3.5).

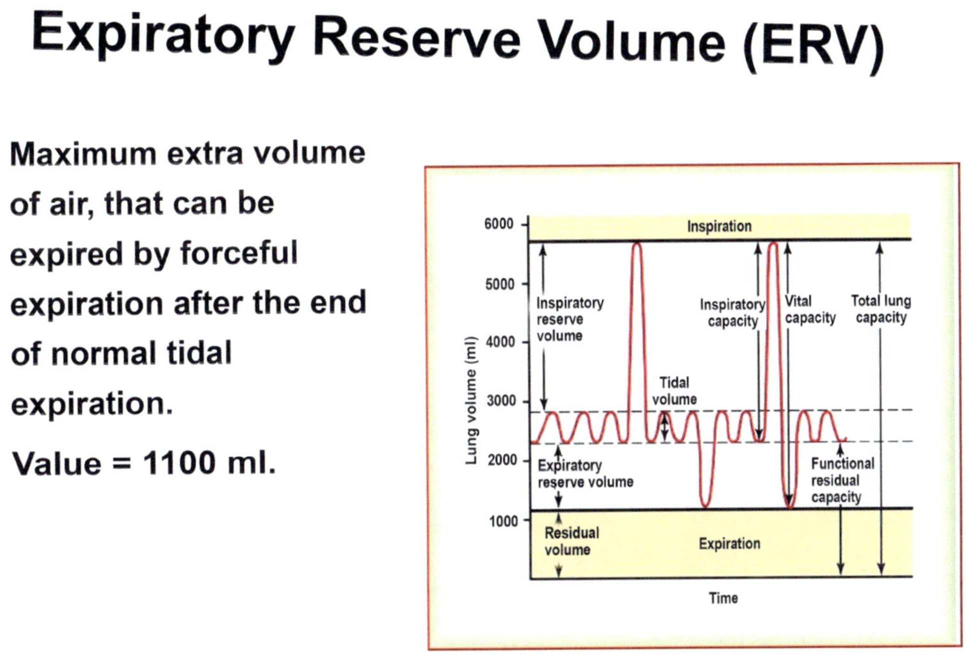

Figure 3.5. Expiratory reserve volume (ERV).

Source: https://image1.slideserve.com/2352295/expiratory-reserve-volume-erv-l.jpg.

3.2. Definitions of Lung Capacities

Knowing the lung capacities helps assess how well the lungs are functioning and helps determine if someone has a pulmonary condition. The lungs are measured by the amount of air they can hold and by the different air compartments that are measured during breathing. The main parts are TV, which is the amount of air taken in or released with a breath, and IRV and ERV, which are extra air that can be brought in or let out during breathing. Altogether, these volumes contribute to functional capacities such as VC and TLC, providing a comprehensive picture of lung health and functionality, essential for both clinical assessments and research (Knutsen et al., 1976). Besides the usual definitions, lung capacity can vary significantly from one person to another due to factors such as age, sex, ethnicity, and overall health. Taller individuals tend to have larger lungs, and females generally have smaller lung volumes than males. Lung compliance decreases with age, which often results in less capacity. Changes in lung capacities can give important information about respiratory diseases; many illnesses can have a significant impact on these measurements. Alterations in lung volumes can occur in COPD and restrictive lung disease, making it more challenging to evaluate patients accurately. As such, appreciating these nuances is vital for accurately interpreting PFTs and tailoring appropriate interventions (Alessandri et al., 2018). Accurate definitions and measurements of lung capacities are essential for both medical care and public health initiatives. The condition of the lungs is a primary indicator of overall health, and it helps us understand how air pollution and workplace hazards can impact us. Researchers utilize lung capacities, as defined by science, in epidemiological studies to understand how various risks affect lung health, which helps inform the development of prevention strategies. Additionally, new technologies such as imaging and spirometry allow doctors to measure lung sizes more accurately. Collectively, these insights underscore the importance of precisely defining and measuring lung capacities not only for individual health but also to promote population-level respiratory health (Knutsen et al., 1976) (Figure 3.6).

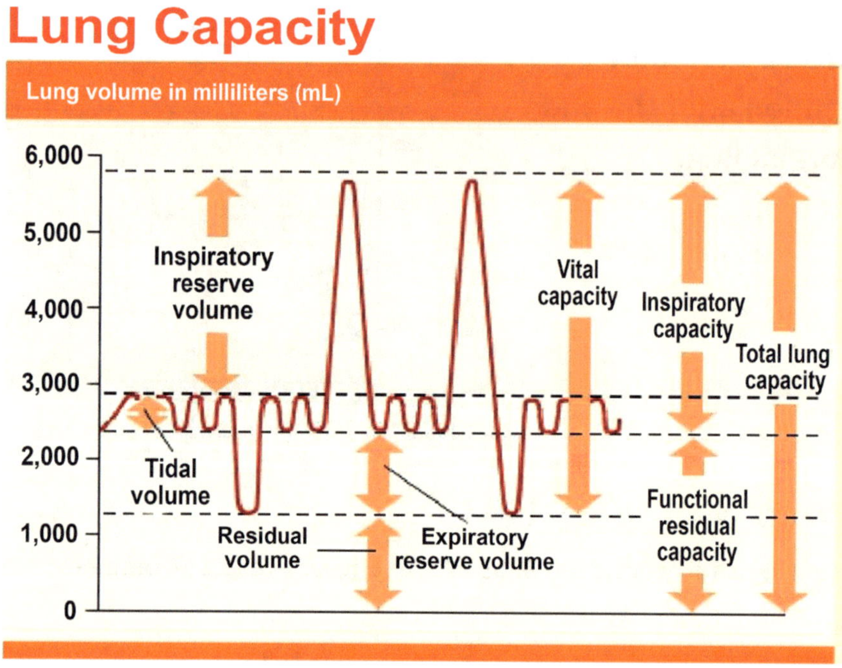

Figure 3.6. Lung capacity.

Source: https://image3.slideserve.com/5627085/lung-capacity-l.jpg.

3.2.1. Total Lung Capacity (TLC)

TLC is important for understanding pulmonary function because it shows the maximum amount of air the lungs can take in. Liters are the usual unit for TLC, which consists of tidal volume, IRV, ERV, and residual volume. TLC measures provide an indication of the general health and efficiency of the lungs. They can reveal if someone has a restrictive lung disease. TLC is especially helpful in distinguishing between various lung diseases, as a low TLC may indicate fibrosis or other disease. TLC analysis by clinicians enables them to assess lung function, predict outcomes, and inform decisions about treatment for patients with long-term respiratory conditions. Studies have shown that TLC is crucial for enhancing patient outcomes, particularly for individuals with restrictive pulmonary disorders. A review of studies suggests that a low TLC is associated with a higher risk of death from any cause, which means clinicians should closely monitor changes in this lung capacity. A meta-analysis showed that individuals with low TLC had a higher risk of death, which highlights TLC's importance in predicting outcomes. These observations underscore the need for rigorous assessment of TLC in clinical practice, as it may serve as a key indicator of disease severity and progression in respiratory conditions, potentially guiding therapeutic interventions and enhancing patient management strategies in a meaningful way (Li et al., 2025). Besides revealing information about restrictive lung disease, TLC measurement can be used to assess the effectiveness of therapies in improving breathing. Studies done recently on benralizumab and lung function in severe eosinophilic asthma patients have reported improvements in other lung volume measures, but changes in TLC have not always been seen. This demonstrates that lung capacities are complex and require doctors to consider Total Lung Capacity, along with other lung volume measurements. Such an integrated analysis helps clinicians formulate a comprehensive picture of a patient's respiratory health and allows for tailored treatment options that address the specific needs of individuals coping with asthma and other chronic lung conditions (António et al., 2024) (Figure 3.7).

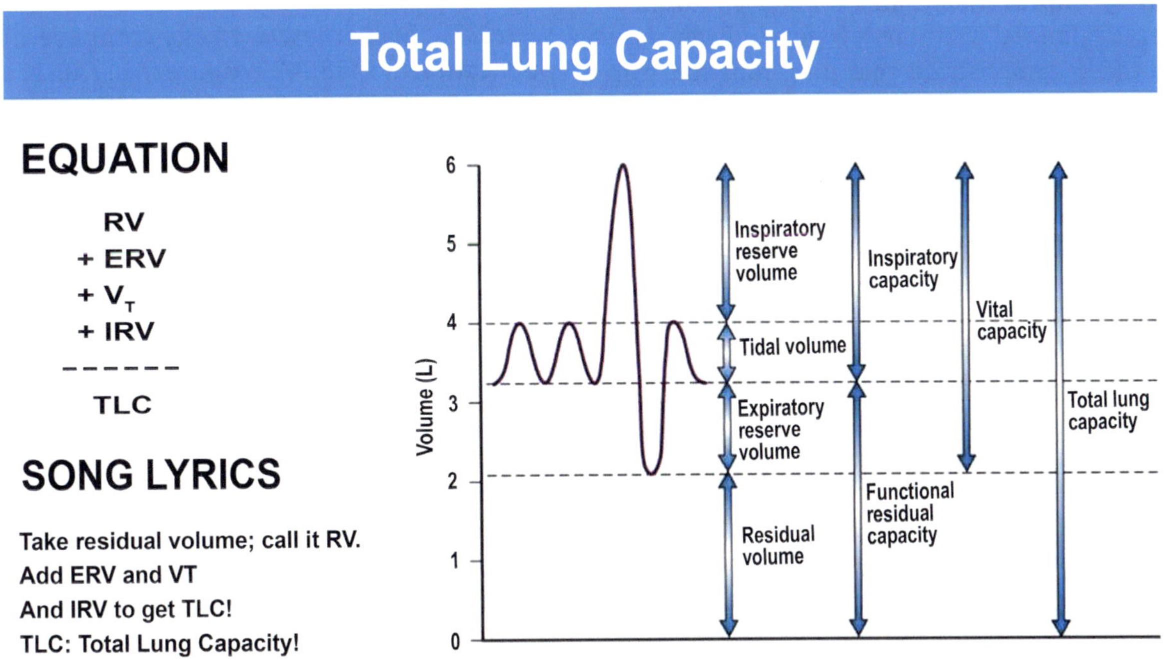

Figure 3.7. Total lung capacity (TLC).

Source: https://i.ytimg.com/vi/trOP49y27JU/maxresdefault.jpg.

3.2.2. Vital Capacity (VC)

VC is an integral part of lung volumes and capacities, indicating the maximum air a person can exhale after inhaling as deeply as possible. Lung capacity is typically assessed during PFTs by asking patients to exhale as forcefully as possible. Because VC indicates how well the lungs are functioning, any changes from the usual values may indicate a respiratory disease or abnormality. A lower VC can suggest that there are lung diseases, but a higher VC can point to other pulmonary conditions. Knowing what affects VC, such as physical fitness, age, and strength of the respiratory muscles, allows healthcare providers to spot and treat respiratory issues early. According to new studies, exercise and especially swimming, has a substantial positive impact on VC. It was discovered that training swimming technical skills increases lung volume and endurance, as seen by improvements in FVC and endurance after a planned training program. Examples like these demonstrate that lung function can adjust to increased physical fitness which means that regular aerobic exercise may increase lung capacity. Also, the results suggest that exercise can play a role in rehabilitation for individuals with breathing problems, mainly when it is controlled. For this reason, incorporating exercise into patient care for better VC may significantly improve health and quality of life. Because PFTs now include tests like VC, they are being used more often in clinics to help detect and control respiratory diseases early. In many medical settings, using spirometry can give important information about a patient's lungs, which helps doctors plan the best treatment. Because these tests are easy to perform, patients with chronic conditions such as asthma can have their health regularly monitored, which helps both patients and doctors manage their breathing issues. Conducting VC assessments in regular clinical practice provides practitioners with a strong tool for evaluating lung function, enabling them to identify both current conditions and potential risks for future problems. As pulmonary capabilities are foundational to overall health, the continued emphasis on VC assessment is vital in advancing respiratory care and promoting optimal lung health in diverse populations (Figure 3.8).

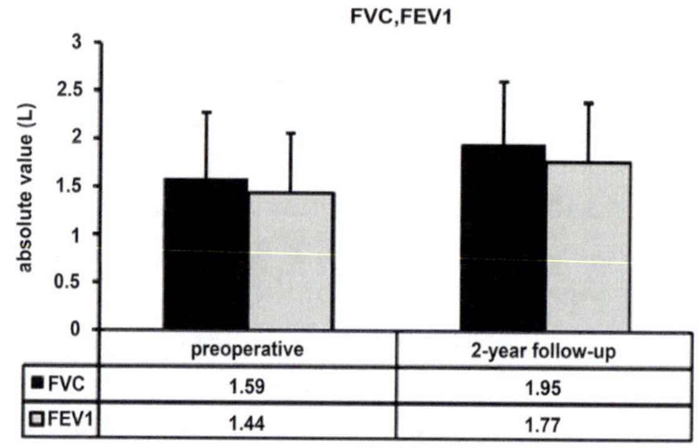

Figure 3.8. Forced vital capacity (FVC), forced expiratory volume in 1 s (FEV1) were significantly improved at 2 years follow-up.

Source: https://www.researchgate.net/publication/357080423/figure/fig1/AS:1185046304174093@1659548464964/Forced-vital-capacity-FVC-forced-expiratory-volume-in-1-s-FEV1-were-significantly.png.

3.2.3. Functional Residual Capacity (FRC)

FRC is the amount of air that is in the lungs after a normal exhalation. It is vital for oxygenation and gas exchange, which are essential for respiratory health. FRC derives from two primary components: ERV and RV. Knowing about FRC is for checking lung mechanics and identifying respiratory problems in many populations. Measuring FRC can help understand obstructive and restrictive lung diseases, as changes in FRC may indicate the severity of the condition or the effectiveness of treatment. Knowing what influences FRC helps us understand individual breathing patterns and plan suitable treatment strategies. Studies done recently have provided more details about how FRC affects children and people with obesity. A well-known study reported that kids with obesity had lower FRC when lying down than kids who were not obese. In particular, FRC decreased more noticeably in children without obesity as they went from a seated to a supine position, which suggests that body position can strongly affect lung volumes. Based on the study, obesity may lead to a higher chance of expiratory flow limitation because of reduced FRC when lying down. This pertains to the necessity of considering body composition and posture when evaluating respiratory function, underscoring the importance of FRC measurements in assessing the health of pediatric populations affected by obesity (Bhammar et al., 2025). In the context of COPD, FRC is also pivotal. Because of airway resistance and lung hyperinflation, those with COPD often have a reduced FRC, which makes it hard for them to expel air completely. Airway changes between full inspiration and full expiration have been studied with multi-volume chest CT-based measurements. Researchers have found that as COPD worsens, there is a decrease in FRC, highlighting the link between lung changes and lung function. By automating the assessment of FRC and related metrics, researchers can gain a deeper understanding of the multifaceted impairments experienced by COPD patients and potentially develop targeted treatments that aim to optimize lung volume and enhance quality of life (Nadeem et al., 2024) (Figure 3.9).

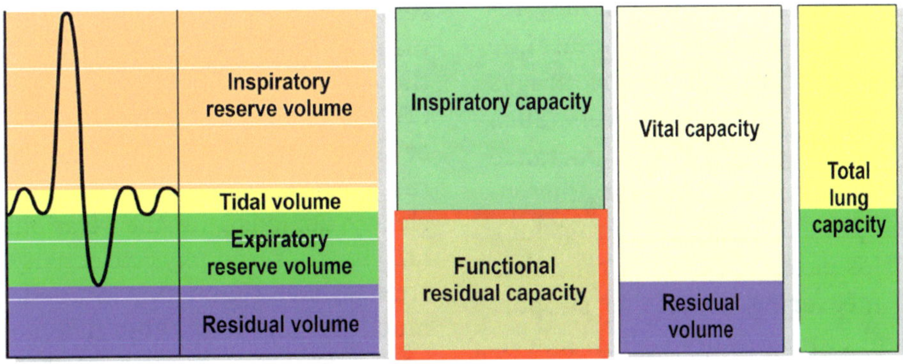

Figure 3.9. Functional residual capacity (FRC).

Source: https://www.respiratorytherapyzone.com/wp-content/uploads/2023/12/Functional-Residual-Capacity-FRC-Lung-Box-Vector.png.

3.3. Measurement Techniques

It is essential to use good measurement methods to find out about lung volumes and capacities which are necessary for diagnosing different respiratory problems. Assessing airflow limitations is a key application of spirometry in pulmonary function testing (PFT), which is often used to diagnose obstructive lung diseases. Still, although spirometry is helpful for diagnosis, using body plethysmography can give a more detailed understanding of lung conditions such as restriction and hyperinflation. New technology in machine learning can now utilize previous spirometry results to estimate lung volumes. Researchers found that using advanced algorithms, the models produced accurate results with minimal errors in predicting lung volumes. These innovations signify potential pathways for improved diagnostic accuracy, especially in clinical settings where traditional measurement modalities may be less accessible or feasible, thereby enriching the clinical utility of spirometry data in respiratory healthcare (Helgeson et al., 2025). Due to the increase in restrictive respiratory diseases following COVID-19, it is now clear that effective ways to measure these conditions are needed to guide treatments. As these lung problems are becoming increasingly common in Colombia, new methods such as lung reexpansion are being employed. It has been demonstrated that incentive physiotherapy is particularly effective in enhancing lung capacity by engaging and motivating patients. The Pontificia Universidad Javeriana Cali and the Universidad del Valle are collaborating on a new project to support this area by developing the Ubicu respiratory incentive system.

The use of gamified software for lung re-expansion helps the initiative provide real-time information on breathing which encourages patients to be involved in their recovery. Such proactive methods highlight the importance of refining measurement techniques to improve overall patient outcomes during lung rehabilitation (Jos et al., 2024). It is crucial to have accurate measuring devices to support the advancement of respiratory care practices. This is demonstrated by the Ubicu respiratory incentive, which utilizes modern sensors and microcontrollers to accurately track respiratory parameters. The research team used TRIZ and Design Thinking to ensure the device is clinically sound and also keeps users interested. The device was validated by comparing it with well-established measuring systems which confirmed its accuracy and reliability in measuring VC. By using this method, the study demonstrates that the device can serve as an alternative and highlights the importance of incorporating new technologies into healthcare systems. Ultimately, such advancements in measurement techniques are integral to enhancing patient management efforts, demonstrating that precision and responsiveness are vital to improving lung health outcomes across diverse populations (Jos et al., 2024).

3.3.1. Spirometry and Its Significance

Spirometry helps doctors in pulmonary medicine by giving important information on lung volumes and capacities. It measures the amount of air moving through the lungs by testing FVC and FEV1. These measurements are vital for detecting and managing asthma and COPD, since these conditions are affected by abnormal lung function. Spirometry matters not only for diagnosis, but also for guiding the treatment given to each patient. This personalized approach aligns with the growing recognition of tailored medical interventions in managing respiratory diseases, as it underscores the complexity of conditions like asthma and COPD that vary markedly among patients (King et al., 2023). Studies examining the spirometric results of athletes and those who are not active clearly demonstrate the relationship between lung function and physical activity. For example, studies have found that trained athletes have much larger lung volumes and capacities and these are related to their improved breathing mechanics. In such studies, athletes displayed mean FEV1 and FVC values that were notably superior to those of their non-active counterparts, emphasizing the positive impact of regular physical training on pulmonary function (Vasantrao et al., 2021). It highlights the importance of maintaining lung health and demonstrates how spirometry can evaluate the impact of exercise on breathing. Therefore, spirometry is a valuable tool for assessing lung function and determining whether lifestyle changes can improve breathing. Additionally, advancements in spirometric equipment have enabled its wider use in both medical and research settings. The software in modern spirometers enables detailed analysis of lung function and the detection of specific breathing problems. The ability to combine spirometry with other lung function tests, such as diffusing capacity assessments, further enriches the understanding of respiratory pathology and guides targeted interventions (King et al., 2023). For this reason, spirometry plays a significant role in healthcare, as it is incorporated into the management of respiratory health. This shift highlights the importance of comprehensive testing and accurate measurement of lung function, which are crucial for optimizing treatment strategies and improving patient outcomes in respiratory diseases (Figure 3.10).

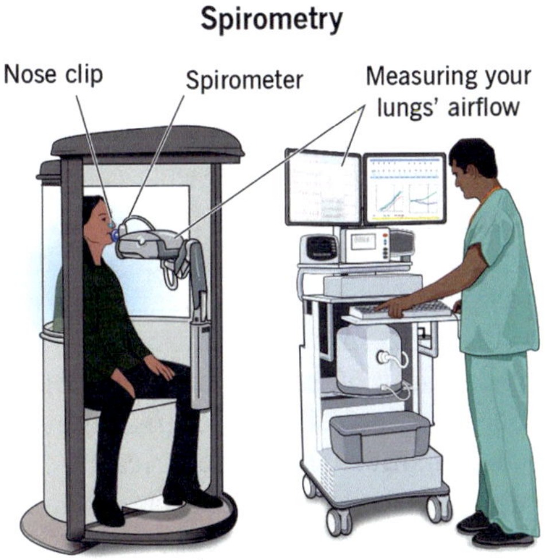

Figure 3.10. Spirometry.

Source: https://my.clevelandclinic.org/-/scassets/images/org/health/articles/17833-spirometry.

3.3.2. Body Plethysmography

Body plethysmography is a helpful way to measure lung volumes and capacities, mainly for people with respiratory disorders. It requires measuring the pressure inside a closed chamber while breathing which helps find out the TLC and FRC with precision. Considering these factors, clinicians can gain insight into various lung diseases, including asthma and COPD. Body plethysmography stands out because it helps identify whether the lung problem is caused by airflow restriction or reduced lung volume, which is helpful in making a diagnosis. It is essential to make this distinction to guide the appropriate treatment and effectively manage chronic respiratory diseases. Besides its usual measurements, body plethysmography is important for learning about airway resistance and compliance. These two aspects are crucial when evaluating individuals with asthma, according to recent studies that emphasize the importance of detailed diagnostic methods. It helps in classifying patients and finding asthma early which makes it easier to use targeted treatments. Additionally, the ability to assess lung regions enables clinicians to identify areas that are not functioning properly. The fact that different patient groups exhibit respiratory conditions differently makes plethysmographic testing crucial for creating individualized treatment plans. Healthcare professionals can use body plethysmography to observe how lung mechanics change, which helps them better understand respiratory diseases. In individuals with COPD, body plethysmography helps measure lung function and track the disease's progression. It provides a detailed examination of lung hyperinflation, a common issue in the advanced stages of the illness. A decrease in lung elasticity can lead to increased difficulties with airflow, which affects both lung function and causes symptoms such as dyspnea and exercise intolerance. This highlights the importance of correct assessment methods, such as body plethysmography, as they demonstrate the relationship between various lung capacities and overall respiratory health. Integrating this technique into healthcare enables providers to assess lung capacities and monitor patients' progress after treatment. Such assessments highlight the potential for enhancing the quality of life in COPD patients, as they inform more effective treatment strategies aimed at reducing hyperinflation and improving functional outcomes (Gagnon et al., 2014; Hadraba et al., 2018) (Figure 3.11).

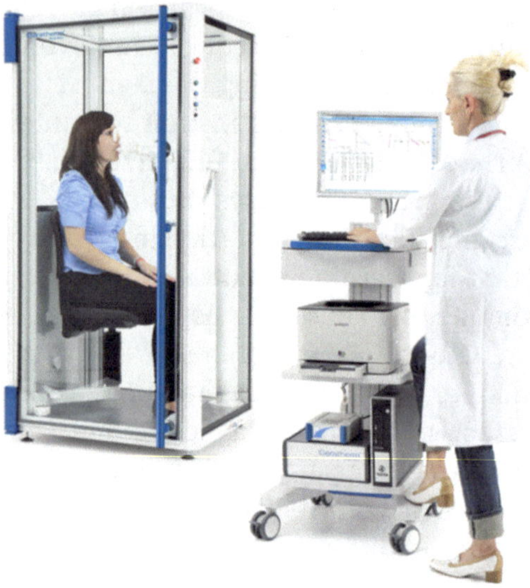

Figure 3.11. Body plethysmography.

Source: https://carnamedicare.com/wp-content/uploads/2020/07/csm_Bodystik_zu_2_1200x853_422a8327e7.png.

3.3.3. Gas Dilution Methods

Evaluating lung volumes and capacities, particularly to assess the respiratory system's function, relies heavily on gas dilution methods. They make use of helium or nitrogen which are inert gases, to calculate the TLC and RV. Measuring the concentration of a gas in the lungs and in the air that is exhaled gives clinicians valuable insights about lung function. One important idea is that the way the gas is distributed shows the different parts and air spaces in the lungs. Because of this, the gas dilution technique is crucial for determining whether a patient has an obstructive or restrictive pattern, which aids in the accurate diagnosis of respiratory diseases. Gas dilution methods are preferred by many because they do not require any invasive steps, which can make patients feel more comfortable and willing to cooperate. Helium dilution is preferred because helium dissolves very little in blood, which minimizes the risk of changes in the body during the test. This method is particularly beneficial in studies involving diverse populations, such as high-altitude natives, where variations in lung volumes can be significant due to genetic and environmental factors (Barker et al., 2012). Researchers can use results from gas dilution methods to find out how altitude affects lung volumes and capacities, which adds to our understanding of how humans adapt to different environments. Although gas dilution methods are helpful, several factors must be considered when evaluating the results. For instance, the accuracy of the measurements can be influenced by factors such as ventilation-perfusion (V/Q) mismatch or inadequate equilibration time, which may lead to errors in estimating lung capacities. Also, the way people breathe and their body structures can make the results less straightforward. Even so, when combined with other PFTs and adjusted for population demographics, gas dilution methods provide helpful information about lung health. Ongoing research continues to explore the implications of genetic and developmental influences on lung function, highlighting the need to consider anthropological factors in respiratory assessments, especially in unique groups (Grobler et al., 2012) (Figure 3.12).

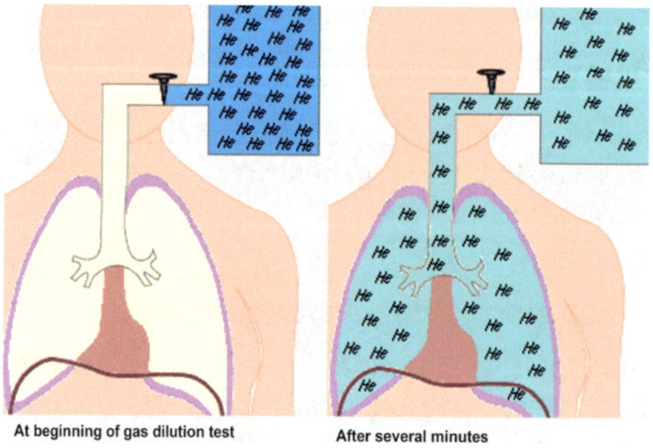

Figure 3.12. Gas dilution.

Source: https://oac.med.jhmi.edu/res_phys/encyclopedia/GasDilution/GasDilutionInhaleExhale.GIF.

3.4. Factors Affecting Lung Volumes and Capacities

Several physiological and environmental factors significantly influence lung volumes and capacities. Both age and gender are important; aging leads to a loss of elasticity in the lungs, and the muscles involved in breathing can become weaker. It causes the lungs to have less space, which is seen in the VC and FEV. It is also found that males tend to have larger lung volumes because their chests and muscles are generally larger. Knowing these differences is important because it enables doctors to make accurate assessments of lung function. Such assessments are crucial for evaluating respiratory health, particularly for vulnerable groups such as the elderly and those with chronic diseases, who are at a higher risk of lung problems. Physical fitness and the body's composition also have a significant impact on lung volumes and capacities. Sticking to regular aerobic exercise can make your lungs work more smoothly by strengthening your breathing muscles. Better lung function enables the lungs to ventilate more effectively, potentially resulting in larger absolute lung volumes. Additionally, the amount of body fat can affect lung volumes; individuals with a high body fat percentage may experience a reduced FRC because their diaphragm is pushed down and cannot contract as fully. Because of this effect, the lungs become less efficient which can cause obesity hypoventilation syndrome. Therefore, assessing physical fitness and body composition is crucial for understanding someone's lung function and determining the most effective way to improve respiratory health. The amount of air in the lungs is greatly affected by things like altitude and the quality of the air we breathe. When at high altitudes, the body's oxygen supply may be lower which encourages the lungs to work harder to get oxygen in. As a result, lung function may change over time such as by increasing TLC and tidal volume, in people who regularly exercise at high altitudes. Breathing polluted air or allergens can harm lung function because it leads to inflammation and reduces the effectiveness of gas exchange. Notably, substances such as volatile organic compounds (VOCs) found in exhaled breath reflect underlying physiological processes and can serve as markers for respiratory health (King et al., 2003; Kupferthaler et al., 2010). Recognizing these environmental factors is crucial for developing public health policies that protect the respiratory health of diverse groups.

3.4.1. Age and Its Impact on Lung Function

As people age, their lungs undergo significant changes, which can impact their overall breathing ability. Lung volumes and capacities tend to decrease significantly as a significant effect of growing older. The VC, which is the highest amount of air you can expel after a deep breath, often drops with age because the lungs and thoracic cavity are not as flexible as they used to be. Lung volumes decrease because the lungs become less compliant and the chest wall becomes stiffer. For this reason, seniors may not be as efficient at breathing, which makes them more susceptible to respiratory illnesses and conditions; therefore, monitoring lung function is important in aging populations. Muscle strength and endurance, which tend to decrease with age, are crucial for efficient breathing. As people age, their muscles often weaken, which can reduce the efficiency of breathing. This problem is especially noticeable in people with chronic conditions such as MS, since respiratory muscle fatigue becomes more noticeable as the disease advances. Research indicates that respiratory muscle training programs can significantly enhance lung volumes and capacities, ultimately improving respiratory performance in aging individuals, as shown in studies exploring interventions for patients with MS (Anisha et al., 2018). These results suggest that specialized rehabilitation programs can help mitigate the negative adverse effects of aging on lung function, which in turn improves the quality of life and health of older individuals. Aging can also alter the composition of our bodies, which may impact our lung function. It is common for the elderly to be obese, and this has been connected to many respiratory disorders. Studies have found that people with obesity often have lung defects, which involve smaller lung volumes and less effective breathing. This is particularly concerning in populations over 50 years, where the accumulation of abdominal fat can impede thoracic expansion and overall respiratory efficiency (Abbruzzese et al., 2023). Understanding the connections between age, obesity, and lung function is crucial for developing effective strategies to support respiratory health. By addressing these contributing factors, healthcare professionals can enhance the management of age-related respiratory issues and promote better lung health across the lifespan (Figure 3.13).

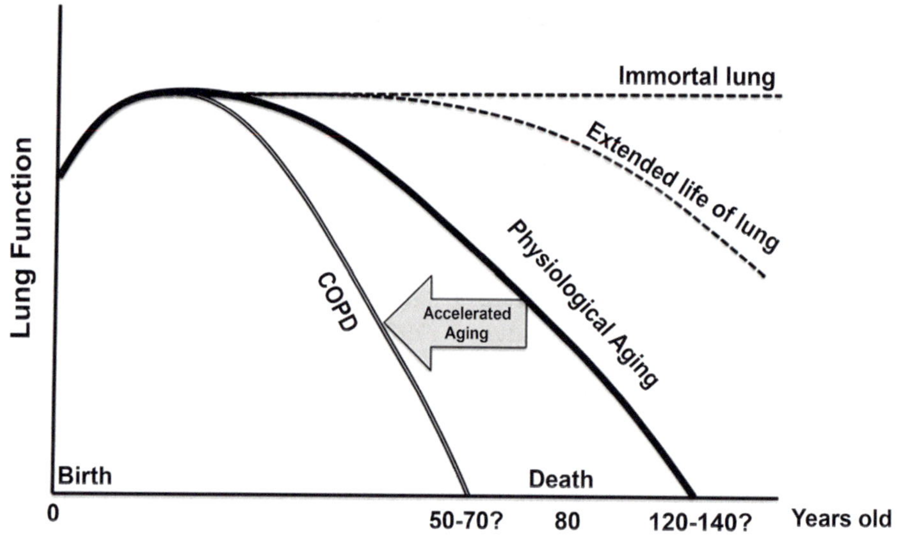

Figure 3.13. Changes of lung function with aging and its possible modification.

Source: https://www.researchgate.net/profile/Nicolas-Mercado/publication/261443085/figure/fig1/AS:608409925713922@1522067638639/Changes-of-lung-function-with-aging-and-its-possible-modification-Lung-function-is.png.

3.4.2. Gender Differences in Lung Volumes

Understanding gender differences in lung volumes is crucial for accurate respiratory assessment and optimal health outcomes. Research has shown that males and females have different lung volumes due to their anatomical and physiological differences. Most males have larger lungs, which is mainly due to their bigger bodies, greater muscle mass, and the structure of their thoracic cavity. For example, males generally have larger FVC and FEV1 values than females, which shows why it is important to use gender-specific reference values in hospitals. Besides the differences in lung function, other factors, such as hormones and the way the lungs function, affect growth and capacity during development. Therefore, it is necessary to use different methods to diagnose and treat respiratory diseases in different groups. Furthermore, due to these differences, certain health conditions have a greater impact on women than on men. Patients who have chronic diseases may show different lung problems depending on their gender. A study conducted on patients with chronic kidney disease (CKD) undergoing hemodialysis revealed significant differences in respiratory function parameters, particularly among those with diabetes. The study found that gender influences the maximal inspiratory pressure (MIP) and maximal expiratory pressure (MEP), with notable decrements observed predominantly in diabetic males on hemodialysis. These findings emphasize that gender must be a critical consideration when assessing lung function among populations at risk for compromised respiratory health, underscoring the need to establish specific risk profiles for both genders in clinical practice (Elizabeth de Daher et al., 2020).

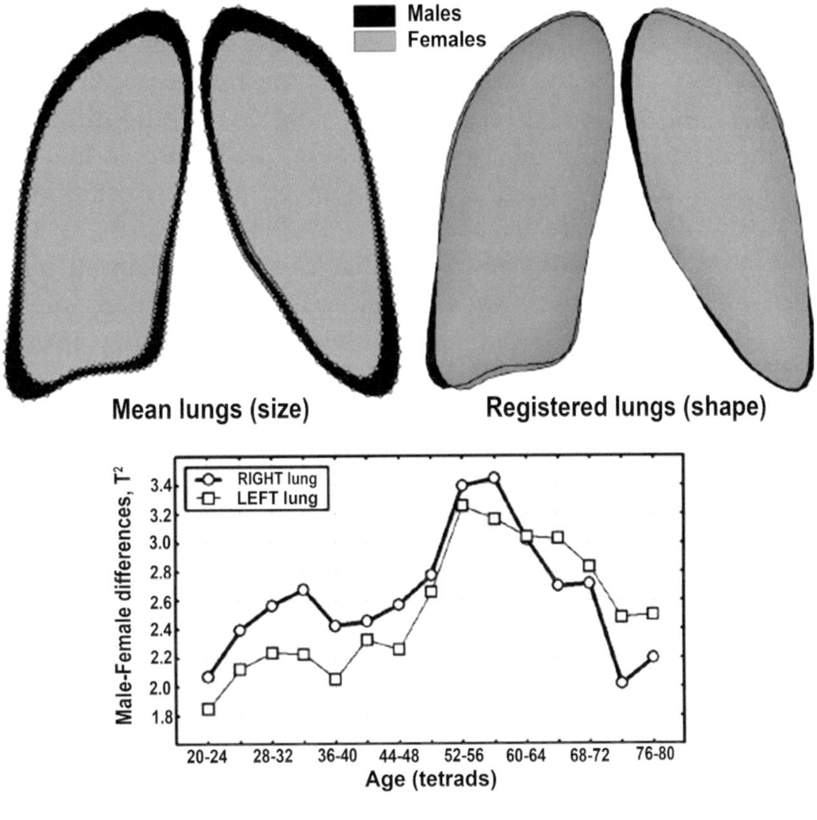

Figure 3.14. Gender-related differences in lung size and lung shape as revealed by comparison of mean (top left) and registered (top right) lung contours of 18000 subjects and the Hotelling's T^2 significance score of gender-related lung shape differences.

Additionally, studies on lung function in various ethnic groups confirm that gender plays a key role in understanding lung volumes. For example, investigations focusing on the Indian population have illustrated that Indian men and women exhibit lower TLC and Diffusing Capacity of the Lung for Carbon Monoxide (DLCO-SB) when compared to European standards. The analysis found that men had 22%–25% less TLC and women had 20% less TLC, indicating significant ethnic differences in lung volumes due to both gender and geographic location. These discrepancies necessitate the development of localized predictive equations to ensure accurate clinical evaluations, particularly as reliance on generic European equations may lead to misdiagnoses or overestimations of lung diseases in specific populations, as indicated in recent studies (Vanjare et al., 2018) (Figure 3.14).

3.4.3. Influence of Physical Fitness and Health Conditions

How fit someone is physically can significantly influence their lung volumes and capacities, which affects their respiratory system. Physically fit people often have more lung capacity which shows as an increase in VC and TLC. Such a relationship is significant in endurance athletes, as they usually have larger lung volumes than those who are sedentary. Regular physical activity strengthens the respiratory muscles, which in turn enables the body to take in more oxygen and remove carbon dioxide during exercise. Additionally, being physically fit can lower the risk of developing COPD and other breathing-related problems. Consequently, maintaining an active lifestyle not only improves lung capacity but also acts as a preventive measure against the decline in pulmonary function associated with aging and various health conditions (Alexander et al., 2022).

Long-term diseases, such as chronic illnesses, can reduce the amount of air the lungs can hold. People with asthma, obesity or pulmonary fibrosis may face many respiratory problems and reduced ability of the lungs to stretch. If someone has asthma, the airways become inflamed and narrow, which can reduce airflow and affect both the lungs' volume and the exchange of gases. Excess weight, similarly, can be a problem; it can limit the movement of the diaphragm, resulting in shallow breathing and reduced lung capacity. Moreover, health conditions can exacerbate the impact of infectious diseases, as seen in individuals recovering from COVID-19, where a significant proportion experiences post-acute sequelae, including persistent respiratory symptoms like shortness of breath and impaired exercise tolerance (Jason et al., 2021). It means that addressing health issues can enhance lung health and function. The relationship between being fit and experiencing health issues highlights the need for multiple approaches to lung health. Assessing and addressing a patient's fitness should be part of managing chronic lung diseases for clinicians. Exercise programs designed for rehabilitation can make lungs function better, which shows that the proper exercise routines can greatly improve lung capacity. Additionally, incorporating aerobic exercises and strength training into rehabilitation programs for patients with chronic lung disease has led to improved physical condition and lung health. As evidence suggests, a proactive approach that combines enhanced physical fitness with effective management of health conditions is vital in promoting optimal lung function, particularly in vulnerable populations affected by chronic diseases and respiratory ailments (Alexander et al., 2022) (Figure 3.15).

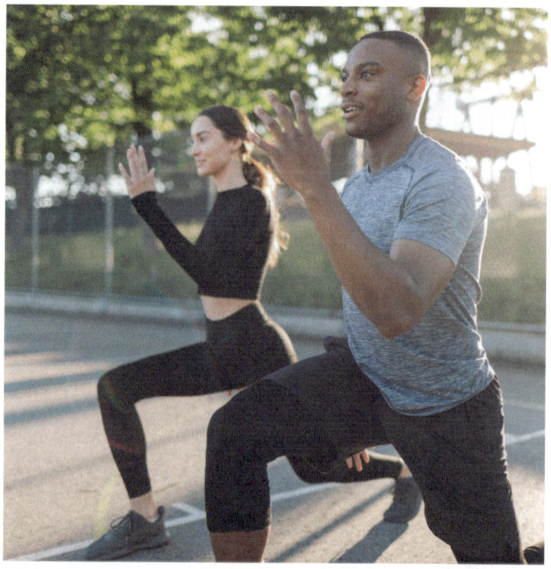

Figure 3.15. Physical exercise and respiratory health.

Source: https://lunghealth.ca/wp-content/uploads/2024/07/Post-on-Jul-18_social-2.png.

3.5. Clinical Relevance

Understanding lung volumes and capacities is crucial for doctors treating and managing these conditions. Healthcare professionals often use spirometry to measure these volumes, which can show important details about breathing and lung function. A change in lung volumes can point to COPD or restrictive lung disease, which should be handled with specific treatments. Looking at FEV1 and FVC lets healthcare professionals measure how severe the disease is and how it is progressing, which helps them choose the best treatment plan. Furthermore, the significance of bronchodilator responsiveness (BDR), as discussed in Anderson et al. (2019), adds a layer of complexity to this analysis, emphasizing the importance of understanding individual patient profiles to accurately predict clinical outcomes. In acute clinical settings, knowledge of lung capacities plays a crucial role in managing conditions such as acute respiratory distress syndrome (ARDS). People with ARDS usually have difficulty breathing, and their lungs do not expand easily, which means their lung volumes need to be carefully monitored to help with ventilation. Prone positioning and high-frequency oscillatory ventilation, which help deliver oxygen better, depend on how much lung volume is present. The management of fluid status also correlates with lung capacities, as restrictive fluid management has shown favorable outcomes without significantly impacting mortality rates in ARDS patients, according to findings from Alessandri et al. (2018). How lung volumes influence clinical care points out the importance of accurate assessments for better patient care and results in critical situations. Measuring lung volumes and capacities helps identify respiratory diseases and supports preventive healthcare. If healthcare providers can identify individuals who are at risk of developing chronic diseases, they can intervene early to help prevent or mitigate the disease or avoid serious complications. The relationship between lung function and comorbidities, such as cardiovascular diseases (CVDs), highlights the importance of comprehensive lung assessments in routine clinical evaluations. Moreover, understanding the significance of BDR in COPD patients, as noted in Anderson et al. (2019), supports the development of personalized management plans. Having these plans can help patients learn more and manage their health better, which leads to a better quality of life. Besides their role in diagnosis, lung volumes and capacities significantly impact the entire process of patient care and contribute to improved overall health outcomes.

3.5.1. Use of Lung Volume Measurements in Diagnosing Respiratory Diseases

Measuring lung volumes accurately is very important for diagnosing lung diseases. Using spirometry and body plethysmography helps measure lung function, particularly in identifying restrictive and obstructive lung problems. Their importance is clear because we need population-specific reference values to correctly interpret each person's results. For example, a study investigating the Global Lung Function Initiative (GLI) reference equations indicated a poor fit within specific populations, leading to the development of tailored equations that enhance diagnostic precision. The findings demonstrated that without applicable reference values, the detection and understanding of conditions such as COPD might be compromised, showcasing the essential role of personalized lung volume measurements in effectively diagnosing respiratory diseases (Mraz et al., 2024). Lung volume measurements play a crucial role in detecting diseases, monitoring disease progression over time, and assessing the effectiveness of treatment. In ARDS, for instance, end-expiratory lung volume (EELV) has emerged as an essential metric. Studies on EELV in people with COVID-19-associated ARDS found significant differences between those who survived and those who did not, proving it is a good indicator of outcomes. According to the study, higher EELV values were associated with better survival, suggesting that regular lung volume checks can be a valuable tool for predicting patient outcomes. Through methods such as the nitrogen washout-wash-in technique, clinicians gain access to dynamic lung function indicators, enabling more informed decision-making in critical care settings (Hao et al., 2024). Including lung volume measurements in routine tests can help identify respiratory illnesses earlier and facilitate prompt treatment. For instance, knowing about TLC and RV, which are static lung volumes, helps clinicians tell apart different lung diseases, which is important for choosing the best treatment. Achieving accurate results from these measurements depends on using reference equations that accurately fit the group being studied. As shown in studies, for example, the Austrian LEAD Study, using custom reference frameworks can greatly enhance the accuracy of lung volume assessments and help manage conditions properly. This case highlights the ongoing need for updating diagnostic criteria in response to evolving demographic data, thereby enriching the field of pulmonary medicine (Mraz et al., 2024).

3.5.2. Importance in Preoperative Assessments

Before a patient undergoes surgery, a preoperative assessment is crucial for evaluating the function of their lungs. Healthcare providers measure lung volumes such as tidal volume and VC to spot any risks of respiratory complications in patients having surgery. With these assessments, healthcare teams can design a care plan that helps the patient's breathing and addresses any weaknesses before surgery. Without thorough preoperative evaluations, there is an increased likelihood of postoperative pulmonary complications (PPCs) that can extend hospital stays and negatively impact patient outcomes, emphasizing the importance of this initial assessment phase. Preoperative assessments enable doctors to implement early strategies to manage identified risks, particularly in patients with lung function issues.

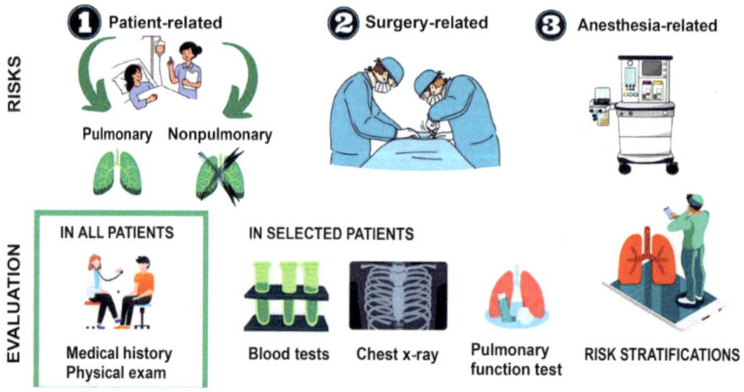

Figure 3.16. Preoperative pulmonary risk evaluation.

Source: https://media.springernature.com/lw1200/springer-static/image/art%3A10.1007%2Fs44254-023-00034-2/MediaObjects/44254_2023_34_Figa_HTML.png.

As an illustration, respiratory muscle training can increase the amount of air you can breathe, which is supported by studies showing that PPCs are much lower after exercise programs before surgery. Research shows that patients who follow tailored exercise programs improve their peak oxygen uptake and MIP, which leads to shorter hospital stays, proving that strong preoperative evaluations improve postoperative recovery. This information highlights the importance of ensuring optimal lung volumes and capacities before surgery, which enables doctors to use the most effective therapies for better outcomes. Also, when evidence-based practices are used in preoperative assessments, patients often recover faster, and healthcare costs are reduced. Reviewing respiratory capabilities through evaluations can help place patients in the appropriate surgical risk category for the procedures they are undergoing. If these assessments guide the selection of anesthesia and surgery, the risk of complications after surgery goes down. Additionally, addressing lung volume and capacity issues prior to surgery facilitates a safe and effective approach to patient care. Thus, establishing a comprehensive preoperative assessment protocol is essential for minimizing complications, improving patient quality of care, and ultimately enhancing surgical success rates, highlighting its paramount importance in the realm of lung health in surgical contexts (Figure 3.16).

3.5.3. Role in Monitoring Chronic Lung Conditions

Evaluating lung volumes and capacities is crucial for managing long-term lung illnesses, particularly in understanding how various factors impact breathing. Checking lung volumes, such as tidal volume, VC, and TLC, provides important information about an individual's lung health. They make it possible to tell apart obstructive and restrictive lung diseases, which helps decide on the best treatment. Research has shown that both social and dietary factors significantly impact lung function in children. Children from lower socioeconomic backgrounds often exhibit reduced lung volumes due to undernutrition or exposure to pollutants, highlighting the need for targeted interventions to improve lung health and effectively monitor chronic conditions (Adeniji et al., 2018). Using various methods demonstrates that monitoring is crucial for managing chronic lung diseases across different groups. Lung function monitoring plays a crucial role in public health efforts to manage and reduce the prevalence of chronic respiratory diseases.

The Centers for Disease Control and Prevention report that chronic lower respiratory diseases significantly contribute to mortality rates, particularly among vulnerable populations (Miller et al., 2017). If lung volume is measured during regular health checks, healthcare providers can identify early changes in breathing and act to prevent problems. Regular checks can also reveal how environmental and lifestyle factors impact lung health, which can lead to community actions to improve air quality and help people quit smoking. Being aware of lung capacities helps guide public health policies to fight chronic lung diseases, which helps the overall health of the population. Additionally, new technology continues to improve the measurement of lung volumes and capacities, making it both easier and more accurate. Thanks to portable spirometers, people can now be screened for lung problems and monitor their lung health. For individuals dealing with chronic health issues, these devices can be highly beneficial because they encourage users to take an active role in their health management. Regular checks using these tools give important information that can be shared with doctors to improve treatment. As our understanding of respiratory diseases grows, the integration of sophisticated monitoring tools into clinical practice can enhance patient outcomes by fostering timely interventions and targeted support for managing chronic lung conditions (Miller et al., 2017). By prioritizing the role of lung volume measurement in patient care, we can achieve improved management of these increasingly prevalent health issues (Figure 3.17).

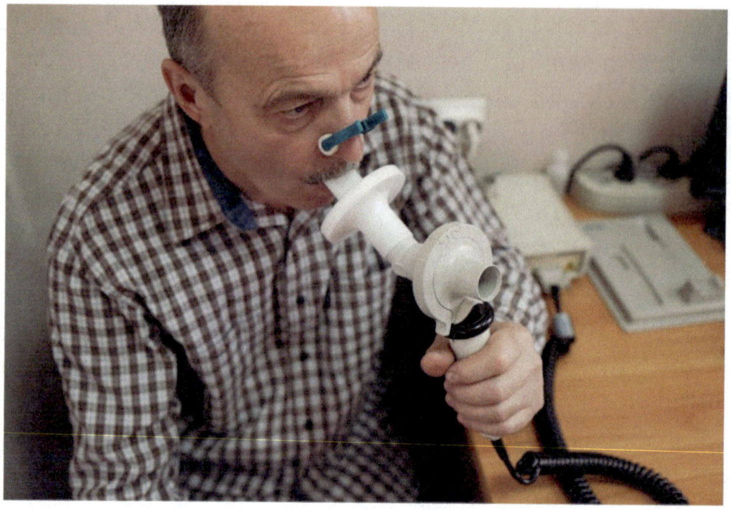

Figure 3.17. A patient undergoing spirometry to assess lung function.

Source: https://www.verywellhealth.com/thmb/ABpRboC45dLUdM5rjeyHC5K5Lpw=/1500x0/filters:no_upscale():max_bytes(150000):strip_icc()/GettyImages-1173957346-a8ebdf0c3e99405bbaf0b3074919dabd.jpg.

SUMMARY

The importance of lung volumes and capacities extends beyond learning; they are crucial in medical settings, particularly for maintaining respiratory health. Assessing lung function accurately allows doctors to choose the best rehabilitation strategies, mainly for people suffering from post-COVID-19 syndrome. It appears that certain breathing exercises can improve lung function and breathing, making it essential to tailor treatments to each patient. As highlighted in contemporary research, improvements in FVC and peak expiratory flow indices are indicative of positive outcomes in rehabilitation endeavors, suggesting that timely interventions can reverse or mitigate the decline in lung function observed in affected individuals (Parisi et al., 2024).

Additionally, the impact of body composition on lung function underscores the multifaceted nature of respiratory health. The research indicates that somatotypes are associated with changes in spirometric measures, demonstrating how body shape influences breathing ability. If endomorphs and mesomorphs experience peripheral airway dysfunction more frequently than ectomorphs, this suggests that healthcare practitioners should pay closer attention. Since mesomorphs tend to have higher FVC, it appears that maintaining a fit body may support strong and healthy lungs. Addressing these differences through tailored approaches could further enhance rehabilitation outcomes, making it imperative to consider individual respiratory assessments in conjunction with somatotype evaluations (Jaiswal et al., 2024). All in all, combining information about lung volumes, capacities, and demographics gives a full picture needed for progress in respiratory care. Although new rehabilitation methods and a better understanding of how lung function varies among individuals have been developed, further research is needed to create effective assessment and intervention strategies. It is essential to continually encourage new ideas in respiratory healthcare and utilize the findings from research to enhance our practices. Understanding lung function and patient profiles more effectively will clearly lead to improved patient outcomes and better care in the field of respiratory medicine.

Assessing lung volumes and capacities is important because they help determine the health of the lungs and any problems. Tidal volume, IRV, and ERV are the main lung volumes that show the air inhaled or exhaled in normal breathing, extra air that can be inhaled, and extra air that can be exhaled forcefully, respectively. These volumes cumulatively contribute to vital capacity (VC), the maximum amount of air that can be exhaled after maximal inhalation. Due to this knowledge, PFTs can be utilized to diagnose and monitor respiratory diseases. Also, TLC and FRC are important lung capacities used to study respiratory mechanics. TLC is the total amount of air in the lungs, providing a comprehensive view of lung size. FRC, which is made up of residual volume and ERV, is the amount of air that stays in the lungs after you exhale.

They are essential for assessing diseases that block or restrict the lungs. COPD patients tend to have higher TLC because of air trapping, while those with restrictive lung diseases have a lower TLC which suggests their lungs do not expand enough. Understanding lung volumes and capacities also helps in selecting effective treatments for various lung diseases. Since ARDS primarily affects the lungs, understanding lung function can help determine how therapies are working. For instance, recruitment maneuvers and cautious fluid management strategies are often employed to mitigate hypoxemia in ARDS patients, as seen in recent studies suggesting potential interventions such as inhaled nitric oxide and extracorporeal membrane oxygenation (ECMO) for severe cases

(Alessandri et al., 2018). Furthermore, research exploring pharmacological interventions, such as the use of captopril to address radiation-induced pulmonary effects, highlights the importance of maintaining optimal lung function and vascular health in critical care settings (Fish et al., 2012). Recognizing these factors aids in treating individual patients and also helps develop general strategies in respiratory medicine.

CLOSER LOOK

FORCED VITAL CAPACITY (FVC)

FVC is the amount of air that can be forcibly exhaled from your lungs after taking the deepest breath possible. It's measured by spirometry, a common breathing test used to assess lung function.

This test may help distinguish obstructive and restrictive lung diseases. Obstructive diseases, such as asthma and COPD, make it difficult to exhale all the air from your lungs. Restrictive lung diseases, such as pulmonary fibrosis and sarcoidosis, cause problems with inhaling air to fill your lungs (Figure 3.18).

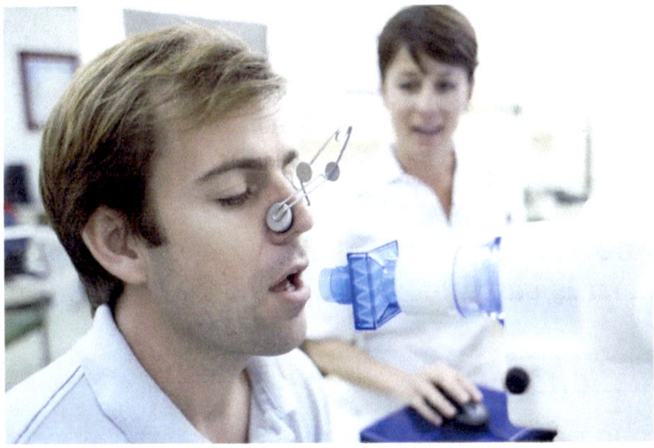

Figure 3.18. Pulmonary function test.

Source: https://www.verywellhealth.com/thmb/WeWypLak3CZ6--DCG-EaLhcBgKM=/750x0/filters:no_upscale():max_bytes(150000):strip_icc():format(webp)/lung-function-test-99310789-76d56899319b4b989ea1b07abee10866.jpg.

FVC can also help healthcare providers assess the progression of lung disease and evaluate the effectiveness of treatment. An abnormal FVC value may be chronic, but sometimes the problem is reversible, and the FVC can be corrected.

Purpose of FVC

FVC is used to evaluate your lung function. It measures the effect that your lung disease has on your ability to inhale and exhale.

While FVC cannot identify which specific lung disease you have, the results can help narrow down potential diagnoses. It can be used, along with other studies, to help determine which type of lung disease you have.

Reasons you may need to have your FVC measured include:

- You have shortness of breath, a persistent cough, or wheezing.
- Your healthcare provider wants to assess your respiratory function when your blood oxygen level is low.

- You are having surgery. It's essential to determine if your breathing is stable before undergoing a procedure, particularly if you are scheduled for lung surgery.
- You have heart disease and need an assessment of its effects on your ability to breathe.
- You and your healthcare provider are planning your lung rehabilitation program.
- You have reached the endpoint in a clinical trial expected to affect lung function.

Associated Tests

You may have other tests done when you go in to have your FVC measured. These include your VC and FEV1.

FVC and VC record similar information. They both measure the amount of air you can exhale after maximally inhaling. But FVC refers to the amount of air you can exhale forcefully. VC records the maximum amount of air exhaled when breathing normally.

FEV1 differs in that it measures the amount of air you can exhale in one second.

Your FVC and other PFTs are used to establish the status of your lung function. They compare your measurements to standards based on your age, gender, race, height, and weight.

Risks and Contraindications

FVC requires your cooperation and effort, but it is a safe procedure. However, be sure to have medical supervision the first time you use a spirometer, the device used to measure your FVC. You could potentially use a spirometer incorrectly, exhausting yourself.

Afterward, you may be instructed on how to use it at home independently. Ensure the spirometer you use has been thoroughly cleaned before each use. That way you won't be exposed to anything that can cause an infection.

REFERENCES

1. Agaba, I. E., Odanaogun, R. A., Odeh, S. O., Sabo, B., et al. (2005). Pulmonary performance in asymptomatic young Nigerian population following the administration of ascorbic acid and salbutamol. *Nigerian Journal of Physiological Sciences.* https://core.ac.uk/download/478375626.pdf (accessed on 31st May 2025).
2. Alessandri, F., Pugliese, F., & Ranieri, M. (2018). *The Role of Rescue Therapies in the Treatment of Severe ARDS.* https://core.ac.uk/download/132156803.pdf (accessed on 31st May 2025).
3. Amann, A., Lumb, A. B., Schrikker, A. C., Mörk, A. K., Amann, A., Amann, A., Anton, A., et al. (2010). A mathematical model for breath gas analysis of volatile organic compounds with special emphasis on acetone. *J. Math. Biol.* http://arxiv.org/abs/1003.4475 (accessed on 31st May 2025).
4. Anderson, W., Arjomandi, M., Barjaktarevic, I. Z., Bhakta, N., et al. (2019). Clinical significance of bronchodilator responsiveness evaluated by forced vital capacity in COPD: SPIROMICS cohort analysis. *Int. J. Chron. Obstruct. Pulmon. Dis.* https://core.ac.uk/download/323062278.pdf (accessed on 31st May 2025).
5. Andrade, A. D. de, Bernardino, S. N., Fernandes, J., Fuzari, M., et al. (2020). Pulmonary capacity of patients with total traumatic injury of the brachial plexus submitted to neurotization with the phrenic nerve: A case series. *Revista Brasileira de Neurologia* https://core.ac.uk/download/477890536.pdf (accessed on 31st May 2025).
6. Andrade, K., Backus, A., Haapanen, K. A., Lindsey, J., et al. (2020). *Aligning Community-Engaged Research to Context.* https://core.ac.uk/download/287622822.pdf (accessed on 31st May 2025).
7. Anisha, T. V. (2018). Effectiveness of respiratory muscle training program (RMT) improves total lung volumes and capacities and reduces fatigue in patients with multiple sclerosis. https://core.ac.uk/download/288215776.pdf (accessed on 31st May 2025).
8. Assouline, B., Cools, E., Elia, N., Kayser, B., et al. (2021). Preoperative exercise training to prevent postoperative pulmonary complications in adults undergoing major surgery: A systematic review and meta-analysis with trial sequential analysis. https://core.ac.uk/download/355099467.pdf (accessed on 31st May 2025).
9. Aydin, G., & Koca, İ. (2014). *Swimming Training and Pulmonary Variables in Women.* https://core.ac.uk/download/32322335.pdf (accessed on 31st May 2025).
10. Azevedo, J. L. M. C., Barbalho, M. C., Costa, D., Forti, E., et al. (2008). *The Impact of Obesity on Pulmonary Function in Adult Women.* https://core.ac.uk/download/pdf/8274863.pdf (accessed on 31st May 2025).
11. Barker, J., Barker, D., Barker, R., Bartlett, M., Beall, C., Beall, C., Beall, C., et al. (2012). Developmental and genetic components explain enhanced pulmonary volumes of female Peruvian Quechua. *American Journal of Physical Anthropology.* https://deepblue.lib.umich.edu/bitstream/2027.42/92086/1/22069_ftp.pdf (accessed on 31st May 2025).
12. Bhammar, D., Wilhite, D., Olojo, T., Alagappan, K., Jones, K., Liu, Y. L., & Babb, T. G. (2025). Effects of obesity and sex on supine functional residual capacity and expiratory flow limitation in children. *Pediatric Pulmonology, 60.* https://www.semanticscholar.org/paper/c415be2f0bda2ea50edd2a9ddc993f953df838c5 (accessed on 31st May 2025).

13. Buras, J. C. (2004). *A Comparison of the Pulmonary Function of Older Endurance Athletes with Age-Matched Sedentary Controls.* https://core.ac.uk/download/216835090.pdf (accessed on 31st May 2025).

14. Crew, J. D., Ferguson, A. R., Kosarchuk, J. J., McKenna, K., et al. (2017). Pulmonary outcomes following specialized respiratory management for acute cervical spinal cord injury: A retrospective analysis. *Spinal Cord.* https://core.ac.uk/download/323063139.pdf (accessed on 31st May 2025).

15. Daher, E. F., Marizeiro, D. F., Mont'alverne, D. G. B., Meneses, G. C., Freitas, T. V. de S., Costa Martins, A. M., & Bezerra da, S. Jr. G. (2020). P0663 – Relationship between endothelial lesion and pulmonary dysfunction among hemodialytic chronic kidney disease patients with and without diabetes mellitus. *Nephrology Dialysis Transplantation.* https://www.semanticscholar.org/paper/572e32c76230f7ae26a9753626b3c245ce3cbfc8 (accessed on 31st May 2025).

16. Fish, B. L., Jacobs, E. R., Medhora, M. M., Molthen, R. C., et al. (2012). Mitigation of radiation induced pulmonary vascular injury by delayed treatment with captopril. *Respirology.* https://core.ac.uk/download/213080178.pdf (accessed on 31st May 2025).

17. Gagnon, P., Guenette, J. A., Langer, D., Laviolette, L., et al. (2014). *Pathogenesis of Hyperinflation in Chronic Obstructive Pulmonary Disease.* https://core.ac.uk/download/77517176.pdf (accessed on 31st May 2025).

18. García, P. J. J., González, M. I., Aguilar, Z. J., Valencia, M., Moncada, E., & García, J. D. (2024). Biomedical equipment for the measurement of inspiratory and expiratory volumes based on the Ubicu respiratory incentive. In *2024 3rd International Congress of Biomedical Engineering and Bioengineering (CIIBBI).* https://www.semanticscholar.org/paper/192c33aad5a53f4191f87499bb7c5ce2e00c4c76 (accessed on 31st May 2025).

19. Gerardo, A. M., Alves, C. da S., Gomes, M., Pardal, C., Sokolova, A., Liberato, H., Mendes, A., et al. (2024). The effects of benralizumab on lung volumes and airway resistance in severe eosinophilic asthma: A real-world study. *Cureus, 16.* https://www.semanticscholar.org/paper/5c8999a91bdaab61bdb44131ac48b15ed4b9da47 (accessed on 31st May 2025).

20. Grobler, C., Maree, D. M., & Irusen, E. M. (2012). *Functional Evaluation in Respiratory Disorders.* https://core.ac.uk/download/322408718.pdf (accessed on 31st May 2025).

21. Hadraba, D., Jelen, K., Koucky, V., Lopot, F., et al. (2018). *Functional Lung Examination in Diagnostics of Asthma and its Phenotypes.* https://core.ac.uk/download/322437794.pdf (accessed on 31st May 2025).

22. Hao, S., Wei, Y., Wang, Y., Muhetaer, Y., Zhou, C., Qiong, S., Jiang, P., et al. (2024). End-expiratory lung volumes as a potential indicator for COVID-19 associated acute respiratory distress syndrome: A retrospective study. *BMC Pulmonary Medicine, 24.* https://www.semanticscholar.org/paper/be97b50f93e99d57be6a878e2dfce1f6aff54fcb (accessed on 31st May 2025).

23. Helgeson, S., Quicksall, Z. S., Johnson, P. W., Lim, K. G., Carter, R., & Lee, A. S. (2025). Estimation of static lung volumes and capacities from spirometry using machine learning: Algorithm development and validation. *JMIR AI.* https://www.semanticscholar.org/paper/c8187a144879df75296d245c2e30a9fb0c335b97 (accessed on 31st May 2025).

24. Jaiswal, K. N., Talwar, A., Vayyat, S., & Bade, G. (2024). Effect of somatotypes on lung volumes, capacities and respiratory impedance: A pilot study. *Lung India: Official Organ of Indian Chest Society, 41,* 3–10. https://www.semanticscholar.org/paper/

a5cf5de4b115522ee1bd4b033d8481f3296b4ffd (accessed on 31st May 2025).

25. Jun, J. (2022). Dying with OSA, or from it: A cautionary note about novel hypoxia metrics. *American Journal of Respiratory and Critical Care Medicine, 206*, 1563, 1564. https://www.semanticscholar.org/paper/390d8a233514a813be93b60f773aa518850ed21e (accessed on 31st May 2025).
26. King, G., Formenti, F., & Petousi, N. (2023). Editorial: Physiological phenotyping in respiratory diseases: New approaches. *Frontiers in Physiology, 14*. https://www.semanticscholar.org/paper/c61eb0679c99f80a3d7d9435ac33f10b187f175a (accessed on 31st May 2025).
27. King, J., Koc, H., Unterkofler, K., Mochalski, P., et al. (2003). *Physiological Modeling of Isoprene Dynamics in Exhaled Breath*. http://arxiv.org/abs/1010.2145 (accessed on 31st May 2025).
28. Knutsen, G. L. (1976). *The Influence of Age, Sex and Weight on Respiratory Function in the Sedate Canine*. https://core.ac.uk/download/212846424.pdf (accessed on 31st May 2025).
29. Kupferthaler, A., Amann, A., Amann, A., Amann, A., Anderson, W., Anderson, W., Anton, A., et al. (2010). *Physiological Modeling of Isoprene Dynamics in Exhaled Breath*. http://arxiv.org/abs/1010.2145 (accessed on 31st May 2025).
30. Li, F., Chen, Y., Zhang, G., Liu, M., Zeng, H., & Dai, H. (2025). Baseline total lung capacity and all-cause mortality in restrictive pulmonary disorders: A meta-analysis. *BMC Pulmonary Medicine, 25*. https://www.semanticscholar.org/paper/b1ab020ee87a0ddfe1901e06e9ca4b0761e4b0cf (accessed on 31st May 2025).
31. Lo Mauro, A., Tringali, G., Codecasa, F., Abbruzzese, L., Sartorio, A., & Aliverti, A. (2023). Pulmonary and chest wall function in obese adults. *Scientific Reports, 13*(1). https://doi.org/10.1038/s41598-023-44222-3Adeniji, E. O., Adeniyi, A. T., Kuti, B. P., Kuti, O. O., et al. (2018). Rural-urban disparity in lung function parameters of Nigerian children: Effects of socio-economic, nutritional and housing factors. *Pan African Medical Journal*. https://core.ac.uk/download/478431377.pdf (accessed on 31st May 2025).
32. Lyon, A. R., López-Fernández, T., Couch, L. S., Asteggiano, R., Aznar, M. C., Bergler-Klein, J., Boriani, G., et al. (2022). 2022 ESC Guidelines on cardio-oncology developed in collaboration with the European Hematology Association (EHA), the European Society for Therapeutic Radiology and Oncology (ESTRO) and the International Cardio-Oncology Society (IC-OS). *European Heart Journal, 43*, 4229–4361. https://doi.org/10.1093/eurheartj/ehac244 (accessed on 31st May 2025).
33. Maley, J. H., Alba, G. A., Barry, J. T., Bartels, M. N., Fleming, T. K., Oleson, C. V., Rydberg, L., et al. (2021). Multi-disciplinary collaborative consensus guidance statement on the assessment and treatment of breathing discomfort and respiratory sequelae in patients with post-acute sequelae of SARS-CoV-2 infection (PASC). *PM&R, 14*, 77–95. https://doi.org/10.1002/pmrj.12744 (accessed on 31st May 2025).
34. Miller, L., Pinkerton, K., Royer, C., Schelegle, E., et al. (2017). *Nonhuman Primate Models of Respiratory Disease: Past, Present, and Future*. https://core.ac.uk/download/323069778.pdf (accessed on 31st May 2025).
35. Miller, W. B., & Torday, J. S. (2016). *The Unicellular State as a Point Source in a Quantum Biological System*. https://core.ac.uk/download/323079765.pdf (accessed on 31st May 2025).
36. Mraz, T., Asgari, S., Karimi, A., Breyer, M., Hartl, S., Sunanta, O., Ofenheimer, A., et al. (2024). Updated reference values for static lung volumes from a healthy population

in Austria. *Respiratory Research, 25*. https://www.semanticscholar.org/paper/b4cc203a181608b2f00631e140e82628c3a72621 (accessed on 31st May 2025).

37. Nadeem, S. A., Comellas, A., Chan, K. S., Hoffman, E. A., Fain, S. B., & Saha, P. K. (2024). Automated CT-based measurements of radial and longitudinal expansion of airways due to breathing-related lung volume change. *Medical Physics, 52*, 2316–2329. https://www.semanticscholar.org/paper/ebb5c6e06ac3dcd6f590458f29d6f46dbffc4804 (accessed on 31st May 2025).

38. Parisi, M. C., Di Corrado, D., Mingrino, O., Crescimanno, C., Longo, F., Pegreffi, F., & Francavilla, V. (2024). SpiroTiger and KS Brief Stimulator: Specific devices for breathing and well-being in post-COVID-19 patients. *Journal of Functional Morphology and Kinesiology, 9*. https://www.semanticscholar.org/paper/592bf98598a5f8395701e170df0c68650626e79e (accessed on 31st May 2025).

39. Salvi, D. J., & Moradia, D. (2020). Effect of obesity on lung function test among adults. *International Journal of Advances in Medicine*. https://www.semanticscholar.org/paper/670c34c5b9b0c0546eead3525d1f52e4ca2badae (accessed on 31st May 2025).

40. Swaminathan, S. (1999). *Pulmonary Function Testing in Office Practice*. https://core.ac.uk/download/83048680.pdf (accessed on 31st May 2025).

41. Vanjare, N., Rasam, S. A., Das, V., Thorat, Y., Jadhav, S., Salvi, S., & Pawar, S. (2018). How different are the lung volumes and diffusing capacities of healthy Indians compared to age & gender-matched Europeans? *Respiratory Function Technologists/Scient*. https://www.semanticscholar.org/paper/df83f55eed1a01c34eeac441f78b832f7962938c (accessed on 31st May 2025).

42. Vasantrao, B., & Jain, M. (2021). Evaluation of respiratory parameters between normal sedentary male control and sportsman persons. *IAR Journal of Medicine and Surgery Research*. https://www.semanticscholar.org/paper/2f96dbefcc34efb4f4a4730cf7f7b5b615b36e87 (accessed on 31st May 2025).

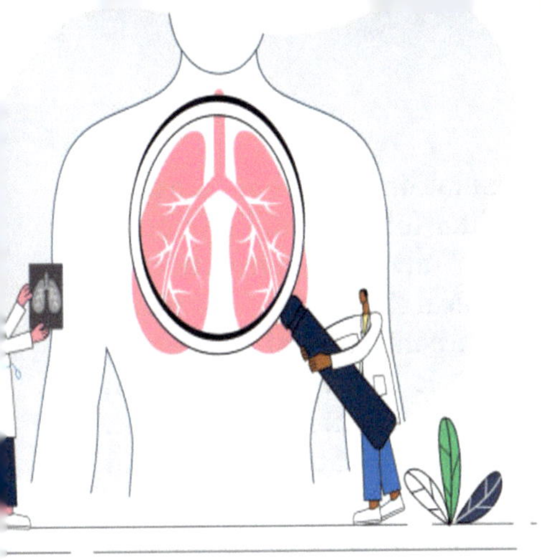

Chapter 4

ALVEOLAR VENTILATION

Contents

Introduction

Alveolar ventilation is essential for explaining the workings of the respiratory system. Alveolar ventilation is the amount of air that arrives at the alveoli, where gas exchange takes place. This value is crucial for ensuring that oxygen is delivered and carbon dioxide is removed properly, both of which are necessary for maintaining homeostasis. The significance of alveolar ventilation becomes especially pronounced in clinical settings, such as acute respiratory distress syndrome (ARDS) and community-acquired pneumonia (CAP), where impaired gas exchange can lead to severe health consequences. Treating these conditions effectively involves understanding how pulmonary mechanics and gas diffusion interact to influence alveolar ventilation and the entire respiratory system. Recently, medical research has helped elucidate the complexities of alveolar ventilation. For example, studies have shown that patients with ARDS respond differently to treatment, making it necessary to use individualized approaches. Contemporary literature stresses that because ARDS patients are so different, it is challenging to develop a single standard drug treatment. Instead, using precision medicine is now being promoted to help doctors achieve better clinical outcomes. By employing biomolecular technologies and bioinformatics, researchers aim to understand better the underlying pathways of diseases affecting alveolar function, thus allowing for more targeted therapeutic approaches that account for individual variations in response to treatment (Calfee et al., 2017). It is now more evident that combining different medical specialties can enhance patient outcomes for diseases affecting alveolar ventilation. One example is physiotherapy, which has received notice for its ability to improve respiratory function in people with CAP. The modified Delphi technique was employed in the research, and it revealed that experts agreed on the best ways to manage physiotherapy in these patients. Specifically, expert panels have identified critical assessment and treatment strategies essential for individuals who are invasively ventilated (Braun et al., 2018). Although insights come from various disciplines, the primary goal is to enhance alveolar ventilation, thereby helping patients recover and improving the effectiveness of treatment.

Definition of Alveolar Ventilation

Alveolar ventilation is important in respiratory physiology because it describes the amount of fresh air entering the alveoli, which are the air sacs in the lungs that allow gas exchange. It is important to measure this because some of the air you breathe does not contribute to ventilation, as it remains in the dead space where gas exchange does not occur. Calculating alveolar ventilation involves subtracting dead space ventilation from minute ventilation, which indicates how effectively the lungs are functioning. In hospitals, it is crucial to make this distinction when assessing various lung disorders, as it affects oxygen supply to the blood and the elimination of carbon dioxide, both of which are vital for maintaining bodily balance. Additionally, alveolar ventilation is crucial in various medical situations, particularly for patients who require mechanical ventilation. When ARDS occurs, it is essential to focus on alveolar ventilation. Mechanical ventilation should help the alveoli breathe better and avoid harm from high pressures or volumes, which is generally known as lung protection. Recent advancements in ventilation techniques underscore the importance of understanding the balance between tidal volume (TV) and positive end-expiratory pressure (PEEP), which together ensure adequate alveolar recruitment.

The ongoing evolution of these approaches underscores the need for precise definitions and methods of calculation in both practical and theoretical frameworks, as misinterpretation can lead to adverse outcomes in patient care, potentially exacerbating pre-existing lung conditions (Blank et al., 2019). Research also shows that inadequate alveolar ventilation can significantly impact overall health, particularly in situations that compromise respiratory function. For example, pulmonary diseases, environmental factors, and systemic illnesses can disrupt normal ventilation, causing less oxygen to reach the body and more carbon dioxide to accumulate. Because of COVID-19, patients usually had severe respiratory problems, which required frequent monitoring and changes to their alveolar ventilation plans. According to studies, pregnant and peripartum women with respiratory diseases such as COVID-19 may be more likely to experience serious complications because their bodies are changing. Understanding the nuances of alveolar ventilation not only enhances the efficacy of treatment strategies but also improves patient outcomes, illustrating its pivotal role in both routine clinical practice and emergency interventions (O'Neil et al., 2021) (Figure 4.1).

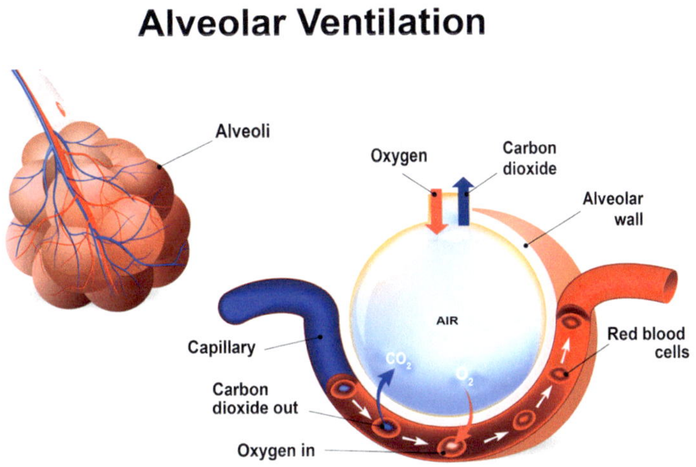

Figure 4.1. Alveolar ventilation.

Source: https://www.respiratorytherapyzone.com/wp-content/uploads/2023/08/Alveolar-Ventilation-Gas-Exchange-Vector-Illustration.png.

Importance in Respiratory Physiology

Respiratory physiology is facilitates gas exchange, which is essential for life. Alveolar ventilation enables gas exchange between the air and the alveoli, which is crucial for maintaining high oxygen levels and removing carbon dioxide. The way alveolar ventilation works allows fresh air to reach the alveoli, increasing the area where gas exchange can occur. Good ventilation improves oxygenation in the blood and also helps regulate the balance of acids and bases in the body by controlling carbon dioxide levels. Tidal volume and respiratory rate, working together, demonstrate the fine balance required to support metabolism. Understanding these principles is vital in fields such as critical care and anesthesia, where even minor deviations can result in significant physiological consequences. Also, the changes in the body during exercise show the importance of adequate alveolar ventilation. As exercise becomes more intense, the body's need for oxygen increases, and it produces more carbon dioxide. Sensory information from group III/IV muscle afferents is essential for adjusting ventilation during exercise so that it matches the body's metabolic needs. Studies indicate that during prolonged bouts of exercise, the inefficacy of ventilatory responses due to attenuated sensory feedback can impede gas exchange efficiency and arterial oxygenation (Iannetta et al., 2023).

Because of this, being able to adapt respiration is vital for maintaining the body's performance and overall health, which emphasizes the key role of alveolar ventilation in respiratory physiology. In hospitals and clinics, knowledge of alveolar ventilation is crucial for both anesthesia and the treatment of critically ill patients. Monitoring end-tidal carbon dioxide ($ETCO_2$) levels, for instance, provides vital insights into a patient's ventilation and metabolic state during anesthesia. By using this method, it is possible to visualize alveolar ventilation and assess gas exchange, which helps prevent many complications in surgical and intensive care settings. Changes in $ETCO_2$ can signal changes in how well a patient is breathing or utilizing oxygen, which helps healthcare providers choose the most effective ventilation support. Therefore, a comprehensive understanding of the principles governing alveolar ventilation is essential for enhancing patient outcomes across various clinical scenarios, ultimately underscoring the fundamental importance of respiratory physiology in health and disease.

4.1. Anatomy of the Respiratory System

The structure of the respiratory system is key to understanding how alveolar ventilation happens which is the leading way gas exchange takes place in the lungs. The trachea, bronchi, bronchioles, and alveoli are part of this system, which allows us to breathe in and out. All the parts are necessary for oxygen to reach the alveoli and be absorbed into the blood. Because bronchioles have many branches, they provide a larger surface area for gases to exchange, which improves the lungs' efficiency. Air passing through the lungs gradually enters narrower airways and finally reaches the alveoli, where air and blood exchange takes place. Besides the airway's elaborate structure, the alveoli are built differently which significantly helps with effective breathing. Because the alveolar sacs have a large surface and the epithelial barrier is very thin, gas can easily move through the alveolar membrane. Additionally, surfactant (a lipoprotein produced by type II alveolar cells) reduces surface tension and helps prevent alveoli from collapsing during exhalation. This interplay of structural and physiological factors is fundamental in maintaining adequate ventilation-perfusion (V/Q) ratios within the lungs, thereby ensuring optimal oxygenation. Recent studies suggest that disruptions in alveolar integrity can lead to compromised gas exchange, highlighting the importance of understanding the anatomy and pathology surrounding the alveoli in conditions such as acute respiratory distress syndrome (ARDS) (Jabaudon et al., 2021). The respiratory system is further demonstrated to be dynamic through the various physiological processes that contribute to alveolar ventilation. The lungs are not merely stationary; they respond to various types of mechanical and chemical changes through complex regulatory systems. For example, the diaphragm and intercostal muscles work together to create the pressure changes necessary for breathing in and out. Apart from that, the nervous system controls breathing to match the body's oxygen needs, such as when we exercise. Advances in understanding lung mechanics and gas exchange, including the development of tools for evaluating pulmonary function, reflect the critical nexus between anatomical structure and biosystem efficiency, particularly in understanding complex respiratory conditions (Gray, 1963).

4.1.1. Structure of the Lungs

The lungs' detailed structure is necessary for alveolar ventilation, which allows gas exchange to happen. There are two lobes in the left lung and three in the right, and the lungs are surrounded by pleural membranes that help control fluid flow. The bronchial tree in each lung branches into many bronchioles, which end in alveoli —the small sacs that facilitate gas exchange. Because of the alveolar surface area and the thin blood-gas barrier, oxygen and carbon dioxide are transferred as efficiently as possible. This unique structural arrangement is particularly significant in light of recent studies indicating that alterations in lung morphology can affect overall pulmonary function, especially in aging populations and those with respiratory diseases (Gremlich et al., 2021). Moreover, the extracellular matrix (ECM) maintains the structural integrity of the lungs, contributing to their mechanical properties and facilitating ventilation processes. In many illnesses, collagen and elastin are remodeled, which can have significant effects on the functioning of the alveoli. For instance, in the context of lung aging, changes can lead to increased airspace and parenchymal volume, as evidenced in research that showcases varying trends in cellular proliferation without accompanying apoptosis (Gremlich et al., 2021). With age, these changes in the lungs may make people more likely to develop COPD or pulmonary fibrosis, which is why understanding lung architecture is important in disease. It is essential to keep the lung structure intact to allow adequate alveolar ventilation for many years. The structure of the lungs also external and internal challenges. For example, if the lungs are damaged by a viral infection such as COVID-19, their structure is essential for proper breathing; any damage can result in inflammation that prevents oxygen and carbon dioxide from being exchanged in the alveoli. Additionally, significant changes in the normal standard lung structure can make it difficult for air to move in and out, which can lead to acute respiratory distress. The structure of the lungs is linked to their ability to fight disease, highlighting the importance of maintaining lung health. Ensuring that alveolar ventilation remains unimpeded by environmental or biological stressors is essential for overall respiratory health, suggesting that both clinical and therapeutic approaches must consider the intricate relationship between lung structure and function in promoting effective gas exchange (Figure 4.2).

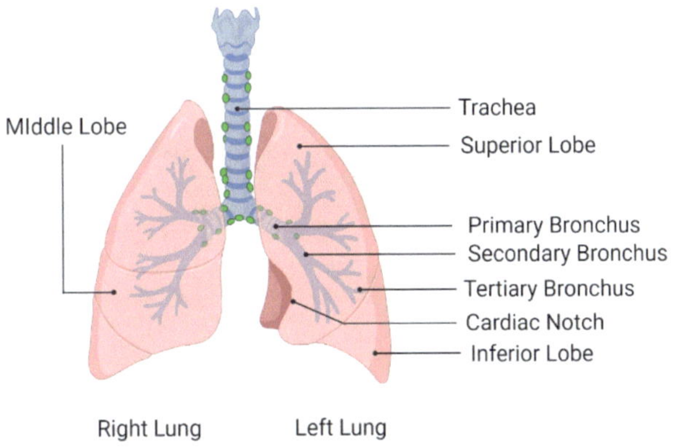

Figure 4.2. Lung structure.

Source: https://microbenotes.com/wp-content/uploads/2022/06/Structure-of-Lungs.jpeg.

4.1.2. Role of Alveoli in Gas Exchange

Gas exchange in the body, which is necessary for homeostasis, happens mainly in the alveoli, the final air sacs in the lungs. Their large surface, which is approximately the size of a tennis court, allows oxygen and carbon dioxide to exchange easily between the air in the lungs and the blood vessels. The alveoli have thin walls and many microvilli, which help gases move easily through them. Surfactant, which coats the alveoli, lessens the surface tension, so the alveoli do not collapse, and proper ventilation is maintained. Thanks to these anatomical and biochemical changes, the alveoli can do their job of exchanging gases to provide oxygen to the blood and remove carbon dioxide which is produced by cells. In instances of mechanical ventilation, protecting alveolar function becomes paramount in mitigating the risks of ventilator-induced lung injury (VILI). Ventilation strategies that work well aim to ensure the air reaching the alveoli is optimal, using smaller volumes to prevent overstretching and preserve the alveolar structure. Such strategies in ventilation allow clinicians to facilitate gas exchange while also avoiding harm to the lungs. The management of positive end-expiratory pressure (PEEP) plays a significant role in this context, helping to maintain alveolar recruitment and preventing atelectasis. As noted, clinicians must not overlook the delicate balance required to ensure that alveoli function effectively during mechanical ventilation, addressing both the physiological demands of gas exchange and the prevention of further lung injury in vulnerable patients (Adrish et al., 2024). New studies suggest that pulmonary perfusion and alveolar ventilation interact, indicating that alveoli can adjust to changes in blood flow. Pulmonary perfusion disorders may lead to atelectasis, as a result of a loop involving the amount of carbon dioxide in the alveolar spaces. A low amount of CO_2 in the alveoli can cause surfactant secretion to decrease, resulting in less air being moved in and out of the alveoli. This indicates that alveoli play a crucial role in maintaining a stable V/Q ratio, highlighting their adaptability in various situations. Understanding this novel CO_2-sensing mechanism may reveal new opportunities for enhancing alveolar function in clinical settings, ensuring the optimization of gas exchange despite potential pulmonary limitations (Goetz et al., 2011) (Figure 4.3).

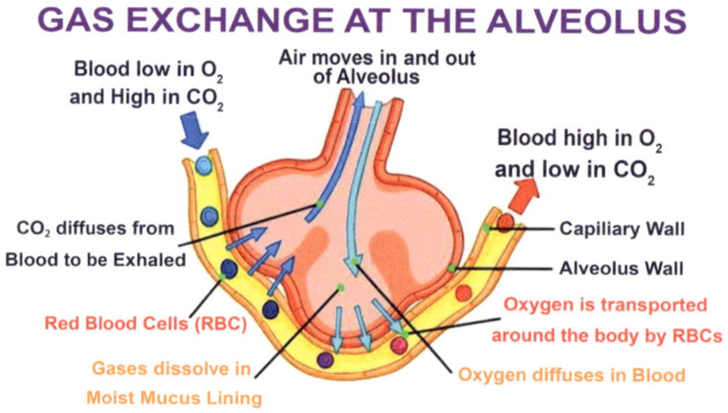

Figure 4.3. Gas exchange at the alveolus.

Source: https://www.vedantu.com/question-sets/0ed42933-a211-44fa-b77d-017490fceed92350581896987932719.png.

4.1.3. Pathway of Air Through the Respiratory Tract

The first part of the air in the respiratory tract is the nasal cavity, where it is warmed, made moist, and filtered. The nasal passages are lined with cilia and mucus, which catch particles and germs, allowing only clean air to reach the lungs. The first filtration step is crucial, as impurities in the air can cause inflammation and damage the delicate parts of the lower respiratory tract. The air continues through the pharynx and larynx, entering the trachea, which helps the air move more smoothly. The trachea's structure and airflow are maintained by its C-shaped cartilage rings, which prevent obstruction even as pressure changes while breathing. Every inhalation moves air into the lungs, and gas exchange happens in the alveoli. The air moves from the trachea to the right and left bronchi, which go to each lung. The bronchi then get smaller and become bronchioles, which end at the alveolar sacs. The numerous branches of bronchi to bronchioles increase the area where gas exchange occurs, demonstrating the effectiveness of the respiratory tract's design. Smooth muscle in each bronchiole lets airflow be controlled by narrowing or widening the airway. It is in the alveoli, which are surrounded by capillaries, that oxygen and carbon dioxide are exchanged. The effectiveness of alveolar ventilation relies heavily on this pathway; obstructions or damage at any level, such as the effects of respiratory pathogens noted in various studies, can lead to significant respiratory compromise, emphasizing the importance of maintaining an unobstructed air pathway (Hendrickson et al., 2013). Conditions like acute lung injury (ALI) can arise when this pathway is disrupted, as seen in scenarios involving viral infections. Acute viral pneumonia leads to significant lung damage, highlighting how pathogens can disrupt the movement of air into the alveoli and, consequently, how gas exchange is carried out. For instance, the severe acute respiratory syndrome (SARS) coronavirus and other viruses can instigate severe damage to the respiratory epithelium, leading to inflammation and altered airflow dynamics (Hu et al., 2023). Such pathogens can cause too much inflammation, which closes the airways and damages the walls of the alveoli. This exacerbates the challenges of adequate ventilation, underscoring the importance of a clear and healthy pathway through the respiratory tract for effective alveolar ventilation and overall pulmonary function (Figure 4.4).

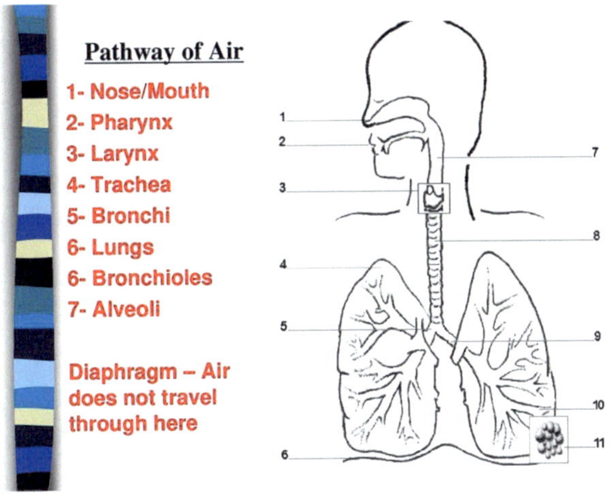

Figure 4.4. Pathway of air.

Source: https://hi-static.z-dn.net/files/d98/88c9db46768008ba82fa7b9c889c5f4b.jpg.

4.2. Mechanisms of Alveolar Ventilation

For gas exchange to occur efficiently, alveolar ventilation mechanisms play a crucial role in the lungs. Alveoli, which are small air sacs in the lungs, allow for the exchange of oxygen and carbon dioxide because they have a large surface and thin walls. Air breathed in fills the alveoli, allowing oxygen to enter the blood and carbon dioxide to leave the body. The process is affected by how easy the lungs can expand, how much resistance there is in the airways, and the rate of breathing. It is crucial to utilize proper mechanical ventilation in clinical settings to maintain optimal alveolar ventilation, even when lung function is compromised by ARDS. Understanding these mechanisms enhances our fundamental knowledge and informs the care of patients experiencing respiratory distress. PEEP is crucial for enhancing alveolar ventilation, particularly for patients with ARDS. PEEP stops alveolar collapse as the patient exhales which helps to overcome the effects of surfactant problems and higher surface tension. By maintaining stability in the alveolar units, PEEP contributes to a higher end-expiratory lung volume (EELV), which enhances the respiratory system's compliance and reduces the driving pressure (ΔP) required for effective ventilation. By using this mechanism, gas exchange is enhanced and the risks of intratidal recruitment and derecruitment, which harm the lungs, are reduced. Nonetheless, the application of PEEP must be carefully balanced against potential adverse effects on hemodynamics, such as reduced cardiac output and increased pulmonary vascular resistance (PVR), prompting ongoing evaluation of its use in mechanistic models of ventilatory support (Rezoagli et al., 2019). It is also essential to prevent VILI when considering alveolar ventilation. Problems with ventilation settings or excessive pressure in the airway easily harm the alveoli. Gaining knowledge of the way alveoli fill and empty helps us find better ways to protect the lungs from mechanical harm. Implementing an optimal mechanical breath profile (MBP) tailored to individual patient needs enhances aeration and helps prevent harmful over-distension of the alveolar units. Applying strategies such as the open lung strategy, which are lung-protective, is supported by evidence that suggests these approaches can significantly lower the risks of ARDS. Prioritizing both the functional and structural integrity of the alveoli while managing ventilation underscores the complexity of supporting patients facing critical respiratory challenges (Nieman et al., 2017) (Figure 4.5).

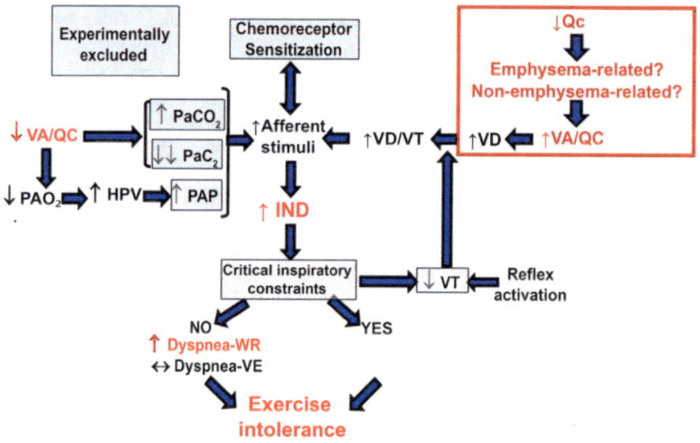

Figure 4.5. Schematic representation of the key mechanisms by which alveolar ventilation.

Source: https://www.researchgate.net/publication/378181802/figure/fig4/AS:11431281300172339@1735289908634/Schematic-representation-of-the-key-mechanisms-by-which-alveolar-ventilation.jpg.

4.2.1. Inspiration and Expiration Processes

The exchange of gases in the lungs, which is necessary for homeostasis, depends on the processes of inspiration and expiration. When we are inspired, the diaphragm and intercostal muscles contract, which expands the chest and draws air into the lungs. The airflow mainly goes to the alveoli, which allow oxygen to enter the blood and carbon dioxide to leave. The smooth functioning of this process depends on the alveoli being healthy; any problem can significantly reduce how well the lungs ventilate. For instance, mechanical ventilation strategies that fail to account for respiratory mechanics can inadvertently induce VILI through mechanisms such as stress concentrations near collapsed alveoli, leading to diminished gas exchange efficacy and further lung compromise (Zimmermann et al., 2024). During normal breathing, the diaphragm relaxes, allowing the thoracic cavity to expand, and causing air to enter the lungs. At this step, carbon dioxide is removed, which helps maintain the blood's pH. Sometimes, such as in patients with ARDS, expiration is not as usual due to the changed conditions. Pulmonary microcirculation changes with each breath, and this is clear when using advanced imaging technology, which shows big differences in perfusion patterns. Studies indicate that during high ΔP conditions, the proportion of perfused vessels is noticeably greater at expiration than during inspiration, suggesting that the mechanics of expiration are intricately linked with pulmonary microcirculation and alveolar function (Yuan et al., 2024). Changes in either inspiration or expiration can affect how the lungs function, which highlights the complexity of alveolar ventilation. If PEEP is very low for long and extended period, it can cause microatelectasis, which blocks proper gas exchange in some parts of the lungs. Because of this balance, optimal pressure in the lungs is maintained, and any disruption can lead to numerous respiratory issues. Being aware of these factors is crucial when selecting therapy to enhance alveolar ventilation and mitigate the adverse effects of mechanical ventilation. Thus, both inspiratory and expiratory mechanics are vital for ensuring efficient gas exchange and lung health (Zimmermann et al., 2024) (Figure 4.6).

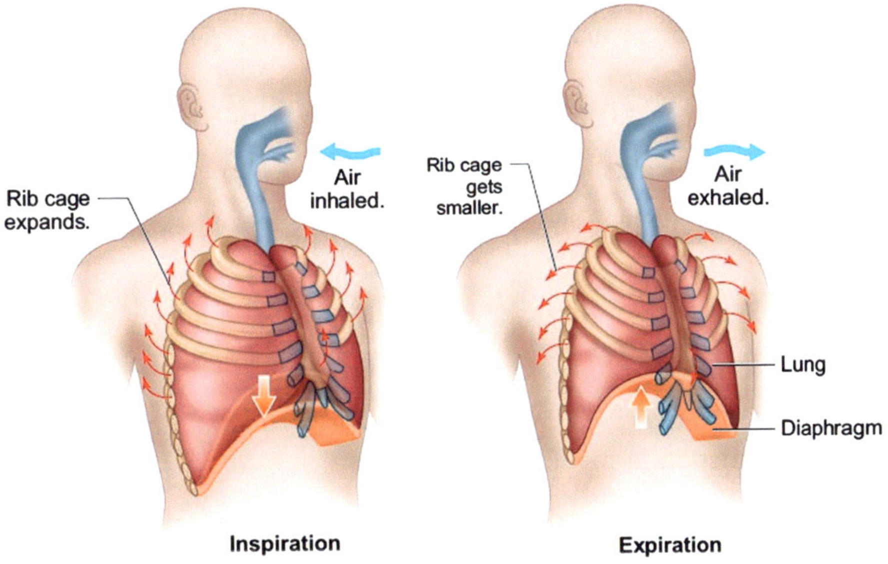

Figure 4.6. Illustration of the processes of inspiration and expiration.

Source: https://img.brainkart.com/imagebk34/QAmtHkM.jpg.

4.2.2. Role of Diaphragm and Intercostal Muscles

The way we breathe relies heavily on the diaphragm and intercostal muscles, which greatly affect alveolar ventilation. The diaphragm (a dome-shaped muscle under the lungs) contracts during inhalation and pulls downward to increase the size of the thoracic cavity. This action decreases the pressure inside the lungs, allowing air to enter. Once the diaphragm contracts, the intercostal muscles, located between the ribs, help raise the rib cage and expand the thoracic cavity. Due to the way the diaphragm and intercostal muscles work together, alveolar ventilation is adequate, and gas can be exchanged efficiently between the blood and alveoli. If the muscles involved in ventilation do not work together, the efficiency of breathing decreases, which can result in breathing problems and reduced oxygen intake. Unlike passive expiration, which just relaxes the diaphragm and intercostal muscles, active expiration also uses the abdominal muscles. Accessory muscles are crucial in heavy breathing or during respiratory distress, as they facilitate the expulsion of air from the lungs and increase both the ventilation rate and alveolar pressure, which are essential for gas exchange. The way these muscles interact is crucial for maintaining balance in the body and illustrating how the respiratory system adapts to different needs. Moreover, research has shown that activating both the diaphragm and the intercostal muscles can reduce fatigue during respiration and improve tidal volumes under certain conditions, indicating their collective importance in respiratory health (Adury et al., 2019). Understanding how these muscles affect alveolar ventilation is crucial in both medical and sports situations. It helps healthcare professionals design approaches to support better breathing, particularly for individuals with weakened lungs. Computational models examining the transition from quiet breathing to active expiration offer further insight into the neural control mechanisms that govern these muscle contractions (Ben-Tal et al., 2014). By analyzing the intricate relationship between diaphragm, intercostal muscles, and overall respiratory dynamics, we gain a deeper appreciation of how these factors contribute to efficient alveolar ventilation, ultimately impacting overall health and performance in various populations (Figure 4.7).

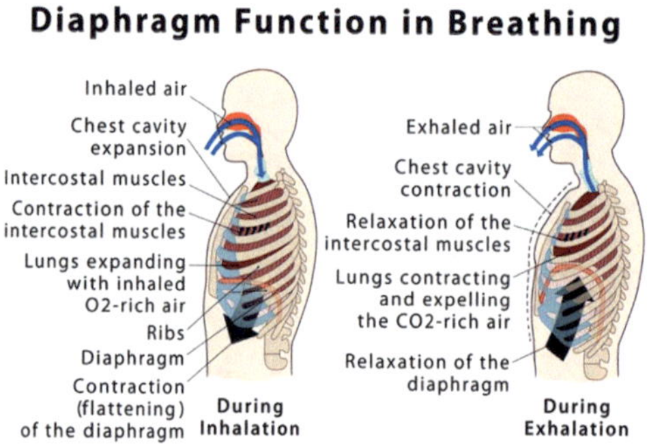

Figure 4.7. Diaphragm function in breathing.

Source: https://energizehealth.ca/uploads/Diaphragm-Function-in-Breathing.jpg.

4.2.3. Factors Affecting Lung Compliance

Lung compliance refers to the lungs' ability to expand when pressure is applied, which is necessary for effective alveolar ventilation. compliance, which affects how easily the lungs expand during breathing. As an example, pulmonary fibrosis can stiffen the lungs, which significantly decreases how much the lungs can expand. Alternatively, emphysema can lessen the elasticity of the lungs, which can change how ventilation occurs. Recent research indicates that changes in lung compliance can significantly impact gas exchange, making it essential to understand these factors to optimize mechanical ventilation. As lung compliance decreases, the work required for breathing increases, ultimately leading to respiratory fatigue, especially in critically ill patients undergoing mechanical ventilation (Humbert et al., 2022). The flexibility of the chest wall is vital for the total compliance of the lungs. The thoracic cavity gets its mechanical features from the ribs, muscles, and connective tissues found in the chest wall. Obesity, kyphosis, and other similar problems can make it harder for the chest wall to expand and contract, which impacts lung inflation. When the chest wall is stiff because of these deformities, even a healthy lung might not be able to fill with enough air, which causes FRC to drop. This impact is particularly relevant in patients requiring mechanical ventilation, as inadequate chest wall compliance can further complicate management strategies (Corp et al., 2021). It is crucial for healthcare professionals to understand these relationships to deliver effective respiratory care. Moreover, the influence of positive pressure ventilation (PPV) on lung compliance cannot be overlooked. Because of the changes in intrathoracic pressure during PPV, compliance can be improved or reduced depending on the type of ventilation used. PEEP is often introduced to help open collapsed areas in the lungs, which improves lung compliance. However, if PEEP is set too high, it can cause the alveoli to overinflate, which harms how well the lungs work and how well blood is distributed. Therefore, it is crucial to carefully adjust ventilator settings to ensure that the benefits and risks of increased lung volume and pressure are balanced during mechanical ventilation. The dynamics of lung compliance thus represent a critical area of focus in optimizing strategies for alveolar ventilation (Humbert et al., 2022).

4.3. Measurement of Alveolar Ventilation

Measuring alveolar ventilation helps to understand how well the lungs are working and how healthy the metabolism is. Alveolar ventilation refers to the amount of air that enters the alveoli and participates in gas exchange, which is crucial for effective breathing. Alveolar ventilation is measured in several ways, but usually by subtracting dead space ventilation from total ventilation. This difference is important because it affects how efficiently gas exchange happens; only the air that joins in gas exchange helps with oxygen and carbon dioxide transport. So, to be accurate, an assessment needs to include the effects of dead spaces in the lungs, which depend on body posture, lung disease, and the effort involved in breathing. Recent studies have begun to explore innovative methods for measuring exhaled gases, particularly volatile organic compounds (VOCs), which reflect underlying metabolic processes.

For example, research on how isoprene affects end-tidal breaths can show how differences in ventilation and perfusion can change the amount of isoprene found in exhaled air during exercise. They help in understanding alveolar ventilation because they show the effect of metabolism on gas exchange at any given time. They not only enhance our understanding of normal body processes but also provide potential applications for diagnosis. As such, the relationship between ventilatory parameters and systemic concentrations of biomarkers remains a promising area for further research (Kupferthaler et al., 2010). Measuring biomarkers in the breath can enhance the management of alveolar ventilation. Technological progress is quickly making it possible to monitor different compounds in breath which can reveal changes in lung function. With clear links between what is in the breath and the body's systemic markers, practitioners can gain a deeper understanding of diseases that affect alveolar ventilation. In addition, understanding these factors enables the development of guidelines for reviewing breath gases, which can impact various areas of clinical care. This information might be used to improve the way respiratory conditions are assessed, help personalize medicine, and make it possible to respond quickly. Such advancements echo the significant role that meticulous measurement of alveolar ventilation plays in advancing both clinical and research domains in respiratory health (King et al., 2003) (Figure 4.8).

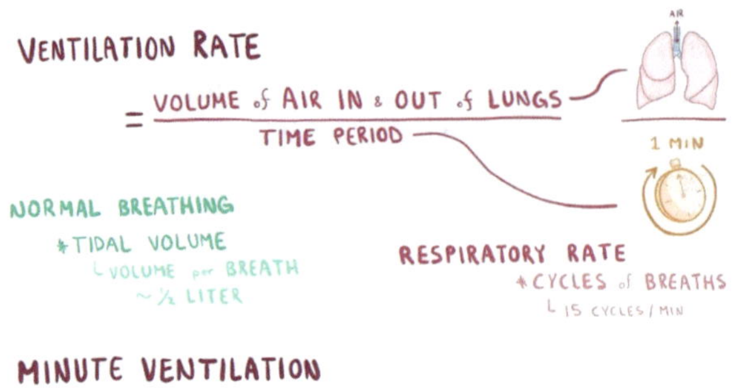

Figure 4.8. Ventilation rate measurement.

Source: https://www.osmosis.org/_next/image?url=https%3A%2F%2Fd16qt3wv6xm098.cloudfront.net%2FWEVjT8weRMeHahzahyGybA1hQ4i9NcR8%2F_.jpg&w=3840&q=75.

4.3.1. Techniques for Assessing Ventilation

Examining ventilation is crucial for maintaining respiratory health, particularly in medical settings where ARDS can impact the exchange of gases. Several techniques are available to assess the effectiveness of ventilation, each with its own set of advantages and disadvantages. Among these, the calculation of physiological dead space (VD/VT) is significant, as it reflects the proportion of air that does not participate in gas exchange. The traditional methods of determining VD/VT are not often applied in clinics, as they are considered too complicated. Recent advances, such as the validation of volumetric capnography (VCap), provide a more accessible and reliable method for measuring the partial pressure of carbon dioxide in alveolar air ($PaCO_2$) and mixed expired air (PeCO2), thereby enhancing the accuracy of VD/VT assessments. Efforts to integrate these technologies can lead to improved patient outcomes in critical care settings (Doorduin et al., 2016). The relationship between carbon dioxide and ventilation is also well supported by the many methods developed to estimate $PaCO_2$. The 1952 Copenhagen polio epidemic showed that when $PaCO_2$ is high, alveolar ventilation drops because of respiratory failure. Blood gas analyses, capnography, and transcutaneous methods are now used to measure $PaCO_2$ and help determine the appropriate treatment. These assessments are helpful in multiple situations, for example, acute and chronic respiratory failure, moving patients and sedation. Recognizing that each technique has unique implications in practice ensures that healthcare providers can utilize complementary approaches for assessing ventilation, ultimately improving diagnostic accuracy and treatment efficacy (Huttmann et al., 2014). Besides providing detailed information about ventilation, these techniques make it possible to track patients in various clinical settings, providing detailed information about ventilation. Since the state of alveolar ventilation can change quickly, monitoring ventilation in real time becomes very important. VCap can immediately indicate whether ventilation and perfusion are functioning properly by detecting changes in $PaCO_2$. In ARDS, real-time data on dead space and adequate ventilation is essential for treating the patient. Clinicians can combine various techniques according to the patient's needs to obtain a comprehensive picture of ventilation. As the landscape of respiratory monitoring continues to evolve, integrating multiple modalities will be critical for enhancing patient care and managing respiratory pathologies effectively, thereby underscoring the importance of ongoing research and development in this field (Figure 4.9).

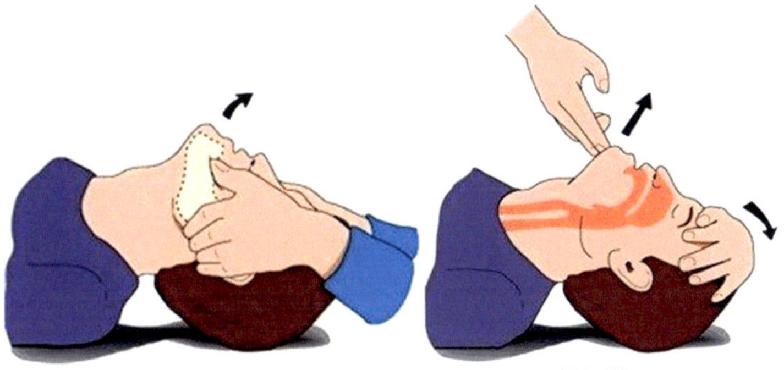

Figure 4.9. Airway opening maneuvers: jaw thrust and chin lift techniques.

Source: https://s3.us-east-2.amazonaws.com/medictests/app/public/ckeditor_assets/pictures/522/content_headtilt_chinlift.jpg.

4.3.2. Importance of Tidal Volume and Respiratory Rate

How much air is breathed in and how often it is breathed out forms the foundation for good alveolar ventilation, which affects how well gas exchange happens in the lungs. Tidal volume describes the quantity of air that is inhaled or exhaled in a normal breath, and the respiratory rate is how many breaths a person takes each minute. The amount of air going in and out of the lungs each minute is called minute ventilation, and both parameters are important in determining it. The right amount of tidal volume and respiratory rate helps oxygen reach tissues and helps remove carbon dioxide from the blood. When either parameter is changed, it can have a significant impact on alveolar ventilation which is why they are important in both medical practice and normal body function. Several clinical cases demonstrate that managing tidal volume and respiratory rate is crucial. For instance, in one-lung ventilation (OLV) used during pulmonary surgery, maintaining a judicious tidal volume is crucial to minimize lung injury and inflammatory responses. Research indicates that different tidal volume settings, ranging from protective to conventional ventilation strategies, do not significantly impact postoperative cytokine responses when proper ventilation techniques are applied (Andreetti et al., 2018). It means that choosing the right tidal volume and respiratory rate can help patients breathe well and also reduce problems after surgery. Therefore, it is essential to understand how to adjust these parameters to enhance the care provided to patients and their outcomes. Besides being important in clinical care, tidal volume and respiratory rate can change the gas content of exhaled air, which is relevant for diagnostic purposes. For example, the concentrations of trace gases and VOCs in exhaled breath reflect the underlying metabolic state and can be influenced by alterations in breathing patterns (Amann et al., 2010). There is a complicated link between alveolar ventilation and the release of certain gases, and both the amount of air inhaled and the rate of breathing can strongly affect breath gas profiles. For this reason, clinicians and researchers have to carefully examine these respiratory parameters to assess lung function and metabolism correctly. They contribute to our understanding of how the respiratory system functions and also support the development of standardized methods for diagnosing respiratory diseases.

4.3.3. Use of Spirometry in Clinical Settings

In hospitals and clinics, spirometry is a primary tool used to test lung function and learn about many respiratory diseases. This non-invasive technique measures vital parameters such as forced vital capacity (FVC) and forced expiratory volume (FEV), which are essential in the diagnosis and management of diseases like asthma, COPD, and pulmonary fibrosis. Spirometry provides doctors with instant information to detect changes in the disease and assess the effectiveness of treatment. Besides, it makes it possible to set a baseline for lung function, which supports the creation of personalized treatment plans for each patient. In this situation, spirometry helps assess the severity of the respiratory disease and improves the accuracy of treatments, highlighting its importance in respiratory medicine. Spirometry is now used not only for diagnosis but also to check how treatments are affecting the patient. Recent research has highlighted the effectiveness of advanced techniques, such as computed cardiopulmonography (CCP), which augments traditional spirometric measurements by evaluating lung inhomogeneity. Research on patients with T2-high asthma has found that CCP can distinguish between those who respond to treatment and those who do not by examining changes in lung metrics. Using both traditional spirometry and innovative assessments together provides a more comprehensive picture of how the patient is responding, enabling clinicians to adjust the treatment plan accordingly. These advancements highlight the use of spirometry alongside new technologies, which improve how chronic lung diseases are managed and monitored. Besides helping with established illnesses, spirometry helps detect early signs of lung issues which is very important for preventive care. For example, in people recovering from severe lung infections, such as COVID-19, spirometry may reveal slight changes in lung function that are not detected by standard exams. With a set of baseline norms, it becomes possible to create equations that can identify changes that may suggest a health problem. Regularly using spirometry results in patient care allows doctors to take action earlier, which helps slow down the development of respiratory diseases. As a result, the implementation of spirometry within clinical frameworks not only informs immediate therapeutic strategies but also contributes to long-term preventive measures, reinforcing its value in promoting optimal alveolar ventilation and overall respiratory health (Figure 4.10).

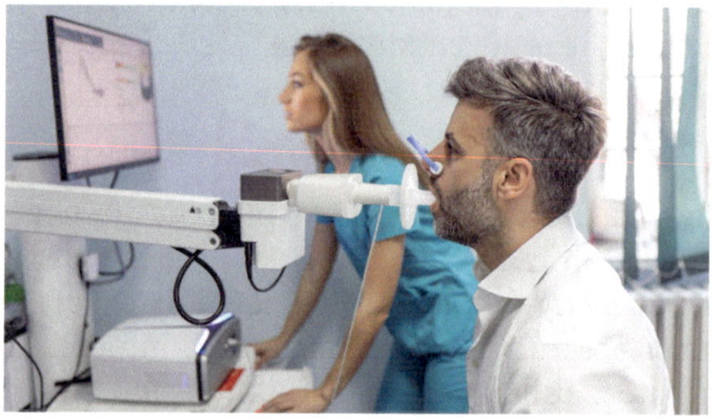

Figure 4.10. Spirometry for assessing lung function.

Source: https://lh7-rt.googleusercontent.com/docsz/AD_4nXejo1IIY18fPFzPQV2QzZemplwJnXVujP2emFtotvfI82bpTGhfvbvzpyGxH9Rp8Eca_cScwFrJrqtBMjYCQXAOB NoQqrHNEE41wyQM6sWWKRLZsoeL3SOTY2z QEeGXrJxbJuk5zA?key=IJ1xlYLelWBlXRXJjrCJGXdW.

4.4. Factors Influencing Alveolar Ventilation

Several factors, including a person's specific anatomy and physiology, influence the effectiveness of alveolar ventilation. The way the lungs are made and their ability to expand or contract can immediately influence gas exchange. Larger lung volumes are associated with greater alveolar ventilation because the person can inhale a larger tidal volume. Additionally, conditions such as COPD or asthma can increase airway resistance, which reduces the lungs' ability to ventilate efficiently. All these elements together control the amount of fresh air that gets to the alveolar sacs, which in turn shapes the respiratory performance of different people and those with health problems. Pollution and allergens, which are present in the environment, can significantly affect how the lungs perform alveolar ventilation. Exposure to ultrafine particles (UFPs) has been recognized as a detrimental factor affecting respiratory health. Recent studies have found that indoor emissions from laser and 3-D printers can contribute to the presence of UFPs in the air, potentially worsening lung problems and causing increased breathing difficulties in sensitive individuals. Exposure to these pollutants can cause inflammation, which interferes with the alveoli's ability to ventilate properly. A deeper understanding of these environmental contributors is essential, as it can guide interventions aimed at minimizing exposure and improving overall pulmonary function, particularly in occupational settings where such exposures are prevalent (Johnson et al., 2018). The body's oxygen and carbon dioxide needs, which are metabolic, greatly influence the rate of breathing through the alveoli. During physical exertion, for example, the demand for oxygen increases concomitantly with elevations in carbon dioxide production, necessitating an increase in respiratory rate and depth (tidal volume). The body uses this mechanism to ensure that the tissues receive enough fresh air for their needs. In neonates suffering from respiratory distress syndrome (RDS), insufficient surfactant production leads to complications that challenge the attainment of adequate alveolar ventilation. The administration of exogenous surfactant has significantly improved outcomes for these patients, demonstrating how targeted interventions can effectively enhance ventilation in critically affected populations (Thorkildsen et al., 2016) (Figure 4.11).

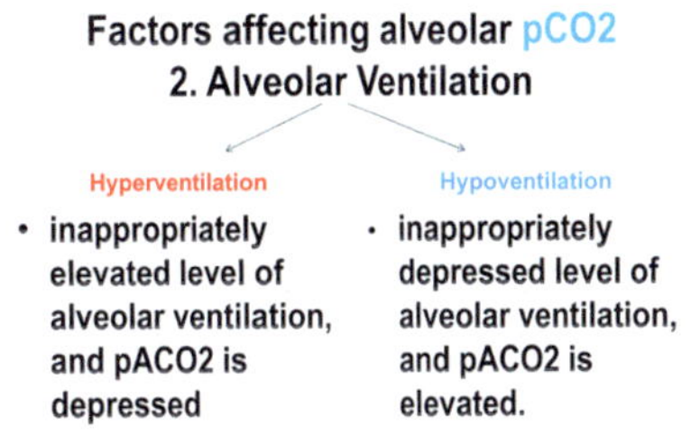

Figure 4.11. Factors affecting alveolar ventilation.

Source: https://slideplayer.com/slide/6343975/22/images/22/Factors+affecting+alveolar+pCO2+2.+Alveolar+Ventilation.jpg.

4.4.1. Physiological Factors (Age, Fitness Level)

The way age and fitness affect the body plays a significant role in determining alveolar ventilation and, therefore, pulmonary function. As people get older, the elasticity of their lungs lessens, which causes their lungs to shrink and makes it harder for them to breathe correctly. Aging leads to changes in the thoracic cage and respiratory muscles, resulting in reduced maximal voluntary ventilation. Therefore, the changes in the body can cause older people to have less alveolar ventilation. It shows that understanding how aging affects the lungs and breathing is crucial, as this leads to changes in oxygen uptake during activities. Therefore, more research should be conducted to find better ways to support the respiratory health of elderly individuals. A person's fitness level is important, fundamental in determining how well their lungs can ventilate. Exercise regularly helps strengthen and improve the endurance of breathing muscles, which enhances how well ventilation occurs. People who are fitter usually have larger lungs which allows more air to move in and out, even when they are resting or working hard. Engaging in aerobic exercise enhances the volume of air you inhale and exhale, as well as your breathing rate. Due to this relationship, public health strategies should incorporate regular physical activity to promote better ventilation and respiratory health. The positive correlation between fitness level and ventilatory function highlights the importance of sustained engagement in physical activities, as demonstrated in studies examining the benefits of dance on fitness levels and conditioning (Warot et al., 2025). It is also possible to observe differences in physiological health based on age and fitness, which are influenced by the environment in which the activities take place. Research demonstrates that adolescents in private schools exhibit better physical fitness, as well as lower stress levels, compared to their counterparts in government and government-aided institutions (Parvathi et al., 2024). It is clear that having access to resources and planned physical education opportunities significantly impacts respiratory health and fitness. For this reason, examining the impact of age and fitness on alveolar ventilation should also consider environmental differences. Helping less resourced populations improve their physical fitness could help reduce these gaps and encourage better respiratory health across different age groups and geographical locations.

4.4.2. Pathological Conditions (Asthma, COPD)

When someone has asthma or COPD, the process of alveolar ventilation is significantly altered. Episodes of asthma involve the narrowing of airways, inflammation, and increased mucus production, which interrupt the normal movement of air and gases in the lungs. These symptoms might be wheezing, difficulty breathing, and chest tightness, which reduce the effectiveness of alveolar ventilation. When someone with asthma has an attack, their breathing rate and tidal volume often fall, which leads to both hypoxemia and hypercapnia. COPD also encompasses various lung diseases, such as emphysema and chronic bronchitis, which make breathing more difficult. Because lung function declines in COPD, it leads to slower airflow during exhalation, making it harder for air to leave the lungs and reducing the area for gas exchange, which causes severe breathing problems.

Research indicates that respiratory support, remarkably non-invasive ventilation (NIV), can ameliorate some of the exercise limitations in patients with COPD, enhancing overall alveolar ventilation. It was found that when patients received ventilatory support before exercising, their peak work rates increased, allowing them to exercise for a longer total time. These findings suggest that prior application of non-invasive ventilatory strategies may optimize not just performance but also the efficiency of oxygen delivery during exercise in COPD patients (Doggett et al., 2006). At the same time, such measures do not affect important metabolic changes, such as peak oxygen uptake or blood lactate levels, during low-intensity efforts, indicating that different mechanisms control performance and breathing at various exercise intensities. Problems related to asthma and COPD are made worse by age-related changes in lung structure and function. The elasticity of lung tissue decreases with age, and the alveoli may also shrink, which can cause a person's ventilatory capacity and reserve to decrease. The presence of COPD is particularly notable in older populations where the risk factors for the disease, including smoking and environmental pollutants, are prevalent (Ebejer et al., 1999). Breathing in harmful particles for a long time, along with the usual decrease in lung function, makes these diseases have a more substantial effect on alveolar ventilation. Clinicians must therefore approach the assessment of lung function in older patients with a nuanced understanding of both age-related physiological changes and the effects of chronic respiratory diseases, ensuring a comprehensive evaluation of respiratory health (Figure 4.12).

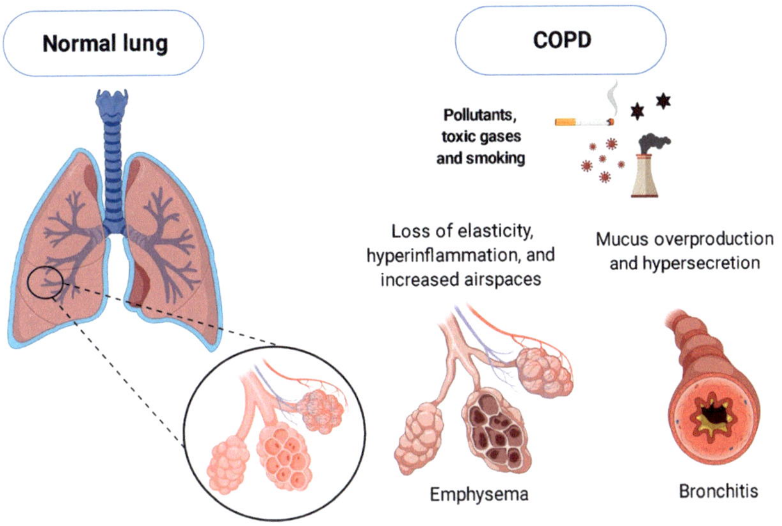

Figure 4.12. COPD phenotypes. Morphological differences exist between a normal lung and a lung with COPD.

Source: https://www.mdpi.com/pharmaceuticals/pharmaceuticals-14-00979/article_deploy/html/images/pharmaceuticals-14-00979-g001.png.

4.4.3. Environmental Influences (Altitude, Pollution)

Altitude and pollution play a significant role in how well alveolar ventilation functions, which is important for respiratory health. At higher altitudes, since there is less oxygen in the air, the body's respiratory rate goes up to help make up for this lack of oxygen in the blood. It increases breathing at first, but if the elevation is severe, the body may not get enough oxygen, which can lead to lasting problems. Additionally, to cope with high altitude, the body increases the production of RBCs, which helps maintain steady oxygen flow in challenging conditions. Because of this, altitude both creates a problem and encourages the body to adjust, which can influence how well oxygen is exchanged in the lungs and overall lung health. Air pollution is another danger to the proper function of alveolar ventilation. Particulate matter and black carbon enter the lungs, potentially causing damage to the alveoli. Research indicates that individuals exposed to high levels of black carbon experience elevated deposition rates of these harmful particles within their lungs, which can exacerbate respiratory issues and reduce ventilation efficiency over time (Madueño et al., 2024). In addition, the air in cities is often polluted by numerous car fumes and emissions from factories, which increases the risk of exposure to harmful airborne substances. As walking is different from riding in open-sided vehicles, the amount of particles people breathe in can vary significantly. Due to the effects of altitude and pollution, there is a need for special policies to protect the lungs of individuals at risk. Stricter air quality rules and measures to help people living at high elevations adapt more effectively can significantly mitigate the adverse effects of these factors. Emerging technologies for monitoring air quality and personal exposure, like the MERDOC system developed for assessing black carbon levels, provide critical data for understanding how environmental influences affect alveolar ventilation (N/A, 2025). Ultimately, a multipronged approach that incorporates education, innovative monitoring, and policy reform is essential to address the respiratory risks posed by both altitude and pollution, thereby promoting healthier living conditions and improved alveolar function (Figure 4.13).

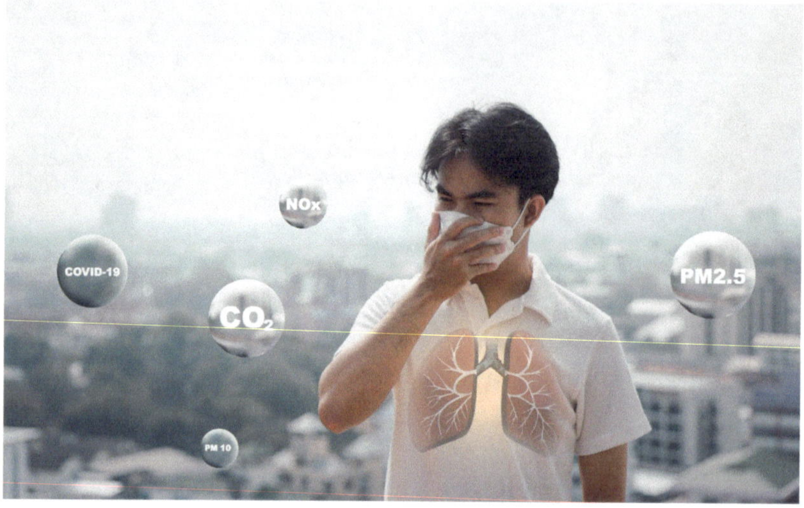

Figure 4.13. Environmental factors affecting alveolar function.

Source: https://medanta.s3.ap-south-1.amazonaws.com/blogs/August2024/jrFyA9PGka9fy3wd5iX490IY6QxaxV-metaUmVzcGlyYXRvcnkgUHJvYmxlbXMuanBn-.jpg.

4.5. Alveolar Ventilation and Gas Exchange

The way alveolar ventilation works is very important for efficient gas exchange in the lungs. Alveolar ventilation is the amount of fresh air that goes into the alveoli, where gas exchange takes place, in a particular time. Several factors affect this process, including tidal volume and respiratory rate, which determine the amount of air taken into the lungs with each breath. When alveolar ventilation is insufficient, it can lead to both hypoxemia and hypercapnia. Different breathing rhythms can alter the amount of air breathed in and out, as well as the levels of gases in the alveoli. Being aware of these factors is crucial for designing treatments that improve breathing, particularly in settings where lung problems are evident, such as hospitals or during sedation. The relationship between ventilation and perfusion (V/Q ratio) plays a pivotal role in optimizing gas exchange. A proper V/Q ratio means the air in the alveoli is matched by blood flow, which helps the body take in oxygen and release carbon dioxide efficiently. A disturbance in this ratio, which can happen in different diseases, reduces the efficiency of gas exchange. If a patient has a pulmonary embolism, some parts of the lung may receive air but no blood, which means the air is wasted. Alternatively, when alveolar atelectasis occurs, ventilation is reduced, but perfusion is not, which results in significant mismatches. To address these issues, targeted therapies such as enhancing alveolar recruitment are necessary to restore proper gas exchange and facilitate patient recovery in respiratory care settings. Additionally, examining trace gases in exhaled breath has become a valuable method for assessing alveolar ventilation and gas exchange. It is now well established that measuring nitric oxide in breath can help diagnose some respiratory issues. Task force recommendations have highlighted the importance of standardizing the measurement of these trace gases, which may also aid in the measurement of other VOCs involved in metabolism. It is critical to understand how alveolar concentrations relate to the amounts of these substances found in the blood to assess alveolar gas exchange accurately. The classical Farhi equation primarily focuses on alveolar concentrations, which may overlook changes resulting from variations in breathing or exercise patterns. Thus, developing comprehensive models that capture these complexities is essential for advancing our understanding of pulmonary physiology and the overall health of the respiratory system (Amann et al., 2010; Auckburally et al., 2017) (Figure 4.14).

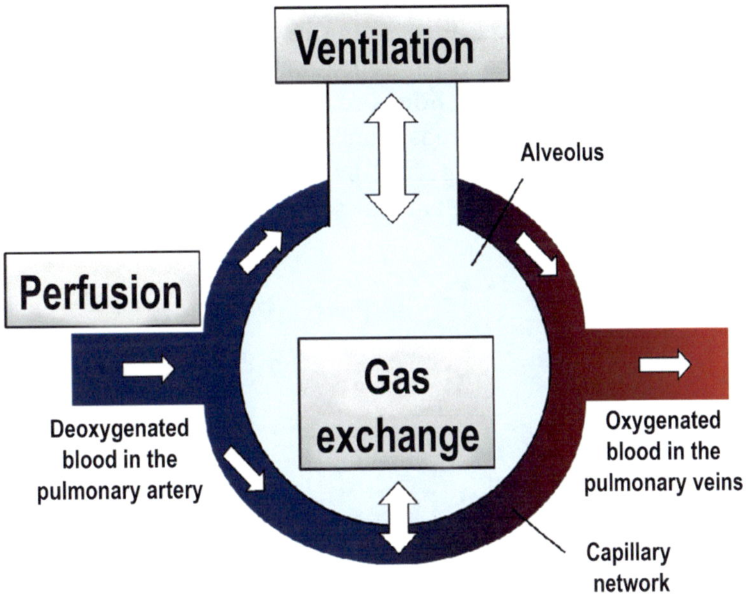

Figure 4.14. Illustrates that gas-exchange in alveoli is a complex interaction between ventilation of air and perfusion of blood to the alveoli.

https://www.researchgate.net/profile/Mads-Mogensen/publication/268249556/figure/fig3/AS:667665668513804@1536195308428/llustrates-that-gas-exchange-in-alveoli-is-a-complex-interaction-between-ventilation-of.png.

4.5.1. Role of Partial Pressures in Gas Exchange

Gas exchange in the lungs depends on the amount of oxygen and carbon dioxide in the air and blood. Each gas in a mixture, according to Dalton's law, acts as if it were alone, so the total pressure is the sum of the partial pressures of all the gases. In the context of alveolar ventilation, the partial pressure of oxygen (PaO_2) in the alveoli needs to exceed that in the pulmonary capillaries for diffusion to occur. This is important for oxygen to go from the alveoli into the blood, where it attaches to hemoglobin in RBCs. Conversely, carbon dioxide ($PaCO_2$) moves from the blood into the alveoli due to the higher partial pressure in the blood compared to the alveolar air. The efficiency of gas exchange depends mainly on the partial pressure differences created during respiration. When the lungs are acutely affected, mechanical ventilation must focus on partial pressure to facilitate gas exchange. In instances of an ALI, the mechanical stretch applied to pulmonary epithelia during ventilation can initiate protective mechanisms, as noted in recent research (Bonney et al., 2013). The stabilization of hypoxia-inducible factor 1A (HIF1A) during mechanical stretch helps improve oxygen uptake and mitigate inflammation in the lungs. These strategies enhance alveolar-capillary gas exchange, which helps to mitigate the adverse effects of mechanical ventilation. Understanding the effects of partial pressures on gas transfer enables the development of innovative ventilation approaches that minimize harm to the lungs during mechanical support. Additionally, the mechanisms by which healthy lungs exchange gases efficiently can cause difficulties in certain clinical cases, such as when horses are anesthetized and become highly sensitive to low oxygen levels. The adaptations that optimize gas exchange during exercise can lead to V/Q mismatches when the animal is recumbent, potentially resulting in impaired oxygenation (Auckburally et al., 2017). Using higher inspired oxygen to treat hypoxemia may not address the primary issues of shunting and discrepancies between blood flow and ventilation. Instead, scientists are looking into new ways to move blood in the lungs to areas where ventilation is better. Exploring these options can improve understanding of the role of partial pressures and enhance approaches to managing gas exchange among different species and clinical scenarios (Figure 4.15).

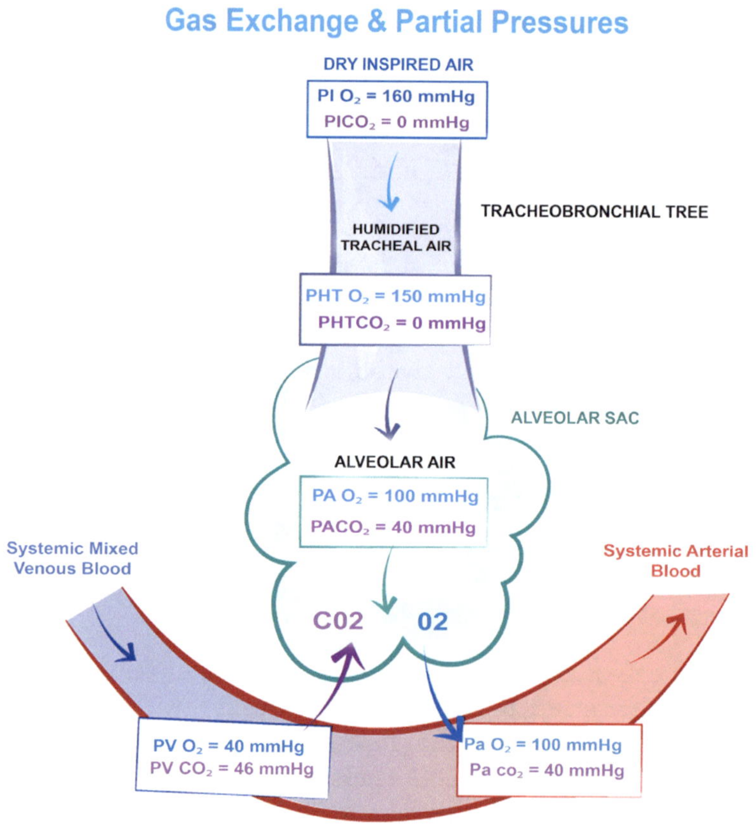

Figure 4.15. Gas exchange and partial pressures.

Source: https://d1j63owfs0b5j3.cloudfront.net/term/images/gas-exchange-partial-pressures-1645.png.

4.5.2. Impact of Ventilation-Perfusion Ratio

The amount of gas the alveoli exchange depends greatly on the V/Q ratio, which is important when discussing alveolar ventilation. This ratio reflects the relationship between the amount of air reaching the alveoli (ventilation) and the amount of blood flowing through the pulmonary capillaries (perfusion). An optimal V/Q ratio (approximately 0.8) ensures efficient oxygen uptake and carbon dioxide elimination. A change in this ratio can cause significant problems in the body. A V/Q ratio that is too low may be found in cases of pulmonary edema or blocked airways, which can result in insufficient oxygen even when breathing is normal. High V/Q ratios are usually caused by a drop in perfusion, which can occur in cases of pulmonary embolism. It is essential to recognize these imbalances, as they can hinder the delivery of sufficient oxygen, potentially leading to issues throughout the body. Additionally, recent advancements in measuring specific gases in breath have underscored the importance of V/Q ratios in evaluating patients.

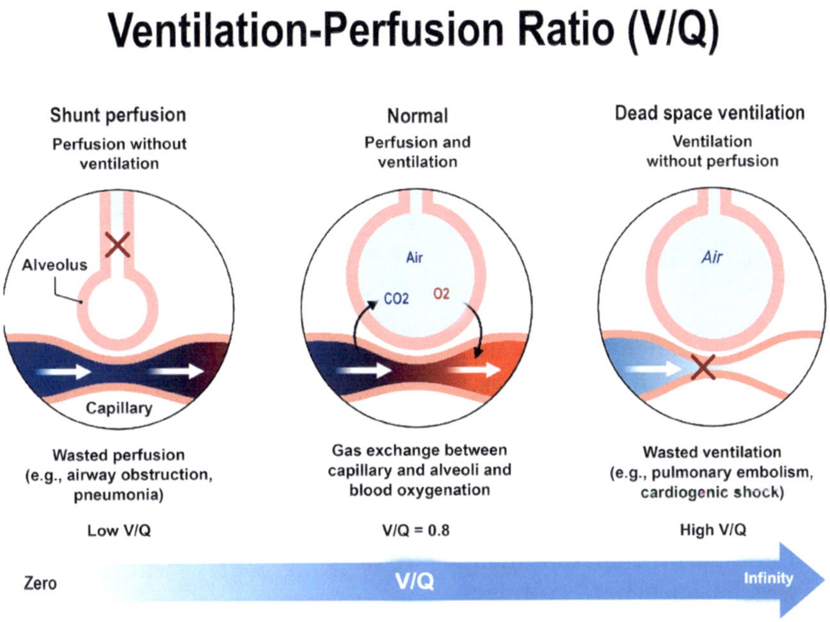

Figure 4.16. Ventilation perfusion ratio.

Source: https://cdn.prod.website-files.com/621e95f9ac30687a56e4297e/65dcff58158b583bb62882e9_V2_1689171520366_8e854bbd-1845-4a18-a592-0d52a456baab_HIGH_RES.png.

It has been suggested that the level of trace gases, such as VOCs, can reveal how well air is exchanged in the lungs and its current health state. It is shown by research that the concentrations are primarily determined by airway actions, the makeup of the lining fluid and the resulting differences in alveolar and general body concentrations. In such cases, traditional equations, for example the classical Farhi equation, might not accurately describe these relationships. The development of more sophisticated compartment models enables a better capture of variability in breath concentrations, ultimately highlighting the intricate connection between the V/Q ratio and both physiological mechanisms and clinical diagnostics (Amann et al., 2010). Additionally, problems with the V/Q ratio can impact more than just gas exchange; these problems can lead to pulmonary edema and various other complications. Recent studies have highlighted that pulmonary edema can be caused by cardiogenic reasons and also by increased permeability of the pulmonary capillaries due to inflammation. The mechanism of pulmonary edema highlights the importance of assessing V/Q ratios to initiate treatment as soon as possible. Increasingly, clinicians are utilizing various tools at the bedside to detect pulmonary edema, including lung ultrasonography and transpulmonary thermodilution, which aid in measuring fluid in the lungs. A nuanced understanding of how V/Q ratios interrelate with these diagnostic approaches enhances clinical management, ensuring timely interventions for conditions that can lead to significant morbidity if left unaddressed (Assaad et al., 2018) (Figure 4.16).

4.5.3. Consequences of Impaired Gas Exchange

Impaired gas exchange can lead to significant issues in both the body and mind of a person. If alveolar ventilation is reduced, the first and most significant effect is hypoxemia, which means there is not enough oxygen in the blood. A lack of oxygen can cause problems throughout the body, for example, anaerobic metabolism and lactic acidosis, which exacerbate cellular dysfunction. Certain animals, such as horses, are very susceptible to hypoxemia due to their specialized body adaptations for physical activity. While the prevalence of hypoxemia in healthy horses during general anesthesia is not fully documented, the recognition of this condition is crucial for preventing potential morbidity and mortality associated with it (Auckburally et al., 2017). Additionally, when oxygen delivery is reduced, clinicians should be aware that it can damage various organs, potentially leading to multi-organ dysfunction syndrome if not promptly addressed. In addition to affecting the body as a whole, impaired gas exchange can lead to significant changes in breathing mechanics. A lack of proper ventilation in the alveoli causes a V/Q mismatch, which makes it difficult for effective gas exchange to occur. Due to this, blood frequently shunts to avoid the ventilated parts of the lung, which exacerbates hypoxia. With age, the lungs do not work as well, which reduces the body's ability to exchange gases. Because of a smaller reserve in their lungs and a greater risk of COPD, elderly patients are more likely to be affected. Understanding these age-related changes is vital, as they complicate the interpretation of respiratory function tests and exacerbate the consequences of impaired gas exchange (Ebejer et al., 1999). Hence, it is essential for clinicians to pay closer attention to respiratory assessment in elderly patients, as numerous factors can contribute to this. It is essential to employ management strategies for impaired gas exchange to mitigate the problems it causes, but these strategies can be challenging to apply. In hospitals, administering extra oxygen or using breathing machines is intended to aid in gas exchange, although their effectiveness can vary significantly. For example, in anaesthetized horses, simply increasing the inspired oxygen fraction may prove ineffective due to underlying shunts and atelectasis, leading to variable outcomes (Auckburally et al., 2017). As a result, various methods to redirect pulmonary blood flow from poorly ventilated to well-ventilated areas have been investigated; however, the results have not been consistent. Additionally, using invasive methods often requires weighing the potential risks against the potential benefits. It is crucial to comprehend the impact of impaired gas exchange in order to develop effective strategies for restoring healthy alveolar ventilation and facilitating patient recovery.

4.6. Clinical Implications of Alveolar Ventilation

Understanding how alveolar ventilation impacts health is crucial for managing various respiratory conditions. For individuals with COPD, ensuring adequate alveolar ventilation is crucial for preventing disease progression and maintaining proper gas exchange. Current literature highlights that the use of inhaled corticosteroids (ICS) in COPD patients has raised concerns regarding pneumonia risk; however, recent studies suggest that the outcomes for pneumonia do not differ significantly between those treated with ICS and those given long-acting bronchodilators (Chang et al., 2024). It means that although the link between alveolar ventilation and bronchodilators is not straightforward, maintaining adequate ventilation remains necessary to help patients and reduce the risk of complications in COPD exacerbations. Additionally, managing critically ill patients often involves optimizing oxygen delivery and carbon dioxide removal by enhancing alveolar ventilation. When someone has acute respiratory failure, mainly because of COVID-19, mechanical ventilation is required. Advanced techniques such as extracorporeal membrane oxygenation (ECMO) offer alternative pathways to support patients whose alveolar ventilation may be severely compromised. The use of ECMO has prompted clinicians to modify their methods when standard ventilation techniques are insufficient. Knowing how alveolar ventilation works in response to these interventions can guide clinicians in acting in ways that are most beneficial to patients, especially when resources are limited. Monitoring and adjusting alveolar ventilation can play a significant role in the clinical care of patients with respiratory problems. If alveolar ventilation is insufficient, hypercapnia and hypoxemia may result, which can then bring about respiratory acidosis or difficulties in several organs. Thus, clinicians are increasingly tasked with utilizing arterial blood gas (ABG) analyses and other diagnostic tools to assess ventilation adequacys" in real-time. If interventions are made early, by adjusting the ventilator or using NIV, it can help patients with respiratory distress avoid serious problems. Researchers continue to study alveolar ventilation and its effects on health, which shows why healthcare professionals should use a team approach to design the best prevention and treatment plans for each patient.

4.6.1. Importance in Critical Care Settings

Alveolar ventilation is crucial in critical care because it directly impacts how patients fare in severe conditions. Alveolar ventilation, which describes the process of exchanging air in the alveoli, is essential for the body to receive sufficient oxygen and eliminate carbon dioxide. In critically ill patients, particularly those with respiratory failure or conditions such as congestive heart failure (CHF), precise management of ventilation becomes crucial. Mechanical ventilation (MV) emerges as a vital therapeutic tool, as it can effectively support patients struggling to breathe independently, thus ensuring essential gas exchange while simultaneously reducing the workload on respiratory muscles. The intricate balance between the benefits and potential complications of MV emphasizes the necessity for ongoing assessment of alveolar ventilation to facilitate timely interventions and optimize patient care in these high-stakes environments (Adams et al., 2016). Moreover, understanding alveolar ventilation in the context of conditions like community-acquired pneumonia (CAP) is integral to developing effective physiotherapeutic strategies. Patients with CAP who need intubation can create unique problems in respiratory care because of issues linked to mechanical ventilation. A review of expert opinions on physiotherapy revealed that there are various approaches to managing patients, underscoring the need for reliable guidelines. It was found that working on alveolar ventilation through physiotherapy can help patients breathe more easily and recover more quickly. By enhancing corporeal mechanics and facilitating clearance of secretions, physiotherapy plays a vital role in ensuring the effectiveness of alveolar ventilation in critically ill individuals, thereby enhancing overall treatment outcomes (Braun et al., 2018). All in all, managing alveolar ventilation in critical care extends beyond simply supporting breathing. Good ventilation practices and patient recovery go hand in hand, especially in cases of CAP. Being able to modify ventilation management according to a patient's needs can significantly impact their recovery rate, which is why strong guidelines are crucial in clinical practice. In light of these insights, fostering a thorough understanding of alveolar ventilation undoubtedly emerges as paramount in critical care, ensuring that healthcare professionals are well-equipped to make informed clinical decisions that advance patient health and recovery in these demanding environments (Adams et al., 2016; Braun et al., 2018) (Figure 4.17).

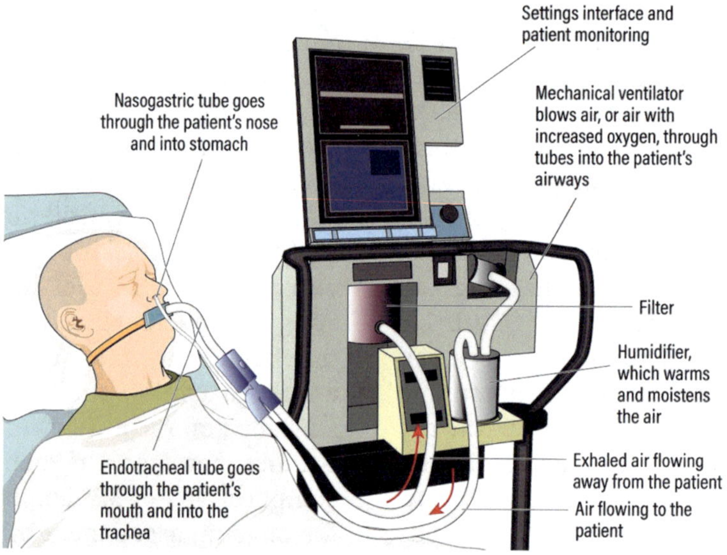

Figure 4.17. Mechanical ventilator for positive pressure ventilation.

Source: https://www.icuanswers.com/images/93fc70cad160638fdf4e3f0d8ebf7d27.jpg.

4.6.2. Management of Respiratory Failure

Treating respiratory failure requires the use of several therapies to help the lungs ventilate adequately. Among the causes are obstructive or restrictive lung diseases, neuromuscular disorders, and lung infections. Promptly identifying the main problem helps doctors take swift action, which can significantly improve patient recovery. In cases where pulmonary issues, such as alveolar proteinosis, lead to severe respiratory compromise, patients may require advanced interventions, including whole-lung lavage, which necessitates meticulous anesthetic management to ensure patient safety during the procedure (Varley et al., 2008). Addressing the main issues and maintaining proper oxygen and air flow helps healthcare professionals improve lung function. Mechanical ventilation is very important for treating severe breathing problems such as those seen in decompensated CHF. PPV helps with gas exchange and also relieves the heart by reducing the pressure on its filling and emptying chambers, which is important for heart failure. This method enables clinicians to enhance oxygen delivery while simultaneously reducing the work of breathing, thereby offering a dual benefit for patients with severe respiratory distress (Adams et al., 2016). Nevertheless, it is essential to select the appropriate mechanical ventilation approach, as volutrauma and barotrauma are potential risks. It is important to regularly check how the patient responds to mechanical ventilation to prepare them to be liberated from ventilation. Besides mechanical and surgical methods, respiratory failure is often managed with drugs that increase alveolar ventilation. These drugs, including bronchodilators, corticosteroids, and mucolytics, can significantly help individuals with obstructive airway diseases by facilitating better airflow and oxygenation. Also, treating any problems like anxiety or pain can help make breathing easier for patients. A comprehensive treatment plan for each patient is developed when pulmonologists, respiratory therapists, and critical care physicians collaborate. As such, a multidisciplinary approach that leverages both medical management and supportive therapies can significantly improve outcomes in patients suffering from respiratory failure, ultimately enhancing their quality of life through better ventilatory support (Figure 4.18).

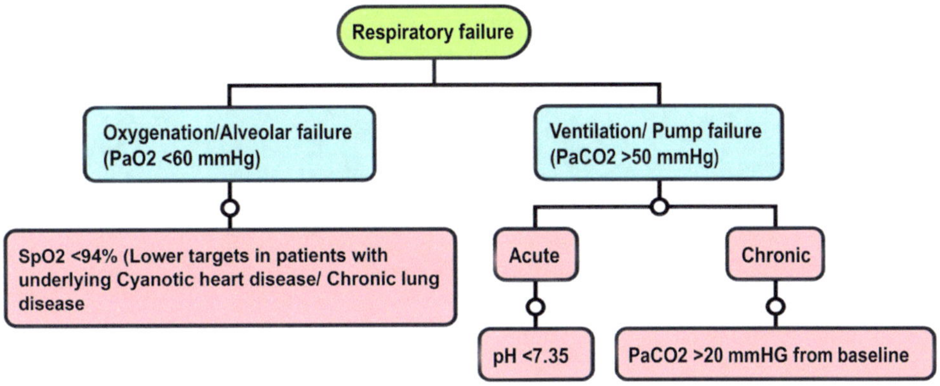

Figure 4.18. Respiratory failure.

Source: https://media.springernature.com/lw1200/springer-static/image/art%3A10.1007%2Fs12098-023-04559-z/MediaObjects/12098_2023_4559_Fig1_HTML.png.

4.6.3. Role in Anesthesia and Surgery

Optimal alveolar ventilation is crucial in anesthesia and surgery to protect patients and achieve favorable outcomes. Proper ventilation is important while using anesthesia to ensure oxygen levels are correct and risks from OLV are reduced during surgery. OLV, commonly used during pulmonary resections, can result in a complex inflammatory response, as observed in studies evaluating the effects of various tidal volumes (VT) on local cytokine production in the lungs. Specifically, the inflammatory cytokine response in the dependent lung showed stability despite variations in ventilation strategies, suggesting that proper ventilation settings could mitigate the risk of postoperative complications, particularly respiratory ones, and enhance recovery rates in surgical patients (Andreetti et al., 2018). The impact of ischemia-reperfusion (I-R) injury during surgery is another critical factor related to alveolar ventilation. Surgery, especially when it stops blood from reaching the lung, can cause serious problems with lung function because of the inflammation caused by I-R injury. Experiments with mouse models have shown that the innate immune system recognizes the inflammation that follows I-R injuries, and alveolar macrophages and toll-like receptors primarily mediate this recognition. Given that surgeries often require brief periods of OLV, understanding the inflammatory dynamics at play can help anesthesia providers develop strategies that circumvent potential complications stemming from I-R injury, thereby safeguarding lung function and overall patient outcomes (Dodd-o et al., 2012). Additionally, the use of new ventilation techniques demonstrates how anesthesia management is evolving during surgery. For example, when protective ventilation is used, such as with lower tidal volumes and the help of PEEP, it has been proven to minimize lung problems and ensure adequate oxygenation. They aim to enhance alveolar ventilation and also show a better understanding of how lung mechanics change under anesthesia. The emphasis on ventilation strategies specifically tailored to maximize alveolar efficiency during surgical procedures illustrates the critical interplay between anesthesia practices and surgical outcomes, ultimately enhancing patient safety and contributing to shorter recovery times (Dodd-o et al., 2012; Andreetti et al., 2018).

SUMMARY

The mechanism of action of alveolar ventilation is very important to keeping the lungs functioning well and promoting the efficient exchange of gases. It is important to understand what influences alveolar ventilation, such as tidal volume, ventilator settings, and various medical conditions, to manage patients well. Research indicates that mechanical ventilation with high tidal volumes can lead to adverse effects, including increased alveolar diameters and reduced septal capillary dimensions, thereby affecting overall pulmonary function (Damiani et al., 2024). It is essential for healthcare professionals to consider these respiratory mechanics as they work with respiratory therapists to benefit patients.

Furthermore, conditions such as severe viral infections, notably COVID-19, underscore the significance of monitoring the alveolar-arterial oxygen gradient ($GAaO_2$). Data reveals that a higher GAaO2 is associated with a greater risk of needing mechanical ventilation sooner, which helps clinicians. Understanding these correlations is vital, as timely intervention can significantly affect morbidity and mortality rates in critically ill patients (Moreno et al., 2023). It therefore highlights the importance of constantly reviewing and adjusting ventilation strategies to suit each patient. In short, alveolar ventilation influences much more than just how the lungs function; it also involves learning about pathophysiology and therapy. It is essential for clinicians to monitor changes in lung function, particularly in individuals at high risk. Using advanced imaging and measurements can help doctors make more informed decisions about mechanical ventilation. When healthcare providers use many approaches, they can improve the way patients breathe, which reduces the risk of complications and helps them recover faster, especially in severe respiratory infections.

It is essential to understand how mechanical ventilation and lung protection strategies interact during the process of alveolar ventilation. Research has shown that utilizing endogenous pathways during mechanical ventilation can significantly impact the outcomes for individuals with ALI. Research indicates that under cyclic stretch conditions, pulmonary epithelia exhibit a transcriptional response akin to hypoxia signaling, ultimately leading to the stabilization of hypoxia-inducible factor 1A (HIF1A) in normoxic environments. This suggests that HIF1A may help reduce ALI by reducing pulmonary edema and inflammation, as well as by enhancing mitochondrial function. Emphasizing the endogenous feedback loops supporting lung health, these findings highlight the necessity of integrating protective strategies during mechanical ventilation to enhance patient recovery outcomes and decrease mortality rates associated with ALI (Bonney et al., 2013). Also, for patients on a ventilator, physiotherapy for CAP should be based on evidence, mainly to ensure proper alveolar ventilation.

A recent study employed a modified Delphi technique to determine what experts consider the best physiotherapy practices for these patients. The consensus was built from the advice of international experts in critical care physiotherapy, who suggested 38 ways to assess and manage patients. There is a strong consensus that specific physiotherapy treatments can significantly enhance respiratory function and improve outcomes for hospitalized patients with CAP who are on a ventilator. This underscores the broader implications of coordinated therapeutic measures aimed at optimizing alveolar ventilation, highlighting how well-structured physiotherapy interventions can play a pivotal role in the recovery trajectory of critically ill patients (Braun et al., 2018). To sum up, linking these key points shows that understanding and applying physiology plays a significant role in improving alveolar ventilation. When healthcare professionals understand the biology of lung protection and the clinical methods for treating respiratory illnesses, they can take the most effective actions during emergencies. Both stabilizing HIF1A and using proven physiotherapy for CAP show the need for a complex approach in caring for critically ill patients with respiratory problems. Such comprehensive strategies not only aim to optimize alveolar ventilation but also to ultimately improve health outcomes and quality of life for those affected by severe respiratory ailments (Bonney et al., 2013; Braun et al., 2018).

CLOSER LOOK

POSITIVE END-EXPIRATORY PRESSURE (PEEP)

PEEP is a mechanical ventilation setting that applies positive pressure to the airway at the end of exhalation, preventing alveolar collapse and improving lung function, especially in patients with ARDS. By keeping the alveoli open, PEEP can improve oxygenation, reduce the work of breathing, and potentially decrease VILI.

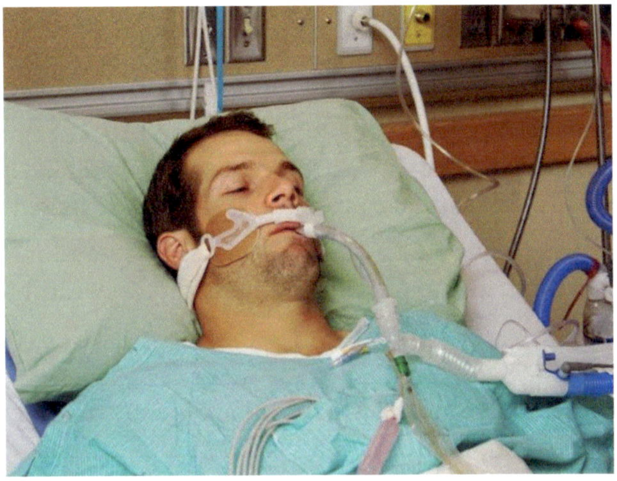

Purpose and Mechanisms

- **Alveolar Recruitment and Prevention of Collapse:** PEEP helps to "recruit" or reopen collapsed alveoli and prevents them from collapsing during exhalation, leading to a more homogeneous distribution of ventilation and improved oxygenation.
- **Increased Functional Residual Capacity (FRC):** PEEP increases FRC, the volume of air remaining in the lungs after a normal exhalation, thereby improving lung compliance and reducing the effort required to breathe.
- **Reduced Work of Breathing:** By improving lung compliance and preventing alveolar collapse, PEEP can reduce the work required by the respiratory muscles, making breathing easier.
- **Potential Reduction of Ventilator-Induced Lung Injury (VILI):** PEEP can help minimize the cyclical opening and closing of alveoli, a known mechanism of VILI.

Types of PEEP

- **Extrinsic PEEP:** This refers to the PEEP applied by the ventilator, a deliberate setting used during mechanical ventilation.
- **Intrinsic PEEP:** This occurs when there is incomplete exhalation, resulting in air being trapped in the lungs, also known as "AUTOPEEP."

Clinical Applications

- **ARDS:** PEEP is commonly used in patients with ARDS to improve oxygenation and reduce VILI.
- **Other Respiratory Failure:** PEEP can also be used in conditions of other respiratory failures to improve lung function and oxygenation.
- **Chronic Obstructive Pulmonary Disease (COPD) and Asthma:** PEEP may be used in these conditions to manage dynamic hyperinflation and improve oxygenation.

Considerations and Potential Complications

- **Optimal PEEP Setting:** Determining the optimal PEEP level is crucial, as excessive PEEP can lead to complications such as pneumothorax (a collapsed lung).
- **Cardiac Effects:** PEEP can impact cardiac output, particularly in patients with heart disease, as it increases intrathoracic pressure, which can restrict venous return to the heart.
- **Intra-abdominal Pressure:** PEEP can also affect intra-abdominal pressure, potentially leading to complications like abdominal compartment syndrome.

Monitoring and Management

- **Arterial Oxygenation:** Monitoring arterial oxygenation is crucial for assessing the effectiveness of PEEP and identifying potential complications.
- **Lung Compliance**: Assessing lung compliance is crucial for determining the appropriate PEEP level and for monitoring potential complications.
- **Patient Assessment:** Careful clinical assessment and monitoring of the patient's response to PEEP are essential to ensure safe and effective management.

REFERENCES

1. Adury, R. Z. (2019). *Synergistic Activation of Inspiratory Muscles by an Adaptive Closed-Loop Controller.* https://core.ac.uk/download/361013486.pdf (accessed on 31st May 2025).
2. Alamoudi, A. (2024). *Assessment of Inhomogeneity in Gas Exchange Using a Novel Methodology.* https://core.ac.uk/download/622442722.pdf (accessed on 31st May 2025).
3. Amann, A., Lumb, A. B., Schrikker, A. C., Mörk, A. K., Amann, A., Amann, A., Anton, A., et al. (2010). A mathematical model for breath gas analysis of volatile organic compounds with special emphasis on acetone. *J. Math. Biol.* http://arxiv.org/abs/1003.4475 (accessed on 31st May 2025).
4. Andreetti, C., Borro, M., Cipolla, F., Defraia, G., et al. (2018). *Short-Term One-Lung Ventilation Does Not Influence Local Inflammatory Cytokine Response After Lung Resection.* https://core.ac.uk/download/158822841.pdf (accessed on 31st May 2025).
5. Assaad, S., Friedman, M. B., Kratzert, W. B., Perrino, A. C., et al. (2018). *Assessment of Pulmonary Edema: Principles and Practice.* https://core.ac.uk/download/145643671.pdf (accessed on 31st May 2025).
6. Auckburally, A., & Nyman, G. (2017). *Review of Hypoxaemia in the Anaesthetized Horse: Predisposing Factors, Consequences and Management.* https://core.ac.uk/download/46558350.pdf (accessed on 31st May 2025).
7. Ben-Tal, A., Molkov, Y. I., Park, C., Rubin, J. E., et al. (2014). *A Closed-Loop Model of the Respiratory System: Focus on Hypercapnia and Active Expiration.* https://core.ac.uk/download/33561889.pdf (accessed on 31st May 2025).
8. Blank, R. S., & Lesh, R. E. (2019). Low tidal volume ventilation in the surgical patient: Not particularly low and perhaps not particularly protective. *Anesthesia & Analgesia.* https://www.semanticscholar.org/paper/50a76d2a278e33f396b569f503c408cfe86f4a9b (accessed on 31st May 2025).
9. Bonney, M., Borchers, C. H., Brodsky, K., Eckle, T., et al. (2013). *HIF1A Reduces Acute Lung Injury by Optimizing Carbohydrate Metabolism in the Alveolar Epithelium.* https://core.ac.uk/download/17028321.pdf (accessed on 31st May 2025).
10. Braun, V., Dennis, D., Hodgson, C., Hsu, C. C., McMillan, S. S., & Portney, L. G. (2018). Expert consensus for respiratory physiotherapy management of mechanically ventilated adults with community-acquired pneumonia: A Delphi study. *Journal of Evaluation in Clinical Practice, Early View.* https://core.ac.uk/download/213607876.pdf (accessed on 31st May 2025).
11. Calfee, C. S., & Meyer, N. J. (2017). *Novel Translational Approaches to the Search for Precision Therapies for Acute Respiratory Distress Syndrome.* https://core.ac.uk/download/323074546.pdf (accessed on 31st May 2025).
12. Chang, M. S., Cho, I. S., Yu, I., Park, S., Lee, S. J., Yong, S., Lee, W., et al. (2024). Inhaled corticosteroids may not affect the clinical outcomes of pneumonia in patients with chronic obstructive pulmonary disease. *Tuberculosis and Respiratory Diseases, 87*, 319–328. https://www.semanticscholar.org/paper/0d0f693f1965c1d24ddd1115cc0b4631900871cd (accessed on 31st May 2025).

13. Corp, A., Thomas, C., & Adlam, M. (2021). The cardiovascular effects of positive pressure ventilation. *BJA Education, 21*, 202–209. https://doi.org/10.1016/j.bjae.2021.01.002 (accessed on 31st May 2025).

14. Crivellari, B., Hosgood, G., Mosing, M., Murphy, K., et al. (2021). Use of electrical impedance tomography (EIT) to estimate tidal volume in anaesthetized horses undergoing elective surgery. *Animals*. https://core.ac.uk/download/428436282.pdf (accessed on 31st May 2025).

15. Damiani, E., Casarotta, E., Di Bella, C., Galosi, M., Angorini, A., Serino, F., Tambella, A. M., et al. (2024). Effects of different ventilatory settings on alveolar and pulmonary microvessel dimensions in pigs. *Scientific Reports, 14*. https://www.semanticscholar.org/paper/5b18859c3ecbf2563a3a6d1f2acfada026a57644 (accessed on 31st May 2025).

16. Dodd-o, J. M., Hellman, J., Mesa, K. R., Prakash, A., et al. (2012). Alveolar macrophages and Toll-like receptor 4 mediate ventilated lung ischemia reperfusion injury in mice. Anesthesiology. https://core.ac.uk/download/323080421.pdf (accessed on 31st May 2025).

17. Doggett, A. (2006). *Effect of Inspiratory Pressure Support on Exercise Performance in Patients with Chronic Obstructive Pulmonary Disease*. https://core.ac.uk/download/11310949.pdf (accessed on 31st May 2025).

18. Doorduin, J., Nollet, J. L., Vugts, M. P. A. J., Roesthuis, L., Akankan, F., Van Der Hoeven, J. G., Van Hees, H. W. H., et al. (2016). Assessment of dead-space ventilation in patients with acute respiratory distress syndrome: A prospective observational study. *Critical Care, 20*. https://www.semanticscholar.org/paper/1b65155466ae17fb7e303af4d40dc38647294ea5 (accessed on 31st May 2025).

19. Ebejer, M. J., & Lesauskaite, V. (1999). *Age-related Changes in the Respiratory System*. https://core.ac.uk/download/46601782.pdf (accessed on 31st May 2025).

20. Goetz, A., Heckel, K., Schulte-Uentrop, L., Kiefmann, M., Tritt, O., Keller, P., Kiefmann, R., et al. (2011). *A Novel Alveolar Krebs Cycle-Triggered CO_2 Sensing Mechanism Regulates Regional Pulmonary Ventilation*. https://core.ac.uk/download/pdf/290175.pdf (accessed on 31st May 2025).

21. Gray, F. (1963). Pulmonary structure and function. *The Yale Journal of Biology and Medicine, 35*, 365. https://www.semanticscholar.org/paper/4faa746d463612c4ffceb95121dadd150e3ecd51 (accessed on 31st May 2025).

22. Gremlich, S., Cremona, T. P., Yao, E., Chabenet, F., Fytianos, K., Roth-Kleiner, M., & Schittny, J. C. (2021). Tenascin-C: Friend or foe in lung aging? *Frontiers in Physiology, 12*. https://doi.org/10.3389/fphys.2021.749776 (accessed on 31st May 2025).

23. Hendrickson, C. M., & Matthay, M. A. (2013). *Viral Pathogens and Acute Lung Injury: Investigations Inspired by the SARS Epidemic and the 2009 H1N1 Influenza Pandemic*. https://core.ac.uk/download/323072736.pdf (accessed on 31st May 2025).

24. Hu, B., Guo, H., Zhou, P., & Shi, Z. L. (2020). Characteristics of SARS-CoV-2 and COVID-19. *Nature Reviews Microbiology, 19*, 141–154. https://doi.org/10.1038/s41579-020-00459-7 (accessed on 31st May 2025).

25. Hu, X., Liu, N., & Xu, J. (2023). Rhubarb alleviates hyperoxia induced lung injury in neonatal rats with bronchopulmonary dysplasia by inhibiting inflammation. *Tropical Journal of Pharmaceutical Research*. https://core.ac.uk/download/553558636.pdf (accessed on 31st May 2025).

26. Humbert, M., Kovács, G., Hoeper, M. M., Badagliacca, R., Berger, R. M. F., Brida, M., Carlsen, J., et al. (2022). 2022 ESC/ERS guidelines for the diagnosis and treatment of pulmonary hypertension. *European Respiratory Journal, 61*, 2200879. https://doi.org/10.1183/13993003.00879-2022 (accessed on 31st May 2025).

27. Huttmann, S., Windisch, W., & Storre, J. (2014). Techniques for the measurement and monitoring of carbon dioxide in the blood. *Annals of the American Thoracic Society, 11*(4), 645–652. https://www.semanticscholar.org/paper/0abc9d742ad4e4e47825c2944e191f621f5e8997 (accessed on 31st May 2025).

28. Iannetta, D., Weavil, J., Thurston, T., Georgescu, V., Laginestra, F., Inglis, E., Jenkinson, R., et al. (2023). On the significance of group III/IV muscle afferent feedback for the control of breathing and gas exchange efficiency during prolonged locomotor exercise. *Physiology*. https://www.semanticscholar.org/paper/0372a7a93fe757473b0b68ac270510495537e222 (accessed on 31st May 2025).

29. Jabaudon, M., Pereira, B., Laroche, E., Roszyk, L., Blondonnet, R., Audard, J., Godet, T., et al. (2021). Changes in plasma soluble receptor for advanced glycation end-products are associated with survival in patients with acute respiratory distress syndrome. *Journal of Clinical Medicine, 10*. https://www.semanticscholar.org/paper/74ed5aa98b892b1d7f4a25deddd445737f3ff8d7 (accessed on 31st May 2025).

30. Johnson, A. R. (2018). *Laser and 3-Dimensional Printers: Characterizing Emissions and Occupational Exposures*. https://core.ac.uk/download/230482479.pdf (accessed on 31st May 2025).

31. King, J., Koc, H., Unterkofler, K., Mochalski, P., et al. (2003). *Physiological Modeling of Isoprene Dynamics in Exhaled Breath*. http://arxiv.org/abs/1010.2145 (accessed on 31st May 2025).

32. Kuhn, B., Bradley, L., Dempsey, T., Puro, A., & Adams, J. (2016). Management of mechanical ventilation in decompensated heart failure. *Journal of Cardiovascular Development and Disease, 3*(4), 33. https://doi.org/10.3390/jcdd3040033Adrish, M., Doppalapudi, S., & Lvovsky, D. (2024). *DRIVING Pressure Decoded: Precision Strategies in Adult Respiratory Distress Syndrome Management*. https://core.ac.uk/download/643777065.pdf (accessed on 31st May 2025).

33. Kupferthaler, A., Amann, A., Amann, A., Amann, A., Anderson, W., Anderson, W., Anton, A., et al. (2010). *Physiological Modeling of Isoprene Dynamics in Exhaled Breath*. http://arxiv.org/abs/1010.2145 (accessed on 31st May 2025).

34. Madueño, L. (2024). *Experimental Quantification of Respiratory Tract Deposition of Black Carbon*. https://core.ac.uk/download/630928008.pdf (accessed on 31st May 2025).

35. Moreno, L. P., Correa, B. J., Rivera Guevara, M. de la L., Vera, L. C., & Mendez de, J. I. A. (2023). Alveolar-arterial oxygen gradient ratio ($GAAO_2$) as a predictor of early mechanical ventilation in a patient with suspected SARS-CoV-2 infection in the adult continuous admission area of the "Dr. Gaudencio González Garza" of the La Raza National Medical Center. *Clinical Medicine and Health Research Journal*. https://www.semanticscholar.org/paper/830869580b0ef93f69af6a650a43040e42d7f4ed (accessed on 31st May 2025).

36. N/A. (2025). *Aerospace Medicine and Biology: A Continuing Bibliography with Indexes, Supplement 125*. https://core.ac.uk/download/pdf/42897953.pdf (accessed on 31st May 2025).

37. Nieman, G., Satalin, J., Kollisch-Singule, M., Andrews, P., Aiash, H., Habashi, N., & Gatto, L. (2017). Physiology in medicine: Understanding dynamic alveolar physiology to minimize

ventilator-induced lung injury. *Journal of Applied Physiology, 122*, 1516–1522. https://www.semanticscholar.org/paper/86b69224a4b1bedc70dcda90e52005dab1da6fad (accessed on 31st May 2025).

38. O'Neil, E., Lin, H., Shamshirsaz, A. A., Naoum, E. E., Rycus, P., Alexander, P., Ortoleva, J., et al. (2021). Pregnant and peripartum women with COVID-19 have high survival with extracorporeal membrane oxygenation: An Extracorporeal Life Support Organization Registry analysis. *American Journal of Respiratory and Critical Care Medicine, 205*, 248–250. https://www.semanticscholar.org/paper/d93168333ddb16ac4efd6223b47a5965e9e9ced1 (accessed on 31st May 2025).

39. Parvathi, A. U., & Sanjith, T. K. (2024). Analysis of selected physical fitness, physiological, and psychological variables among government, government-aided, and private school boys in Chennai District. *International Journal of Innovative Science and Research Technology (IJISRT)*. https://www.semanticscholar.org/paper/083e751145ee2e7f5f73cef138c7919c8583f64a (accessed on 31st May 2025).

40. Rezoagli, E., & Bellani, G. (2019). How I set up positive end-expiratory pressure: Evidence- and physiology-based! *Critical Care, 23*. https://www.semanticscholar.org/paper/7420a86c0ddf34b53d5b0467f35f47b5e7d32ca0 (accessed on 31st May 2025).

41. Thorkildsen, K. (2016). *The Utilization of Exogenous Surfactant in the Neonate*. https://core.ac.uk/download/58827079.pdf (accessed on 31st May 2025).

42. Varley, A. J., Evans, A. J. R., Klein, A. A., Trapnell, B. C., Ramirez-Rivera, J., Moutafis, M., Nadeau, M., et al. (2008). *Anaesthesia for Serial Whole-Lung Lavage in a Patient with Severe Pulmonary Alveolar Proteinosis: A Case Report*. https://core.ac.uk/download/pdf/8232298.pdf (accessed on 31st May 2025).

43. Warot, J., & Żukow, W. (2025). Impact of sport dance on physical fitness and condition in the opinion of dancers from [N] Club in [City]. *Journal of Education, Health and Sport*. https://www.semanticscholar.org/paper/21f4b8f1eb6beb2cf2e8840d82d5dcea7d78635e (accessed on 31st May 2025).

44. Yuan, S., Chen, X., Mi, L., Chi, Y., Huang, H., Liu, B., Yue, C., et al. (2024). Effect of fluid and driving pressure on cyclical "on–off" flow of pulmonary microcirculation during mechanical ventilation. *Intensive Care Medicine Experimental, 12*. https://www.semanticscholar.org/paper/6886346fcaccaa2154b104b4954f9aafd420bb30 (accessed on 31st May 2025).

45. Zimmermann, R., Roeder, F., Ruppert, C., Smith, B. J., & Knudsen, L. (2024). Low volume ventilation of pre-injured lungs degrades lung function via stress concentration and progressive alveolar collapse. *American Journal of Physiology: Lung Cellular and Molecular Physiology*. https://www.semanticscholar.org/paper/9bd8a746aee99d1dab68be3c51b778d0362a40eb (accessed on 31st May 2025).

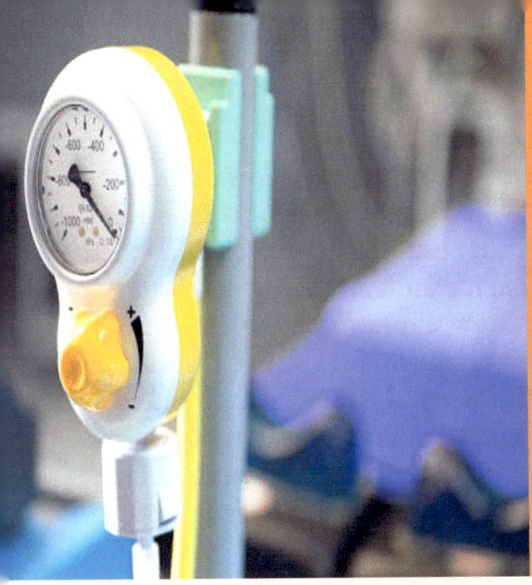

Chapter 5

GAS LAWS AND PULMONARY PRESSURES

Contents

Introduction

Gas laws help explain the physiological processes that control breathing. At the heart of respiratory physiology is Boyle's Law, which says that at a fixed temperature, the pressure and volume of a gas are inversely related. It is important to explain the effects of lung volume changes on the pressure of gases in the alveoli. Air entering the lungs causes the lungs to expand, which lowers the pressure within the air sacs and facilitates air movement. During exhalation, the lungs shrink, increasing pressure and pushing air out of the lungs. This basic idea sets the stage for examining how various external conditions and diseases can impact the pressures in the lungs and the overall health of the respiratory system. For gas exchange to work well, pulmonary pressures such as atmospheric, intra-alveolar, and intrapleural pressures are very important and significant. Several factors influence the way these pressures operate, including altitude, body position, and the surrounding environment. The study of how these pressures operate parallels physiological responses to different stimuli, such as water immersion, highlighted in Dorchak et al. (2025). It is essential to know about these pressures, because they can seriously influence breathing in normal and abnormal situations. For example, in exercise physiology, changes in lung function and gas exchange are significant. Changes in pressure during these activities enable the body to adapt for improved oxygen delivery and carbon dioxide removal, highlighting the importance of gas laws in regular body functions and sports. In addition to the mechanical aspects, there are also critical implications of gas laws and pulmonary pressures in specialized contexts, such as extravehicular activity (EVA). As discussed in Furr et al. (2025), various physiological aspects, including oxygen levels and carbon dioxide accumulation, demand careful examination to ensure safety and efficiency in space environments. Due to these circumstances, it is essential to understand how gas behaves under varying pressures and volumes, which may differ significantly from those found on Earth. Mismanagement of these variables can severely affect human health in situations where people are exposed for an extended period. Therefore, combining gas laws with knowledge of pulmonary pressures is important for medical, sports science, and aerospace research, and it improves our understanding of the human body in different situations.

Definition of Gas Laws

Gas laws explain the actions and properties of gases in different conditions, which is important in both physical chemistry and respiratory physiology. These laws are Boyle's Law, Charles's Law, and the Ideal Gas Law, which all show how pressure, volume, and temperature relate in gases. Boyle's Law states that, for a gas at a fixed temperature, pressure and volume are inversely related, so a rise in volume means the pressure will fall. In the same way, Charles's Law shows that gas volume increases as its absolute temperature rises, as long as the pressure does not change. The fundamental gas laws form the basis for exploring breathing and gas exchange in the lungs, which are important in many pulmonary medical practices. Understanding the gas laws is crucial for understanding pulmonary pressures, as they explain how ventilation works. Respiratory mechanics can be studied well by using the Ideal Gas Law, which blends the effects of pressure, volume, and temperature. Recognizing how gas laws affect gases is crucial in understanding why intrapulmonary pressure changes during inspiration and expiration. The ability to predict changes in gas behavior due to modifications in temperature and volume has implications for understanding conditions like asthma and chronic obstructive pulmonary disease (COPD). Gas laws contribute to the development of improved methods for diagnosing and treating respiratory diseases, underscoring their importance in respiratory health. Additionally, gas laws are explored not only for their fundamental concepts but also for their clinical applications, such as measuring the gases a patient exhales to assess their respiratory system.

The development of standardized procedures for measuring trace gases, including nitric oxide, exemplifies the intersection of gas law theory and practical diagnostics (Amann et al., 2010). Healthcare professionals use information about these gases to assess a patient's metabolic condition and determine how well they can breathe. Increased carbon dioxide in the blood reveals the connection between gas laws, pulmonary pressures, and the possible outcome of respiratory acidosis. The literature emphasizes the crucial need for ongoing research to understand these physiological aspects and refine measurement techniques (Furr et al., 2025). This ongoing inquiry underscores the importance of gas laws as essential tools in both basic science and clinical practice (Figure 5.1).

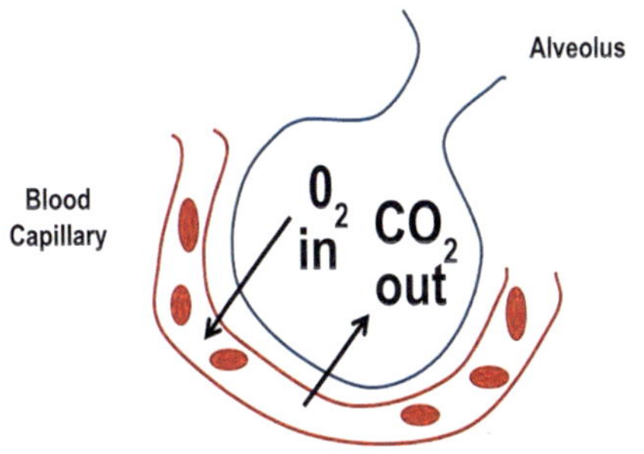

Figure 5.1. Diffusion of gases.

Source: https://upload.medbullets.com/topic/117017/images/diffusion.jpg.

Importance of Gas Laws in Respiratory Physiology

Gas laws are important in respiratory physiology because they demonstrate how gases behave in various temperature and pressure conditions. For example, the ideal gas law explains how volume, pressure, and temperature are related in the alveoli, which are the small air sacs in the lungs. The law states that when the lungs fill with air, the pressure inside drops, allowing oxygen to enter the blood. When exhaling, the lungs contract, increasing pressure and facilitating the removal of carbon dioxide. Knowing these principles is crucial for healthcare professionals in critical care and anesthesiology, as managing respiratory functions is essential to properly care for patients. In addition, gas laws help explain conditions such as pulmonary edema and emphysema, which are not limited to normal breathing. They can change the way breathing works and the efficiency of oxygen and carbon dioxide exchange. In emphysema, damage to the alveolar walls reduces the area where gas exchange occurs, affecting the partial pressures of oxygen and carbon dioxide and disrupting regular gas exchange. Gas laws help healthcare workers understand how these changes will influence the lungs, which guides their approach to treatment. Additionally, understanding how gases move in and out of the lungs under various conditions highlights the importance of maintaining pulmonary pressures in balance, as imbalances can lead to severe breathing problems that may compromise a patient's health. In addition, gas laws are important for public health, not just for individual health conditions. Understanding how pollution and other environmental issues influence gas exchange helps develop policies to stop respiratory diseases, which are standard worldwide. This is particularly pertinent considering the growing burden of non-communicable diseases (NCDs) that can be exacerbated by poor air quality and respiratory health issues. Understanding how gas laws relate to respiratory physiology enables stakeholders to improve air quality and effectively educate the public. Thus, the integration of gas laws into respiratory physiology emphasizes not only the biological aspects of breathing but also the ethical considerations involved in health management and policy-making, highlighting the need for holistic approaches to respiratory health management and disease prevention, as suggested in contemporary reviews on these subjects like those discussing lifestyle management and societal awareness (Budrevi et al., 2020) and considerations of medical ethics in patient care (Varkey, 2020).

Overview of Pulmonary Pressures

Assessing respiratory function and how efficiently gases are exchanged in the lungs depends on knowing pulmonary pressures. Pulmonary pressures refer to the pressures within the pulmonary circulation, encompassing those in the pulmonary arteries and pulmonary capillaries, which help maintain proper lung function. The alveolar-capillary membrane allows oxygen and carbon dioxide to move between the lungs and blood because of the pressure gradient. Although gas laws govern how gases behave in the lungs, the interaction between pressure and volume is significant. When examining the Farhi equation, which is based on alveolar concentrations, we should acknowledge its limitations. For instance, this equation does not account for the complexities arising from the dynamic nature of gas exchange, which can be more accurately captured using advanced models that take into account airway gas exchange, such as those described in recent studies (Amann et al., 2011). Measuring pulmonary pressures and gas concentrations has improved the ways doctors diagnose patients. For instance, standardized procedures developed by task forces from the European Respiratory Society and the American Thoracic Society (ATS) have established protocols for determining exhaled nitric oxide levels. Due to these improvements, it is now possible to assess lung function non-invasively and to diagnose many respiratory diseases. However, it is equally imperative to expand these methods to include the analysis of volatile organic compounds (VOCs) in exhaled breath. Research indicates that concentrations of hydrophilic VOCs, like acetone, are influenced by multiple factors, including breathing patterns and systemic concentrations (Amann et al., 2010).

Being aware of these components can enhance our understanding of the pressures in the lungs and the mechanisms by which gases are exchanged in the alveoli. In addition, the way pulmonary pressures respond is significant for the body's reaction to exercise and stress. Physical activity causes the body to breathe differently, which changes how efficiently gases are exchanged and the amount of pressure in the lungs—monitoring breath profiles as people exercise or rest shows how airway gas exchange changes the amounts of gases in their breath. For example, during moderate exercise, fluctuations in breath acetone concentrations can be observed, highlighting the limitations of relying solely on traditional models, such as the Farhi equation (Amann et al., 2011). It highlights the importance of creating compartment models that account for exercise-related changes in airway gas exchange, which would help us better understand pulmonary pressures and the health of the respiratory system. All of this helps improve how clinical assessments related to gas exchange in the lungs are carried out.

5.1. Basic Principles of Gas Laws

You need to understand gas laws to understand how pressure works in the lungs. Gas laws, mainly Boyle's Law, Charles's Law, and Gay-Lussac's Law, explain the changes in gases when pressure, volume, and temperature change. Boyle's Law, which explains that pressure decreases as volume increases at the same temperature, is important in the way respiration works. The diaphragm contracts downward during inhalation, allowing more air into the lungs and reducing pressure in the chest. Because of this pressure difference, air enters the lungs, illustrating how gas laws are applied in the body. Considering how these laws affect gases helps healthcare professionals understand normal breathing and the effects of any breathing disorders. Pulmonary physiology also depends on Charles's Law and Gay-Lussac's Law in addition to Boyle's Law. When the pressure is constant, the volume of a gas increases as its absolute temperature rises. This relationship becomes significant in the lungs as the air is warmed, since it helps the air expand and promotes good gas exchange in the alveoli. Gay-Lussac's Law also explains that as temperature increases, pressure increases, which is important to know when dealing with hyperthermia or changes in lung pressures. They prove that when temperature and volume change, how well the lungs function can be affected which is helpful in deciding on ventilatory assistance in different diseases. As elucidated in the literature, a comprehensive understanding of these principles enables practitioners to diagnose and manage respiratory conditions effectively, underscoring the importance of gas laws in clinical practice.

Gas laws and the pressures in the lungs are closely linked, and this has major consequences in critical care situations, for example, mechanical ventilation. The shortage of artificial ventilators during the COVID-19 pandemic illuminated the underlying principles of gas laws that dictate the design and function of these crucial devices (Santos et al., 2020). Mechanical ventilators use gas laws to control airflow, pressures and volumes which helps patients with breathing difficulties. Understanding these principles enables individuals to operate ventilators safely and also enhances the design of new and more advanced ventilators. Due to constant improvements in technology, the safety standards of ventilators can be met by enhancing the interface and operation. Because of this, having a basic understanding of gas laws and pressures forms the foundation for both learning and doing work in respiratory healthcare.

5.1.1. Boyle's Law and Its Implications

Boyle's Law states that for a gas in a container, the pressure decreases as its volume increases, provided the temperature remains constant. This happens is very significant when considering pulmonary pressures and the way breathing works. The diaphragm and intercostal muscles contract when someone inhales, which increases the space in the thoracic cavity. As the lungs expand, Boyle's Law explains that air pressure in the alveoli drops, which helps air enter the lungs. This law is particularly important for doctors in fields such as respiratory therapy and anesthesiology, as it explains many aspects of gas exchange and lung function. Boyle's Law is used in medicine for purposes other than respiratory mechanics.

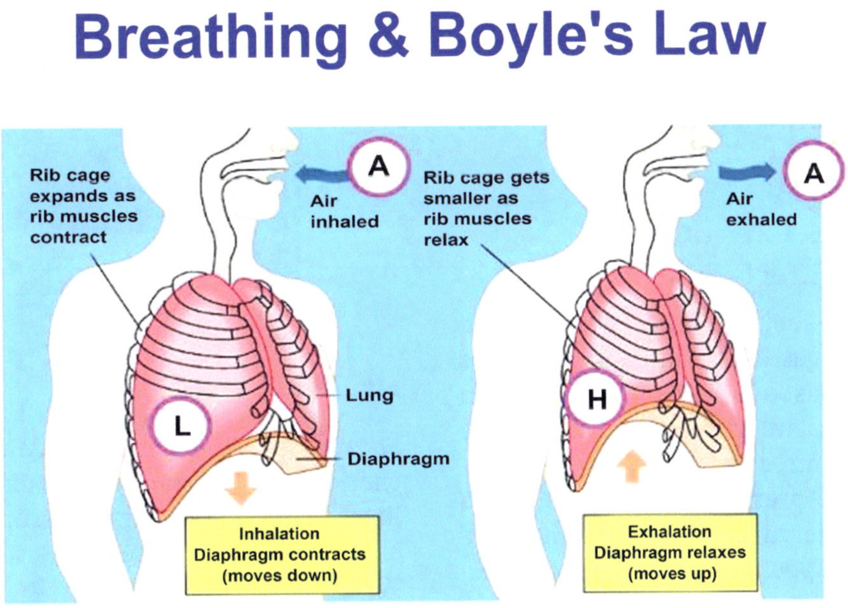

Figure 5.2. Breathing and Boyle's law.

Source: https://image.slideserve.com/670197/breathing-boyle-s-law-l.jpg.

For example, the effectiveness of inhaled medications can be examined using this approach. Anderson et al. (2024) highlight that a knowledge gap persists regarding the optimal delivery of inhaled medications to pediatric populations. Examining airflow patterns using computational fluid dynamics can reveal how changes in pressure affect the distribution of therapeutic agents in the lungs. It is essential for safe and effective dosing, mainly in children and adolescents, so that respiratory drugs work effectively. In occupational health, Boyle's Law is important for controlling airborne substances, for example, radon. The National Institute for Occupational Safety and Health (NIOSH) recommendations emphasize ventilatory measures to mitigate risks associated with radon progeny exposure found in underground mines. The National Institute for Occupational Safety and Health (NIOSH), Division of Health Development and Technology Transfer, outlines that proper ventilation directly influences gas concentrations, in alignment with Boyle's Law principles, to maintain safe working environments. Managing the amount of pressure and volume in the system can help keep the lungs safe. Consequently, Boyles Law is not merely a theoretical construct but a crucial framework for practical applications in both therapeutic and environmental settings (Figure 5.2).

5.1.2. Charles's Law and Temperature Effects

The relationship between the volume and temperature of a gas is explained by Charles's Law, which is based on gas principles. In other words, this law states that the volume of a gas increases directly with its temperature, provided that the pressure remains constant. It is essential to learn Charles's Law in terms of physiology, especially for understanding pulmonary pressures. Changes in body temperature lead to changes in the amount of gases in the lungs. During physical activity, the rise in body temperature can cause you to breathe in more air, which facilitates gas exchange. For athletes and those who are physically active, this principle is particularly important because it describes the changes in the lungs that enable more oxygen to reach the body when it is working hard. Examples such as space exploration reveal how temperature changes can affect gas behavior, and Charles's Law plays a key role in keeping astronauts safe. As documented in the scientific literature, understanding how gas volumes change with temperature is crucial when designing life support systems that manage oxygen levels and carbon dioxide removal during extravehicular activities (EVA) (Furr et al., 2025). Temperature differences may impact gas mixtures which can be dangerous unless handled correctly.

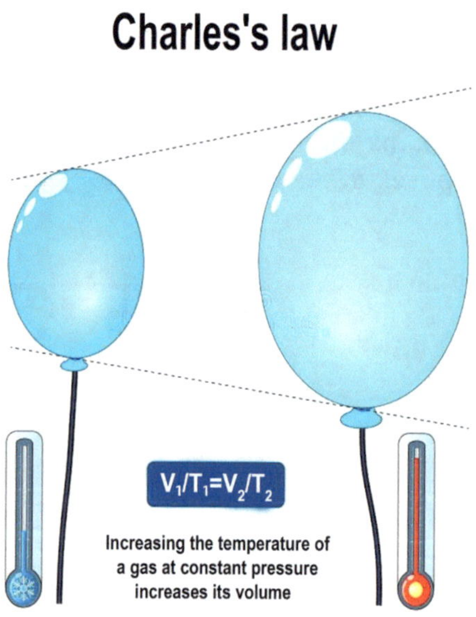

Figure 5.3. Charles's law.

Source: https://thumbs.dreamstime.com/b/charles-s-law-relationship-volume-temperature-increasing-gas-constant-pressure-increases-its-explanation-273845430.jpg.

Maintaining these systems at optimal performance in changing environmental conditions demonstrates how gas laws are applied in the body. Gas laws are used in both medical science and aviation because they relate temperature, volume, and pressure. Additionally, incorporating Charles's Law into pulmonary pressure dynamics reveals why ongoing research is essential to help us understand respiratory health. Scientific studies on how temperature affects gas in the lungs can inform changes in medical care for individuals with breathing difficulties. For instance, individuals experiencing conditions such as asthma or chronic obstructive pulmonary disease (COPD) may be particularly sensitive to temperature changes that affect lung gas volumes and pressures. The need for comprehensive literature reviews in this area is exemplified by reports detailing physiological aspects of EVA, which underscore the necessity for ongoing examination of the interplay between gas laws, temperature effects, and pulmonary function. As researchers seek to bridge theoretical knowledge with clinical applications, the insight gained could guide future innovations in respiratory care and therapeutic strategies (Figure 5.3).

5.1.3. Dalton's Law of Partial Pressures

It is important to know Dalton's Law of Partial Pressures when studying gas behavior in the lungs. The law states that when non-reacting gases are mixed, the total pressure is equal to the sum of the partial pressures of each gas.

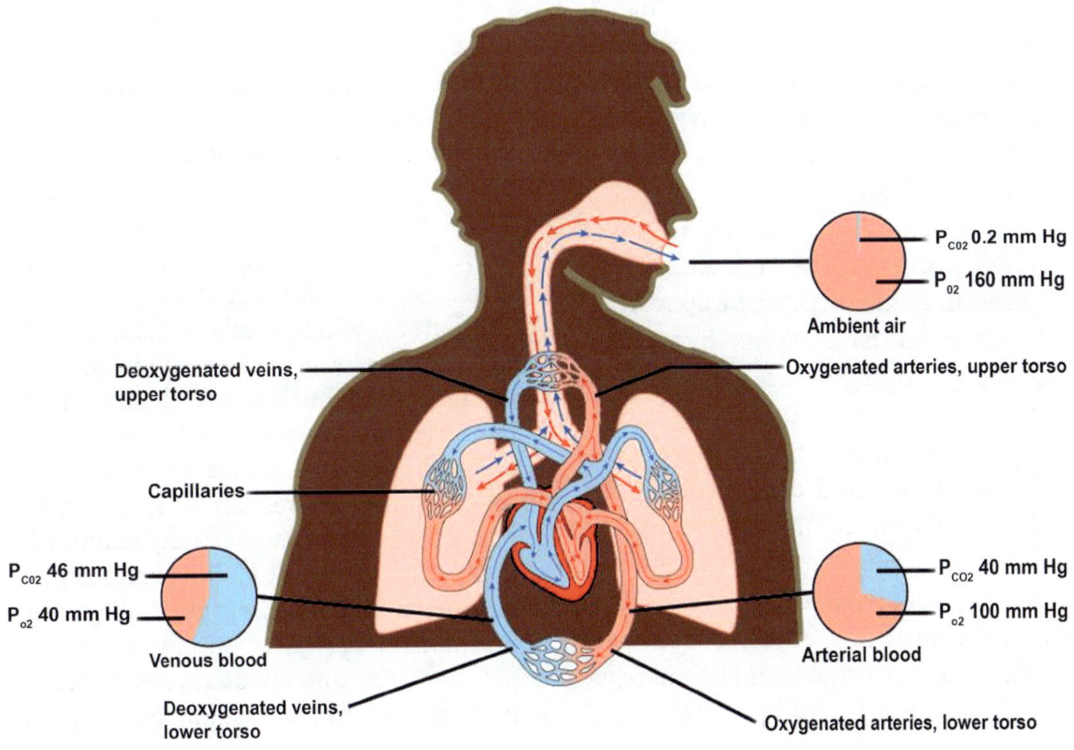

Figure 5.4. The partial pressures of oxygen and carbon dioxide change as blood moves through the body.

Source: https://files.mtstatic.com/site_4463/67460/0?Expires=1746694510&Signature=c1FOrXAn-g3TIxLSESXvTCAlkhoQJLkyLCdZZw5s5iXLuB~6Jiwf910UWy5U0vYfK5wGJlnVfMnmkOo0qlV1hYKfK7VzmMVwFRRKY3aDiuaPj7aX6AeUiBiwbeiNf-hhmlQo5zPmrGhUjmdW31490--zBUQzq8-1nb8L~rblDno_&Key-Pair-Id=APKAJ5Y6AV4GI7A555NA.

This principle in the lungs explains how oxygen and carbon dioxide exchange during breathing. The partial pressure of each gas is necessary, as it helps determine the gradient for gas diffusion, which brings oxygen into the blood and removes carbon dioxide. Not only does this idea demonstrate how the lungs function normally, but it also provides insight into various diseases in which lung pressures are disturbed. Dalton's Law is also applicable for explaining how altitude changes the way gases are exchanged and pressures in the lungs. The total pressure in the atmosphere decreases as you go higher, which also reduces the partial pressure of oxygen. A lack of oxygen (hypoxia) can occur leading to reduced performance and altitude sickness. Seeing the significance of Dalton's Law in clinical practice helps healthcare professionals choose the right interventions, such as offering supplemental oxygen. For patients with breathing problems or those at high altitudes, understanding the effects of altered pressures on oxygen delivery is crucial for proper treatment. Moreover, Dalton's Law of Partial Pressures has practical applications in medical treatments, such as hyperbaric oxygen therapy (HBOT). It utilizes gas laws to enhance oxygen uptake by tissues under controlled pressure, which may be beneficial for soft tissue injuries and certain infections. As noted in the review commissioned by City Football Services, understanding the efficacy and parameters required for utilizing HBOT is paramount in designing effective treatment strategies for conditions that could be managed through optimized gas pressures (Goodwin et al., 2015). The ability of HBOT to alter partial pressures in a therapeutic setting underscores the importance of Dalton's Law not only in theoretical frameworks but also in real-world clinical applications, emphasizing its relevance in modern medicine (Institution WHO, 1982) (Figure 5.4).

5.2. The Role of Gas Laws in Respiration

Understanding how gas laws affect respiration is essential for the proper functioning of the lungs. Boyle's Law explains how the lungs expand during inhalation and contract during exhalation, which involves changes in both volume and pressure. When the diaphragm tightens and the thoracic cavity expands, the pressure in the lungs decreases, allowing air to move in from areas of higher pressure. During exhalation, the diaphragm relaxes, which reduces the space in the lungs, increasing the pressure inside and pushing air out. They explain the physical processes and also underline the importance of predictable gas behavior which links physics and physiology in human respiration. When a patient is critically ill and their respiratory mechanics are impaired, using artificial ventilation is crucial. Modern ventilators operate based on gas laws to deliver the correct amount of air and adjust pressures for each patient. It has been most noticeable during sudden global health crises, such as the recent surge in demand for ventilators, which made it clear that they are essential and that technology is not yet perfect in their distribution and design. Technology is always developing which demonstrates the ongoing effort to enhance these medical devices. As explained by researchers, devices need to pass strict tests to meet safety standards, which highlights the need to follow rules set by groups like the ISO. This integration of gas laws into mechanical design is paramount for ensuring patient safety and adequate respiratory support in various clinical scenarios (Santos et al., 2020). Additionally, understanding how gas laws influence the body's reactions to various conditions, such as being underwater, can help explain how humans can survive in extreme situations. Many studies have examined how bodies adjust to changes in pressure such as when people are underwater. Higher external pressure can alter the amount of air the lungs can hold and reduce the efficiency of gas exchange, as dictated by the gas laws. Such responses can be applied in medicine to understand how the body adapts in various situations. The summarized research contributions include findings related to the effectiveness of respiration under varying conditions, emphasizing the influence of external pressures on human physiology (Dorchak et al., 2025). Learnings from these studies can enhance our understanding of both natural and artificial respiration, connecting the gas laws taught in textbooks to their practical applications in medicine.

5.2.1. Mechanism of Inhalation and Exhalation

The diaphragm and intercostal muscles primarily work together to facilitate inhalation. When you inhale, the diaphragm tightens and goes down, and the intercostal muscles lift and move the rib cage outward. Because of this, there is less air pressure in the lungs, which causes air to be drawn into the lungs. Boyle's Law from the gas laws shows that as the thoracic volume goes up, the pressure inside the lungs goes down. Due to the negative pressure, oxygen-rich air from the atmosphere can flow into the lungs, facilitating gas exchange. As the lungs enlarge, oxygen moves through the alveolar walls into the blood, which helps cells use oxygen and supports the body's main functions, allowing life to continue and homeostasis to be maintained. The diaphragm and intercostal muscles relax, allowing most of the air in our lungs to escape. As the muscles relax, the thoracic cavity shrinks, which increases the pressure inside the lungs.

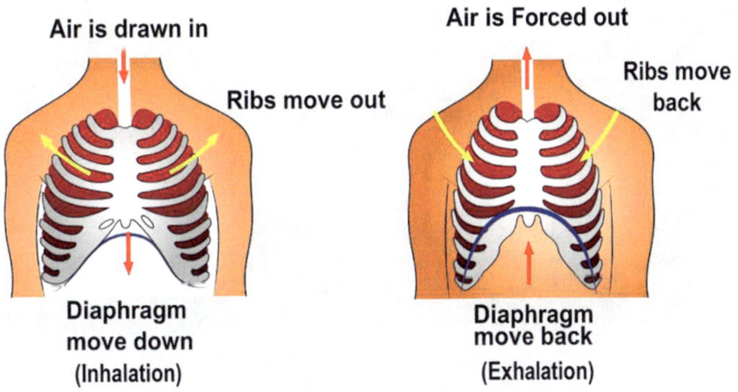

Figure 5.5. Inhalation and exhalation mechanism.

Source: https://www.olabs.edu.in/userfiles/1/Breathing_TheoryIMG2.png.

The gas laws and specifically Boyle's Law, state that when the volume of a space decreases, the pressure inside that space goes up. The extra pressure in the chest causes air to leave the lungs and enter the surrounding air. At the same time, the abdominal and internal intercostal muscles work together to further compress the thoracic cavity, which helps expel air even faster. Since breathing is a rhythmic process, carbon dioxide is released from the blood and oxygen is absorbed, which helps the body maintain its normal functions and respiratory balance. It is crucial for the cardiovascular and respiratory systems to work together for proper gas exchange and to ensure proper pulmonary pressure. A comprehensive understanding of these interactions can be gained through models like the integrated cardiopulmonary model (CP Model), which mathematically describes how respiratory mechanics relate to cardiovascular functions. This model clearly illustrates how blood flow and the need for oxygen in tissues influence the entire process of respiration. If the body is exercising or at high altitude, the system responds by speeding up and deepening the breath, which demonstrates the link between these systems. These adaptations are crucial for maintaining adequate oxygenation and carbon dioxide removal, particularly in challenging environments, ensuring that homeostatic mechanisms function effectively under various physiological stresses (Albanese et al., 2015; Joachim et al., 2021) (Figure 5.5).

5.2.2. Gas Exchange in the Alveoli

Most gas exchange in the human respiratory tract occurs in the alveoli, which are highly efficient due to their large surface area and thin walls. The process of taking in oxygen and releasing carbon dioxide depends on gas laws, mainly Henry's Law, which says that the amount of gas dissolved in a liquid increases with the rising pressure of that gas above the liquid. The gases in air entering the alveoli have different partial pressures. The higher partial pressure of oxygen in the alveoli compared to the pulmonary capillaries allows oxygen to diffuse into the bloodstream. In contrast, carbon dioxide, having a higher partial pressure in the blood, moves in the opposite direction, promoting effective gas exchange, which is crucial for cellular respiration and metabolic activity (Harch, 2020).

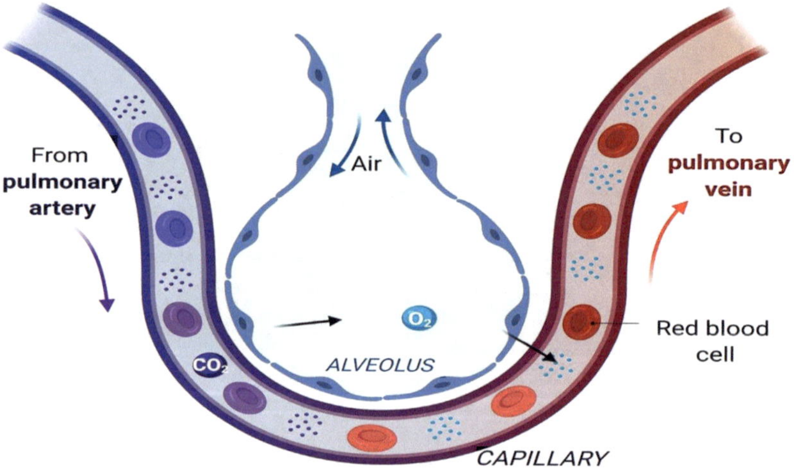

Figure 5.6. Gas exchange in the alveoli.

Source: https://blob-static.studyclix.ie/cms/media/r1jp0l5x/eisitkjucnxfk-xb_cgmnf2sgztijcqk0.jpg.

Things that can affect how well gas exchange happens are environmental factors, lung diseases and how much pressure is in the lungs. If someone has pulmonary edema or pneumonia, the alveolar-capillary membrane thickens, and breathing patterns become abnormal, which can reduce gas exchange. For this reason, these conditions make it more difficult for oxygen and carbon dioxide to pass between the alveoli and the blood. Furthermore, based on Henry's Law, increasing the pressure of oxygen in the alveoli — as seen in HBOT — can enhance the transport of oxygen into the blood, addressing hypoxemia arising from various respiratory illnesses, including COVID-19 pneumonia, which exemplifies how systemic inflammatory responses can obstruct effective gas exchange (Richard et al., 2018). Exploring how gas exchange occurs in the alveoli also involves examining the physiological processes involved in breathing. Factors such as ventilation-perfusion (V/Q) ratio, which reflects the relationship between air reaching the alveoli and the blood flow in the capillaries, play a critical role in determining overall gas exchange efficiency. If the ratio is not correct, oxygen may not reach the body properly, and carbon dioxide will not be eliminated properly. Furthermore, various factors may influence the diffusion of the alveolar-capillary membrane, such as inflammation or changes in the lungs caused by sarcoidosis. Thus, a comprehensive grasp of these variables informs the clinical approaches to optimize gas exchange and maintain effective pulmonary pressures, illustrating the complex interplay between the gas laws and pulmonary function (Harch, 2020) (Figure 5.6).

5.2.3. Impact of Altitude on Gas Laws and Respiration

With higher altitude, air pressure drops. This is a phenomenon which has a big impact on gases, according to Boyle's law. It means that when temperature stays the same, the volume of a gas decreases as its pressure increases. Due to lower barometric pressure at higher altitudes, the partial pressure of oxygen is reduced. Thus, there is less oxygen for breathing – which is a problem for organisms, especially humans, who need adequate oxygen in their blood. Due to this, it is essential to understand gas laws when in high-altitude areas, as they impact how efficiently the lungs exchange gases. In addition, altitude changes not only the amount of oxygen, but they also affect breathing and the adjustments made to it. As people ascend higher, their bodies naturally increase their breathing rate and the amount of air they take in to compensate for the reduced oxygen. It is necessary for this response to keep oxygen levels in the tissues high because a lack of oxygen can cause serious health problems such as altitude sickness. Furthermore, research has demonstrated that prolonged exposure to high altitudes may result in physiological adaptations, including enhanced red blood cell (RBC) production and alterations in hemoglobin affinity for oxygen. These adaptations highlight the dynamic interplay between gas laws and pulmonary pressures, underscoring the need for further exploration into how altitude uniquely challenges respiratory function (Furr et al., 2025). In addition to the physical changes at high elevations, understanding how gas exchange works according to gas laws is crucial for adventurers and athletes in these areas. Oxygen becomes so scarce in the death zone, which is above 8,000 meters, that it puts life in danger. At high altitudes, the body does not receive enough oxygen, which reduces the amount of exercise it can perform and increases the risk of serious altitude-related illnesses. So, it is common to advise acclimatization and oxygen use to help prevent the adverse effects of hypoxia. The knowledge gained from investigating the relationship between gas laws and respiratory mechanisms is invaluable, not only for those in extreme environments but also for policymakers and health professionals aiming to ensure safety and well-being at high altitudes.

5.3. Pulmonary Pressures Explained

Pulmonary pressures rely on the fundamental gas laws, which describe how gases behave as pressure and volume change. Boyle's Law demonstrates that pressure and volume are inversely related in closed systems, which is crucial for understanding how the respiratory system functions. When the diaphragm contracts, the thoracic cavity expands, resulting in lower pressure in the lungs. This negative pressure allows air to enter, demonstrating that changes in pressure are necessary for breathing. Understanding these pressures is crucial for medical professionals, as improper pulmonary pressures can lead to complications such as atelectasis or pneumothorax, highlighting the importance of maintaining optimal lung function to ensure effective gas exchange in living organisms (Febrianti et al., 2024).

Besides Boyle's Law, the rules that affect how much gas is dissolved in the lungs, especially at different partial pressures, are also critical in lung function. Dalton's Law states that the total pressure of a gas mixture is made up of all the partial pressures of the gases in it. Oxygen and carbon dioxide are exchanged in the alveoli during pulmonary gas exchange, which is why this law is important in that context. Due to the partial pressure gradient, oxygen moves from the alveoli to the blood, and carbon dioxide moves from the blood to the alveoli. Understanding these dynamics is essential, especially in clinical settings where gas exchange abnormalities can manifest in diseases such as COPD and pulmonary embolism (Alamé et al., 2024). Additionally, understanding the relationships between pulmonary pressures and ventilation mechanics can be enhanced by examining various physiological situations. When someone exercises intensely, their body requires more oxygen, so both their breathing rate and depth change, which in turn influences intrapulmonary pressure. To get the best results from ventilation, thoracic pressure, airway resistance, and lung compliance should be managed together. If this does not happen, hypoxemia or hypercapnia may result, which are conditions with low oxygen or high carbon dioxide in the blood. Research has shown that understanding these principles can lead to improved management strategies in respiratory therapy, thereby aiding patient recovery in critical medical situations with compromised pulmonary function (Febrianti et al., 2024) (Figure 5.7).

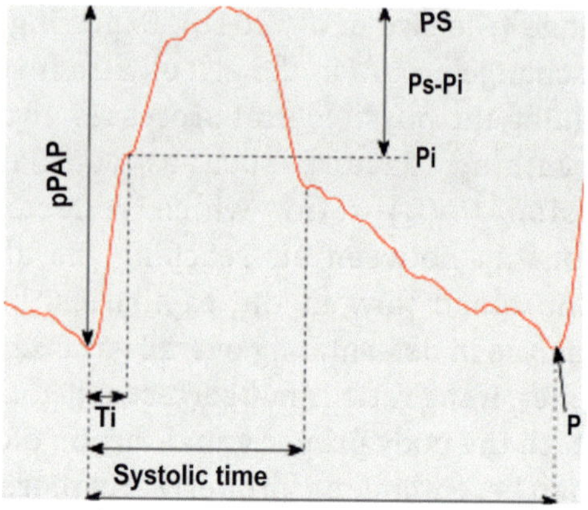

Figure 5.7. Typical pulmonary artery pressure tracing showing the PA waveform analysis.

Source: https://www.researchgate.net/profile/Juan-Grignola/publication/49802961/figure/fig2/AS:341660279033859@1458469566221/Typical-pulmonary-artery-pressure-tracing-showing-the-PA-waveform-analysis.png.

5.3.1. Definition of Intrapulmonary Pressure

Intrapulmonary pressure, or the pressure within the thoracic cavity during breathing, plays a crucial role in pulmonary function. Pressure changes that occur and allow the important gas exchange between the alveoli and the air are a result of the mechanical process of breathing. While resting and breathing quietly, the intrapulmonary pressure is usually equal to atmospheric pressure. When you inhale, the diaphragm contracts, which increases the size of your chest cavity and lowers the pressure inside your lungs to a level lower than the pressure outside. The negative pressure gradient helps air reach the lungs, allowing oxygen to move to the alveoli for exchange, which is necessary to maintain adequate blood oxygen levels. Besides being defined, intrapulmonary pressure is important for understanding several physiological conditions. In forced expiration, the lungs contract and increase pressure inside them, which pushes air from the alveoli. Due to this relationship, the gas laws (specifically Boyle's law, which states that pressure and volume are inversely related in a closed system) are followed. Changes in lung volume during respiration are directly related to changes in intrapulmonary pressure, which is why understanding this concept is crucial for respiratory mechanics and diagnosing lung diseases. The intricacies of intrapulmonary pressure are not only crucial for respiratory physiology but also for comprehending the implications of various pathophysiological states that can alter these pressures, such as restrictive lung disease or obstructive airway conditions (Schramm et al., 2022).

The clinical use of intrapulmonary pressure is evident in tests that measure lung function. Measuring intrapulmonary pressure provides information on lung function and the efficiency of gas exchange. Healthcare professionals use measurements of this pressure to assess how well the respiratory system is functioning and to identify any potential issues. Understanding intrapulmonary pressure is crucial in critical care, as ventilation strategies using machines are employed to assist patients with breathing difficulties. As the relationship between intrapulmonary pressure and overall respiratory efficiency becomes clearer, it becomes imperative for both clinicians and researchers to examine how alterations in this pressure can serve as indicators of pulmonary disease progression and treatment efficacy (Nairn et al., 1966).

5.3.2. Definition of Intrapleural Pressure

To grasp pulmonary mechanics and gas laws, intrapleural pressure is significant. It is about the pressure inside the pleural cavity, which is the small space between the visceral and parietal pleura around the lungs. Usually, intrapleural pressure is always lower than the surrounding atmospheric pressure during normal breathing. Maintaining lung inflation depends on negative pressure, which creates a pressure difference that allows the lungs to expand as the thoracic cavity enlarges during inhalation. A clear understanding of intrapleural pressure helps explain many respiratory problems and their underlying causes, emphasizing its role in pulmonary physiology. Additionally, intrapleural pressure plays a crucial role in breathing, as it influences lung compliance and the effort required to breathe. As the diaphragm contracts and the thoracic cavity gets bigger, the intrapleural pressure goes down, which lets air enter the lungs because the pressure outside is higher. It means that changes in intrapleural pressure can have a significant impact on how easily the lungs expand which is called lung compliance. It has also been studied how intrapleural pressure changes in individuals with diseases such as COPD and pulmonary fibrosis.

Understanding these alterations is crucial, as it can inform treatment strategies and enhance patient outcomes, particularly for individuals with chronic respiratory conditions (Barnes et al., 1949). Intrapleural pressure affects more than breathing and also plays a role in treating and managing diseases. As an example, tuberculosis often leads to persistent pleural cavities, which cause issues due to the way intrapleural pressure changes. While therapeutic measures aim to manage these cavities and their associated pressures, insufficient resolution may still lead to ongoing issues such as hemoptysis or disease spread (Barnes et al., 1949). Better models of the cardiopulmonary system have helped predict and control intrapleural pressure. Such models enable personalized medicine approaches, allowing clinicians to tailor interventions based on individual patient parameters, thereby optimizing both diagnosis and therapeutic strategies (Albanese et al., 2014). Understanding intrapleural pressure thus emerges as essential for both basic physiology and clinical practice in respiratory health (Figure 5.8).

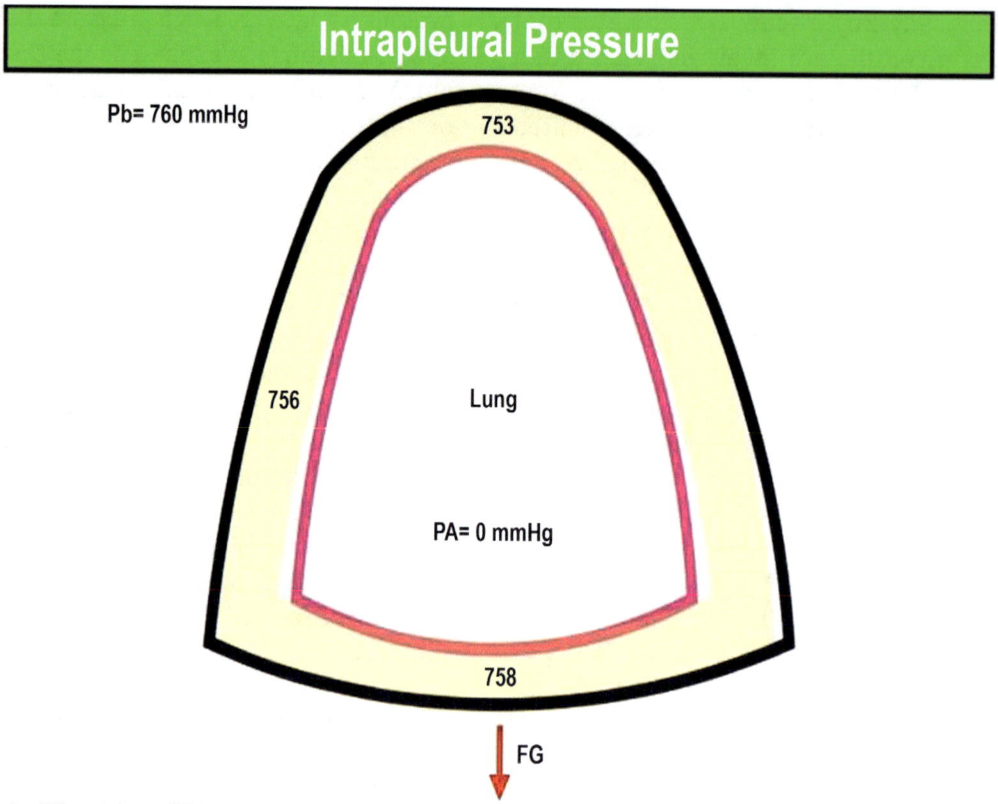

Figure 5.8. Intrapleural pressure.

Source: https://i.ytimg.com/vi/lUhGx26YGi8/maxresdefault.jpg.

5.3.3. Importance of Transpulmonary Pressure

To understand how the lungs and respiratory system function, transpulmonary pressure plays a crucial role. The difference between intrapulmonary pressure and pleural pressure is known as transpulmonary pressure, which maintains the alveoli's open state as air is inhaled and exhaled. Increasing the pressure gradient allows the lungs to expand more, thereby supporting better gas exchange. When someone has COPD or asthma, alterations in transpulmonary pressure can significantly impact how the lungs function and how air moves through them. Studying the role of this pressure gradient helps predict when someone may experience respiratory distress, which is crucial for diagnosing and managing lung diseases that impair breathing effectiveness and reduce the area for gas exchange. The link between transpulmonary pressure and airway resistance makes it even clearer why it matters for respiratory health. When there is increased airflow resistance in the lungs, such as from constriction or inflammation, the pressure required to ventilate the lungs increases. Asthma and COPD are conditions where the airways become more resistant, making it very difficult for the respiratory system to handle. In fact, airway changes and muscle contraction in the airways cause resistance, which requires more pressure to keep effective breathing. Understanding these interactions clarifies how changes in pulmonary pressures impact the mechanical properties of the lungs, highlighting the crucial role that transpulmonary pressure plays in mitigating the adverse effects of increased airway resistance, particularly in obstructive lung diseases (McNulty et al.,

2014). Additionally, transpulmonary pressure plays a crucial role in maintaining lung health in various medical conditions, influencing both gas exchange and the progression of respiratory diseases. Changes in transpulmonary pressure during mechanical ventilation may influence how well the lungs are recruited and how evenly ventilation is distributed among them, which is particularly important for patients with weakened respiratory systems. In such situations, a nuanced understanding of transpulmonary pressure can guide clinicians in optimizing ventilatory strategies to minimize ventilator-induced lung injury (VILI). Ongoing research into the relationship between lung volume, airway resistance, and transpulmonary pressure seeks to advance therapeutic methods for addressing these complex interactions (Boss et al., 2010). Ultimately, appreciating the significance of transpulmonary pressure is vital for advancing our understanding of gas laws and pulmonary pressures, leading to improved clinical outcomes in patients with diverse respiratory conditions (Figure 5.9).

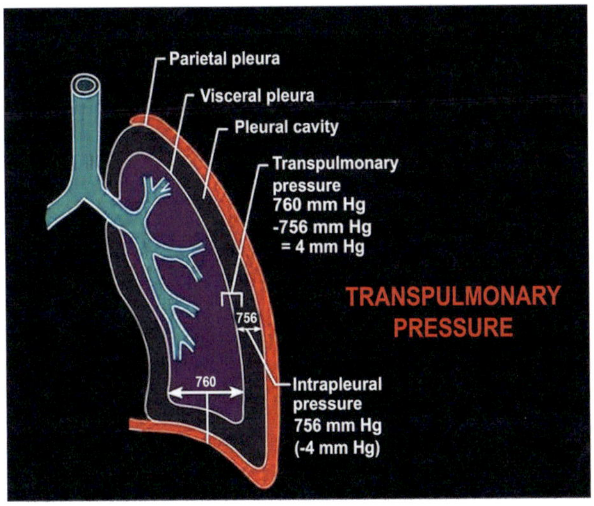

Figure 5.9. Transpulmonary pressure.

Source: http://img.medscape.com/thumbnail_library/ih_160923_transpulmonary_pressure_diagram_800x600.jpg.

5.4. Clinical Applications of Gas Laws

Understanding how gas laws are applied in medicine helps improve the diagnosis and treatment of lung diseases. Gas laws and pulmonary pressures, working together, provide us with important information about respiratory physiology. Gas laws can be used to measure VOCs in breath, which is important for finding out about metabolic functions and health-related issues. Especially, isothermal rebreathing approaches are now considered a method to measure the alveolar concentration of hydrophilic VOCs, such as acetone. This application highlights the role of breathing patterns and airway gas exchange in determining observable breath outputs, which diverges from traditional pulmonary inert gas elimination theories (Amann et al., 2011). Therefore, applying gas laws in clinical situations enhances both the accuracy of measurements and the ability to diagnose respiratory problems. Additionally, gas laws are crucial for non-invasive tests that measure inflammation and other changes in the respiratory system. Standardized practices for measuring exhaled nitric oxide levels, as recommended by the European Respiratory Society and the American Thoracic Society (ATS), exemplify how gas laws can be leveraged for impactful clinical applications (Amann et al., 2010). The presence of nitrogen oxides in breath can indicate whether the airways are inflamed, demonstrating that gas behavior in the body is helpful in diagnosis. These guidelines enable the examination of other trace gases, such as VOCs, which may reveal changes in metabolism. Consequently, applying gas laws to different respiratory gases can help us gain a deeper understanding of respiratory conditions, enabling us to diagnose and treat them more effectively. The way gas behaves is also significant for understanding how respiratory mechanics affect the body, especially in situations where pulmonary pressures are altered. The classical Farhi equation typically accounts for alveolar concentrations but fails to address the complexities introduced by airway gas exchange and individual breathing patterns (Amann et al., 2010). New developments, for example, compartment models, are designed to address these missing points by including factors that determine the volatility and solubility of gases in biological systems. They can make it more straightforward how end-tidal levels relate to the systemic levels of compounds such as acetone. With more research into these details, medical professionals will gain a clearer understanding of respiratory gas exchange, which will improve both their ability to diagnose and provide treatments in pulmonary medicine.

5.4.1. Understanding Respiratory Diseases

It is essential to understand respiratory diseases in relation to gas laws and pulmonary pressures, since these concepts explain the causes of various conditions. Restrictive and obstructive lung disorders, which are respiratory diseases, can disrupt the everyday workings of the lungs and result in both impaired gas exchange and altered lung movements. An example of a restrictive disorder is congenital myopathy, which causes patients to have difficulty breathing, with hypoventilation syndrome and type II respiratory failure.

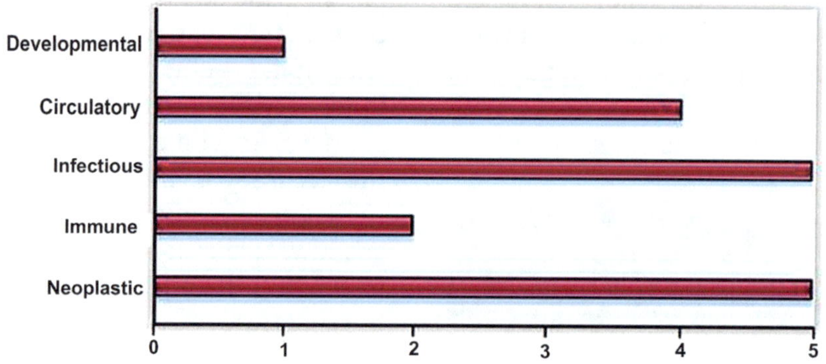

Figure 5.10. The relative clinical significance of various pulmonary diseases.

Source: https://basicmedicalkey.com/wp-content/uploads/2016/10/B9781416002291500087_f05-01-9781416002291.jpg.

This dysfunction arises from weakness in respiratory muscles, resulting in an inability to maintain adequate ventilation and effective gas exchange (Chen et al., 2024). Due to the increased pressure in their pulmonary system, such patients commonly have pulmonary hypertension, which adds to their breathing difficulties. Understanding these relationships highlights the importance of using clinical measures that can mitigate respiratory problems and promote overall health. Respiratory diseases can also cause additional complications, illustrating the interconnectedness of different body systems. For instance, severe respiratory infections, such as those caused by the SARS-CoV-2 virus, can lead to secondary pulmonary fibrosis (SPF). The dysregulated immune response and aberrant repair processes following COVID-19 can significantly alter pulmonary function, further compromising gas exchange efficiency (Lv et al., 2024). Using MUC1, CEA, and CXCL10 as biomarkers can help determine how severe PF is and show the link between inflammation and breathing. Because of these findings, further research is needed to understand how respiratory diseases develop, enabling healthcare professionals to design treatments for both acute and chronic lung problems. Gas laws and pulmonary pressures together help explain the best ways to treat respiratory diseases. For instance, the application of non-invasive ventilation (NIV) has shown promise in managing patients with restrictive ventilatory dysfunction, allowing for improved oxygenation and reduced work of breathing. In cases such as RYR1-related myopathy, where patients face significant respiratory challenges, NIV can lead to substantial improvements in cardiopulmonary function over time (Chen et al., 2024). Additionally, understanding how changes in pulmonary pressures affect thoracic mechanics enables the selection of the most effective treatment, whether through medication or ventilation. By fostering a comprehensive understanding of respiratory diseases through the lens of gas laws, healthcare practitioners can better predict outcomes, personalize treatment regimens, and ultimately enhance the quality of life for affected individuals (Figure 5.10).

5.4.2. Use of Gas Laws in Mechanical Ventilation

Gas laws are essential in mechanical ventilation for providing the best respiratory support to patients with lung problems. understand Boyle's Law and Charles's Law because they use these principles when managing air pressure and volume during ventilation. Boyles Law means that when the temperature of a gas stays the same, its pressure rises as its volume decreases. Because of this, clinicians can manage the amount of air entering the lungs, which improves the exchange of gas. Because Charles's Law relates gas volume to temperature, changes in the temperature of inhaled air can be addressed by adjusting ventilator settings, which helps the patient during mechanical ventilation. Additionally, understanding the gas laws helps improve patient safety when treated with mechanical ventilation. Because mechanical ventilation requires precise pressure and volume, not following the gas laws can result in complications such as barotrauma or volutrauma.

Not paying attention to Boyle's Law during ventilation and applying too much pressure could cause the lungs to stretch too far, which could potentially harm the patient. Furthermore, during resuscitation efforts, particularly highlighted in the recent European Resuscitation Council Guidelines, these principles take on added significance, demonstrating how adherence to gas law principles can improve outcomes in emergencies where mechanical ventilation is employed in cardiac arrest scenarios, highlighting the vital importance of such knowledge in high-stakes environments (Gavin et al., 2021). Advances in gas laws have significantly aided in addressing the challenges posed by respiratory diseases, particularly during the COVID-19 pandemic. SARS-CoV-2 can be easily spread, which causes severe breathing problems that may require patients to be put on ventilators. In such cases, it is clear that gas exchange and pulmonary pressures play a significant role, and understanding gas laws is crucial in helping the patient survive and recover. Understanding the effects of alveolar pressure changes on ventilation enables doctors to improve oxygenation and prevent complications associated with ventilators. As evidenced in contemporary research, understanding these principles is essential, not only for individual patient care but also for addressing broader public health challenges in vulnerable populations that are adversely impacted by respiratory infections (Donald, 2020).

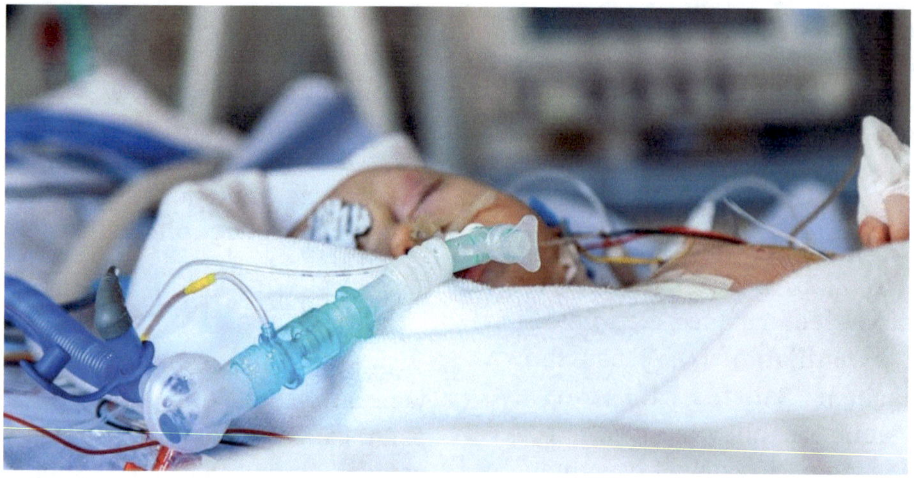

Figure 5.11. Gas laws guide mechanical ventilation, helping tailor pressure, volume, and flow to deliver safe and effective respiratory support for patients with compromised lungs.

Source: https://respiratory-therapy.com/wp-content/uploads/2020/06/nicu-infant-intubation-ettube-2k-1280x640.jpg.

5.4.3. Implications for Anesthesia and Surgery

The implications of gas laws and pulmonary pressures on anesthesia and surgery are profound, particularly concerning the administration of thoracic epidural anesthesia (TEA). Previous studies illustrate how TEA serves as an effective intervention for reducing driving pressure (ΔP) during mechanical ventilation in surgical patients. Lower ΔP values are associated with a decreased incidence of postoperative pulmonary complications (PPCs), highlighting the critical role that variations in airway pressures play during and after surgery. Patients having major upper abdominal surgery had a lower ΔP when TEA was used with general anesthesia compared to those who only received general anesthesia. This finding suggests that maintaining appropriate pulmonary pressures through TEA could enhance lung protection, drive optimal ventilation strategies, and ultimately mitigate the incidence of PPCs, illustrating an essential consideration in anesthetic management (Li et al., 2024). In addition, understanding how lung compliance changes during laparoscopic surgery provides further insight into the role of anesthesia. It has been found that pneumoperitoneum and the positioning of patients can decrease lung compliance, leading to higher airway pressures and less efficient gas exchange. Studying laparoscopic gynecological procedures found that compliance was much lower during setup and did not recover to its original level after the surgery. Still, using an alveolar recruitment maneuver after surgery improved the lungs' function and the exchange of gases. These findings underscore the importance of monitoring pulmonary pressures and the necessity of maneuvering techniques that can optimize lung function during anesthetic management (Griva et al., 2024). The management of pulmonary pressures and adherence to gas laws significantly impact the outcome of patients undergoing anesthesia and surgery. TEA combined with alveolar recruitment maneuvers helps to prevent many postoperative issues. It is essential for anesthesia providers to closely monitor changes in respiratory function to deliver the appropriate anesthetic care for each patient. Understanding how gas laws affect pulmonary pressures enables anesthetists to promote a better recovery and shorter hospital stays. This speaks to a broader commitment within surgical practice to improve procedural safety and enhance clinical outcomes for patients (Griva et al., 2024; Li et al., 2024) (Figure 5.12).

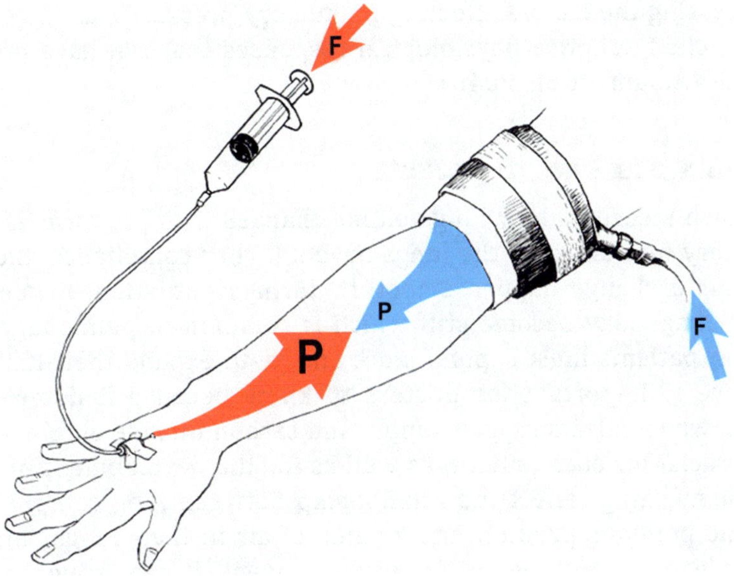

Figure 5.12. Regional anesthesia: Bier block.

Source: https://www.pharmacology2000.com/physics/Chemistry_Physics/bier_pressure.gif.

5.5. Factors Affecting Pulmonary Pressures

Many physiological and environmental factors play a significant role in changing pulmonary pressures which affects the way the lungs work. The interaction between airways and blood circulation is crucial in determining pulmonary pressure. The size of the bronchi and any accompanying inflammation can alter airway resistance, which may impact airflow and the pressures within the lungs. For example, asthma or COPD can cause the airways to narrow, increasing resistance and raising pulmonary pressure. Changing body position from standing to lying down can alter venous return and the pressure in the lungs, illustrating the relationship between airway mechanics and pulmonary pressure. The way gas exchange occurs in the lungs is crucial for influencing pulmonary pressures. As shown by examining rebreathing, the rate at which gases are exchanged has a significant effect on the VOC levels in exhaled breath. Changes in how we breathe, both when we are resting and when we exercise, can cause acetone from the blood to reach the alveoli, which affects pulmonary pressure. They demonstrate that changes in physiological states directly affect gas exchange efficiency and the pressures which shows the link between metabolism and how the lungs function. Understanding these mechanisms helps highlight the variability inherent in pulmonary pressures under differing physiological conditions (Amann et al., 2011). In addition to internal factors, altitude and the surrounding pressure also play a significant role in influencing pulmonary pressures. At higher elevations, the decreased atmospheric pressure alters the partial pressures of gases in the lungs, leading to reduced oxygen availability and potential changes in pulmonary vascular resistance (PVR). This may lead to the body trying to compensate, such as by breathing faster, which can change the pressure in the lungs. Additionally, if animals are exposed to low oxygen levels for an extended period, the pressure in their lungs can increase, a condition known as pulmonary hypertension. Therefore, understanding these external factors is crucial for comprehensively assessing the factors affecting pulmonary pressures, as they not only modify gas composition but also elicit adaptive physiological responses that can have profound implications for respiratory health (Amann et al., 2010).

5.5.1. Lung Compliance and Its Effects

Lung compliance, which measures how lung volume changes with pressure, is very important and essential for respiratory mechanics. If the lungs have a higher compliance, they can expand more easily, which helps air exchange happen smoothly during ventilation. If people do not breathe deeply enough, their lungs may become stiff which is common in pulmonary fibrosis and ARDS. Due to these diseases, patients must expend more energy to expand their lungs with each breath fully. Lung compliance is important for doctors to know because it determines how well gas exchange takes place, which affects oxygen supply and carbon dioxide elimination. Management of lung compliance is crucial for each patient, as well as for the development of respiratory therapy and rehabilitation. Many things affect the relationship between lung compliance and pulmonary pressures, such as the patient's position, the volume of air in their lungs, and any diseases they may have. For example, when intrapleural pressure changes, it can straight away influence lung compliance. In circumstances where positive end-expiratory pressure (PEEP) is applied, studies have shown that while it can improve ventilation in specific lung units, excessive levels can lead to overdistension and increased intrapulmonary shunt, thereby complicating gas exchange (Wittenstein et al., 2024). The application of PEEP during one-lung ventilation (OLV) can enhance lung aeration, but it also increases the risk of further impairing compliance if not carefully monitored. Therefore, maintaining good lung compliance is crucial to facilitate V/Q matching in various clinical scenarios. Helping the lungs to expand and contract more easily is a key part of treating severe pneumonia or ARDS. A recent study highlighted that comprehensive nursing approaches based on specific therapeutic theories can significantly enhance lung function metrics in pediatric patients, including forced vital capacity (FVC) and oxygen saturation levels (Liu et al., 2025). Using proper supportive care, such as positioning the patient or using drugs, healthcare providers can help the lungs expand and become more flexible. As a result, gas exchange becomes more efficient, allowing the patient to recover more quickly and achieve better outcomes. Therefore, it is crucial to understand and improve lung compliance for effective respiratory care, as it plays a vital role in gas laws and pulmonary pressures.

5.5.2. Airway Resistance and Its Implications

Airway resistance is significant in pulmonary mechanics and affects both gas exchange and how the lungs function. It is when airflow is resisted in the airways, controlled mainly by the size of the airways and how viscous the air is. Changes in airway resistance may cause different pressures in the lungs, which can impair the effectiveness of ventilation. Asthma or COPD causes the airways to narrow, forcing the lungs to work harder, so the respiratory system must generate stronger intrathoracic pressures to breathe. A greater effort can result in more severe hyperinflation, which can complicate the patient's condition and make it difficult for the body to maintain normal oxygen levels in the tissues. Airway resistance also affects the way mechanical ventilation is performed, particularly in newborns. As infants are thought to have fragile airways, uncuffed endotracheal tubes are usually used to prevent injury during protective movements. Recent studies suggest that gas leaks from such tubes can alter normal lung function by reducing tidal volume, compliance, and resistance, particularly when the patient's head position or breathing cycle changes. These findings emphasize the necessity for clinicians to reassess their ventilation strategies, as the unanticipated consequences of airway resistance might lead to inadequate ventilation and compromised oxygen delivery, further complicating patient outcomes in critical care situations (Sinha, 2012). In addition, knowing how airway resistance works supports both practical care and the scientific basis for gas laws relevant to lung pressure. When gas composition is altered, such as adding helium-oxygen to the air during ventilation, it reduces the resistance to breathing and makes breathing easier. For example, helium's low density makes it easier for air to move, which could help with oxygen exchange in people with obstructive lung diseases. As a result, changes in gas properties play a significant role in designing methods to manage airway resistance. Therefore, further research and clinical trials are imperative, particularly focusing on innovative interventions such as gas mixtures and revised respiratory techniques to optimize pulmonary pressures and enhance patient care across various clinical contexts (Figure 5.13).

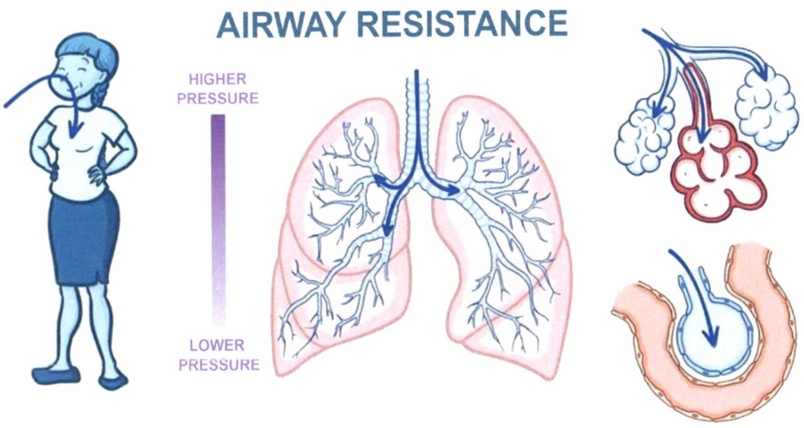

Figure 5.13. Airway resistance.

Source: https://d16qt3wv6xm098.cloudfront.net/1F6F9tpSR0OLV1Po0pFec3g2Se2pdZgt/_.jpg.

5.5.3. Role of Surfactant in Pulmonary Function

Surfactant plays a crucial role in maintaining the lungs' function and stability. Type II alveolar cells produce surfactant, which is a mixture of lipids and proteins, to lessen the tension between air and liquid in the alveoli. Due to the presence of surfactant, the alveoli do not collapse as they empty, which helps the lungs stretch and lowers the effort needed for breathing. This function is vital, especially in premature infants who may be deficient in surfactant, leading to conditions such as respiratory distress syndrome (RDS). Recognizing the role of surfactant helps explain how it facilitates gas laws, particularly by managing pressure changes that enable the exchange of oxygen and carbon dioxide in the lungs. For this reason, enough surfactant is important for healthy and efficient breathing. Surfactant is crucial in preventing lung problems by serving as the first line of defense in the alveoli. It helps to keep the air sacs stable and helps clear out pathogens and irritants inhaled by the lungs. In conditions such as bronchopulmonary dysplasia (BPD), which occurs predominantly in premature infants, surfactant deficiency leads to a cascade of pulmonary injuries and impaired lung development. Because BPD remains a problem, it highlights the need for medical treatments that help manage surfactant and support better breathing in affected babies. Studies have found that when surfactant is used correctly, it can significantly help premature babies breathe better and so reduce the risk of BPD and other chronic lung diseases. It emphasizes the key role played by surfactant and gas laws in determining pressures inside the lungs and how breathing is affected when someone is ill. A deeper understanding of surfactant's biomechanical features can be gained by studying the stability of nanobubbles in the alveolar space. Nanobubbles are able to change how surfactants behave and this behavior goes against traditional views of the stability at liquid-gas interfaces. In particular, the role of Laplace pressure in bubble stability highlights the differences between what is expected by thermodynamics and what actually occurs in the lungs. This investigation can reveal how surfactants facilitate the movement of gases in and out of the lungs, influencing the pressures within the lungs and thereby helping to maintain balance in the respiratory system. As observations on emerging technologies in pulmonary medicine continue to expand, integrating knowledge of both surfactant development and nanobubble dynamics could present new avenues for improving respiratory support in clinical practice, ultimately aiming to mitigate the risks associated with respiratory dysfunction (Figure 5.14).

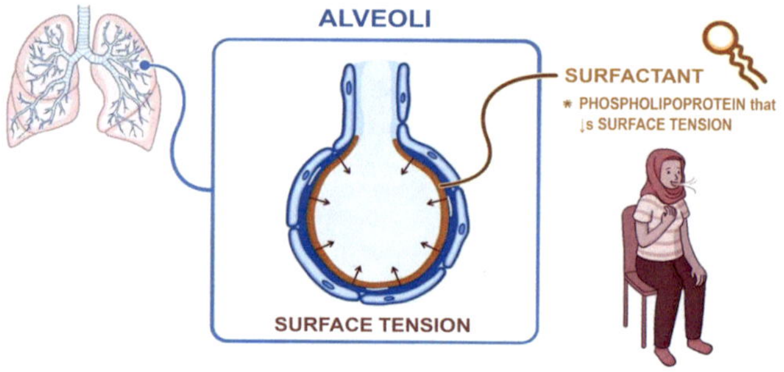

Figure 5.14. Alveolar surface tension and surfactant.

Source: https://d16qt3wv6xm098.cloudfront.net/yrVdywkZQbGwh6XAdG_qKA68QcWgahii/_.jpg.

5.6. Experimental Methods to Measure Pulmonary Pressures

Studying experimental techniques to measure pulmonary pressures shows that both physiology and mathematics are involved. Many approaches exist, but isothermal rebreathing is popular because it allows for the measurement of alveolar VOC concentrations in breath. By using acetone as a prototype, researchers have demonstrated that breath profiles obtained from isothermal rebreathing can challenge some of the theories about inert gas elimination in the lungs, such as those proposed by Farhi. Using this approach, it is evident that physiological outcomes may differ significantly from predictions, which calls for further study of gas exchange in the airway. With this approach, detailed studies of rebreathing protocols can reveal the exact ways gas is ventilated and transported in the lungs. Special ways of analyzing pulmonary pressures have been developed, and mathematical models have helped explain how airway gas exchange affects breathing. They provide a framework that helps explain the differences in blood-breath ratios between experiments conducted in the lab and in living organisms. Including air flow rates, the solubility of gases, and physiological responses in these models, they provide useful and valid numbers that can inform how experiments are designed and understood. A good understanding of how isothermal rebreathing works helps ensure that pulmonary pressure measurements are more accurate, making the data more useful and reliable in various settings. It highlights the importance of using experimental methods that acknowledge physiological differences. Additionally, new technology has expanded the methods for measuring pulmonary pressures experimentally. Using non-invasive monitoring devices enables real-time data collection, allowing for a more detailed assessment of pulmonary function. New studies using advanced respiratory equipment have found strong correlations between pulmonary pressures and patient outcomes during various medical procedures. In this case, gas laws are crucial because they explain how gases behave under various pressure conditions. In this way, experiments can confirm theories and also provide valuable insights for enhancing medical care and discovering new therapies. Combining theory and experimental results is likely to increase our knowledge of pulmonary mechanics and their relevance to medicine and respiratory health.

5.6.1. Techniques for Measuring Intrapulmonary Pressure

Intrapulmonary pressure needs to be measured to fully understand how gases are exchanged and how the lungs function, which follows the gas laws. Several methods have been created to measure this pressure in the lungs, which helps doctors interpret the patient's breathing condition. A common technique involves inserting a balloon into the esophagus using a catheter, which enables the measurement of intrapulmonary pressure by monitoring pressure changes. The esophagus is similar to intrapulmonary pressure because it is adjacent to the thoracic cavity and is influenced by diaphragm movements during breathing. However, this procedure must be practiced carefully by clinicians, as variations in the body can influence the findings. Another method is to use ultrasound, which enables the examination of respiratory mechanics without the need for invasive procedures. With real-time imaging, ultrasound follows changes in the diaphragm to show the activity of breathing in and out. It is beneficial for patients who are very sick or have impaired lung function, as invasive procedures might be dangerous for them. Additionally, new developments in modeling and real-time monitoring tools are expected to provide a clearer picture of intrapulmonary pressure, enabling clinicians to adjust ventilator settings according to each patient's specific needs. The ongoing development in pulmonary medicine suggests that incorporating advanced monitoring may benefit patients. Understanding intrapulmonary pressures is crucial for treating ARDS, as gas exchange in this condition is significantly impaired. The severity of lung injury can be judged, and proper treatment can be set by measuring pressure accurately. Using esophageal balloon monitoring and ultrasound is very useful in this situation, as they provide information on the patient's breathing and allow for interventions to prevent further harm. Ultimately, these evolving methodologies underscore the necessity for precision in measuring intrapulmonary pressure, thereby fostering a better understanding of the intricate relationships between gas laws and pulmonary function in clinical scenarios such as ARDS (Radermacher et al., 2017). Additionally, as therapies like HBOT gain traction, understanding how these pressures interact with treatment outcomes becomes increasingly pertinent (Heyboer et al., 2017) (Figure 5.15).

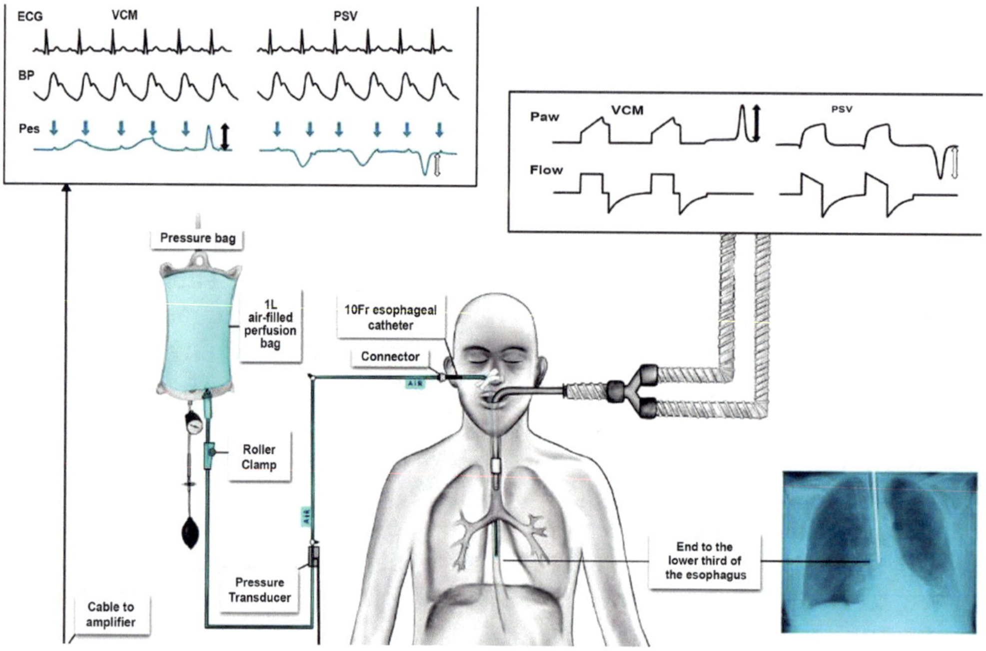

Figure 5.15. Air-filled catheter without balloon method.

Source: https://media.springernature.com/full/springer-static/image/art%3A10.1186%2Fs40635-021-00411-w/MediaObjects/40635_2021_411_Fig1_HTML.png?as=webp.

5.6.2. Methods for Assessing Intrapleural Pressure

Examining intrapleural pressure is essential for understanding lung conditions and optimizing lung therapy. Different ways can be used to measure this pressure, and each has its own strengths and weaknesses. For example, direct measurement methods typically involve inserting pressure transducers into the pleural space through a tube thoracostomy. It enables continuous monitoring of intrapleural pressures, which is crucial for patients with pneumothorax or pleural effusions. Additionally, using ultrasonic or imaging methods, it is possible to estimate intrapleural pressure by considering the patient's anatomy and the principles of fluid movement. Since both methods are useful, the assessment method should be tailored to the situation and the treatment goals. Hyperpolarized gas diffusion MRI is now considered a good alternative for measuring lung mechanics and indirectly measuring intrapleural pressure. The use of hyperpolarized ^129Xe gas enables this method to visualize how different areas of the lungs are functioning and how air moves through them. In particular, hyperpolarized ^129Xe gas MRI enables us to visualize how the pleural space changes in relation to lung function, thereby enhancing our understanding of diseases such as pulmonary fibrosis. By correlating these MRI findings with traditional pulmonary function tests (PFTs), researchers can develop a more holistic understanding of a patient's respiratory mechanics, ultimately leading to improved diagnostic accuracy and therapeutic strategies (Zhang et al., 2024). Additionally, anesthesia and surgical procedures can alter the pressure within the chest cavity, which should be considered. Studies done recently investigate how anesthetic agents influence the lungs' blood flow which can be used to measure intrapleural pressure during complex surgeries like cardiopulmonary bypass indirectly. For example, anesthetics such as propofol may adversely affect lung function and compliance, leading to increased intrapleural pressures postoperatively. In contrast, inhalational agents like sevoflurane have been shown to maintain functional lung parameters during surgery (Taranov et al., 2024). Understanding these interactions helps select the most suitable anesthetic, which may lead to improved lung function and more accurate measurements of pressure within the chest cavity during surgery. Combining these approaches provides a comprehensive method for respiratory care, enhancing the accuracy of measuring pulmonary pressure.

5.6.3. Use of Spirometry in Pulmonary Function Tests

Spirometry is a key part of PFTs for examining how well the lungs are working. Spirometry measures the amount of air the lungs take in and the rate at which it is exhaled, providing important insights into lung function. By employing parameters such as FVC and forced expiratory volume in one second (FEV1), healthcare providers can assess the presence of obstructive or restrictive pulmonary diseases. It is essential to understand Boyle's Law to explain the results, as it demonstrates that pressure and volume in the lungs are inversely related. This relationship is particularly important for asthma or COPD, as spirometric data can accurately measure the amount of air a patient can exhale. So, spirometry is helpful in diagnosing the disease and also for tracking its progress and the effects of treatment. Besides diagnosis, spirometry is helpful in tracking how the lungs are working over an extended period. Regular spirometry tests can indicate if the pressure or volume in the lungs is changing, which may reflect a worsening health issue or the effectiveness of treatment. In individuals who exercise, spirometry can reveal the effects of training on the efficiency and capacity of their lungs during physical activity. Recent studies have utilized spirometry in conjunction with other methods, demonstrating its application in comprehensive lung function tests. The research demonstrating the impact of carrying additional weight on respiratory mechanics reinforces this point; understanding ventilatory responses to increased load not only illuminates pulmonary function but also sheds light on exercise efficacy and safety in various populations (Aliverti et al., 2014). They confirm spirometry's essential function in clinical and sports medicine. New technology in spirometry has improved the accuracy and reliability of checking pulmonary health. Due to handheld spirometers and mobile applications, patients can conduct tests at their convenience, allowing them to take a more active role in managing their health. Additionally, such technologies enable patients to send their spirometric readings to doctors in real-time from anywhere, helping personalize their care. This aligns with the growing understanding that focusing on patients is crucial for treating chronic respiratory diseases. In addition, scientists are looking into the reasons behind ventilatory limits during strenuous exercises, mainly in athletes who have trained. Understanding these intricacies through refined spirometric assessments enables the development of tailored training regimens and improved athletic performance, highlighting the multifaceted applications of spirometry in both clinical and athletic settings (Layton et al., 2013). In this way, incorporating spirometry into routine pulmonary function testing is crucial for enhancing respiratory medicine.

SUMMARY

The interaction between gas laws and pulmonary pressures is crucial for both respiratory function and medical treatment. Boyle's Law and Henry's Law, which are gas laws, help explain how gases behave in the lungs under different pressures and volumes. They explain the processes by which oxygen is taken up and carbon dioxide is removed, which are necessary for maintaining balance and ensuring a good blood supply to body tissues. In addition to physiology, these principles are also useful in the clinical setting for managing conditions such as COPD and ARDS. Following these guidelines, healthcare workers can make sure treatments help patients exchange gases properly, which reduces the risk of complications and death. Additionally, HBOT and other emerging treatments demonstrate how gas laws can be applied to address hypoxemia and the associated issues. It has been shown in recent research that HBOT uses Henrys Law to increase the amount of oxygen in the blood when pressure is raised. It has been successful in treating severe COVID-19 pneumonia, as traditional oxygen therapy was not effective. Those who received HBOT showed improved oxygen saturation, indicating that gas laws are successfully applied in clinical settings. Furthermore, the mechanism by which HBOT impacts mitochondrial function and downstream inflammatory processes demonstrates the profound implications of gas dynamics in therapeutic settings, reinforcing the necessity for an integrated understanding of pulmonary pressures and gas behavior in modern medicine (Harch, 2020). Ultimately, understanding gas laws and pulmonary pressures enables a deeper understanding of respiratory physiology and facilitates the development of innovative treatment methods. Using science in healthcare shows how gas behavior is linked to lung health. With more research being conducted on pulmonary pathophysiology, healthcare professionals should stay informed to provide evidence-based care. The ongoing exploration of gas laws in a clinical context will undoubtedly yield new insights and potential therapies aimed at improving patient outcomes, particularly in an era marked by the increasing prevalence of pulmonary diseases and global health challenges (Budrevi et al., 2020).

To understand how the lungs and metabolism work, it is essential to recognize the connection between gas laws and pulmonary pressures. Gas laws explain that the actions of gases such as oxygen and carbon dioxide are affected by changes in pressure and temperature inside the lungs. Boyle's Law shows that when the temperature is held constant, the pressure and volume of a gas are inversely related. Changes in thoracic volume during breathing cause pressure changes that facilitate the movement of air in and out of the lungs. All respiratory phases adhere to this rule, demonstrating that gas laws play a crucial role in facilitating efficient pulmonary ventilation and gas exchange in the alveoli to meet metabolic demands. The control of pulmonary pressures by gas laws can reveal important insights about the heart and the body's energy utilization. If oxygen or carbon dioxide partial pressures change, it can have a significant effect on cell activity and the blood flow in the brain. Research indicates that proper matching between metabolic demands and physiological delivery mechanisms is essential for maintaining critical brain functions, as highlighted in Claassen et al. (2021). If there are changes in these pressures, hypoxia or hypercapnia may result, which can seriously harm both health and mental function. It is crucial to understand these factors in clinical practice, especially when evaluating patients with breathing difficulties or issues with gas exchange. The link between gas laws and pulmonary pressures shows that good ventilation and perfusion are essential for life support. Last but not least, recent guidelines on emergency care and resuscitation stress that these principles should be followed when choosing treatments for patients with respiratory failure. The 2021 European Resuscitation Council Guidelines reflect a synthesis of current evidence demonstrating how effective emergency response hinges on understanding the underlying gas laws that influence pulmonary pressures (Gavin et al., 2021). They stress that immediate actions are needed to correct gas exchange problems that happen during cardiac arrest or trauma. People trained in resuscitation learn how to perform basic and advanced life support, and also understand how gas movement affects outcomes in critical situations. Therefore, applying gas laws in managing pulmonary pressure is crucial for everyday care and for making informed decisions in emergency situations.

CLOSER LOOK

PULMONARY EDEMA

Pulmonary edema is a condition in which the lungs become filled with fluid, making it difficult to breathe. This fluid buildup can occur in the air sacs (alveoli) or the lung tissue itself. The fluid interferes with the regular exchange of oxygen and carbon dioxide, leading to various symptoms (Figure 5.16).

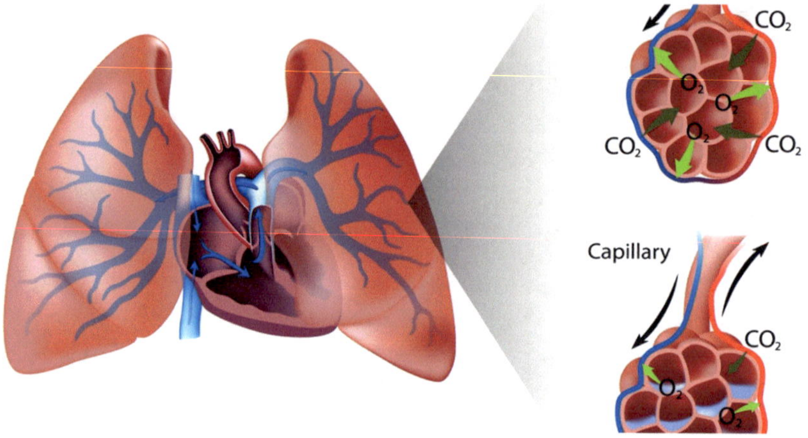

Figure 5.16. Pulmonary edema.

Source: https://cdn-epico.nitrocdn.com/mBHJEeYkdSseARCwzDBzsrjorjknQwQh/assets/images/optimized/rev-19dce78/sukino.com/wp-content/uploads/2024/02/Vital-Role-of-Respiratory-Rehab-in-Treating-Pulmonary-Edema.png.

Causes

- **Cardiogenic:** Heart problems, such as heart failure, can cause fluid to accumulate in the lungs.
- **Non-cardiogenic: Other conditions, such as pneumonia, high-altitude exposure, or certain medications, can also cause** pulmonary edema.

Symptoms

- **Shortness of Breath**: This is a common symptom, often described as difficulty breathing or a feeling of breathlessness.
- **Orthopnea**: Difficulty breathing while lying down.
- **Coughing**: A persistent cough, sometimes with frothy or pink-tinged sputum.
- **Wheezing**: Abnormal breathing sounds.

- **Rapid Breathing**: The body may attempt to compensate for low oxygen levels by increasing its breathing rate.
- **Cyanosis**: Bluish discoloration of the skin, particularly around the lips and fingertips.
- **Anxiety or Restlessness**: Due to difficulty breathing.
- **Fatigue**: The body may become easily tired.
- **Swelling**: Fluid retention may cause swelling in the legs, ankles, or feet.
- **Elevated Heart Rate**: The heart may beat faster to compensate for the lungs.

Diagnosis

- **Physical Exam:** A doctor will listen to your lungs for crackles and rapid breathing, and examine your heart for abnormal rhythms.
- **Blood Tests:** To check oxygen levels, electrolyte levels, kidney function, liver function, blood counts, and heart failure markers.
- **Imaging Studies:** Chest X-rays or CT scans can help visualize the fluid buildup.

Treatment

- **Improve Respiratory Function:** This may involve using medications to reduce fluid buildup, oxygen therapy, or mechanical ventilation.
- **Treat the Underlying Cause:** Addressing the underlying heart problem or other condition that causes pulmonary edema is crucial.
- **Prevent Further Damage:** To prevent future episodes, measures such as medication adherence, lifestyle changes, and follow-up care may be recommended.

Pulmonary edema can be a serious condition, and prompt medical attention is crucial, especially for acute cases, which can be life-threatening.

REFERENCES

1. Alamé, K., & Mahesh, K. (2024). Effect of gas content on cavitation nuclei. *Journal of Fluid Mechanics, 982*. https://doi.org/10.1017/jfm.2024.79Albanese, A. (2014). *Physiology-Based Mathematical Models for the Intensive Care Unit: APPLICATION to Mechanical Ventilation*. https://core.ac.uk/download/161447562.pdf (accessed on 31st May 2025).
2. Albanese, A., Cheng, L., Ursino, M., & Chbat, N. W. (2015). An integrated mathematical model of the human cardiopulmonary system: Model development. *AJP Heart and Circulatory Physiology, 310*, H899–H921. https://doi.org/10.1152/ajpheart.00230.2014 (accessed on 31st May 2025).
3. Alcendor, D. J. (2020). Racial disparities-associated COVID-19 mortality among minority populations in the US. *Journal of Clinical Medicine, 9*, 2442. https://doi.org/10.3390/jcm9082442 (accessed on 31st May 2025).
4. Alheshibri, M., Qian, J., Jéhannin, M., & Craig, V. S. J. (2016). A history of nanobubbles. *Langmuir, 32*, 11086–11100. https://doi.org/10.1021/acs.langmuir.6b02489 (accessed on 31st May 2025).
5. Aliverti, A., Harms, C. A., Shirley, D., Ross, E., Borg, G. A., et al. (2014). *Thoracic Load Carriage-Induced Respiratory Muscle Fatigue*. https://core.ac.uk/download/77059990.pdf (accessed on 31st May 2025).
6. Amann, A., Hinterhuber, H., King, J., Koc, H., et al. (2011). A modeling-based evaluation of isothermal rebreathing for breath gas analyses of highly soluble volatile organic compounds. *J. Breath Res.* http://arxiv.org/abs/1105.0864 (accessed on 31st May 2025).
7. Amann, A., Lumb, A. B., Schrikker, A. C., Mörk, A. K., Amann, A., Amann, A., Anton, A., et al. (2010). *A Mathematical Model for Breath Gas Analysis of Volatile Organic Compounds with Special Emphasis on Acetone*. http://arxiv.org/abs/1003.4475 (accessed on 31st May 2025).
8. Anderson, N. V. E. (2024). Progress towards the integration of experimental and computational techniques to better understand the delivered dose of aerosolized medication. https://core.ac.uk/download/613908463.pdf (accessed on 31st May 2025).
9. Barnes, E. G. (1949). Persistent cavities in pulmonary tuberculosis: A critical inquiry into the principles underlying causation and means of treatment; with a study of four cases. https://core.ac.uk/download/429724518.pdf (accessed on 31st May 2025).
10. Bossé, Y., Riesenfeld, E., Paré, P. D., & Irvin, C. G. (2010). It's not all smooth muscle: Non-smooth-muscle elements in control of resistance to airflow. *Annual Review of Physiology, 72*, 437–462. https://doi.org/10.1146/annurev-physiol-021909-135851 (accessed on 31st May 2025).
11. Budrevičiūtė, A., Damiati, S., Sabir, D. K., Önder, K., Schuller-Goetzburg, P., Plakys, G., Katileviciute, A., et al. (2020). Management and prevention strategies for non-communicable diseases (NCDs) and their risk factors. *Frontiers in Public Health, 8*. https://doi.org/10.3389/fpubh.2020.574111 (accessed on 31st May 2025).
12. Chen, Y., Zhang, S., Lu, X., Xie, W., Wang, C., & Zhai, Z. (2024). Unusual cause of muscle weakness, type II respiratory failure and pulmonary hypertension: A case report of ryanodine receptor type 1 (RYR1)-related myopathy. *BMC Pulmonary Medicine, 24*. https://www.semanticscholar.org/paper/d28441aa92e9020299980330340f46fdaa9370c9 (accessed on 31st May 2025).

13. Claassen, J. A. H. R., Thijssen, D. H. J., Panerai, R. B., & Faraci, F. M. (2021). Regulation of cerebral blood flow in humans: Physiology and clinical implications of autoregulation. *Physiological Reviews, 101*, 1487–1559. https://doi.org/10.1152/physrev.00022.2020 (accessed on 31st May 2025).

14. Dorchak, K. J., Greenleaf, J. E., Kollias, J., Vanderveer, J. B., et al. (2025). *Physiologic Responses to Water Immersion in Man: A Compendium of Research.* https://core.ac.uk/download/pdf/42884411.pdf (accessed on 31st May 2025).

15. Febrianti, W., Hendriansyah, E., Imani, K. A., Harielpaniadi, M. A., Sari, N. N., & Hartini, T. I. (2024). Understanding the interaction between pressure and volume in gas systems through Boyle's law practicum. *Islamic Journal of Integrated Science Education (IJISE)*. https://www.semanticscholar.org/paper/b675d2d109d29945c0399a97858781389cae1538 (accessed on 31st May 2025).

16. Furr, P. A., Monson, C. B., Peterson, D. H., Santoro, T., et al. (2025). Extravehicular activities limitations study. *Physiological Limitations to Extravehicular Activity in Space* (Vol. 1). https://core.ac.uk/download/pdf/42829415.pdf (accessed on 31st May 2025).

17. Goodwin, P. C., & Sanderson, P. (2015). *Evidence for the Use of Hyperbaric Oxygen Therapy (HBOT)*. https://core.ac.uk/download/161890001.pdf (accessed on 31st May 2025).

18. Griva, P., Talliou, C., Rougeris, L., Samara, D., Panagouli, K., Varvarousi, G., Papa, M., et al. (2024). Restoration of pulmonary compliance after laparoscopic gynecologic surgery using a recruitment maneuver. *Journal of Personalized Medicine, 14*. https://www.semanticscholar.org/paper/4ff6098bec318271dc133ad8cfacf21dbc2ba032 (accessed on 31st May 2025).

19. Harch, P. (2020). Hyperbaric oxygen treatment of novel coronavirus (COVID-19) respiratory failure. *Medical Gas Research, 10*, 61, 62. https://www.semanticscholar.org/paper/83e6ea0a322c63e667a942395c4af3f0287a58f2 (accessed on 31st May 2025).

20. Harch, P. G. (2020). Hyperbaric oxygen treatment of novel coronavirus (COVID-19) respiratory failure. *Medical Gas Research, 10*, 61. https://doi.org/10.4103/2045-9912.282177 (accessed on 31st May 2025).

21. Heyboer, M., Sharma, D., Santiago, W., & McCulloch, N. (2017). Hyperbaric oxygen therapy: Side effects defined and quantified. *Advances in Wound Care, 6*, 210–224. https://doi.org/10.1089/wound.2016.0718 (accessed on 31st May 2025).

22. Kalikkot, T., R., Cuevas, G. M., & Shivanna, B. (2017). Bronchopulmonary dysplasia: A review of athogenesis and pathophysiology. *Respiratory Medicine, 132*, 170–177. https://doi.org/10.1016/j.rmed.2017.10.014 (accessed on 31st May 2025).

23. Layton, A. M. (2013). *Ventilatory Mechanics in Endurance Athletes*. https://core.ac.uk/download/161444077.pdf (accessed on 31st May 2025).

24. Li, X., Yang, Y., Zhang, Q., Zhu, Y., Xu, W., Zhao, Y., Liu, Y., et al. (2024). Association between thoracic epidural anesthesia and driving pressure in adult patients undergoing elective major upper abdominal surgery: A randomized controlled trial. *BMC Anesthesiology, 24*. https://www.semanticscholar.org/paper/c97d8ab8cb4d348938af7053751a148eeddaf798 (accessed on 31st May 2025).

25. Liu, X., Jin, J., Lin, C., Ye, W., Xu, X., & Chen, X. (2025). Impact of comprehensive nursing based on the "3H" theory on blood gas, recovery speed and lung function in children with severe

pneumonia. *Signa Vitae*. https://www.semanticscholar.org/paper/310d602ad0698f7fff948ca5b494dac111d55590 (accessed on 31st May 2025).

26. Lv, J., Chen, L., & Wang, H. (2024). The diagnostic and predictive value of biomarkers for pulmonary fibrosis in patients with Coronavirus Disease 2019. *Journal of Global Infectious Diseases, 16*, 45–53. https://www.semanticscholar.org/paper/cfec21bd9a93f069d90718f5a6028ef6c8dae20d (accessed on 31st May 2025).

27. McNulty, W., & Usmani, O. S. (2014). Techniques of assessing small airways dysfunction. *European Clinical Respiratory Journal, 1*, 25898. https://doi.org/10.3402/ecrj.v1.25898 (accessed on 31st May 2025).

28. Nairn, J. R. (1966). *Mainly About Emphysema of the Lungs: A Study on Different Aspects of a Disease* (Vo. I). https://core.ac.uk/download/286351682.pdf (accessed on 31st May 2025).

29. National Institute for Occupational Safety and Health Division of Standards Development and Technology Transfer. (2025). *Radon Progeny in Underground Mines*. https://core.ac.uk/download/144184123.pdf (accessed on 31st May 2025).

30. Perkins, G. D., Gräsner, J. T., Semeraro, F., Olasveengen, T. M., Soar, J., Lott, C., Van de Voorde, P., et al. (2021). European Resuscitation Council Guidelines 2021: Executive summary. *Resuscitation, 161*, 1–60. https://doi.org/10.1016/j.resuscitation.2021.02.003 (accessed on 31st May 2025).

31. Pleil, J. D., Geer Wallace, M. A., Davis, M. D., & Matty, C. (2021). The physics of human breathing: Flow, timing, volume, and pressure parameters for normal, on-demand, and ventilator respiration. *Journal of Breath Research, 15*, 042002. https://doi.org/10.1088/1752-7163/ac2589 (accessed on 31st May 2025).

32. Radermacher, P., Maggiore, S. M., & Mercat, A. (2017). Fifty years of research in ARDS: Gas exchange in acute respiratory distress syndrome. *American Journal of Respiratory and Critical Care Medicine, 196*, 964–984. https://doi.org/10.1164/rccm.201610-2156so (accessed on 31st May 2025).

33. Rissmiller, R. W., & Ennis, J. W. (2018). *Pulmonary Function Testing and Sarcoidosis: A Review* (Vol. 2). https://www.semanticscholar.org/paper/eb9c1ee550a195faa22a89fe65086c3590e548b6 (accessed on 31st May 2025).

34. Santos, J. (2020). *Ventilator: An Analysis of the History, Design, and Current World Implications*. https://core.ac.uk/download/479046406.pdf (accessed on 31st May 2025).

35. Schramm, W. (2022). *The (Human) Respiratory Rate at Rest*. http://arxiv.org/abs/2210.01673 (accessed on 31st May 2025).

36. Sinha, S. (2012). Endotracheal tube leakage in babies receiving mechanical ventilation: A bane or a boon? *Journal of Pediatric Intensive Care, 1*, 47–48. https://www.semanticscholar.org/paper/42e2ef8ae207a3619bac641b297401246018cd25 (accessed on 31st May 2025).

37. Taranov, E. V., Pastukhova, N. K., Pichugin, V., Fedorov, S. A., Brichkin, Y. D., Nezabudkin, S. N., ZhIlyaev, S. A., et al. (2024). Comparative assessment of the effect of anesthetics (propofol, sevoflurane, desflurane) on hemodynamics and gas exchange in the lungs during operations for acute pulmonary embolism. *Messenger of Anesthesiology and Resuscitation*. https://www.semanticscholar.org/paper/3f990607f6b756d6e9ff6cafb0f383ea45ae0f7d (accessed on 31st May 2025).

38. Varkey, B. (2020). Principles of clinical ethics and their application to practice. *Medical Principles and Practice, 30*, 17–28. https://doi.org/10.1159/000509119 (accessed on 31st May 2025).

39. Wittenstein, J., Scharffenberg, M., Fröhlich, J., Rothmann, C., Ran, X., Zhang, Y., Chai, Y., et al. (2024). Effects of positive end-expiratory pressure on pulmonary perfusion distribution and intrapulmonary shunt during one-lung ventilation in pigs: A randomized crossover study. *Anesthesiology, 141*, 44–55. https://www.semanticscholar.org/paper/da8c0493c78e477cf7c79fcaf39168649a9c666e (accessed on 31st May 2025).

40. Woods Hole Oceanographic Institution. (1982). *Oceanus*. https://core.ac.uk/download/pdf/4513626.pdf (accessed on 31st May 2025).

41. Zhang, M., Li, H., Xiao, Y., Li, H., Liu, X., Zhao, X., Zheng, Y., et al. (2024). Assessment of global and regional lung compliance in pulmonary fibrosis with hyperpolarized gas MRI. *Journal of Magnetic Resonance Imaging: JMRI*. https://www.semanticscholar.org/paper/af9902f463dda7560b601d525e6e665999f14b09 (accessed on 31st May 2025).

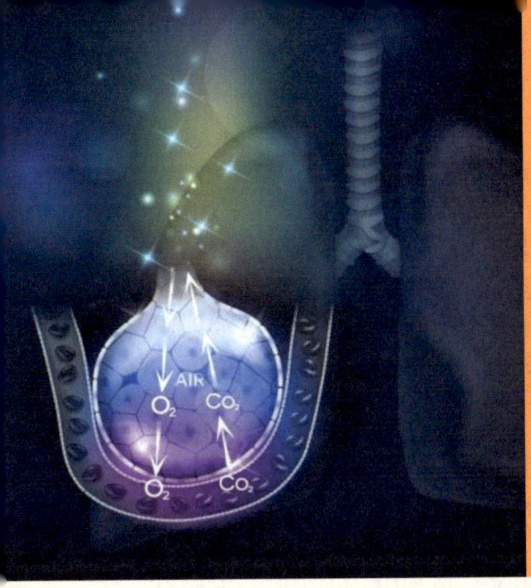

Chapter 6

DIFFUSION OF GASES IN THE LUNGS

Contents

Introduction

Gas diffusion in the lungs is very important for the exchange of oxygen and carbon dioxide between the alveoli and blood. Fick's Law of Diffusion is the basis for this mechanism, which means that the rate of diffusion depends on the surface area, the difference in partial pressures, the diffusivity of the gas, and the inverse of the membrane thickness. Understanding how these variables interact can reveal how gas exchange is facilitated, and this process can be altered by conditions such as COPD or pulmonary fibrosis. If the alveolar-capillary membrane thickens or the surface area is reduced, the lungs' ability to exchange gases can be significantly impaired, leading to reduced oxygen uptake and increased carbon dioxide retention in the blood. The diffusion capacity of the lung, often measured via the diffusing capacity of the lung for carbon monoxide (DLCO), serves as a pivotal indicator of pulmonary function. DLCO tells us about the size of the alveolar surface and the condition of the alveolar-capillary membrane, which gives information about a patient's lung health. It is essential in clinical settings because it helps doctors diagnose several lung diseases. If the alveolar membrane is damaged, it may cause a drop in DLCO which means the lungs are not exchanging gases properly. Advances in imaging technologies, such as hyperpolarized 129Xe MRI, enable non-invasive assessments of lung function and can reveal changes in the lung microstructure that impact gas diffusion (Dregely et al., 2010). The combination of imaging and physiological data provides a more comprehensive picture of an individual's lung health. Factors affecting gas exchange go beyond the mechanical properties of the lung and include physiological aspects such as blood flow distribution and ventilation-perfusion (V/Q) matching. Any change that disrupts this balance can cause gas exchange to work less effectively, which may be seen clinically as hypoxemia or hypercarbia. When someone has pulmonary embolism or regional lung disease, the V/Q ratio can become very imbalanced, which can result in a major drop in arterial oxygen levels. Additionally, factors such as age, altitude, and exercise can also affect how gases are diffused in the body. So, using various methods to understand gas diffusion is necessary to develop good strategies for treating respiratory diseases. An enhanced understanding of these mechanisms is crucial, as outlined in contemporary educational resources on human physiology, which aim to bridge the gap between theoretical knowledge and clinical application (Shokr et al., 2016).

Definition of Gas Diffusion

Gas diffusion occurs when gas molecules move from areas of higher concentration to areas of lower concentration due to the concentration gradient. This tendency is significant in biological systems (mainly in the lungs) where air and blood exchange gases efficiently. Gas diffusion is crucial for understanding how oxygen enters the blood and carbon dioxide is removed. The process can be explained using Fick's Law of Diffusion, which says that the rate of diffusion depends on the difference in concentration, the surface area involved, and the diffusion coefficient of the gas. They not only change the rate at which gases are exchanged but also the effectiveness of breathing in keeping the body's balance and providing energy. Another key aspect of gas diffusion is the DLCO—Diffusing Capacity of the Lung for Carbon Monoxide, which measures the lungs' ability to diffuse gases. It shows how easily gases can move through the alveolar-capillary membrane. Special breathing tests are conducted, and patients are asked to inhale a small amount of non-toxic carbon monoxide for a short period, then hold their breath. Research indicates that measuring DLCO is integral to diagnosing various pulmonary conditions, as highlighted in a study that shows differences in DLCO values across patient populations, including individuals with COPD and interstitial lung disease (ILD) (Magro et al., 2012). Also, how much gas can be exchanged depends on how many alveoli there are and how much gas space is available, which underlines the importance of gas diffusion in respiratory physiology. The efficiency of gas diffusion in the lungs is affected by several things, such as temperature, the levels of respiratory gases, and any abnormalities in the lungs. As an illustration, oxygen and carbon dioxide move through diffusion because their partial pressure gradients cause them to move from areas of high to low pressure. Various conditions, such as COPD, can alter these gradients and lead to inadequate gas exchange, emphasizing the clinical relevance of understanding gas diffusion in respiratory health (Lindenmaier et al., 2015). Additionally, the thickness of the alveolar-capillary membrane and the degree of lung structure also play a significant role in the diffusion process. Therefore, a comprehensive understanding of gas diffusion mechanics is imperative for both clinical assessments and the development of therapeutic strategies in pulmonary medicine (Figure 6.1).

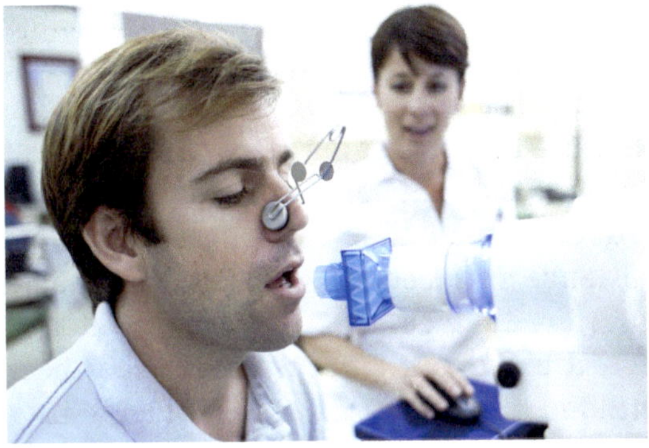

Figure 6.1. Patient undergoing a lung diffusion capacity test.

Source: https://cdn-prod.medicalnewstoday.com/content/images/articles/325/325484/man-having-lung-diffusion-test.jpg.

Importance of Gas Exchange in Respiration

Respiration relies on effective gas exchange, which facilitates the entry of oxygen into the blood and the removal of carbon dioxide. It is mainly in the alveoli that oxygen molecules move into the pulmonary capillaries due to the differences in their partial pressure. This process is clarified by Fick's Law of Diffusion, which states that the speed of gas transfer depends on the surface area and the difference in partial pressures of the gases. When gas exchange is at its best, the body's tissues get enough oxygen and efficiently get rid of carbon dioxide. The importance of maintaining this balance is underscored in various pathophysiological contexts, such as chronic heart failure, where impaired gas transfer can significantly hinder an individual's respiratory efficiency and overall health, as noted in research addressing the condition's impact on diffusing capacity (Binks, 2022). There are many and varied elements that influence gas exchange, and understanding them is necessary to assess how the lungs are working. How much the alveolar membrane thickens, the space for gas exchange, and any lung diseases can all influence how efficiently gas exchange takes place. When membranes thicken, as in fibrosis, oxygen absorption and carbon dioxide removal are reduced, which may result in hypoxemia. COPD and similar conditions also reduce the amount of surface area available for gas diffusion, which can lower the effectiveness of exchanging gases. As highlighted in pulmonary physiology literature, optimizing these factors can lead to improved respiratory function and patient outcomes, particularly in pre-clinical environments where future medical professionals are trained (Binks, 2022).

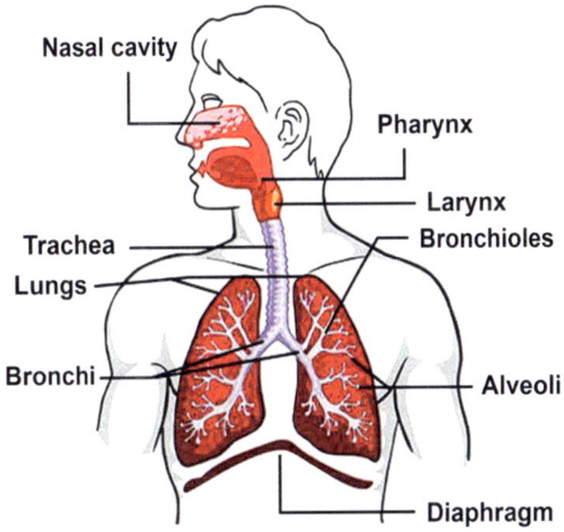

Figure 6.2. Gas exchange in humans.

Source: https://o.quizlet.com/zhSW9-iObLkyuNFypCFqcw.jpg.

The assessment of diffusing capacity, often measured through the diffusion capacity of the lung for carbon monoxide (DLCO), is a vital diagnostic tool in evaluating respiratory health. A low DLCO can suggest that some underlying problems are affecting the exchange of gases, such as emphysema or diseases of the pulmonary vessels. Measuring the efficiency of gas transfer across the alveolar-capillary membrane helps healthcare providers determine the severity of lung damage and select the appropriate treatment. Also, knowing how partial pressures work in gas exchange helps us appreciate the delicate balance needed for good respiration. Ultimately, maintaining optimal gas exchange is imperative not only for individual health but also for overall physiological homeostasis, reinforcing the critical role it plays in respiration and clinical outcomes (Guazzi, 2000) (Figure 6.2).

6.1. Fick's Law of Diffusion

To understand how gases move in and out of the lungs, Fick's Law of Diffusion is very important. law that the rate of diffusion of a gas through a membrane depends on how much area is available and the difference in partial pressures of the gas on both sides of the membrane. It is essential in respiratory physiology because the large surface area of the alveolar-capillary membrane helps the body take in oxygen and release carbon dioxide. As gases exchange, the partial pressures of oxygen (PaO_2) and carbon dioxide ($PaCO_2$) play vital roles, driving the movement of these gases down their concentration gradients. Therefore, knowing Fick's Law makes it easier to see how the lungs work and how any disturbance in this balance can affect breathing and gas exchange. In clinical practice, the measurement of the lungs' diffusion capacity (DLCO) provides critical insights into alveolar function, as it closely relates to Fick's Law of Diffusion. Clinicians use the assessment of gas exchange at the alveolar-capillary interface to detect if lung diseases are affecting this function. The usual way to measure DLCO is by having patients inhale a mixture of carbon monoxide, hold their breath for a few seconds and then exhale. Studies indicate that lung diseases can significantly alter the diffusion capacity of the lungs, leading to decreased DLCO values, particularly in patients with conditions such as COPD and interstitial lung disease (ILD) (Magro et al., 2012). Subsequently, understanding Fick's Law aids in interpreting pulmonary function tests (PFTs) and informs decision-making in patient care and treatment. Moreover, the fact that diffusion-related issues in extremely premature babies last for a long time shows the effects of Fick's Law on gas exchange. Research has documented that such individuals often experience reduced lung diffusion capacities and altered alveolar structures, which can affect their overall respiratory health into adulthood (Satrell et al., 2022). Fick's Law is linked to developmental respiratory problems, therefore it is essential to monitor and assist affected individuals early. As medical science continues to evolve, comprehending the intricate relationship between Ficks Law of Diffusion and conditions resulting from compromised lung function remains pivotal for improving health outcomes and enhancing respiratory rehabilitation strategies across diverse patient demographics (Figure 6.3).

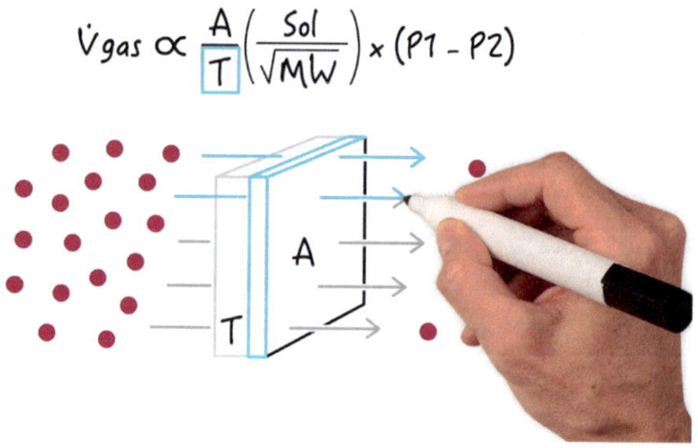

Figure 6.3. Fick's law of diffusion.

Source: https://i.ytimg.com/vi/tDsK0eyuhAk/maxresdefault.jpg.

6.1.1. Explanation of Fick's Law

Fick's Law explains how gases pass through membranes, which is especially important for understanding how the lungs function. It is stated in this law that the speed of diffusion of a gas is connected to its surface area, the difference in partial pressures, the solubility in the membrane and inversely to the thickness of the membrane. At the alveolar-capillary interface, these factors are crucial for efficient gas exchange, allowing oxygen to enter the blood and carbon dioxide to leave the body. Increasing the surface area of the alveoli, for instance, enhances the rate of diffusion, which is especially important during periods of increased metabolic demand, such as exercise or heightened physical activity, confirming the relevance of Fick's Law in pulmonary physiology as outlined in Binks (2022). Also, different physical and medical conditions can strongly affect how Fick's Law is used in the lungs. As an example, chronic heart failure can change the lungs and their function, which may make it harder for gas exchange to take place. Stress failure at the alveolar-capillary interface, which describes the changes there, means that when pulmonary capillary pressure rises, the interstitium becomes thicker and the capillaries become more permeable.

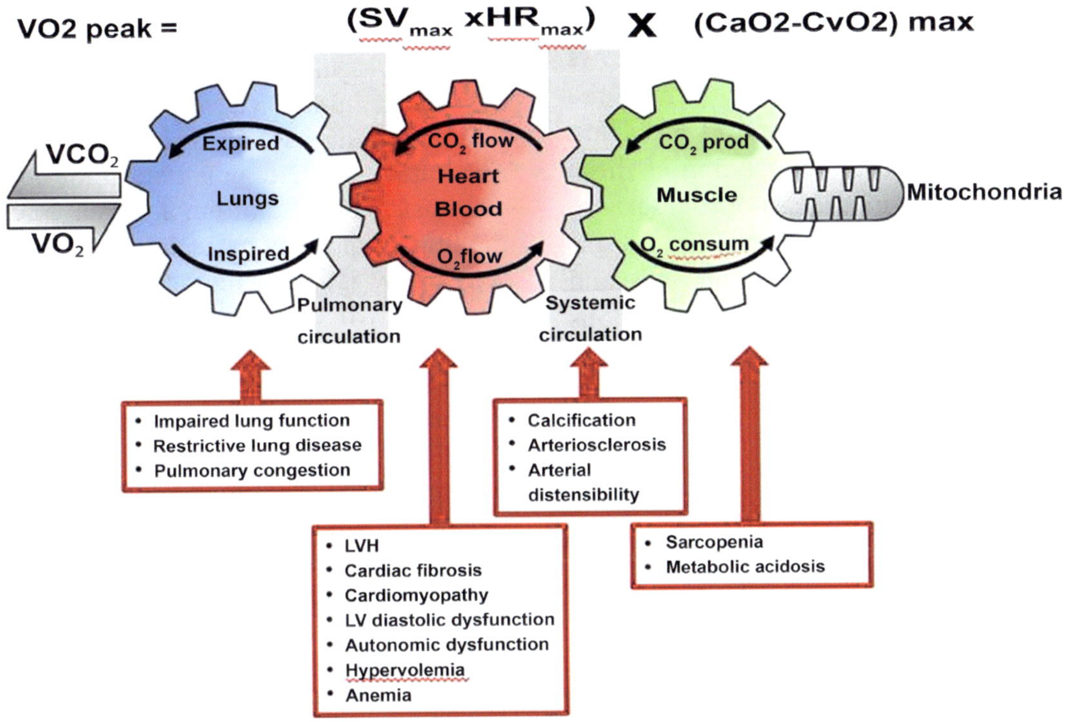

Figure 6.4. The Fick equation and the coupling of external and cellular respiration. The three interlinked gears represent the functional interdependence between the lungs, circulation and muscle.

Source: https://www.researchgate.net/publication/344296785/figure/fig2/AS:11431281255801640@1719440083578/The-Fick-equation-and-the-coupling-of-external-and-cellular-respiration-The-three.tif.

Because of these changes, gas transfer becomes more difficult, which reduces the efficiency of oxygen uptake and carbon dioxide removal. When these alterations disrupt the delicate balance described by Fick's Law, the body may experience reduced exercise tolerance and ventilatory complications, emphasizing the law's critical implications for understanding lung pathology as exemplified in Guazzi (2000). Furthermore, the diffusion capacity of the lungs (DLCO) serves as a clinical measure that encapsulates the principles outlined in Fick's Law by evaluating the efficiency of gas transfer across the alveolar-capillary membrane. The diffusion capacity of the lung (DLCO) depends on the surface area for diffusion, the gas being exchanged, and the condition of the alveolar-capillary membrane. If the DLCO is reduced in clinical work, it usually suggests that the lungs are affected by a respiratory disease, and further tests should be conducted to determine the cause. It shows that Fick's Law is necessary for guiding the diagnosis and treatment of respiratory problems. Ultimately, a nuanced understanding of these principles enables healthcare providers to appreciate how various conditions impact gas exchange, thereby enhancing patient care and outcomes associated with respiratory conditions linked to diminished lung function and impaired gas diffusion (Figure 6.4).

6.1.2. Application of Fick's Law to Respiratory Physiology

How gases diffuse in the lungs is explained by applying Fick's Law to respiratory physiology. Fick's Law describes the way the rate of diffusion, the change in concentration, and the properties of the medium are related. In the lungs, it explains the movement of oxygen and carbon dioxide through the alveolar-capillary membrane. The partial pressure of gases is significantly higher in alveolar air than in the blood; this makes gas exchange is efficient, allowing oxygen to move into the blood and carbon dioxide to move out. Based on physiological literature, measuring these gradients helps healthcare professionals evaluate respiratory function and identify any potential problems. So, Fick's Law is applicable for explaining the process and also for measuring how well the lungs exchange gases in clinical situations. Fick's Law plays a major role in influencing the DLCO, which is also an important factor. It demonstrates how effectively the lungs can exchange gases between the alveoli and the blood. The surface area, thickness of the membrane, and the ease with which respiratory gases dissolve all play a role in affecting DLCO. Advanced imaging tools, for example, those used in hyperpolarized 129Xe, have been created to observe changes in lung microstructure that might influence gas diffusion. By utilizing multiple exchange time xenon magnetization transfer contrast (MXTC), researchers can obtain localized information about tissue-to-alveolar volume ratios and wall thickness, highlighting how alterations in these ratios can impact gas exchange capabilities. Understanding how diffusion capacity impacts respiratory physiology is crucial for accurately diagnosing COPD and emphysema. Because of the impact of many variables on gas exchange, Fick's Law is more important in respiratory physiology. If there is inflammation, changes in surface tension or edema, gas diffusion will be significantly affected. Such changes in the body can make the membrane thicker or smaller, which reduces the amount of oxygen that gets into the blood and the amount of carbon dioxide that leaves. Additionally, the interaction between oxygen and carbon dioxide partial pressures illustrates the active nature of respiratory actions. With advancements in medical understanding and imaging, it has become imperative to keep abreast of these developments to enhance diagnostic and therapeutic strategies in medicine further (Dregely et al., 2010; Shokr et al., 2016). Such knowledge of gas exchange biometrics can lead to the development of new non-invasive methods that accurately assess lung function and aid in the treatment of respiratory diseases.

6.1.3. Limitations of Fick's Law in Complex Biological Systems

Fick's Law of diffusion is useful for learning about gas exchange, but it does not work well for understanding how gases move in the lungs.

It is often not true that the concentration gradient is uniform in the alveolar architecture, which is a primary limitation. There are many different-sized airspaces and blood vessels in the lungs, which cause partial pressures to change unevenly. In a heterogeneous environment, the straightforward Fick's Law model might not accurately show how gases such as oxygen and carbon dioxide diffuse. For this reason, such a limitation can cause errors in assessing gas exchange efficiency and might impact the understanding of respiratory diseases where the exchange of gases is affected. Besides variations in structure, blood flow, and any pathophysiological problems can make it difficult to use Fick's Law. When we exercise, the body requires more oxygen, which can alter blood flow.

This change in blood flow can affect the rate of diffusion and lead to results that do not follow Fick's predictions. Additionally, conditions such as pulmonary fibrosis or COPD can alter the area where gas exchange occurs, making Fick's Law less accurate. Dynamic physiological changes are crucial in gas exchange, which makes the use of advanced methods necessary. These methods can handle lung conditions that differ which helps to better represent varying gas diffusion characteristics within the lungs. Using hyperpolarized 129Xe MRI is a recent example of a promising approach to addressing these issues. This imaging modality enables a non-invasive examination of gas exchange dynamics by characterizing parameters such as the tissue-to-alveolar volume ratio and alveolar wall thickness, which are crucial for understanding diffusion efficiency in pathological states (Dregely et al., 2010). Additionally, supported liquid membranes (SLMs) offer a novel filtration perspective that could further elucidate the mechanisms of diffusion under complex conditions, enhancing our understanding of gas transport at both macro and micro levels. When researchers use these advanced techniques, they can link the traditional Fickian models with the complexities of gas exchange in the body, which helps improve ways to diagnose and treat different lung diseases.

6.2. Mechanism of Gas Diffusion

The rate of gas diffusion in the lungs is mainly controlled by Fick's Law, which says that the rate increases as the concentration of gas becomes greater on one side of the membrane than the other. Here, the process helps oxygen move from the alveoli to the blood and carbon dioxide move in the opposite direction. The alveoli, which have a large surface area and thin walls, facilitate efficient gas exchange. Oxygen moves from the alveoli (which have a high concentration) to the blood (a low concentration). Carbon dioxide, which is more concentrated in the blood, moves out of the lungs and is breathed out. Due to this process, the pulmonary system demonstrates its ability to adjust and meet the body's changing energy needs. Some other physiological effects also play a role in how gas diffusion works. The surface area of the alveolar membrane, which helps with gas exchange, can be decreased by diseases such as emphysema, which damages the alveolar walls. In addition, the alveolar-capillary membrane's thickness is critical; if it becomes thicker, for example, due to pulmonary fibrosis, it affects how well oxygen and carbon dioxide can be exchanged. The exchange of gases is facilitated by the pressure gradients of carbon dioxide and oxygen, known as partial pressures. Greater differences in partial pressures across the alveolar-capillary membrane facilitate faster diffusion, illustrating the link between structure and function in breathing. Understanding these concepts is essential to comprehend how various factors can impact lung function and gas exchange. Also, if the lung's ability to exchange oxygen and carbon dioxide is reduced, this can directly affect how efficiently gases are exchanged. By measuring DLCO, we can assess how efficiently oxygen and carbon dioxide exchange between the lungs and blood at the alveolar level, which can help identify potential lung diseases. DLCO measurement is clinically important because it facilitates the diagnosis of lung conditions, such as emphysema and pulmonary hypertension. As highlighted by the mechanisms underlying hypercapnic ventilatory failure, an increased carbon dioxide level can stem from impaired diffusion or reduced ventilation efforts, leading to severe physiological repercussions (Amílkar et al., 2022). Therefore, factors such as ventilation-perfusion (V/Q) mismatch, anatomical abnormalities, and various lung diseases must be recognized as they significantly impede the optimal functioning of gas diffusion in the lungs, underscoring the complexity and importance of maintaining respiratory health.

6.2.1. Role of Alveoli in Gas Exchange

Oxygen enters the blood and carbon dioxide leaves it at the alveoli, which are the main air sacs in the lungs. The thin layer of epithelial cells in their structure allows gases to move across easily, according to Fick's Law of Diffusion, which states that the greater the surface area and pressure difference, the faster the gas transfer. The surface area of each alveolus is large, which allows oxygen to reach the pulmonary capillaries and carbon dioxide to leave them.

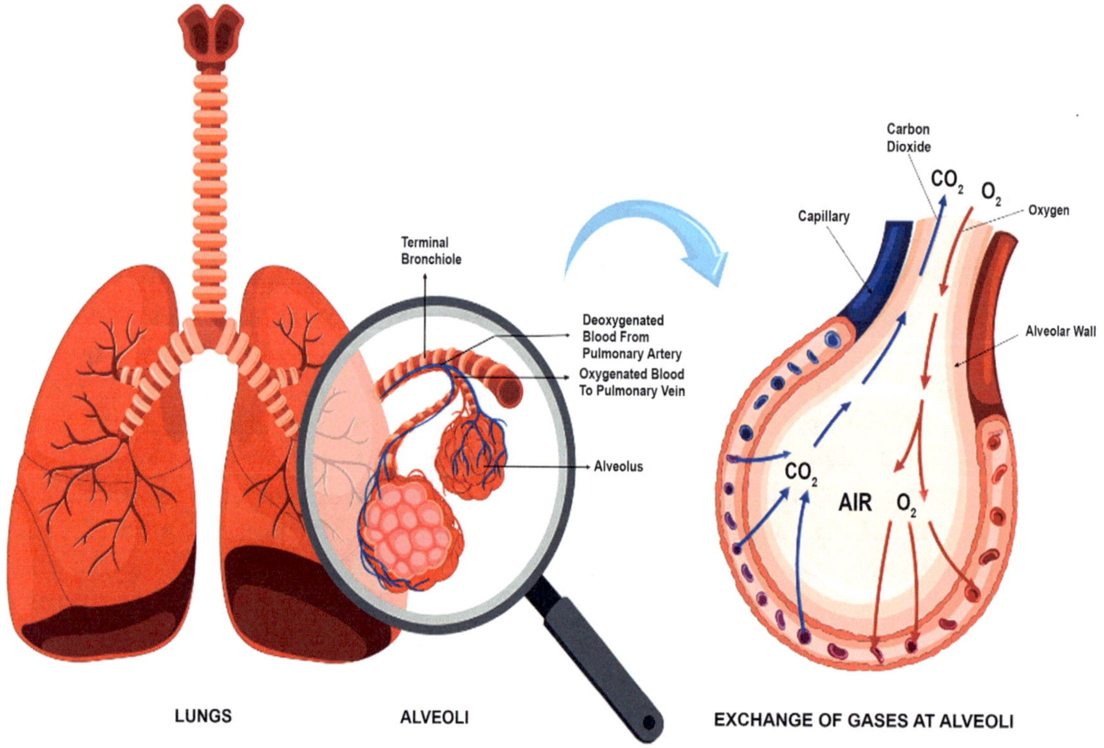

Figure 6.5. Exchange of gas s at alveoli.

Source: https://welcare.com.au/wp-content/uploads/2024/08/lung-function-image.png.

The many capillaries surrounding each alveolus help by maintaining a low oxygen partial pressure in the blood, which encourages oxygen to diffuse from the alveolus into the blood. The DLCO test and similar measures help demonstrate how well the lungs exchange gases, highlighting the importance of healthy alveoli. Alveoli are not merely passive participants in gas exchange; their interaction with red blood cells (RBCs) underscores the complexity of respiratory physiology. It has been found that the way hemoglobin captures oxygen once it diffuses into the capillaries also affects alveolar gas exchange. Notably, studies suggest that gas exchange is affected by both volume absorption in the RBC and surface absorption characteristics, which can vary between gases such as oxygen and carbon monoxide (Min-Kang et al., 2017). Therefore, maintaining the physical and chemical properties of the alveolar-capillary barrier in a healthy state is crucial for both oxygenation and lung health. affect alveolar gas exchange, and these include both normal and abnormal conditions. For instance, endurance-trained athletes exhibit distinct advantages in diffusion capacity, with research indicating that exercise training enhances the lung membrane diffusing capacity without necessarily altering lung structure itself (Tedjasaputra et al., 2016). These adaptations include an increased pulmonary capillary blood volume, which promotes a higher maximal oxygen uptake ($\dot{V}O_2$ max) during physical exertion. Pulmonary edema or fibrosis can also severely affect gas exchange by making the alveolar-capillary membrane thicker or reducing its surface area. Understanding these diverse influences on alveolar function is crucial for developing effective interventions for respiratory diseases, thus highlighting the alveoli's integral role in maintaining oxygen homeostasis within the body (Figure 6.5).

6.2.2. Process of Oxygen and Carbon Dioxide Diffusion

It is essential for maintaining homeostasis in the body that oxygen and carbon dioxide can diffuse through the lungs. Oxygen moves from the alveoli into the blood, and carbon dioxide moves from the blood into the alveoli through the alveolar-capillary membrane. Fick's Law of Diffusion describes this by claiming that the rate of gas diffusion depends on the surface area, the difference in partial pressures, and the diffusion coefficient of the gas, and is inversely related to the thickness of the membrane. So, how well gas exchange happens also depends on the condition of the lung architecture, such as the walls of the alveoli and the nearby capillaries. DLCO, which measures the diffusion capacity of the lungs, provides information about how effectively oxygen and carbon dioxide are exchanged.

The amount of gas exchange in the lungs can be measured by DLCO, which depends on the lungs' surface area and the partial pressures of the gases. If DLCO is high, it means gas transfer is working well; if it is low, it may suggest illnesses such as pulmonary fibrosis or emphysema, which can reduce the surface area and function of the alveoli. This quantifiable assessment of lung function is crucial for diagnosing and monitoring various respiratory disorders, as it reflects the interplay between ventilation and perfusion (Pace, 2015). Besides the structure of the lungs, many other things, such as body conditions and the environment, play a role in gas exchange. For example, changes in height, age, and the presence of lung disease can significantly impact the partial pressures of gases in the airways and the lungs' ability to exchange gases. Due to the fact that there is less air pressure at high altitudes, oxygen becomes less available, which affects the diffusion process. Besides, long-term illnesses like asthma may cause airway blockage and swelling, which makes it harder for gases to move in and out of the lungs. Understanding these factors is critical for developing effective treatment strategies and improving patient outcomes in individuals with respiratory conditions (Pace, 2015) (Figure 6.6).

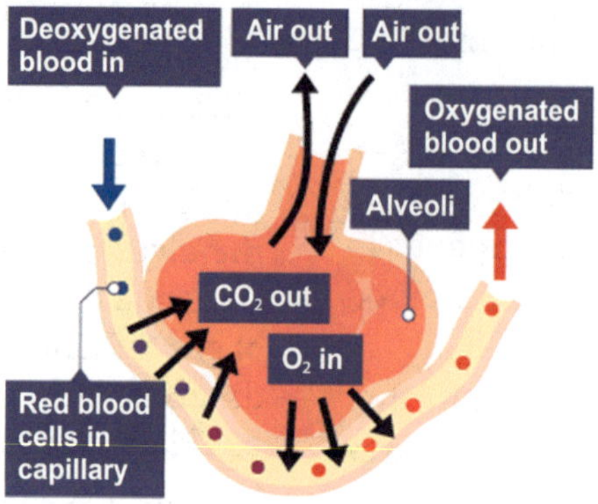

Figure 6.6. Oxygen and carbon dioxide diffusion.

6.2.3. Importance of Surface Area and Membrane Thickness

The efficiency with which gas moves in and out of the lungs depends mainly on the surface area and thickness of the alveolar membrane. Based on Fick's Law of Diffusion, the faster particles move across a membrane, the larger its surface area and the thinner the membrane is. More oxygen and carbon dioxide molecules can move in and out of the body simultaneously through the larger surface area, which is important because tissues require a constant supply of oxygen. This becomes particularly important when the body is working harder, as better gas exchange can significantly impact how the body functions. For this reason, the alveolar structure, which has many small sacs, gives a large surface area, aids in breathing, and helps prevent hypoxemia when oxygen is used more. The thickness of the alveolar-capillary membrane is also critical in controlling how fast substances can move. As the membrane is thinner, gases can move through it more easily, which increases the rate of oxygen uptake and carbon dioxide release. A proper thickness of the membrane is necessary, as too much thickness can occur in diseases such as ILD or pulmonary fibrosis, which makes it harder for gases to pass through the lungs.

As noted in the study of diffusing capacity (DLCO), even slight increases in membrane thickness can lead to significant reductions in lung function, particularly under stressors such as exercise or exacerbations of COPD (Magro et al., 2012). Thus, it is imperative that the membrane is intact and the right size for proper breathing. COPD and similar conditions significantly amplify the influence of surface area and membrane thickness on the lungs. Testing diffusing capacity in the clinic typically reveals the extent to which the structure affects the lungs' functioning. Investigations into pulmonary vessel morphology, including three-dimensional (3D) quantification of the pulmonary arteries, have shown that changes in pulmonary artery size can correlate with decreased lung function and exacerbations of airway limitations (Lindenmaier et al., 2015). This indicates that both the surface area and the thickness of the membrane play important roles in gas exchange. Grasping these connections is important for creating therapies that help restore normal breathing and deal with respiratory diseases, which stresses the importance of thorough assessments in respiratory medicine.

6.3. Diffusion Capacity of the Lung (DLCO)

The DLCO (diffusion capacity of the lung) is an important test that measures the efficiency of gas exchange in the alveoli. This metric evaluates the transfer of carbon monoxide (CO) from the air sacs of the lungs into the bloodstream, serving as an indirect indicator of the alveolar-capillary membranes' integrity and surface area available for gas exchange. Most often, assessing DLCO involves the patient inhaling a CO-laden gas mixture and then holding their breath for a short period. Previous research indicates that while this method can accommodate patients with varying degrees of pulmonary impairment, such as those with severe COPD, reduced breath-hold times significantly impact the results in these populations, reflecting decreased DLCO values when compared to healthier individuals (Magro et al., 2012). It is critical to understand these details when using DLCO in clinical settings. Also, the results from DLCO testing can reveal the effects of different health problems, especially in individuals who were born extremely prematurely. Several studies suggest that people born preterm have a higher risk of lung function problems, which can lead to lower DLCO as time goes on. The underlying mechanisms involve thinner alveolar membranes and decreased surface area, leading to compromised gas diffusion capacity (Satrell et al., 2022). These studies have shown that breathing problems can persist into adulthood, raising concerns about their ongoing respiratory health. Due to this, doctors should take these points into account when assessing lung function in patients born before full term, since it affects their overall breathing care. Overall, DLCO measurement is a valuable tool for assessing lung function in various conditions and populations. Since the alveoli are crucial for both lung function and disease, this highlights the close connection between lung physiology and pathology. In specific groups, such as babies born prematurely or those with long-term lung issues, understanding what affects DLCO can help doctors make more informed decisions and provide better care for patients. Future research should aim to refine DLCO testing protocols and explore its predictive value in various patient populations, aligning with findings that suggest differential responses to gas exchange based on underlying clinical characteristics (Magro et al., 2012; Satrell et al., 2022). This continued exploration will ultimately inform strategies for mitigating respiratory dysfunction and optimizing health outcomes (Figure 6.7).

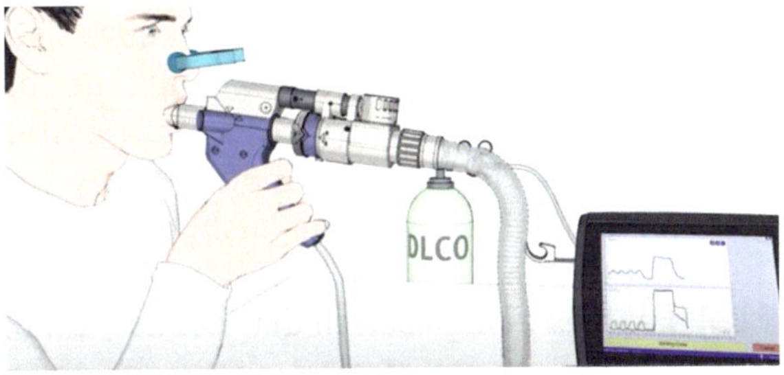

Figure 6.7. DLCO respiratory testing.

Source: https://ioh.health/wp-content/uploads/DLCO-Image-1-1024x466.png.

6.3.1. Definition and Significance of DLCO

The diffusion capacity of the lung for carbon monoxide (DLCO) is a crucial measure in pulmonary medicine, capturing the efficiency of gas exchange across the alveolar-capillary membrane. In particular, DLCO measures how quickly carbon monoxide moves from the alveoli to the blood, which is a way to judge the health of the lungs indirectly. It is important for checking emphysema, pulmonary fibrosis, and various types of ILD. A low DLCO might indicate that either the alveolar surface area is smaller or the alveolar membranes are thicker, which can both prevent gases from moving properly. Because DLCO helps explain how the lungs are working, it is important for both diagnosing and monitoring different respiratory illnesses. DLCO measurement has attracted interest because it helps explain how the lungs work and how diseases develop. Typically, patients inhale a carbon monoxide mixture and hold their breath for a short time to allow diffusion to occur. The combination of these methods allows us to measure both the lung's ability to diffuse gases and its ability to vent air. It has been found that people with advanced pulmonary diseases, for example, COPD, often have lower DLCO values, especially when they are asked to hold their breath for a shorter time. Specifically, research indicates that individuals with severe COPD exhibit significant discrepancies in measured DLCO when breath-hold times are shortened, whereas individuals with normal lung function maintain stable measurements even when breath-hold periods vary, highlighting the clinical utility of DLCO in distinguishing between different pulmonary conditions (Magro et al., 2012). Besides being used in diagnostics, DLCO provides helpful information about the long-term respiratory health of people, mainly those born early. Research has shown that extremely preterm (EP) infants, who experience disrupted alveolar growth and thickened membranes, often exhibit reduced DLCO levels into adulthood. The decrease in oxygen level can persist into childhood and may indicate potential problems, such as pulmonary hypertension and a reduced ability to exercise. Thus, DLCO should be understood because it guides both short-term and long-term care for people at risk. Ultimately, the character and significance of DLCO underscore its role as a fundamental component in the broader landscape of gas exchange mechanisms within the lungs, while serving as a vital tool for both prevention and treatment planning in pulmonary medicine (Satrell et al., 2022).

6.3.2. Methods for Measuring DLCO

Measuring the diffusing capacity of the lung (DLCO) is crucial for evaluating respiratory function and can aid in diagnosing various pulmonary conditions. One of the standard methods is the single-breath technique, which involves a patient breathing in a mixture of gas with a tracer, such as carbon monoxide. It is based on the belief that the difference in carbon monoxide concentration between the air you breathe in and the air you breathe out directly shows how well the lungs move gases across the alveolar-capillary membrane. If patients cooperate and the procedure is performed precisely, it can significantly impact the accuracy of the results, so following the same procedures helps minimize differences. Additionally, this method provides rapid results and is relatively straightforward, thus making it a common choice in clinical settings for evaluating potential lung disease complications (Binks, 2022). The steady-state method is often used to measure DLCO. Rather than a single breath, steady-state measurements require the patient to breathe a gas mixture until the system reaches equilibrium. After that, the amount of carbon monoxide in the breath is measured to find the DLCO. Because of this technique, it is easier to assess patients who are unable to perform the single-breath maneuver due to age or breathing difficulties. Nevertheless, more advanced instruments are needed, and getting to a steady state takes more time, which can make the testing process harder. Nonetheless, this method remains a valuable alternative when individual patient factors preclude the use of single-breath testing, ensuring that comprehensive assessments of lung function can be performed across diverse patient populations (Guazzi, 2000). Lately, new technologies have introduced innovative ways to measure DLCO, such as with portable devices. With these new tools, DLCO can be quickly and easily checked and measured by both patients and doctors. Having portable devices makes it possible to test more often, which helps manage lung conditions. Additionally, such innovations can feature automated systems that help reduce errors in collecting and interpreting data. Although these techniques appear promising, it is necessary to verify their accuracy by comparing them with traditional methods. As research continues to evaluate these next-generation devices, it will be crucial to integrate findings into clinical practice to streamline the assessment of lung diffusion capacity while maintaining robust standards of care (Binks, 2022) (Figure 6.8).

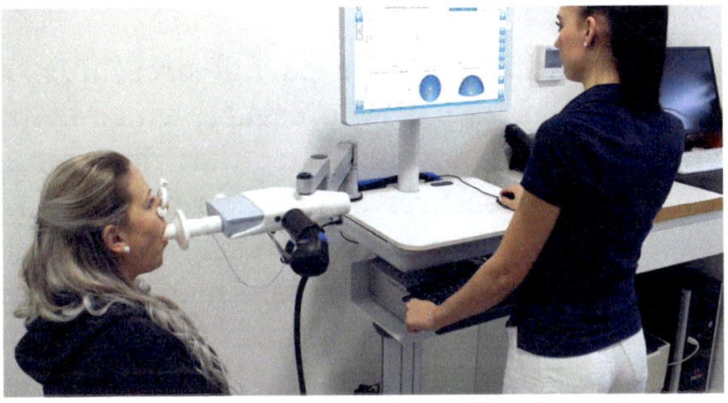

Figure 6.8. Measuring DLCO.

Source: https://i0.wp.com/schillerus.com/wp-content/uploads/2025/03/DLCOPOWERCUBE-DIFFUSION.jpg?fit=1200%2C630&quality=89&ssl=1.

6.3.3. Clinical Implications of Altered DLCO Values

The measurement of diffusion capacity of the lungs for carbon monoxide (DLCO) is a critical diagnostic tool, particularly in assessing various pulmonary conditions. If the DLCO value changes, it can indicate major changes in the body, suggesting that gas exchange at the alveolar-capillary membrane is not functioning properly. Many cases of emphysema, ILD, and pulmonary vascular disease have lower DLCO, which helps doctors tell them apart from other respiratory conditions. For example, a decrease in DLCO in COPD may indicate the extent of emphysema, which helps doctors determine the best treatment. The correlation between DLCO values and clinical symptoms underscores their importance in monitoring disease progression and treatment response, thereby aiding in the management of patients with chronic respiratory illnesses (Satrell et al., 2022). Additionally, a lower DLCO can indicate issues beyond the lungs, as it may be a sign of systemic health problems. For example, in individuals born extremely preterm, research has shown that compromised diffusion capacity persists from childhood into adulthood, revealing potential long-term health effects and necessitating early intervention strategies (Satrell et al., 2022). A decrease in DLCO may be linked to less exercise ability and ongoing symptoms, which means observing this number could help with prognosis. It is recommended that clinicians use DLCO measurements in the regular assessment of individuals at risk, as it can reveal changes in lung function that spirometry alone may miss. Due to DLCO testing, doctors can gain a more comprehensive understanding of how the lungs are functioning.

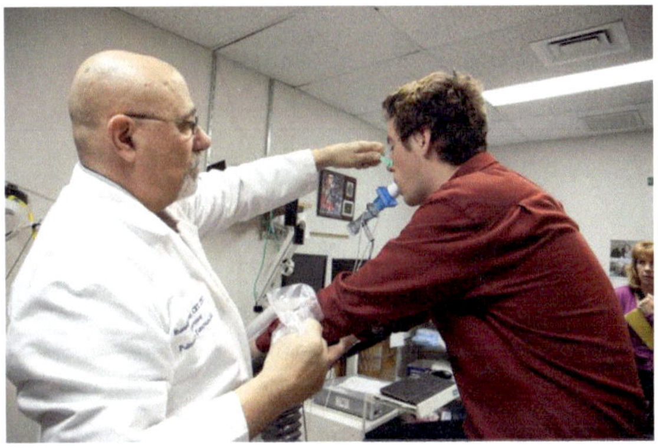

Figure 6.9. Cardiopulmonary exercise testing (CPET) in a clinical setting.

Source: https://scicalgas.com/wp-content/uploads/bfi_thumb/pulmonary_function_laboratory-2v5kynn1yb1s04nyn7rjsw.jpg.

The effects of abnormal DLCO values are especially clear in people with chronic diseases such as COPD. The utility of hyperpolarized gas magnetic resonance imaging (MRI) has emerged as a valuable tool in assessing lung structure and function longitudinally in these patients. Studies have indicated that even in ex-smokers with normal spirometry but reduced DLCO values, functional impairments persist, which are linked to poorer exercise tolerance and more pronounced symptoms (Kirby et al., 2013). It underlines the importance of healthcare providers being aware of how changes in DLCO can show the state of a person's lungs. The inclusion of DLCO assessment in routine evaluations not only enhances diagnostic accuracy but also informs therapeutic strategies and patient education, fostering a more proactive approach to managing chronic respiratory conditions (Figure 6.9).

6.4. Partial Pressures of Respiratory Gases

The process of gas exchange in the lungs depends on understanding the partial pressures of respiratory gases. The pressure of a gas in a mixture is known as its partial pressure, which helps determine how gases move through the alveolar membranes. Dalton's law states that the overall pressure of a gas mixture is the result of adding up the partial pressures of its different parts. In human respiration, this principle is crucial because the differences in partial pressures between the alveoli and the blood facilitate the exchange of oxygen and carbon dioxide. Analyzing these gradients provides insight into how effectively gas exchange is functioning and how different pressures impact respiratory health.

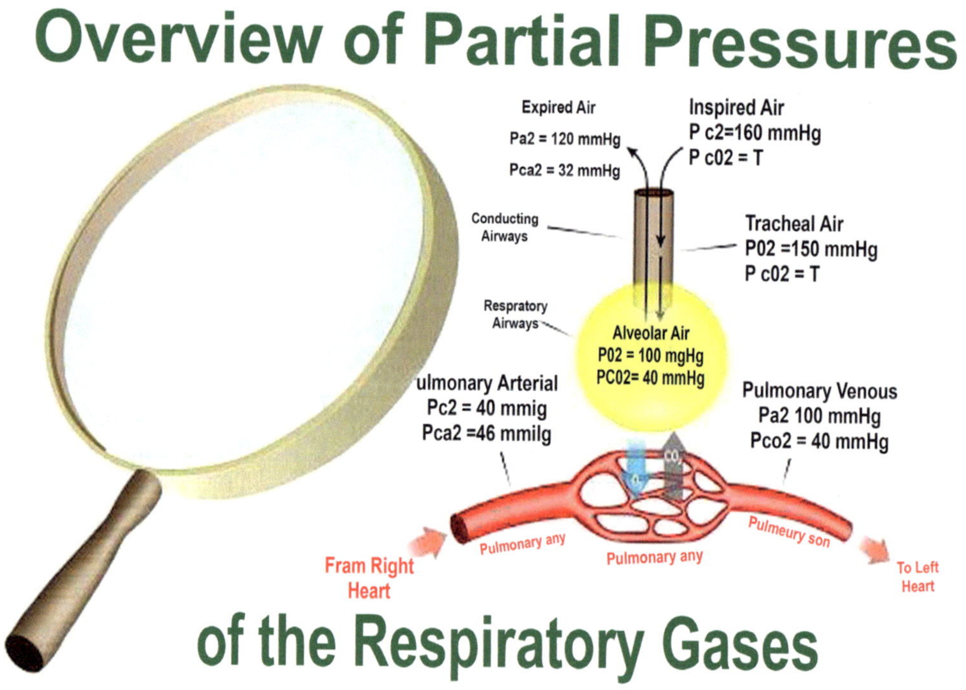

Figure 6.10. Partial pressures of the respiratory gases.

Source: https://i.ytimg.com/vi/cBx955XZVfs/sddefault.jpg.

Additionally, measuring partial pressures is crucial to understanding how effectively gas exchange occurs in the lungs. A clinical methodology involves evaluating the diffusing capacity of the lungs for carbon monoxide (DLCO), which reflects the efficiency of gas exchange across the alveolar-capillary membrane. To do this measurement, you need to know the partial pressure of each gas, as DLCO includes taking up carbon monoxide, which is compared to its partial pressure in the blood. The established relationship indicates that in conditions such as chronic obstructive pulmonary disease (COPD) or ILD, abnormalities in DLCO readings may result from disruptions in the partial pressure gradients. Thus, proper interpretation of DLCO values requires a firm grasp of how partial pressures influence gas exchange and the overall functionality of the lungs (Magro et al., 2012). Many physiological and pathological factors can change the partial pressures, which can affect how well gases diffuse. A change in altitude significantly affects the amount of oxygen in the air we breathe, which in turn alters the oxygen level in our arteries. It is crucial to understand these factors, especially in individuals with respiratory conditions, as their symptoms may worsen with changes in partial pressures. In addition, COPD often leads to changes in the blood vessels of the lungs, as evidenced by the widening of the pulmonary arteries, which can disrupt normal blood flow and alter the partial pressures in the alveoli. By exploring these connections, it becomes evident that a thorough understanding of partial pressures is essential not just for physiological modeling, but for clinical assessment and the management of respiratory diseases (Lindenmaier et al., 2015) (Figure 6.10).

6.4.1. Explanation of Partial Pressure Concept

To understand how gases function in the respiratory system, it is essential to comprehend partial pressure. In a mixture of gases, partial pressure refers to the pressure exerted by one gas on the others. By Dalton's Law, the total pressure of a mixture of gases is made up of the partial pressures of each gas. Air entering the lungs from the outside contains several gases, and every gas adds to the total pressure. The partial pressures of oxygen and carbon dioxide are different, which controls their diffusion through the alveolar membrane. Gas exchange is made possible because oxygen moves from the alveoli (with high partial pressure) to the capillaries (with lower partial pressure), following Fick's Law of diffusion. It is essential for maintaining oxygen levels in the body and for eliminating carbon dioxide, a waste product of metabolism. The pressure of gases in the lungs can be affected by things outside the body, for example, altitude, temperature and what is inhaled. As we ascend higher, atmospheric pressure decreases, and consequently, the partial pressure of oxygen also decreases. A lack of oxygen can occur because of this which may cause hypoxia and reduce how well the body works. Additionally, the temperature of the air plays a role, as it holds less oxygen when warmer, according to the concept of partial pressures. It is essential to have adaptive mechanisms, such as increased ventilation or altered hemoglobin, to maintain a balanced oxygen pressure in the body as conditions change. Understanding these factors contributes to a more comprehensive understanding of how partial pressures affect gas exchange efficiency in the respiratory system (Singh et al., 2023). Additionally, understanding how partial pressure affects lung diffusion is crucial. Diffusion capacity is about how gases cross the alveolar-capillary membrane, and this process is mainly controlled by the partial pressures of the gases. For example, during exercise, the partial pressure of carbon dioxide ($PaCO_2$) in the blood can increase due to enhanced metabolism, creating a gradient that facilitates its diffusion into the alveoli. Also, there must be enough oxygen partial pressure for proper diffusion into the blood. Anything that disrupts the balance in the lungs, such as disease or environmental causes, may make it harder for gas exchange, leading to breathing problems. By measuring partial pressures and their variations, clinicians can infer the efficiency of gas exchange in patients, guiding therapeutic interventions (Singh et al., 2023).

6.4.2. Role of Partial Pressures in Gas Exchange

The mechanism by which respiratory gases cross the lung membrane is primarily explained by the concept of partial pressures. A gas in a mixture exerts a partial pressure, and this is important for understanding how gases move from regions with more gas to regions with less gas, as stated in Fick's Law of Diffusion. In the lungs, the diffusion of oxygen (O_2) and carbon dioxide (CO_2) occurs based on their respective partial pressures. During inhalation, the fresh air has a higher partial pressure of oxygen, which goes into the alveoli, and the blood returning to the lungs has a higher $PaCO_2$. The gradient enables oxygen to enter the blood and carbon dioxide to exit, which is crucial for the body to maintain a stable state. One must understand the things that influence the partial pressures in the lungs to understand gas exchange. Many health conditions can change the partial pressures of respiratory gases, which influence how efficiently gas exchange occurs. COPD or ILD may cause changes in the way the lungs function, limiting airflow and impeding gas exchange. According to significant studies, the diffusion capacity of the lungs (DLCO) serves as an indirect measure of alveolar-capillary function, indicating harm to gas exchange processes in patients with impaired lung function (Magro et al., 2012). Altitude, the chemicals in the air, and the presence of surfactant in the lungs can also alter the partial pressures of gases. Additionally, the presence of surfactant in the lungs can affect the partial pressures of gases, which can impact how oxygen is delivered and carbon dioxide is removed in several clinical cases. The lungs and breathing of some people (e.g., those born extremely early) are often not fully developed, therefore it is important to watch their partial pressures carefully. Research indicates that individuals born prematurely exhibit reduced gas exchange capabilities that can last into adulthood due to underdeveloped lung structures and altered diffusion capacities (Satrell et al., 2022). Assessing how well gas exchange works in these populations by examining partial pressures both explains the body's functions and highlights the lasting effects of early breathing issues. For this reason, it is important to understand partial pressures well to design effective treatments and manage long-term lung problems which benefits patients and improves their respiratory care.

6.4.3. Impact of Altitude on Partial Pressures

A rise in altitude causes air pressure to decrease, making it more difficult for the lungs to absorb oxygen and eliminate carbon dioxide. This happens most clearly when the lungs take up oxygen. According to Fick's law, the pressure gradient is very important in gas movement, so when the atmospheric pressure decreases, the partial pressure of oxygen drops as well. Because of this reduction, there is less oxygen available for diffusion from the alveoli to the blood, which may cause hemoglobin to have lower oxygen saturation, mostly when at high altitudes. As a result of these changes, the body continues to require the same amount of oxygen, yet receives less, which exacerbates altitude sickness symptoms. Because both altitude and lung function are crucial for gas exchange, we must consider how gases are exchanged under low-oxygen conditions. As the pressure difference for oxygen is less at high altitudes, the lung's diffusion capacity is reduced, which makes it harder for the lungs to exchange gases. At higher altitudes, the amount of oxygen in the air is less, which can reduce the oxygen concentration in the alveoli and cause the body to breathe more rapidly and take in more air. They are meant to compensate for the lower oxygen levels present. However, if ascent is rapid or the altitude is very high, the body may not be able to maintain proper balance which shows the significant problems altitude can cause for gas exchange. Additionally, understanding how the body responds to higher altitudes enables the creation of strategies to mitigate the effects of lower partial pressures. Increased production of RBCs is a key factor, triggered by higher erythropoietin levels due to an oxygen shortage. By doing this, the blood can carry more oxygen, which prevents the arterial oxygen levels from falling during environmental changes. Still, such adaptations may not be sufficient to prevent high-altitude cerebral edema and high-altitude pulmonary edema, as the body's balance and homeostasis can become disrupted in individuals who are not accustomed to high altitudes. The changes in the body show that a fine balance exists between the effects of altitude and how well the body can exchange gases, which is key to understanding altitude's impact on breathing.

6.5. Factors Affecting Gas Exchange

Several important things affect how efficiently gas exchange happens in the lungs, such as the area of the alveoli, the thickness of the alveolar-capillary membrane, and the partial pressures of the gases involved. Fick's Law of Diffusion shows that a larger surface area helps more oxygen get into the blood and more carbon dioxide be removed from it. A condition such as emphysema can decrease the area that allows gas exchange, which affects breathing. A thicker alveolar-capillary membrane, which can occur in diseases such as pulmonary fibrosis, makes it harder for gases to exchange, reducing the efficiency of gas exchange. It highlights the importance of healthy lungs for good breathing and overall health. Another significant aspect affecting gas exchange is the diffusion capacity of the lungs, often quantified through measurements of DLCO (diffusion capacity of the lung for carbon monoxide). It measures how well the lungs can move gases, which depends on surface area and the condition of the membrane. An abnormal DLCO may suggest a person has COPD or pulmonary hypertension. A patient may exhibit symptoms of shortness of breath and experience difficulty exercising if gas exchange is not functioning efficiently. By understanding the details of DLCO measurements, clinicians can identify the causes of breathing problems and select suitable treatments to improve patients' breathing and overall well-being, emphasizing their importance in treating lung diseases. Additionally, factors outside the body, such as air pressure and temperature, can influence the exchange of gas. Air quality, the amount of moisture in the air, and altitude can all change the partial pressure of gases in the alveoli. For example, at high altitudes, oxygen pressure is lowered, which can result in hypoxemia and make it difficult for the body to supply enough oxygen to tissues.

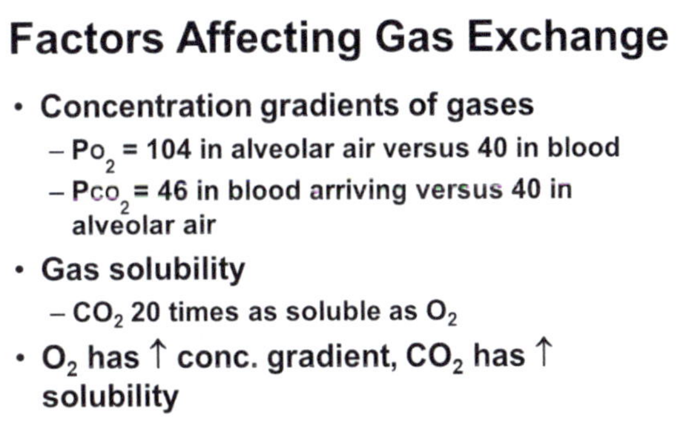

Figure 6.11. Factors affecting gas exchange.

Source: https://slideplayer.com/slide/273487/1/images/60/Factors+Affecting+Gas+Exchange.jpg.

Additionally, air pollutants and allergens can exacerbate existing respiratory problems, reducing the lungs' ability to exchange gases efficiently. In this regard, technologies such as hyperpolarized 129Xe (HXe) MRI have emerged as promising non-invasive tools for evaluating gas exchange dynamics in various lung conditions, providing vital insights into factors impacting lung health and addressing the challenges posed by environmental influences on respiratory function (Dregely et al., 2010; Shokr et al., 2016). Ultimately, a comprehensive understanding of these factors is crucial for optimizing lung function and developing effective clinical strategies for enhancing gas exchange (Figure 6.11).

6.5.1. Influence of Ventilation and Perfusion Ratios

To understand how well gas exchange occurs in the lungs, ventilation and perfusion ratios are very important. Ventilation means that air enters the alveoli, and perfusion is the term for blood moving through the capillaries around these alveoli. A perfect V/Q ratio takes place when ventilation and perfusion are equal, which is best for exchanging oxygen and carbon dioxide.

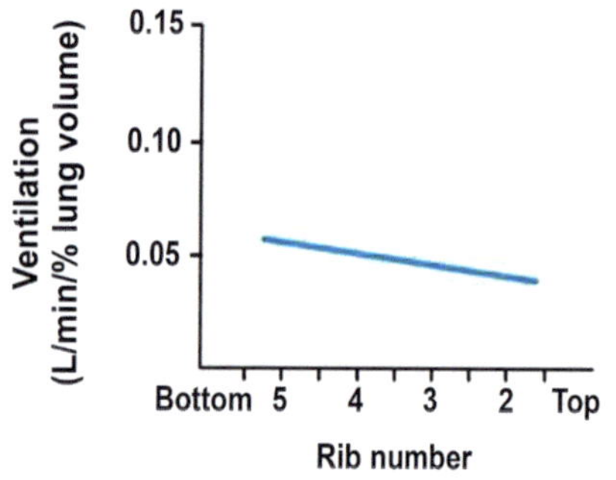

Figure 6.12. Ventilation of the lung decreases as the rib number decreases to the apex lung.

Source: https://d25iein5sonfaj.cloudfront.net/v1/public-drupal-medmastery-assets-production/migrated-images/ventilation-lung-rib-number-relationship.png?cfg=eyJ3aWR0aCI6NjAwLCJoZWlnaHQiOjMxOSwib3V0cHV0Ijoid2VicCJ9.

If this ratio is not right, it may result in shunting or dead space, which stops proper gas exchange and causes blood to be poorly oxygenated. A mismatch often seen in various pulmonary pathologies emphasizes the importance of maintaining a balanced V/Q ratio for effective respiratory function, as it directly impacts the overall ventilation effectiveness and oxygen delivery to tissues, underscoring the significance of studying these ratios in clinical settings (Binks, 2022).

Fick's Law of Diffusion explains how the V/Q ratios show the processes involved in gas exchange. Fick's Law states that how fast a gas will diffuse across a membrane depends on its surface area, the difference in partial pressure, and how thick the membrane is. Therefore, if V/Q ratios are altered, the partial pressures of oxygen and carbon dioxide in both alveolar and arterial blood may be significantly affected. When V/Q ratios are low, the lungs have too much blood and not enough air, so oxygen levels drop and carbon dioxide is not removed properly. On the other hand, when V/Q ratios are high, too much air is used for not enough blood, which leads to wasted ventilation. These dynamics demonstrate that an optimal V/Q ratio is crucial not only for maintaining adequate gas diffusion but also for ensuring efficient respiratory physiology (Schulze, 2020). Applying knowledge of V/Q ratios can influence the treatment of various respiratory disorders. Pulmonary embolism, COPD, and pulmonary hypertension are usually associated with changes in the way V/Q matching takes place. Pulmonary embolism usually blocks a part of the pulmonary blood vessels, so there is breathing but very little blood flow in those areas. Alternatively, COPD can cause low V/Q ratios because airflow is reduced and gas exchange is impaired. Noticing these patterns is important to choosing treatments that help with ventilation and perfusion. Therefore, a nuanced understanding of V/Q ratios not only enhances our grasp of respiratory mechanics but also enriches clinical diagnostic and treatment modalities aimed at ameliorating respiratory efficiency in affected populations (Binks, 2022) (Figure 6.12).

6.5.2. Effects of Lung Diseases on Gas Exchange

Lung diseases primarily impair gas exchange by altering the structure of the alveolar-capillary membrane. COPD, pulmonary fibrosis, and ARDS lead to inflammation and fibrosis, which may cause the alveolar walls to thicken. Due to this thickening, gases have a harder time moving in and out of the lungs, which reduces the ability to take in oxygen and expel carbon dioxide. The rate of gas transfer is related to the surface area, the difference in concentration, and is inversely related to how thick the barrier is, as Fick's Law of Diffusion states. Any illness that leads to thickening of the alveolar walls reduces gas exchange, thereby increasing the risk of hypoxemia and hypercapnia, which are common in individuals with chronic lung diseases. Due to these changes, doctors must use comprehensive management plans to help patients maintain their lung health and enhance the way their lungs exchange gases.

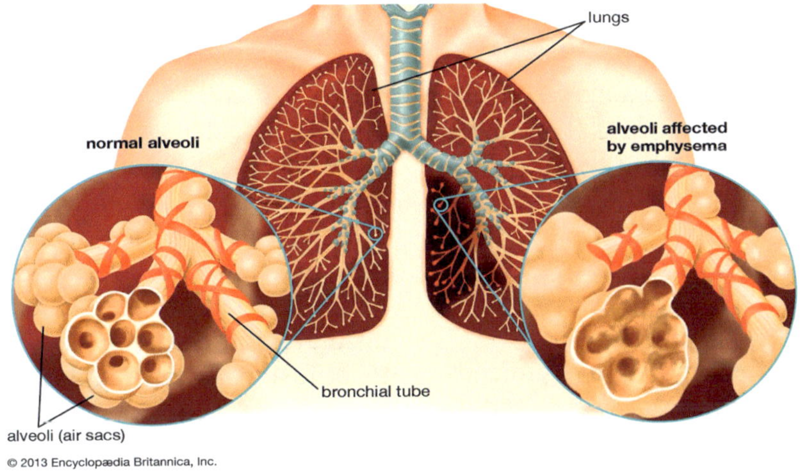

Figure 6.13. Abnormal gas exchange.

Source: https://cdn.britannica.com/04/100104-050-9C3C04EB/Emphysema-walls-alveoli-oxygen-intake-loss-lungs.jpg.

The diffusion capacity of the lung (DLCO) offers a quantifiable measure of the lung's ability to facilitate gas exchange and can be profoundly affected by lung diseases. If someone has pulmonary embolism or heart failure, pulmonary capillary pressure can go up, which can lead to changes at the alveolar-capillary interface. For example, these diseases may cause the interstitium to thicken and the capillaries to become more open, which upsets the balance needed for gas exchange. Due to these changes, the membrane in the lungs may fail, thereby affecting its ability to exchange gases. Research indicates that a reduced DLCO correlates with ventilatory limitations and reduced exercise tolerance in individuals with chronic heart failure, highlighting the significance of monitoring this parameter as a predictor of overall respiratory function and patient prognosis in clinical settings (Guazzi, 2000). Also, the impact of lung diseases on the partial pressures of respiratory gases makes gas exchange more difficult. Oxygen and carbon dioxide in healthy lungs move between the air and blood as their partial pressure gradients direct them, which is necessary for proper respiration. However, if someone has lung disease, the gradients between the blood and alveoli may be altered, resulting in lower oxygen levels in the alveoli and higher carbon dioxide levels in the blood. For example, emphysema patients lose a significant portion of their alveoli, which decreases the surface area for gas exchange, resulting in less oxygen and more carbon dioxide in their blood. For this reason, recognizing the effects on gas exchange, such as V/Q mismatch and changes in compliance, is crucial in selecting the most effective treatment options. This multifaceted approach not only targets symptom relief but also aims to restore optimal gas diffusion and improve the quality of life for affected individuals (Binks, 2022) (Figure 6.13).

6.5.3. Role of Environmental Factors on Gas Diffusion

Many environmental factors play a significant role in how efficiently gases are exchanged in the lungs. A leading environmental factor is the partial pressure of the gases, which leads to differences in gas concentrations on both sides of the alveolar-capillary membrane. At greater altitudes, the amount of oxygen in the air is less which makes it harder for oxygen to move into the blood. As a result, tissues may not receive enough oxygen, indicating that changes in the atmosphere can directly impact how the lungs exchange gases. Besides, changes in humidity and temperature can alter the density and viscosity of air, which Fick's Law explains can influence the rate of diffusion. Such differences point out the strong link between environmental conditions and the way gas moves through the lungs. Besides altitude, the presence of pollutants and particles in the air can negatively impact the way gases move. If you inhale smoke or industrial emissions, the respiratory system may react with inflammation, which thickens the alveolar walls and makes it harder for gases to move. This increased diffusion distance negatively affects the lungs' diffusion capacity (DLCO), resulting in a decrease in the efficiency with which oxygen and carbon dioxide exchange occurs (Mulroney et al., 2023). Also, long-term exposure to such environmental factors often causes chronic respiratory diseases such as COPD, which makes the exchange of gases in the lungs more difficult. Recognizing these external influences highlights the importance of air quality and environmental health in maintaining lung health and facilitating gas exchange. Understanding how temperature affects gases is crucial in comprehending diffusion. The kinetic molecular theory explains that higher temperatures speed up the movement of gas molecules, which can increase the rate of diffusion. However, how much this happens depends on humidity which can affect the rate at which gases diffuse from the lungs into the alveoli. Increased humidity can lead to the condensation of water vapor, ultimately increasing the effective barrier to diffusion as it occupies space that would otherwise be filled with oxygen and carbon dioxide (Mulroney et al., 2023). Therefore, as temperatures go up, the way temperature, humidity, and gas act together becomes very important for efficient gas exchange in the lungs. Examining these interactions is crucial for understanding how various environmental factors impact breathing and health, particularly in many parts of the world.

6.6. Diffusing Capacity of the Lungs

The concept of diffusing capacity of the lungs, often quantified as the diffusion capacity of the lung for carbon monoxide (DLCO), plays a pivotal role in evaluating pulmonary gas exchange efficiency. It is important to measure this value because it reflects the state and performance of the alveolar-capillary membranes, which are needed for proper gas exchange. DLCO is assessed mainly by having the subject inhale a gas mixture and then holding their breath. This technique measures carbon monoxide in the blood to determine DLCO. Research has shown that while this method is effective, alterations in breath-hold time can significantly impact measurements in patients with COPD compared to those with healthier lung function (Magro et al., 2012). Due to these observations, we should interpret DLCO values with caution in clinical settings. Additionally, changes in the environment and within the body can significantly impact how well the lungs exchange oxygen. The amount of surface where gas exchange takes place, the thickness of the alveolar-capillary membrane, and the pressures of the gases are very important for diffusion. Any changes in these factors, such as chronic inflammation or remodeling in lung diseases, can impair the effectiveness of diffusion. Individuals born extremely preterm (EP) are particularly susceptible, as studies suggest they experience ongoing reduced diffusing capacity into young adulthood due to incomplete alveolar development (Satrell et al., 2022). Additionally, conditions such as premature rupture of membranes (PPROM) can exacerbate these deficits, underscoring the interplay between developmental factors and lung function. It is crucial to understand how these variables interact to obtain accurate results for pulmonary health in various groups. It is also critical to assess the lungs' ability to diffuse oxygen to diagnose and monitor various respiratory conditions. If DLCO values are not typical, it can suggest that someone has ILD, pulmonary hypertension, or severe emphysema, which reduces gas exchange. In the clinic, checking DLCO gives important information about a patient's condition and guides the selection of treatments. Moreover, longitudinal studies have demonstrated that patients with conditions such as severe COPD exhibit marked differences in DLCO when subjected to various breath-hold times, emphasizing the need for tailored assessment methods (Magro et al., 2012). Therefore, integrating DLCO into routine PFTs is essential for comprehensive pulmonary assessments and enhancing our understanding of gas exchange dynamics within the lungs (Figure 6.14).

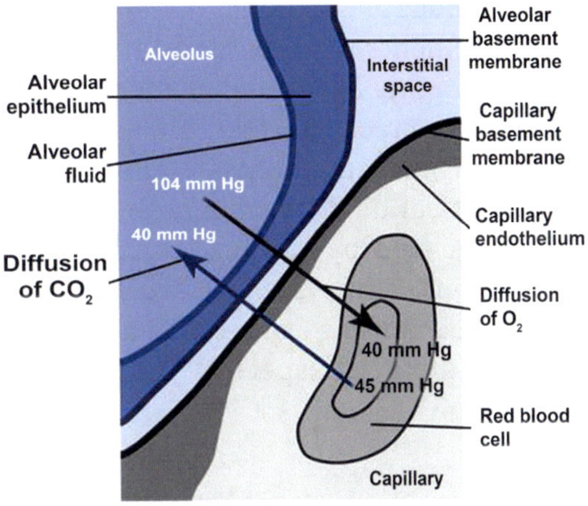

Figure 6.14. Diffusing capacity is performed to evaluate the alveolar capillary interface where gas exchange occurs.

Source: https://clinicalgate.com/wp-content/uploads/2015/06/B9780323085052000034_f03-01-9780323085052.jpg.

6.6.1. Definition and Measurement of Diffusing Capacity

The concept of diffusing capacity of the lungs (DLCO) is essential for understanding gas exchange in the respiratory system. DLCO quantifies how effectively gases, particularly carbon monoxide (CO), transfer from the alveoli to the pulmonary capillaries, reflecting the lungs' functional ability. It is important for diagnosing and assessing conditions in the lungs, such as emphysema and ILD. The usual method for measuring DLCO involves having the person inhale a gas mixture, hold it for a specified period, and then exhale it. Clinicians can measure the amount of diffused gas by comparing the alveolar and capillary concentrations, which helps them judge the health of the alveolar-capillary membrane and estimate gas transfer in the lungs. The steps for measuring DLCO have been revised to ensure better accuracy and reliability. A 10-second breath hold is typically part of the single-breath method, which helps accurately measure gas exchange. However, studies have found that this time may not be suitable for everyone, mainly those with severe lung problems who find it hard to breathe. A study that included different patient groups found that lowering the breath-hold time from 10 seconds to 6 seconds did not significantly affect DLCO measurements for control subjects or patients with ILD. However, in patients with severe COPD, a reduction in breath-hold time led to a marked change in DLCO values, underscoring the necessity for standardized protocols that accommodate individual patient capabilities (Magro et al., 2012). In addition to the standard gas measurements, new methods are being employed to analyze trace gases present in the breath, providing insights into metabolism and lung health. In this way, examining exhaled nitric oxide can help doctors detect and monitor changes in airway inflammation. Similar recommendations for standardizing measurements of other trace gases, such as volatile organic compounds (VOCs), could enhance clinical diagnostics and understanding of lung function. Significantly, these assessments can be influenced by various factors, including breathing patterns, tracheobronchial lining fluid concentrations, and systemic levels of gases (Amann et al., 2010). As the understanding of gas exchange mechanisms expands, an accurate and comprehensive approach to lung diffusing capacity will remain a crucial aspect of pulmonary function evaluation (Figure 6.15).

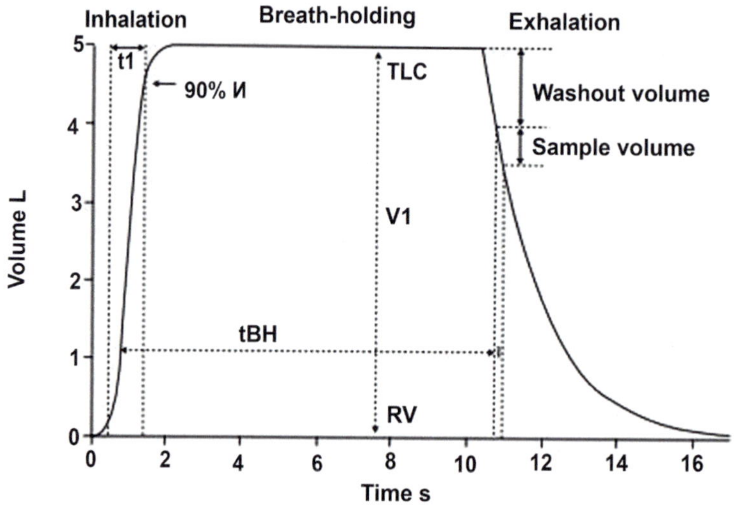

Figure 6.15. Single breath method of measuring DLCO.

Source: https://derangedphysiology.com/main/sites/default/files/sites/default/files/CICM%20 Primary/G%20Cardiovascular%20system/single%20breath%20DLCO%20measurement%20 ytechnique%20from%20the%20ERS-ATS%20statement.jpg.

6.6.2. Factors Influencing Diffusing Capacity

The DLCO can be affected by different factors related to the body and diseases, which can change how well gas exchange occurs. An important element is how much surface area the alveoli have which is mostly influenced by their structure and density. A larger surface area in the lungs facilitates gas exchange, allowing more oxygen to enter the blood and more carbon dioxide to leave. When emphysema occurs, the alveolar walls are damaged, so the total surface area for oxygen exchange is reduced which leads to a decline in DLCO. Also, thickening of the alveolar-capillary membrane can make it more difficult for gases to pass, which reduces the body's ability to exchange gases and may lead to respiratory distress in those affected. The pressure of the gases in the alveoli and capillaries matters a great deal, as it is what drives the diffusion process. It is stated by Fick's Law that the rate of gas diffusion depends on the difference in partial pressures between both compartments. When lungs are healthy, the oxygen in the alveoli has a higher partial pressure than the oxygen in the blood, making it easier for oxygen to enter the bloodstream. For example, if the air pressure is low, as at high altitudes, the partial pressure of oxygen can decrease, which lowers the DLCO. In addition, diseases such as pulmonary edema can disrupt the partial pressure balance, making it harder for gases to move through the lungs, which demonstrates how both internal and external factors can affect diffusion. In addition, respiratory diseases significantly reduce how well the lungs can perform their functions. COPD and ILD are examples of how lung diseases can significantly alter the structure and function of the respiratory system. Research indicates that in severe COPD, even a slight reduction in breath-hold time can lead to a notable decrease in measured DLCO values, reflecting the compromised gas exchange capability in these patients (Magro et al., 2012). Additionally, the changes in lung mechanics and compliance observed in ILD can also impede gas diffusion, highlighting the complex relationship between lung structure, the disease, and gas exchange. Understanding these factors is essential for both diagnosing and managing respiratory conditions, as it informs therapeutic strategies aimed at optimizing diffusing capacity and overall respiratory function (Matharoo et al., 2016).

6.6.3. Clinical Relevance of Diffusing Capacity Assessments

The clinical relevance of diffusing capacity assessments, particularly through the measurement of the diffusion capacity of the lung for carbon monoxide (DLCO), provides critical insights into respiratory health and disease. It helps show how well gas exchange is happening in the lungs and how healthy the alveolar-capillary membrane is. Evaluating DLCO is important for finding out about pulmonary fibrosis, emphysema, and pulmonary hypertension because it can point out changes in gas exchange that may suggest these diseases. Analyzing the connection between gas diffusion, alveolar surface area, and hydraulic permeability allows clinicians to understand how diseases can affect breathing. This diagnostic tool not only helps identify the severity of lung diseases but also aids in monitoring the effectiveness of treatments, making it indispensable in clinical practice (Patel et al., 2023).

Additionally, by assessing diffusing capacity, clinicians can investigate how various factors impact the lungs' functioning. The amount of oxygen and carbon dioxide in the alveoli, which depends on their partial pressures, is important for efficient gas exchange. Evaluating DLCO in different circumstances such as variations in hemoglobin, helps healthcare providers understand a patient's oxygen levels and how well oxygen is being used by the blood. In critical care, it is critical to monitor respiratory status since patients may have different breathing needs or lung problems. Therefore, understanding the nuances surrounding diffusing capacity assessments enhances clinical decision-making and personalized patient care (Binks, 2022). Diffusion capacity is crucial for understanding the impact of various lung diseases on the body, which in turn influences the treatment approach for those diseases. For patients with COPD, a low diffusing capacity often indicates a significant decline in lung function, which requires actions to improve oxygenation. As a result, clinical tests on gas diffusion give details that help choose the best therapies for a patient, such as oxygen or bronchodilator treatments. Ultimately, integrating diffusing capacity assessments into standard pulmonary evaluations represents a comprehensive approach to diagnosing and managing respiratory disorders, effectively bridging the gap between clinical findings and therapeutic interventions (Patel et al., 2023).

SUMMARY

To understand how gases move in the lungs, it is clear that Fick's Law of Diffusion is very important. The law describes how oxygen and carbon dioxide move through the alveolar-capillary membrane and highlights that concentration differences drive diffusion. The concept of diffusion capacity, particularly as measured by DLCO (Diffusion Capacity of the Lung for Carbon Monoxide) , serves as a crucial indicator of pulmonary function. Evaluating DLCO enables us to assess how effectively alveolar-capillary diffusion is functioning, which is crucial for proper gas exchange. In addition, linking DLCO results to reduced surface area in the lungs or poor blood flow can help diagnose different lung conditions, which demonstrates why accurate gas diffusion checks are necessary in medicine. Understanding how the partial pressures of respiratory gases interact is crucial for comprehending how the lungs function. The fact that the partial pressures of oxygen differ in alveolar air, arterial blood and venous blood helps gases pass through the alveolar wall. Due to the pressure gradient, oxygen is carried into the blood, and carbon dioxide is removed for exhalation. Additionally, when factors such as altitude and respiratory rate are altered, it becomes evident that external and bodily changes can affect the way gases diffuse. When at a higher altitude, the lower oxygen in the air can cause hypoxemia, which can make it harder for a person to exercise. Knowing these details is crucial for planning how to optimize oxygen supply, particularly in patients with breathing problems. All the factors that affect gas exchange in the lungs are interrelated and cannot be examined separately. Pulmonary fibrosis, COPD, and heart failure are examples of how problems with diffusion capacity can significantly reduce the health of the lungs. Advanced imaging techniques, such as hyperpolarized 129Xe MRI, provide a non-invasive means to assess lung microstructure and its correlation with gas diffusion efficiency (Dregely et al., 2010). Similarly, studies examining oxygen delivery limitations in heart failure patients emphasize the need for accurate diagnostic tools to assess exercise intolerance and overall cardiac function (Hampson et al., 2018). For this reason, combining knowledge from diffusion mechanics, clinical exams, and imaging technology is crucial for advancing pulmonary care and achieving better patient outcomes.

A key concept in understanding gas diffusion in the lungs is Fick's Law of Diffusion, which explains how gases move through membranes. In other words, the law says that the rate of diffusion depends on the surface area used for gas exchange and the difference in the partial pressures of the gases. The primary importance of Fick's Law is evident in its application to the lungs when they are affected by disease. Emphysema and other diseases can change the surface area of the alveoli, which can significantly reduce the body's ability to transfer gases, showing the importance of having enough alveoli. The insights garnered through imaging techniques, particularly those employing hyperpolarized gases, have enhanced our understanding of these dynamics by providing real-time assessments of the diffusion processes occurring within the pulmonary system (Kaushik et al., 2025). Moreover, the diffusion capacity of the lung (DLCO) plays a crucial role in evaluating pulmonary function. Changes in the size of the alveoli and the thickness of their membrane have a substantial effect on DLCO. Studies using hyperpolarized gas MRI are now connecting these measurements to changes in the lungs, which gives a clearer picture of COPD and pulmonary fibrosis. Recent studies have demonstrated that individuals with reduced DLCO often exhibit significantly different apparent diffusion coefficients (ADC) when assessed with hyperpolarized gases, adding a layer of sensitivity to the identification of lung function impairments and facilitating earlier clinical interventions (Kirby et al., 2013). Additionally, several factors that affect gas exchange make it more challenging to understand lung diffusion. Such factors are V/Q mismatch, the gases' solubility, and the mechanics of the lung tissues. How much oxygen and carbon dioxide are exchanged depends a lot on the partial pressures of these gases, which are affected by the air and a person's body. Recent methods, for example, diffusion-weighted imaging of hyperpolarized gases, provide new insights into how gas exchange occurs in the lungs in various diseases. Such advancements not only enhance diagnostic accuracy but also pave the way for targeted therapies that address specific pathophysiological alterations within the lungs' gas-exchanging surfaces (Kaushik et al., 2025).

CLOSER LOOK

VENTILATION-PERFUSION MISMATCH

A V/Q mismatch occurs when the amount of air reaching the alveoli (ventilation) is not matched by the amount of blood flowing past them (perfusion), resulting in inefficient gas exchange. Various factors, including lung conditions, heart problems, or blood clots can cause this mismatch.

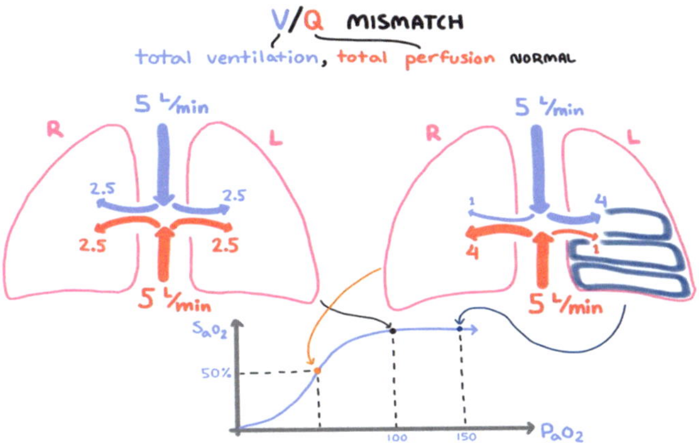

Figure 6.16. Illustration of Ventilation-perfusion (V/Q) mismatch.

Source: https://i.ytimg.com/vi/49YIGySYAtA/maxresdefault.jpg.

V/Q Mismatch

- **V/Q Ratio:** The V/Q ratio represents the relationship between ventilation (V) and perfusion (Q) in the lungs. A normal V/Q ratio is generally around 0.8, meaning for every 4 liters of air entering the lungs, there are 5 liters of blood flowing through the capillaries surrounding the alveoli.
- **Mismatch:** A V/Q mismatch occurs when the ratio of ventilation to perfusion is not properly matched, meaning that some areas of the lungs receive too much air without sufficient blood flow, or vice versa.

Causes of V/Q Mismatch

- **Lung Conditions:** Chronic lung diseases, such as asthma, COPD, and ILDs, can impair ventilation or perfusion, leading to a ventilation-perfusion mismatch.
- **Blood Clots:** Pulmonary embolism (a blood clot in the lung) can obstruct blood flow, causing a V/Q mismatch.
- **Heart Problems:** Heart failure can reduce blood flow to the lungs, resulting in a V/Q mismatch.

- **Other factors, such as infections, pneumonia, or other conditions affecting the airways or blood vessels,** can also disrupt ventilation or perfusion.

Consequences of V/Q Mismatch

- **Hypoxemia:** Inefficient gas exchange can lead to lower oxygen levels in the blood (hypoxemia), causing symptoms such as shortness of breath, lightheadedness, or even loss of consciousness.
- **Hypercapnia:** Reduced ventilation in some areas of the lung can also lead to increased levels of carbon dioxide in the blood (hypercapnia).
- **Other Complications:** Severe V/Q mismatch can worsen lung injury and may be an indicator of poor prognosis in certain conditions like ARDS.

Impact on Oxygen Levels

- **Low V/Q:** In areas with low V/Q, alveolar oxygen is taken up by blood at a high rate, but it is refreshed by ventilation at a slow rate, resulting in poor oxygenation.
- **High V/Q:** In areas with high V/Q, alveolar oxygen levels are increased, but this doesn't fully compensate for the low oxygen levels in areas with low V/Q.
- **Supplemental Oxygen:** While supplemental oxygen can increase oxygen delivery to areas with low V/Q, it may have a limited effect in areas with high V/Q because those areas are already well-oxygenated.

Diagnosis and Treatment

- **V/Q Scan:** A V/Q scan, also known as a V/Q lung scan, is a specialized imaging test that helps diagnose V/Q mismatch by assessing airflow and blood flow in the lungs.
- Treatment for V/Q mismatch depends on the underlying cause and may include medications to address lung disease or heart problems, removal of blood clots, or other interventions to improve ventilation or perfusion.

REFERENCES

1. Almanza-Hurtado, A., Guerra, C. P., Martínez-Ávila, M. C., Borré-Naranjo, D., Rodríguez-Yanez, T., & Dueñas-Castell, C. (2022). Hypercapnia from Physiology to Practice. *International Journal of Clinical Practice, 2022*, 1–10. https://doi.org/10.1155/2022/2635616Amann, A., Amann, A., Lumb, A. B., Schrikker, A. C., Mörk, A. K., Mörk, A. K., Amann, A., et al. (2010). *A Mathematical Model for Breath Gas Analysis of Volatile Organic Compounds with Special Emphasis on Acetone*. http://arxiv.org/abs/1003.4475 (accessed on 31st May 2025).
2. Binks, A. (2022). *Pulmonary Physiology for Pre-Clinical Students*. https://doi.org/10.21061/pulmonaryphysiology (accessed on 31st May 2025).
3. Claassen, J. A. H. R., Thijssen, D. H. J., Panerai, R. B., & Faraci, F. M. (2021). Regulation of cerebral blood flow in humans: Physiology and clinical implications of autoregulation. *Physiological Reviews, 101*, 1487–1559. https://doi.org/10.1152/physrev.00022.2020 (accessed on 31st May 2025).
4. Da Silva, F. O., Camargo, A. F., & Treichel, H. (2023). *Antibiotics Found in Water Bodies and Treatment Methods*. https://doi.org/10.22533/at.ed.559231212 (accessed on 31st May 2025).
5. Dregely, I. (2010). *Hyperpolarized Xenon-129 Magnetic Resonance Imaging of Functional Lung Microstructure*. https://core.ac.uk/download/215517345.pdf (accessed on 31st May 2025).
6. Ferretti, G., Fagoni, N., Taboni, A., Vinetti, G., & di Prampero, P. E. (2022). A century of exercise physiology: Key concepts on coupling respiratory oxygen flow to muscle energy demand during exercise. *European Journal of Applied Physiology, 122*, 1317–1365. https://doi.org/10.1007/s00421-022-04901-x (accessed on 31st May 2025).
7. Guazzi, M. (2000). Impedance to gas transfer across the alveolar-capillary membrane in chronic cardiac failure. *Ital Heart J, 1*(3), 169–173. https://ifcardio.org/pdf/italian-heart-journal/2000/03/20000040.pdf (accessed on 31st May 2025).
8. Hampson, S. A. (2018). *Mechanisms of Exercise Intolerance in Heart Failure*. https://core.ac.uk/download/237179458.pdf (accessed on 31st May 2025).
9. Kang, M. Y., Grebenkov, D. S., Guénard, H., Katz, I., & Sapoval, B. (2017). The Roughton-Forster equation for DL CO and DL NO re-examined. Respiratory *Physiology & Neurobiology, 241*, 62–71. https://doi.org/10.1016/j.resp.2016.12.014 (accessed on 31st May 2025).
10. Kaushik, S. S. (2025). *Translational Imaging of Pulmonary Gas-Exchange Using Hyperpolarized 129Xe Magnetic Resonance Imaging*. https://core.ac.uk/download/pdf/37750571.pdf (accessed on 31st May 2025).
11. Kirby, M. (2013). Pulmonary structure and function in chronic obstructive pulmonary disease evaluated using hyperpolarized noble gas magnetic resonance imaging. *Electronic Thesis and Dissertation Repository*. https://core.ac.uk/download/61637203.pdf (accessed on 31st May 2025).
12. Lindenmaier, T. J. (2015). *Three-Dimensional Computed Tomography Measurements of Pulmonary Artery Volumes: Development and Application*. https://core.ac.uk/download/61658072.pdf (accessed on 31st May 2025).
13. Magro, E. (2012). *Effect of Reduction of Breath-Holding Time in the Single-Breath Method to Assess Carbon Monoxide Diffusing Capacity*. https://core.ac.uk/download/301307415.pdf (accessed on 31st May 2025).

14. Matharoo, H. (2016). Development of a microfluidic oxygenator as an oxygenating unit of a lung assist device for term and pre-term neonates with respiratory distress syndrome. https://core.ac.uk/download/639170923.pdf (accessed on 31st May 2025).

15. Mulroney, S., & Myers, A. (2023). *Netter's Essential Physiology – E-Book*. Elsevier Health Sciences. https://play.google.com/store/books/details?id=35rxEAAAQBAJ&source=gbs_api (accessed on 31st May 2025).

16. N/A. (1993). *Supported Liquid Membranes in Flow Systems*. https://core.ac.uk/download/638451666.pdf (accessed on 31st May 2025).

17. Pace, N. (2015). *Basic and Advanced Sciences for Anesthetic Practice: Prepare for the FRCA*. Elsevier Health Sciences. https://play.google.com/store/books/details?id=i_MACwAAQBAJ&source=gbs_api (accessed on 31st May 2025).

18. Patel, N., & Patel, K. (2023). Mathematical study of the pulmonary gas exchange for the respiratory system under normal and abnormal conditions. *Indian Journal of Science and Technology, 16*(SP4), 1–7. https://doi.org/10.17485/IJST/v16iSP4.ICAMS10 (accessed on 31st May 2025).

19. Satrell, E. (2022). *Alveolar Function Following Extremely Preterm Birth*. https://core.ac.uk/download/548732691.pdf (accessed on 31st May 2025).

20. Schulze, K. M. (2020). *Nitric Oxide Donor Reveals Alterations in Interstitial Oxygen Pressures During Skeletal Muscle Contractions in Rats with Pulmonary Hypertension*. https://krex.k-state.edu/bitstream/handle/2097/40775/KianaSchulze2020.pdf?sequence=2 (accessed on 31st May 2025).

21. Shokr, E. (2016). *Introduction to Human Physiology for Medical Students*. https://core.ac.uk/download/322470167.pdf (accessed on 31st May 2025).

22. Singh, S., Pelosi, P., & Conway, M. A. (2023). *Oxford Textbook of Respiratory Critical Care*. Oxford University Press. https://play.google.com/store/books/details?id=_WHjEAAAQBAJ&source=gbs_api (accessed on 31st May 2025).

23. Tedjasaputra, V., Bouwsema, M. M., & Stickland, M. K. (2016). Effect of aerobic fitness on capillary blood volume and diffusing membrane capacity responses to exercise. *The Journal of Physiology, 594*, 4359–4370. https://doi.org/10.1113/jp272037 (accessed on 31st May 2025).

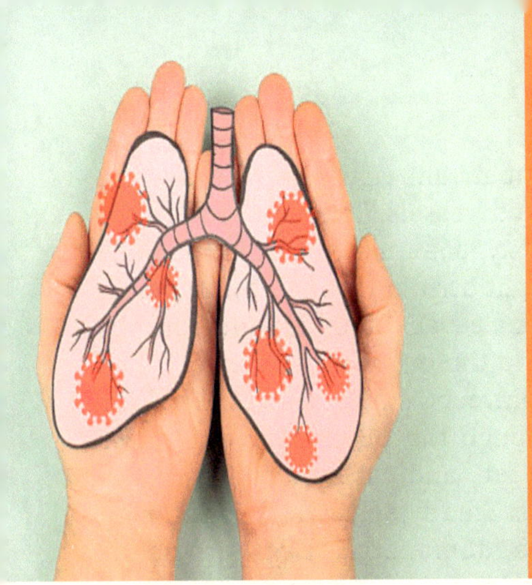

Chapter 7
PULMONARY CIRCULATION

Contents

Introduction

Cardiovascular physiology relies on the detailed structure of pulmonary circulation, which brings deoxygenated blood from the right heart to the lungs. In this system, gas exchange happens, and the body swaps out carbon dioxide for oxygen. At the start, the right ventricle sends deoxygenated blood into the pulmonary artery which carries it to the lungs to be oxygenated. It highlights the importance of blood flow and the specific changes in the body that enhance gas exchange. Pulmonary circulation has special traits, including flexible vessels and the special design of the lungs which support the breathing needed for human survival. Studying pulmonary circulation also encourages a deeper examination of physiology, particularly when considering diseases that can disrupt the process. For instance, the application of Veno-venous extracorporeal membrane oxygenation (V-V ECMO) illustrates the complexity of pulmonary circulation in clinical scenarios. Blood from the central veins is oxygenated outside the body and then sent back to the right heart which proves the important relationship between ECMO and the lungs. To perform such interventions, one must understand both how blood flows and the patient's current condition. Paying attention to the physiology of pulmonary circulation helps improve clinical approaches and treatment, mainly for patients with severe respiratory failure. Besides its role in the structure of the lungs, the pulmonary circulation is involved in many aspects of heart health and disease. The discussion is also aided by new findings on cardiac looping, which describe how the heart's structure affects its ability to function well in the circulatory system. Cardiac looping during embryonic development significantly impacts the relationship between the systemic and pulmonary circulatory pathways. Due to this evolution, the heart is able to pump blood well, and both the pulmonary and systemic circuits work as they should. Having this basic knowledge is essential for guiding the clinical care of pulmonary diseases and for future studies seeking to understand circulatory processes, which leads to a better-coordinated healthcare system.

Definition of Pulmonary Circulation

It is essential to understand the role of the pulmonary circulation in the cardiovascular system to comprehend its intricacies. The pathway of pulmonary circulation is how blood, which is low in oxygen, moves from the right ventricle of the heart to the lungs. It is important because it enables carbon dioxide to be exchanged for oxygen in the alveoli, thereby increasing the oxygen content of the blood before it returns to the heart. The pulmonary arteries and veins ensure that the exchange occurs smoothly, and any problems with this circulation can result in health issues such as pulmonary hypertension and respiratory distress. Essentially, pulmonary circulation is a vital component of systemic circulation, whose primary function is to oxygenate blood and eliminate waste gases from the body. Several key components of pulmonary circulation include the right atrium, right ventricle, and the pulmonary blood vessels. The first step in the cycle is the deoxygenated blood from the body entering the right atrium through the superior and inferior vena cavae. Blood is sent from the right ventricle to the pulmonary arteries when the ventricle contracts. Oxygen enters the blood as it flows through the pulmonary capillaries around the alveoli, and carbon dioxide moves out of the blood. This system, which is carefully designed, both demonstrates its efficiency and highlights its weaknesses; any issue in this process could result in oxygen transport or gas exchange problems. Understanding these dynamics is crucial for addressing and treating conditions like pulmonary arterial hypertension, which showcases the interplay between cardiovascular health and pulmonary function, as seen in studies examining their relationship (Charalampopoulos et al., 2014).

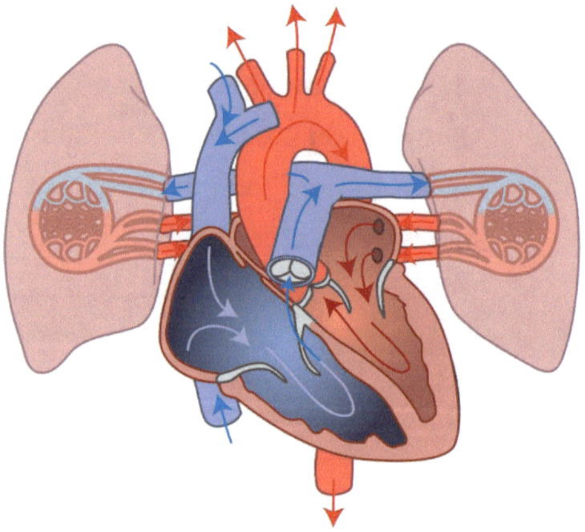

Figure 7.1. Cardiopulmonary circulation.

Source: https://anatomytool.org/sites/default/files/Hartfalen4.NT_.jpg.

Pulmonary circulation is not just about gas exchange; it also helps maintain stable blood pressure and enables the heart to function correctly. The way blood moves and pressure are different in the pulmonary circulation than in the systemic circulation, which affects how atrial fibrillation is managed. Research has found that arrhythmias can originate in the lungs, and premature atrial contractions are often observed in the pulmonary veins. It demonstrates that cardiac rhythm and pulmonary health are linked, which means patients with both conditions should be managed by a team of specialists. Thus, the definition of pulmonary circulation not only encompasses its fundamental physiological roles but also reflects its complex interactions with broader systemic health (Harvey et al., 2017) (Figure 7.1).

Importance of Pulmonary Circulation in the Cardiovascular System

Gas exchange in the lungs is facilitated by pulmonary circulation, which enables the cardiovascular system to function properly. Whereas systemic circulation sends oxygen-rich blood to the body's tissues, pulmonary circulation carries blood low in oxygen from the right ventricle to the lungs. The blood in the capillaries of the lungs is oxygenated, and carbon dioxide is removed while oxygen is added. The oxygen saturation in the blood, which is important for cellular metabolism, is directly affected by this process. For this reason, the health of the pulmonary circulation significantly affects how well the body's organs function and their longevity, making it an important and necessary part of cardiovascular physiology that should be well understood and closely monitored. Pulmonary circulation must be efficient to support gas exchange and also to help control blood pressure in the cardiovascular system. As pulmonary arteries have less pressure than systemic arteries, delicate gas exchange in the alveoli is protected. To maintain the lower pressure, various mechanisms in the body, such as vasodilation and vasoconstriction, respond to things like hypoxia. Due to these processes, the lungs receive enough blood and oxygen, and pulmonary hypertension – which could lead to serious heart problems – is avoided. If circulation in the lungs is interrupted by thromboembolic disorders or congenital anomalies, the right ventricle must work harder, which can lead to heart failure. Thus, understanding pulmonary circulatory dynamics is crucial for preventing and managing cardiovascular diseases (CVDs). Additionally, pulmonary circulation plays a crucial role in the body's response to illnesses and infections, including sepsis. There is much evidence that both the pulmonary and systemic circulatory systems cooperate to support homeostasis. In sepsis, the body's reactions are not appropriately controlled, which changes how blood flows and reduces oxygen to tissues. New findings about sepsis have clarified that poor lung function can make sepsis outcomes more severe. New definitions and clinical criteria have emerged to enhance the recognition and management of this condition, highlighting the necessity of effective pulmonary circulation in maintaining systemic health (Ponikowski et al., 2016; Singer et al., 2016). Therefore, understanding pulmonary circulation well benefits both our general cardiovascular understanding and the way clinicians handle severe conditions, such as sepsis.

7.1. Anatomy of the Pulmonary Circulation

The pulmonary circulation system is essential to the cardiovascular system, facilitating the exchange of gases between the lungs and blood. Deoxygenated blood, which begins in the right ventricle, is carried through the pulmonary arteries to the lungs. Once in the lungs, the blood flows through many capillaries, where it undergoes a vital transformation: it releases carbon dioxide and picks up oxygen. In the alveoli, which are tiny sacs lined with epithelial cells, there is a significant increase in the area for gas exchange. Understanding the intricacies of this system not only highlights its critical role in sustaining life through oxygen delivery but also underscores its significance in various health conditions that may impair respiratory function (Elmaghawry et al., 2015). The unique structure of the pulmonary vessels is essential for efficient gas exchange. The walls of pulmonary arteries are thinner than those of systemic arteries, and their structure allows them to change with the changes in air pressure during breathing. They are important because they keep blood flow steady in the lungs, which change pressure frequently. Also, because alveolar capillaries are very close to alveoli, gases can be exchanged quickly. The composition of pulmonary tissue, particularly the elastic fibers in the walls of the arteries and veins, facilitates this unique flexibility and adaptability, ensuring that the lungs can accommodate varying volumes of air in response to the body's metabolic demands (Danduran et al., 2012). Understanding the structure of pulmonary circulation is crucial for both diagnosing and managing lung-related illnesses. Problems such as pulmonary hypertension or congenital heart defects can significantly disrupt how blood circulates, which can lead to inadequate oxygenation and health complications throughout the body. For example, changes in the pulmonary arteries can lead to increased pressure in the lungs, resulting in symptoms such as shortness of breath and fatigue. Advanced imaging techniques and assessments, such as near-infrared spectroscopy (NIRS), have become invaluable in evaluating these disorders by providing real-time delineation of patterns of blood flow and oxygenation. Thus, a comprehensive grasp of pulmonary circulation anatomy not only enriches the understanding of basic physiology but also informs therapeutic strategies aimed at restoring homeostasis in patients suffering from pulmonary dysfunction (Danduran et al., 2012) (Figure 7.2).

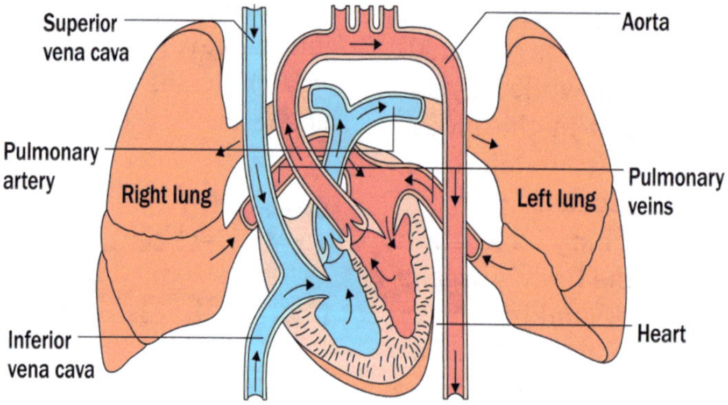

Figure 7.2. Pulmonary circulation.

Source: https://www.shutterstock.com/image-vector/pulmonary-circulation-vector-illustration-on-260nw-436019533.jpg.

7.1.1. Key Components: Heart, Lungs, and Blood Vessels

Pulmonary circulation can only be understood by looking at the relationship between the heart, lungs, and blood vessels. The heart pumps blood to the pulmonary circuit, which carries blood that needs oxygen to the lungs. The blood in the lungs passes through the pulmonary arteries, which branch into numerous smaller vessels to facilitate gas exchange in the alveoli. The exchange means carbon dioxide leaves the blood and oxygen enters it, which is then carried back to the heart through the pulmonary veins. It is essential that this cycle is both efficient and effective, supporting cellular respiration and maintaining the body's overall balance, which underscores the strong connection between these components of the circulatory system. Moreover, the structural integrity and functional capacity of blood vessels are pivotal during pulmonary circulation (Figure 7.3).

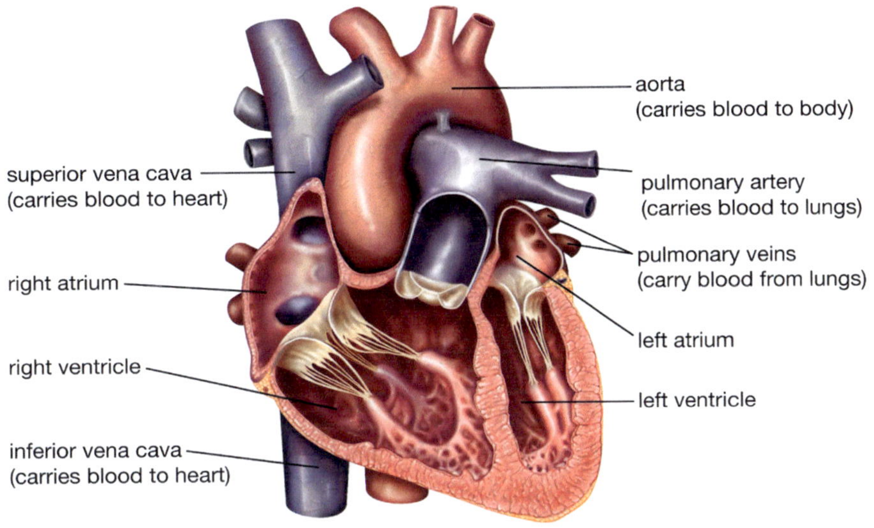

Figure 7.3. Human heart.

Source: https://cdn.britannica.com/05/85505-050-44E1AD82/Cross-section-human-heart.jpg.

The special features of pulmonary arteries and veins enable the lungs to handle a large amount of blood without increasing pressure excessively. If someone has a pathological condition, changes in the vascular system's flexibility, such as fibrosis, can have a significant effect on hemodynamics. Recent research has found that fibrosis in the lungs can lead to increased circulation of additional factors, which in turn increases blood vessel permeability and affects the exchange of gases. Such changes not only sustain tissue oxygenation but also influence tumor organotropism, suggesting that the vascular response is crucial for both normal physiology and disease pathology (Fletcher et al., 2016).

Additionally, techniques like specific ventilation imaging (SVI) have emerged as valuable tools for assessing pulmonary function within this complex system. SVI utilizes oxygen-enhanced magnetic resonance imaging (MRI) to evaluate specific ventilation patterns within the lungs, capturing detailed insights into regional blood flow and oxygen exchange. Research has shown that imaging a single lung slice can reliably represent overall pulmonary function, while also highlighting the influence of venous blood on oxygen measurements within these slices (Burrowes et al., 2018). Understanding such dynamics is fundamental in identifying potential disruptions in pulmonary circulation and can facilitate targeted interventions for various respiratory and cardiovascular diseases (CVDs). As we explore the intricacies of the heart, lungs, and blood vessels, it becomes evident that a comprehensive understanding of pulmonary circulation is paramount for advancing clinical practices and improving patient outcomes (Figure 7.4).

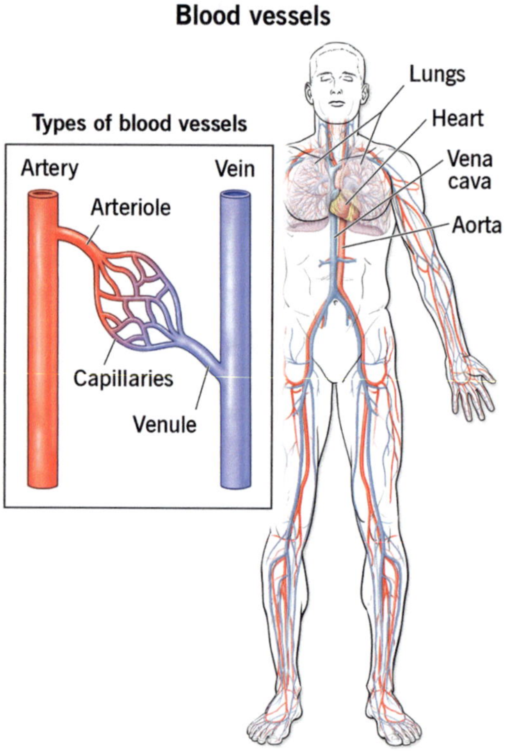

Figure 7.4. Blood vessels.

Source: https://my.clevelandclinic.org/-/scassets/images/org/health/articles/blood-vessels.

7.1.2. The Role of the Right Ventricle

The right ventricle (RV) plays a pivotal role in pulmonary circulation, primarily responsible for pumping deoxygenated blood into the pulmonary arteries, where gas exchange occurs in the lungs. The thin walls of this chamber are necessary so that it can accommodate different amounts of blood with less pressure than the left ventricle, which is responsible for systemic circulation. When it is functioning properly, the RV moves blood smoothly through the lungs, allowing oxygen to enter and carbon dioxide to exit the blood. Still, different problems can disrupt RV function, which can harm both lung circulation and the heart's health. It is crucial to understand RV dynamics to accurately diagnose and treat diseases that impact pulmonary pressures and flow. Increased proper ventricular pressure can significantly affect how the lungs receive blood, as is clear from studies on patients with fluid overload during hemodialysis. Research has shown that patients with higher interdialytic weight gain (IDWG%) demonstrate increased proper ventricular systolic pressure (RVSP), indicating an overload on the pulmonary circulation system (Anastasiou et al., 2023). It proves that the RV must be able to handle rising blood volume and pressure without failing.

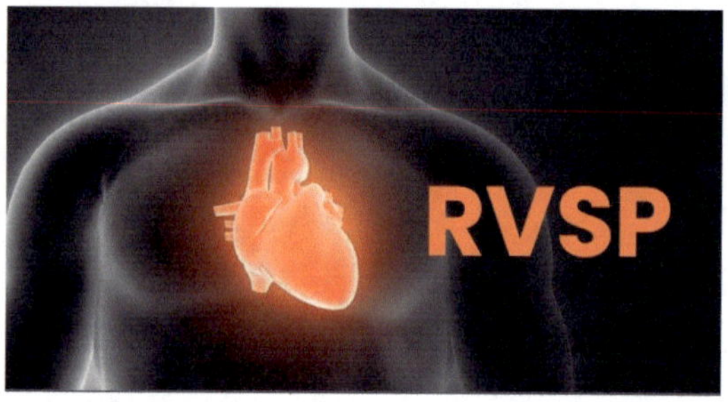

Figure 7.5. Right ventricular systolic pressure (RVSP).

Source: https://aclsnow.com/wp-content/uploads/2024/11/RVSP-%E2%80%93-Right-Ventricular-Systolic-Pressure-post-img.webp.

The heart chambers in these patients are enlarged, which suggests that long-term overload could lead to heart disease. For this reason, clinicians need to track these signs in patients to reduce the chances of complications from pulmonary hypertension and RV dysfunction. In certain cases, such as pre-eclampsia, the health of the right ventricle is particularly crucial. The presence of anti-angiogenic factors in this condition contributes to increased pulmonary vascular resistance (PVR), affecting the functioning of the RV (Zaky et al., 2021). Researchers have seen that women who develop early pre-eclampsia have higher mean pulmonary artery pressure, which shows the RV has to work harder to maintain normal blood flow. Due to this strain, the RV exhibits subtle changes in its function, indicating that it is easily influenced by changes in the body. As such, echocardiography serves an essential role in assessing RV function and identifying potential pulmonary hypertension, allowing for early intervention and improved management strategies in at-risk populations (Figure 7.5).

7.1.3. The Structure of Pulmonary Arteries and Veins

The pulmonary arteries and veins are crucial components of the pulmonary circulation system, as they transport blood from the heart to the lungs. Deoxygenated blood is carried by the pulmonary arteries, which come from the right ventricle, to the lungs for oxygenation. As the pulmonary arteries differ from systemic arteries (they have thinner walls and a larger opening), they allow low-pressure blood to flow without compromising their structure. This is very important since the pressure in the pulmonary circulation is much lower than in the rest of the body. The pulmonary artery branches into two parts, one for each lung, and this is where gas exchange happens in the alveoli, preparing the blood for the body's general circulation. Pulmonary veins are responsible for returning oxygenated blood to the heart. The veins are thicker and stronger than the pulmonary arteries, which helps move blood back to the left atrium when the pressure is higher. Every lung has two pulmonary veins, which, together with the other two, help deliver oxygen-rich blood into the heart. Because the pulmonary veins are arranged in a certain way, blood flow is efficient, and the resistance is low. These veins are composed of smooth muscle and elastic fibers, which enable them to adjust and support varying amounts of blood. It is necessary for this structural change to maintain flexible blood flow, regardless of whether the body is active or at rest. Studying the structure of pulmonary arteries and veins is helpful because it lets us understand the causes and symptoms of diseases in the pulmonary system. For example, in cases of congenital corrected transposition of the great arteries (ccTGA), the anomalies in structural connections between these vascular components can lead to severe physiological complications. This disorder illustrates how the right atrium connects to the left ventricle via the mitral valve, which complicates blood flow dynamics and potentially leads to systemic issues due to inadequate oxygenation (Sümeyye et al., 2025). When a single ventricle defect is present, special surgical techniques that utilize shunts are required, emphasizing the need to understand the biomechanics of these vessels. Recent studies advocate for the use of autologous umbilical vessels as alternatives for palliative shunts, indicating that further analysis of the pulmonary blood vessel structure is crucial for enhancing patient outcomes (Murtada et al., 2023) (Figure 7.6).

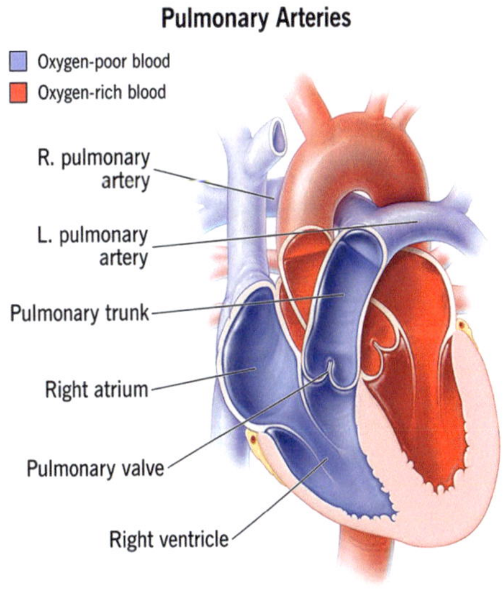

Figure 7.6. Pulmonary arteries.

Source: https://my.clevelandclinic.org/-/scassets/images/org/health/articles/21486-pulmonary-arteries-anatomy.ashx?io=transform:fit,width:780.

7.2. The Process of Pulmonary Circulation

The main job of pulmonary circulation is to carry deoxygenated blood from the heart to the lungs, which is a key function in the cardiovascular system. The circuit starts when the right atrium receives blood from the superior and inferior vena cavae, which are part of the systemic circulation. After the atria squeeze, blood is pushed into the right ventricle by the tricuspid valve. Then, the right ventricle contracts, forcing blood across the pulmonary valve and into the pulmonary arteries. This step is crucial because it prepares the blood for oxygen, enabling the exchange of oxygen and carbon dioxide in the lungs. Understanding this flow is vital as any disruption could lead to significant clinical conditions, such as pulmonary hypertension, which is characterized by progressive narrowing of pulmonary vessels, resulting in increased pressure and potential heart failure (Heydari et al., 2025).

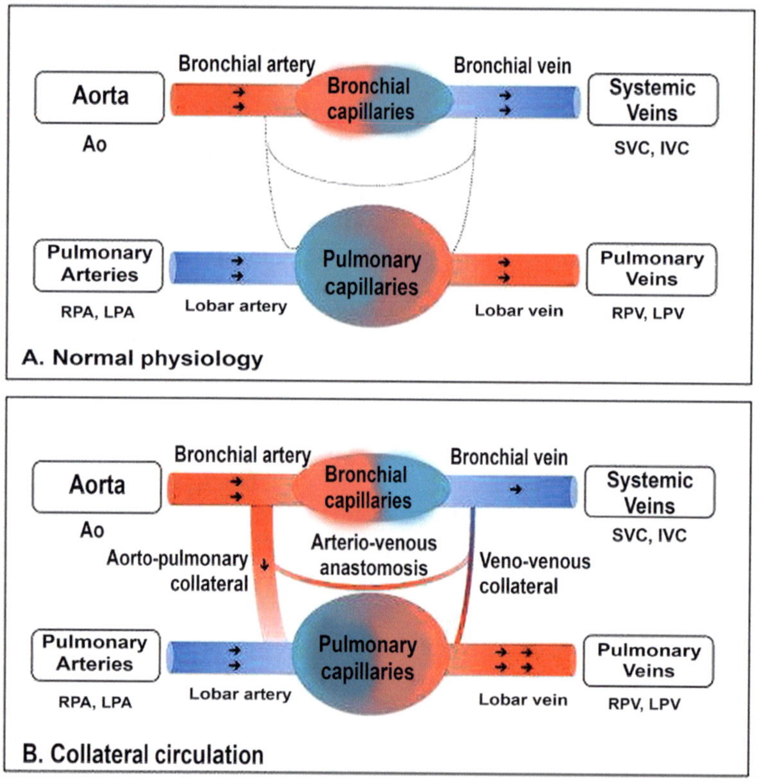

These shunting connections are 1) the aortopulmonary collaterals (between the bronchial artery and the pulmonary artery), 2) the veno-venous collaterals (between the bronchial vein and the pulmonary vein) and 3) the arterio-venous shunts (direct connections between the bronchial artery and vein bypassing the capillary network).

Figure 7.7. Scheme of systemic and pulmonary circulation. (A) Normal physiology: The virtual network connections are present but are not permeable; and (B) Collateral circulation.

source: https://www.researchgate.net/profile/Philipp-Beerbaum/publication/224864994/figure/fig1/AS:213809940701185@1427987670892/Scheme-of-systemic-and-pulmonary-circulation-A-Normal-physiology-The-virtual-network.png.

As blood reaches the pulmonary arteries, it is directed to the lungs and then branches into smaller arterioles, which in turn branch into capillaries close to the alveoli. This transition is pivotal for efficient gas exchange. Oxygen moves from the air into the blood, and carbon dioxide is sent from the blood to the alveoli to be breathed out. The efficiency of this gas exchange process is influenced by several factors, including ventilation-perfusion (V/Q) coupling and the surface area available for diffusion. Pulmonary hypertension causes the blood vessels to narrow, which can significantly affect gas exchange and lead to low oxygen levels in the blood, as well as added strain on the right side of the heart. It highlights the importance of maintaining regular pulmonary circulation for overall well-being. The blood that has taken in oxygen in the lungs is then carried back to the heart by the pulmonary veins. From the veins, the oxygenated blood goes to the left atrium, and after atrial contraction, it travels through the mitral valve into the left ventricle. After leaving the right ventricle, blood is sent into the aorta, which pumps it into the systemic circulation to supply oxygen and nutrients to the body's tissues. The way pulmonary circulation is organized helps to remove carbon dioxide and also provides oxygen for the body to use in metabolism. Furthermore, it underscores the critical interplay between pulmonary and systemic circulation, illustrating how disturbances in one can lead to complications in the other, necessitating a comprehensive understanding of both systems in the realm of cardiovascular health (Heydari et al. 2025) (Figure 7.7).

7.2.1. Blood Flow From the Heart to the Lungs

The movement of blood from the heart to the lungs is crucial for pulmonary circulation, which enables the gas exchange necessary for life. The right ventricle pumps deoxygenated blood through the pulmonary valve into the pulmonary artery. Blood is directed from the pulmonary artery, which has branches on the left and right, to the proper lung. Blood moving through the arteries gives off carbon dioxide and picks up oxygen in the pulmonary capillaries near the alveoli in the lungs. It helps to replace oxygen in the blood, so that tissues everywhere in the body receive enough oxygen. Several physiological factors, including vascular resistance and pressure gradients, influence the flow of blood through the lungs. The pressure in the right ventricle is much lower than in the left ventricle which keeps the delicate capillaries in the lungs safe. If pulmonary circulation is examined, there is a chance of finding pulmonary hypertension, a condition in which the pressure in the pulmonary vessels is higher than usual. Such abnormalities may cause the blood to receive less oxygen, which worsens breathing problems. In this context, advanced techniques like right heart catheterization provide critical insights into pulmonary arterial pressure and help determine the underlying causes of suspected pulmonary hypertension, ultimately guiding effective treatment strategies (Pagnamenta et al., 2017).

Extracorporeal membrane oxygenation (ECMO) has emerged as an important intervention in managing severe cases of pulmonary dysfunction. Patients with acute respiratory distress are helped by ECMO, which takes blood from the right ventricle and enriches it with oxygen. A recent study highlighted the advantages of pulsatile flow in ECMO, indicating that it promotes better oxygenated pulmonary flow while minimizing vascular complications. This method demonstrates that proper hemodynamics in the lungs are crucial for facilitating patient recovery and overall well-being. Understanding the intricacies of blood flow from the heart to the lungs not only illuminates the mechanics of pulmonary circulation but also underscores the implications for clinical practice in treating respiratory conditions effectively (Figure 7.8).

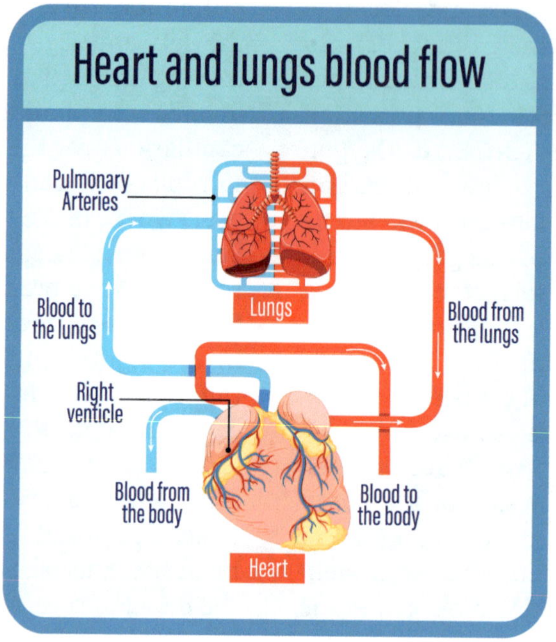

Figure 7.8. Heart and lungs blood flow.

Source: https://nursingwithlight.com/wp-content/uploads/2024/04/25540125_5rqk_2rrq_220303-scaled.jpg.

7.2.2. Gas Exchange in the Alveoli

In the lungs, gas exchange in the alveoli is critical because this is where oxygen goes into the blood and carbon dioxide leaves it. The alveoli, which are at the end of the bronchioles, have fragile walls that help gases diffuse easily. Capillaries, which are small blood vessels, surround each alveolus and facilitate the exchange process. Due to this structure, the lungs have a large surface area for gas exchange, as they contain approximately 300 million alveoli. The movement of gases depends on their partial pressure; oxygen, which is more concentrated in the alveoli, is taken up by the blood, and carbon dioxide, present in greater amounts in venous blood, moves into the alveoli for exhalation. Also, gas exchange in the alveoli depends on ventilation and perfusion. Ventilation means air entering the alveoli, and perfusion describes blood passing through the nearby capillaries. Gas exchange works best when the two processes are coordinated, a phenomenon often referred to as the V/Q ratio. If one part of the lung is well-ventilated but poorly perfused, or vice versa, it may lead to less oxygen being taken in or less carbon dioxide being removed. The body employs various mechanisms to adjust to changes, such as exercise or exposure to high altitude, in order to maintain a good V/Q ratio for effective gas exchange. This indicates that alveolar health and function are crucial for the effective functioning of the lungs. The way respiratory diseases affect the body can make it difficult for oxygen to enter the blood, which puts stress on the heart. Conditions like chronic obstructive pulmonary disease (COPD), pneumonia, and pulmonary edema negatively impact the alveolar-capillary membrane, reducing its surface area and increasing its thickness. When the lungs deteriorate, the process of diffusion is slowed, making it harder for the lungs to oxygenate the blood and remove carbon dioxide. If the virus is severe, for example, MERS-CoV, it can cause severe damage to the lungs, which complicates breathing and often leads to serious consequences. Although no specific antiviral treatments for such infections are universally established, exploring therapeutic options like remdesivir can offer insights into potential interventions as research continues, highlighting the critical interplay between infections and gas exchange efficiency in the alveoli.

7.2.3. Return of Oxygenated Blood to the Heart

Pulmonary circulation relies on oxygenated blood returning to the heart, which helps keep gases exchanged and the heart functioning properly. When the lungs oxygenate the blood, it goes through the pulmonary veins to the left atrium of the heart. The extra oxygen in the blood helps meet the needs of the tissues in the body's periphery. Atrial contraction, together with ventricular relaxation, makes sure the left atrium receives the maximum amount of blood. The blood then moves into the left ventricle, which pumps it into the body's main artery, the aorta. This process ensures that tissues receive enough oxygen to perform cellular respiration and also allows carbon dioxide, produced during metabolism, to be eliminated through the lungs. The proper return of oxygenated blood to the heart depends on several physiological processes that regulate venous flow and enable the heart to function effectively. The changes in thoracic pressure during breathing help blood move back to the heart. Additionally, due to the presence of one-way valves in the veins and the contraction of skeletal muscles, blood is pushed upward against gravity by the heart. Most importantly, all these mechanisms should cooperate to prevent the mixing of blood with deoxygenated blood. This is particularly critical in specialized circulatory variations, such as in patients with single ventricle physiology, where the proper management of systemic venous return becomes integral to maintaining adequate cardiac function and preventing complications associated with Fontan circulatory failure. It is also important to understand how blood returns to the heart with oxygen in clinical settings, particularly when managing fluid for patients with poor circulation. The kidneys, which are easily affected by blood flow changes, can significantly affect the body's overall fluid balance. If venous return is low, it can reduce the amount of oxygenated blood reaching the heart and also cause acute kidney injury due to congestion, illustrating the interconnectedness of these systems. This means that clinicians should carefully manage fluid therapy for patients with heart failure or poor lung function by paying close attention to pressure in the body and how the kidneys are working. This interdependence highlights the intricate balance that exists within the pulmonary circulation and its ultimate impact on systemic health (Figure 7.9).

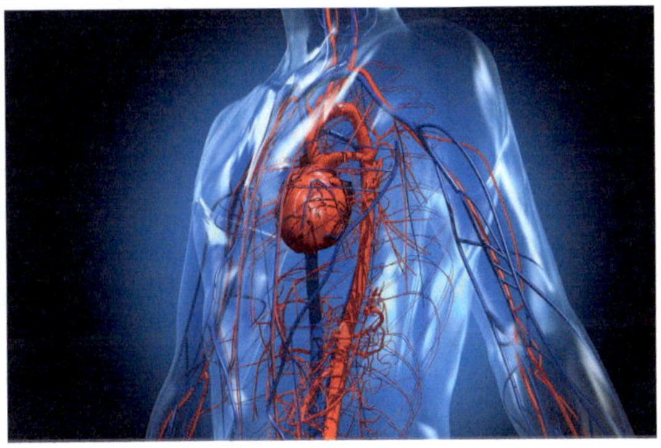

Figure 7.9. Visualization of the human cardiovascular system.

Source: https://www.verywellhealth.com/thmb/q-DE1yH8q4m1eG34Yy4YKntzt2Q=/1500x0/filters:no_upscale():max_bytes(150000):strip_icc()/GettyImages-626974567-defc9220866c4e679c8d244dfbb997bb.jpg.

7.3. Physiological Significance

Pulmonary circulation is not only about moving blood; it is important for gas exchange, which allows oxygen to enter the blood while carbon dioxide is removed. Gas exchange occurs in the alveolar-capillary membrane, which is thin enough to allow gases to diffuse easily. The right ventricle of the heart pumps blood to the lungs for oxygenation, a crucial role in pulmonary circulation. It demonstrates that the cardiovascular and respiratory systems are closely linked, so that changes in one system can affect the other, mainly when the body is working harder or exercising. As advancements in understanding these interactions unfold, particularly concerning heart-lung coupling and its implications on hemodynamics at rest or during physical activity, it has become evident that optimizing pulmonary circulation contributes significantly to overall cardiovascular health (Cheyne et al., 2020). Additionally, the role of pulmonary circulation is crucial in treating various respiratory and cardiovascular problems. Illnesses such as COPD and pulmonary hypertension demonstrate the consequences of poor pulmonary circulation, as they lead to additional health problems. Here, the connection between the lungs and the heart becomes very clear, and it significantly affects how patients fare. Adverse cardiopulmonary interactions are significant because heart problems can be worsened, and exercise can become very difficult. Knowing about these conditions helps doctors choose better treatments and avoid complications which highlights how crucial it is to maintain strong lung circulation. Besides examining pulmonary circulation in specific contexts, research helps us understand its role in the overall health of the body. Pulmonary hemodynamics are linked to several metabolic processes which means that proper pulmonary blood flow is important for controlling inflammation and metabolism throughout the body. Because of this, there is now more interest in the cardiovascular effects of lung diseases, as poor gas exchange may result in systemic hypoxia and organ failure. As the field advances, understanding the impact of pulmonary circulation on both local lung health and the rest of the body is crucial. Engaging with this multidisciplinary perspective can foster innovative solutions to prevent and manage cardiovascular complications associated with respiratory insufficiency, highlighting pulmonary circulation as a cornerstone of holistic health management strategies (Cheyne et al., 2020).

7.3.1. Role in Oxygenation of Blood

The pulmonary circulation enables oxygen to enter the blood and carbon dioxide to exit the blood in the lungs. Deoxygenated blood, which comes from the right side of the heart through the pulmonary arteries, enters the lungs to carry out the primary function of gas exchange. This starts in the alveoli, where oxygen moves into the blood through the walls of tiny capillaries and carbon dioxide moves out in the opposite direction. Pulmonary circulation then delivers oxygen-rich blood from the lungs to the left atrium of the heart, which is ready to be pumped into the body's primary blood system. Proper oxygen exchange is necessary to maintain the right levels of patience, energy, and metabolism in the body, demonstrating the key role of pulmonary circulation in maintaining good health. Additionally, several factors can impact the delivery of oxygen during this crucial stage. As an example, when someone has pulmonary hypertension, a respiratory disease, or weak lung tissue, this can disrupt the regular exchange of oxygen. Additionally, diseases like acute respiratory distress syndrome (ARDS) can severely alter the dynamics of pulmonary circulation, requiring advanced interventions such as ECMO to support oxygenation when traditional methods fail. ECMO, which has become an important treatment, helps support lung-protective ventilation and highlights the connection between artificial support and the body's own mechanisms. Emerging research highlights the importance of understanding these complexities to enhance patient outcomes, particularly in cases of severe respiratory failure, establishing the need for both medical insight and advanced technologies in optimizing oxygenation in pulmonary circulation (Finney et al., 2014). Besides helping individuals, adequate oxygenation is important for many different areas such as veterinary medicine. It has been found in studies on anaesthetized horses that hypoxemia can be very risky, mainly because of the species' special ways of dealing with exercise. Treating hypoxemia in this manner requires meticulous methods to enhance lung oxygen transfer, although these methods may also pose unexpected risks to the heart and lungs. This study highlights the challenges of achieving proper oxygenation in certain settings and underscores the crucial role of pulmonary circulation in facilitating gas exchange across all species and conditions. Understanding the dynamic interplay of pulmonary circulation and oxygenation is therefore an essential part of both medical practice and scientific inquiry, bridging knowledge across fields and enhancing our collective ability to address respiratory challenges effectively (Auckburally et al., 2017) (Figure 7.10).

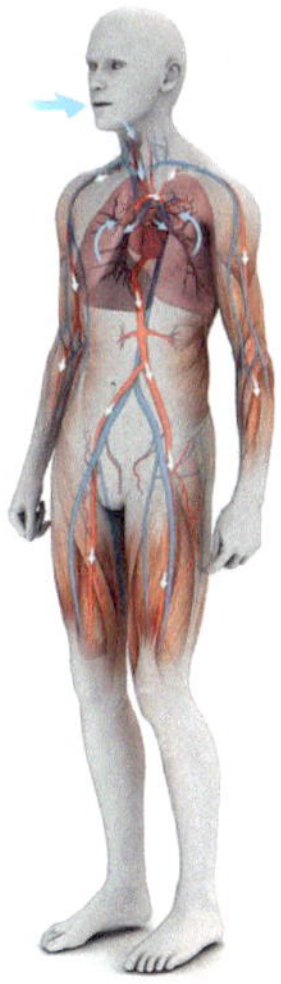

Figure 7.10. Oxygenation of the blood illustration.

Source: https://media.sciencephoto.com/image/c0250678/800wm/C0250678-Oxygenation_of_the_blood,_illustration.jpg.

7.3.2. Impact on Overall Cardiovascular Health

Many pathological processes are key to the important relationship between pulmonary circulation and the overall cardiovascular system. Oxygenating blood and getting it into the systemic circulation depend on pulmonary circulation. When pulmonary hypertension (PH) arises, typically due to chronic lung disease such as COPD, the heart must work harder to pump blood through the narrowed pulmonary arteries. Because of this extra workload, the right ventricle may thicken, which can eventually cause right heart failure and seriously affect the whole cardiovascular system. The consequences of PH not only undermine the efficiency of pulmonary circulation but also cascade into broader cardiovascular issues, deteriorating the health-related quality of life (HRQOL) of affected individuals. These intricacies underscore the necessity for an integrated understanding of the pulmonary and cardiovascular systems in both diagnostic and therapeutic approaches (Bailey et al., 2024). Also, persistent lung issues can significantly reduce a person's ability to exercise, which can make heart problems worse. Patients who get pulmonary hypertension from chronic lung disease are less active because they feel tired and out of breath. Because of this lifestyle, many people experience obesity, hypertension, and diabetes, which are all well-known risk factors for CVD. Because of this cycle, it becomes clear that special actions are needed to help preserve the daily abilities of people with heart disease. Having exercise rehabilitation programs designed specifically for patients with pulmonary hypertension can reduce these risks by improving their physical abilities, mental health, and cardiovascular health. Such multifaceted approaches are essential in breaking the cycle and fostering a healthier cardiovascular system in patients with compromised pulmonary circulation (Bailey et al., 2024). Exploring new areas, such as space, provides additional insights into the interaction between the heart and lungs. The environment of microgravity in space can cause health problems for astronauts, especially with their lungs and hearts. Research has shown that prolonged exposure to microgravity can cause fluid shifts and reduce the heart's fitness, affecting heart rhythms and the body's ability to function properly after landing on Earth. These changes may exacerbate previous issues with pulmonary circulation, adding further stress to the heart. Additionally, being in space means astronauts are exposed to cosmic radiation, which can impact heart health and increase the likelihood of cardiovascular events. Since space travel is being done more often, it is now more important than ever to understand the effects on the pulmonary and cardiovascular systems.

7.3.3. Relationship with Systemic Circulation

The interaction between pulmonary and systemic circulation is significant in cardiovascular physiology because it helps maintain the body's blood pressure and blood flow. Pulmonary circulation takes blood from the systemic veins to the lungs for gas exchange, and systemic circulation carries oxygenated blood to the other parts of the body. Since these two systems are so closely connected, any problem in either one can significantly impact the other. Raised pressure in the pulmonary arteries can cause the right ventricle to function poorly, which may result in problems with the systemic circulation.

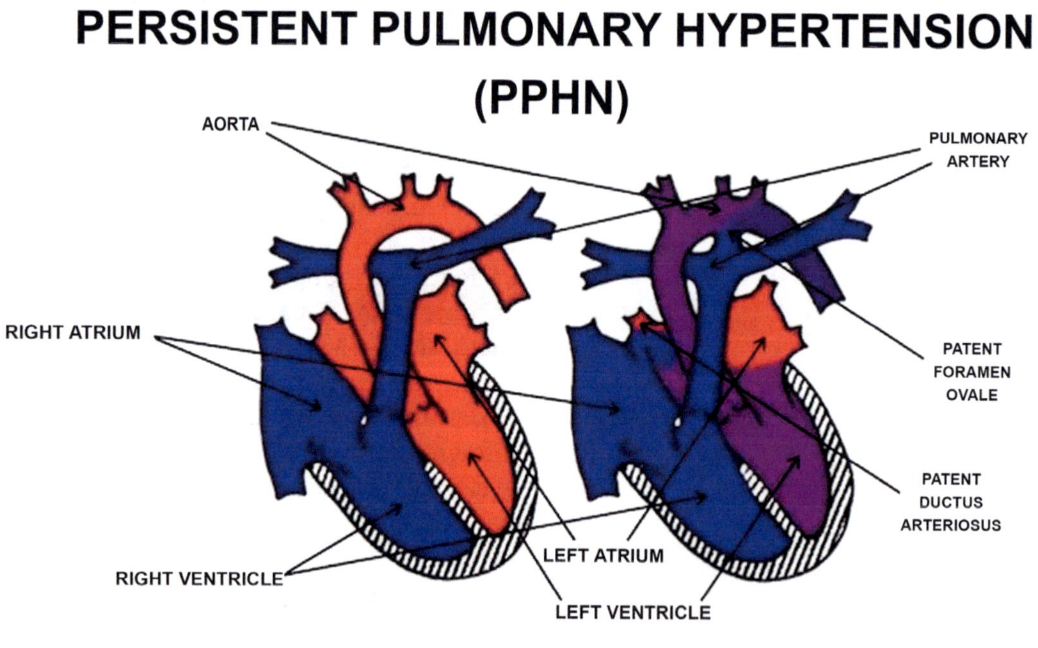

Figure 7.11. Persistent pulmonary hypertension of the newborn (PPHN).

Source: https://cdn.credihealth.com/production/system/blog/uploads/74999/original/pphn20241018-272276-ogpba.webp?1729229177.

This relationship is particularly evident in cases like persistent pulmonary hypertension of the newborn (PPHN), where increased resistance in the pulmonary vasculature can lead to critical hemodynamic alterations and systemic complications (Van de Bruaene et al.). It is crucial to understand how these circulatory systems interact when managing and diagnosing cardiopulmonary issues. The Fontan procedure highlights the close relationship between the pulmonary and systemic circulations in individuals with single-ventricle physiology. The purpose of this surgery is to help blood flow by redirecting it from the veins to the pulmonary arteries, skipping the heart. Even though this arrangement helps separate oxygenated and deoxygenated blood, it can cause high venous pressure throughout the body and lower the heart's output, which is part of the Fontan physiology.

These difficulties happen because the body's blood flow and pressure are changed which affects how much blood the heart receives and how it pumps it. As suggested in recent studies, understanding these systemic venous return dynamics is crucial for improving long-term outcomes in Fontan patients (Van de Bruaene et al.). It demonstrates that changes in pulmonary circulation can have a significant impact on the health of the entire circulatory system and the body's overall balance.

Besides surgery, this relationship also exists in many illnesses that affect both the pulmonary and systemic circulations, such as heart failure. When the heart cannot pump effectively in heart failure, pulmonary venous pressures rise, which in turn affects the pulmonary circulation. As a result, the heart has to work harder, which worsens its function. Furthermore, conditions like PPHN illustrate how pulmonary disorders can detrimentally influence systemic hemodynamics, leading to significant morbidity and mortality in affected neonates (Soni et al., 2021). Thus, understanding this interdependence is crucial for healthcare professionals. It allows for targeted interventions that address the complexities of both circulatory systems, ultimately improving patient care outcomes in populations with cardiopulmonary dysfunction (Figure 7.11).

7.4. Regulation of Pulmonary Circulation

Regulating pulmonary circulation is essential to maintain effective gas exchange and ensure the lungs function properly in oxygenating the blood. It utilizes several processes that respond to different needs in the body, such as when posture changes, the body moves, or when more oxygen is required. This regulation depends significantly on how the blood vessels in the lungs expand and contract. Hypoxia, which means not enough oxygen, can result in pulmonary vasoconstriction, which redirects blood to the lungs that are better ventilated. Adjusting in this way helps protect the alveolar-capillary membrane and boosts the effectiveness of gas exchange. Understanding these mechanisms enables clinicians to identify when pulmonary circulation may be compromised, potentially leading to respiratory failure or other health issues. Pulmonary artery hypertension and congenital heart defects can make it difficult for the pulmonary circulation to be adequately regulated. For instance, patients with Fontan circulation often experience significant challenges, including arrhythmias and the development of pulmonary arteriovenous malformations (PAVM), which suggest impaired hemodynamics within the pulmonary vasculature. Studies have indicated that such conditions may be associated with elevated levels of biomarkers, such as Angiopoietin-2 (Ang-2), which reflects endothelial dysfunction and abnormal angiogenesis. In the cohort of Fontan patients, a higher Ang-2 was connected to recent arrhythmic events, which might point to problems in how pulmonary circulation is regulated. Identifying these biomarkers facilitates an understanding of the pathophysiology of compromised pulmonary circulation and informs therapeutic strategies aimed at mitigating associated risks, such as systemic hypoxia and right heart failure (Aboulhosn et al., 2019). Besides affecting blood vessels, pulmonary circulation regulation also involves the immune system's contribution to pulmonary well-being. The Marginal Pool, which holds a large number of leukocytes in the blood, is very important here. They are located in strategic areas to respond to inflammation and injury, which often occur together with lung diseases. The rules that determine when immune cells are retained or released while moving through the pulmonary circulation illustrate the complexity of managing the pulmonary circulation. Understanding the relationship between immune responses and pulmonary blood flow not only sheds light on potential treatment avenues but also highlights the intricate interplay between respiratory physiology and immune function (Goetz et al., 2002).

7.4.1. Neural Control Mechanisms

The mechanisms that control blood flow in the lungs are crucial for maintaining stable blood pressure and ensuring proper gas exchange. The autonomic nervous system (ANS), comprising both sympathetic and parasympathetic components, plays a complex role in regulating pulmonary vascular tone through adrenergic and cholinergic receptors. Due to this dual innervation, pulmonary blood flow can rapidly adjust to match changes in the local environment, such as pressure and oxygen levels. If pulmonary arterial pressure rises, local nerves are stimulated, triggering a reflex that narrows the pulmonary blood vessels. By doing this, the body can reduce pulmonary edema and also raise systemic vascular resistance, proving the strong link between the nervous system and the lungs. Understanding neural control is especially important in the context of chronic conditions, such as pulmonary hypertension, affecting the lungs. Recent clinical studies have highlighted the potential benefits of targeting autonomic regulation as a therapeutic approach for various diseases. Pulmonary artery denervation and vagal nerve stimulation are ways to control excessive changes in the pulmonary vasculature. Such methods utilize the natural features of the nervous system to help the pulmonary vasculature return to normal balance. These techniques work by directly influencing the sympathetic outflow, which may help patients with elevated pulmonary pressures feel better and live more comfortably. Furthermore, this research contributes to a broader understanding of how the nervous system can be harnessed therapeutically in managing complex pulmonary disorders (Michael et al., 2024). How neural control fits into the overall systemic homeostasis is especially striking, especially when the body is under stress. During exercise, the ANS supervises several body systems to help with oxygen supply and maintain the balance of energy use. Blood pressure has to be controlled because the heart has to pump more blood to meet the extra needs of the lungs. When exercising, the body needs to work harder and this makes it clear that the pulmonary and systemic circulations are carefully regulated. New research on neurovascular transduction reveals that these neural pathways are not merely reactive, but also enable us to make adjustments in advance to perform well under stress. Overall, a comprehensive examination of these neural mechanisms enriches our knowledge of pulmonary circulation and its vital responsiveness (Figure 7.12).

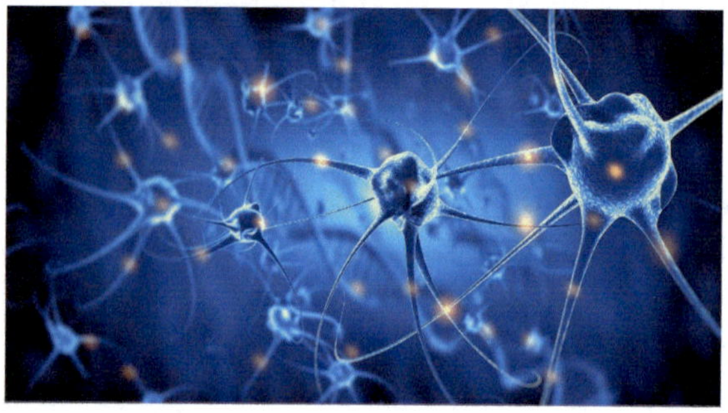

Figure 7.12. Neural control mechanisms.

Source: https://www.biologyonline.com/wp-content/uploads/2020/02/Neural-Control-Mechanisms.jpg.

7.4.2. Hormonal Influences on Pulmonary Blood Flow

Pulmonary blood flow is strongly affected by hormones, which in turn have a major impact on cardiovascular physiology. Vascular tone and blood flow in the lungs are primarily controlled by adrenaline, norepinephrine, and angiotensin II. When a person is stressed or exerts themselves, adrenaline is released, causing the pulmonary arteries to widen, which improves blood flow and facilitates gas exchange. Additionally, the renin-angiotensin system (RAS) plays a pivotal role in regulating pulmonary circulation by promoting vasoconstriction and fluid retention, which ultimately affects the dynamics of circulation. Understanding how hormones influence blood flow in the lungs helps explain the condition and aids in developing new treatments for pulmonary hypertension and heart failure. Besides, hormones in the blood react to oxygen changes, which trigger adaptations within the pulmonary circulation. Hypoxia triggers the release of certain hormones, which help improve blood flow to organs. For instance, elevation of erythropoietin not only stimulates red blood cell (RBC) production but also influences PVR, allowing for enhanced oxygen transport. At the same time, nitric oxide and other vasodilatory substances are released in response to these hormones, which helps blood flow increase by expanding the vessels. regulates. The body's regulation of pulmonary blood flow with hormones when oxygen is lacking is a good example of homeostasis. Ensuring this balance helps the tissue get enough oxygen, and it may be a valuable area to study when these adaptive responses fail in pulmonary diseases. Additionally, hormones play a crucial role in regulating blood flow to the lungs under specific circumstances, such as in space. NASA's Space Physiology and Countermeasures Program has demonstrated that prolonged exposure to microgravity can alter fluid levels and hormone levels in the body, potentially impacting both cardiovascular fitness and pulmonary function. The findings suggest that alterations in hormonal levels can lead to significant changes in pulmonary hemodynamics, potentially compromising oxygen delivery and overall health during space missions (Dickson et al., 2025). The development of predictive models for physiological responses, based on hormone-driven changes, may serve as a basis for ensuring crew safety and performance during spaceflight Therefore, further study of how hormones are regulated in the pulmonary system will increase our understanding of human physiology in various contexts.

7.4.3. Effects of Physical Activity on Circulation

Physical activity significantly affects circulation, particularly pulmonary circulation. Frequent exercise enhances heart health, allowing blood and oxygen to flow efficiently to all parts of the body. People with heart problems, such as those who have had the Fontan procedure, notice a substantial impact from exercise. Research suggests that regular exercise increases your ability to exercise and your blood's oxygen level, which are important for healthy lungs. While some interventions, such as inspiratory muscle training, have shown mixed results in improving lung function, they suggest clinically relevant benefits, emphasizing the need for regular monitoring and tailored exercise programs to optimize pulmonary outcomes in these patients (Neidenbach et al., 2023, pp. 11–24). In addition, those with chronic conditions like a Fontan circulation usually find it more challenging to be active which often means they have less ability to exercise than their peers without health problems. Due to this difference, it is evident that personal programs should concentrate on the unique health-related issues of each individual. Awareness of these restrictions allows healthcare providers to design workouts that help patients become physically fit and also enjoy a better quality of life. Tailored programs that incorporate dietary advice and psychological counseling may help mitigate fears related to exercise, thereby further enhancing participation in physical activity and its associated benefits for pulmonary circulation (Scheffers et al., 2022). In short, physical activity significantly improves circulation, especially for pulmonary health. In many studies, it has been found that regular exercise improves lung circulation, as indicated by increased oxygen saturation and greater exercise capacity. For individuals with specific heart conditions, incorporating exercise into their rehabilitation is crucial. They are designed to help people become stronger and also to enable them to manage their own health. As the importance of tailored and sustained physical activity becomes clearer, it is vital for healthcare systems to foster environments that encourage such behaviors, ultimately enhancing pulmonary circulation and overall patient well-being (Figure 7.13).

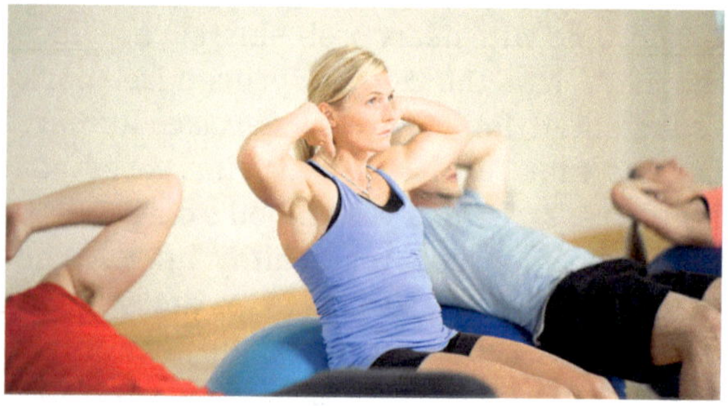

Figure 7.13. Group exercise session promoting core strength and physical fitness.

Source: https://unitedveincenters.com/wp-content/uploads/2025/02/1-9.png.

7.5. Common Disorders Affecting Pulmonary Circulation

The lungs work efficiently at gas exchange due to the important role of pulmonary circulation. Still, several disorders can cause problems with this system, which can seriously harm a person's health. One prominent condition affecting pulmonary circulation is pulmonary embolism (PE), often resulting from venous thromboembolism (VTE). In patients with conditions such as COVID-19, the incidence of PE has notably increased due to underlying hypercoagulability and immobility, complicating patient outcomes and therapeutic management (Wichmann, 2020, pp. 1030–1030). Typically, PE is treated by administering anticoagulation therapy promptly to prevent the formation of additional blood clots and their associated complications. Even so, choosing the right anticoagulation regimen for critically ill patients is still a problem, which suggests that personal evaluations and additional research are necessary. Another common disorder affecting pulmonary circulation is pulmonary hypertension (PH), characterized by increased blood pressure in the pulmonary arteries. This condition can stem from various etiologies, including left heart disease, chronic lung diseases, or idiopathic pulmonary arterial hypertension (IPAH). As a result of PH, the vessels in the lungs change, which causes the blood to flow more slowly, overloads the right ventricle, and leads to heart failure. Good management of PH depends on finding it early and making an accurate diagnosis. clinicians to confirm diagnoses and guide the appropriate treatment. Therapeutic options may encompass endothelin receptor antagonists, phosphodiesterase-5 inhibitors, and pulmonary vasodilators aimed at improving patient outcomes and quality of life, highlighting the importance of a multidisciplinary approach in managing this complex disorder (Zheng et al., 2020, pp. 492–506). In addition to PE and PH, chronic thromboembolic pulmonary hypertension (CTEPH) presents a unique challenge within pulmonary circulation disorders. CTEPH develops when pulmonary emboli are not adequately treated which gradually increases PVR. Patients with CTEPH often exhibit symptoms similar to those of other forms of PH, such as fatigue, shortness of breath, and exercise intolerance (Wichmann, 2020, pp. 1030–1030). Typically, diagnosis involves V/Q scans and pulmonary angiography to identify blockages and assess blood flow in the lungs. Importantly, CTEPH is distinct from other pulmonary disorders in that it can be treated through surgical intervention, such as pulmonary endarterectomy, or medical therapies aimed at managing symptoms and improving functional capacity (Zheng et al., 2020, pp. 492–506). Thus, knowing exactly what these disorders are helps clinicians choose the most effective treatment and reduce the likelihood of long-term health problems for their patients.

7.5.1. Pulmonary Hypertension

PH involves high pressures in the pulmonary artery, which cause many difficulties for the cardiovascular system. The condition can be caused by left heart disease, lung diseases, and thromboembolic events, which shows that it has many different causes. The pathophysiology of PH involves complex interactions among vascular endothelial cells, smooth muscle cells, and the extracellular matrix (ECM), resulting in vascular remodeling and increased resistance to pulmonary blood flow. Recently, scientists have discovered that neurotransmitters play a crucial role in regulating the tone of the blood vessels in the lungs.

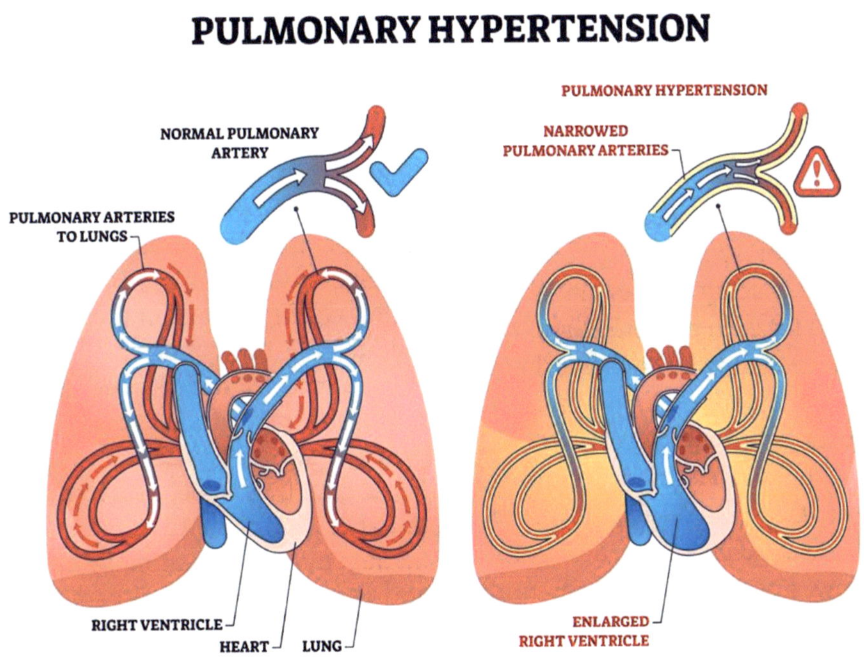

Figure 7.14. Pulmonary hypertension.

Source: https://chroniclungdiseases.com/wp-content/uploads/2024/07/pulmonary-hypertension-respiplus-1024x683.jpeg.

The pulmonary vessels are strongly affected by the actions of the sympathetic and parasympathetic nervous systems. These insights have spurred clinical interest, potentially paving the way for innovative therapeutic approaches for PH patients, such as targeting neural pathways to alleviate symptoms and improve outcomes (Michael et al., 2024). In the search for new treatments for pulmonary hypertension, scientists are interested in understanding the molecular mechanisms by which platelets and blood vessels interact, especially under conditions of low oxygen. The discovery of NEDD9, which helps platelets stick to pulmonary artery endothelial cells, highlights the close link between thrombosis and PH. NEDD9 is increased in the endothelial cells of pulmonary arteries from patients with CTEPH due to hypoxia, and this contributes to vascular changes. Researchers have shown that stopping the NEDD9-P-Selectin interaction may prevent excessive blood clot formation and the complications it causes in PH. By using this method, researchers may restore endothelial function and slow the progression of PH, which underscores the importance of targeting specific molecular pathways in managing this disease.

Additionally, new approaches to treating pulmonary hypertension are shifting towards personalized medicine, placing greater emphasis on individualized care for each patient. Currently, doctors use several medications to help vasodilate blood vessels and lower pulmonary artery pressure. Still, using new experimental methods such as pulmonary artery denervation and cholinergic potentiation is being considered more often by researchers. In addition, understanding how autonomic control and systemic homeostasis work together provides a foundation for creating targeted treatments that address the specific condition of PH. As clinicians and researchers delve deeper into the complexities of pulmonary circulation, the future holds promise for innovative therapies that can significantly impact the lives of those living with pulmonary hypertension (Michael et al., 2024) (Figure 7.14).

7.5.2. Pulmonary Embolism

In the case of pulmonary circulation, PE is a serious condition resulting from blocked pulmonary arteries, typically caused by clots originating from the veins. Due to this disruption, blood flow is abnormal, resulting in insufficient oxygen exchange and hypoxemia. Several factors can cause PE, such as being immobile for a long time, certain illnesses like cancer, and blood clotting disorders. Depending on the location and size of the blood clot, PE can cause a range of symptoms, from mild to serious and potentially fatal conditions, which is why it is crucial to diagnose and treat it promptly. Syncope, or a sudden loss of consciousness, is a common symptom of pulmonary embolism because the blood flow to the brain is not sufficient. Patients with both syncope and acute PE have a more serious prognosis than those with only PE, which means syncope is a sign of a more urgent case. It is now clear that presyncope, which means almost fainting, can also be a serious risk. Research has identified that patients experiencing presyncope display comparable rates of intensive care unit (ICU) admissions to those with syncope, with adjusted odds ratios confirming their predictive significance for adverse outcomes. This critical realization necessitates a heightened awareness among clinicians regarding the implications of both syncope and presyncope in patients with acute PE, urging a comprehensive assessment during initial evaluations (Abraham et al., 2020). Proper management of pulmonary embolism requires addressing hemodynamic instability and trying to avoid serious long-term effects. The primary approach to treatment is anticoagulation, which helps prevent further clot formation and supports the body's natural fibrinolysis process. Sometimes, if PE is very severe or life-threatening, more intense treatments such as thrombolysis or surgery to remove clots may be needed. Because PE can cause serious illness, it is essential to consider this diagnosis in patients who display risk factors or concerning symptoms. Additionally, ongoing studies are necessary to enhance our understanding of how PE develops and how it can be effectively treated. As our comprehension of the disease evolves, improved clinical algorithms for diagnosis and management can be developed, ultimately aiming to reduce the burden of pulmonary embolism on public health and improve outcomes in affected patients (Kitsiou et al., 2013) (Figure 7.15).

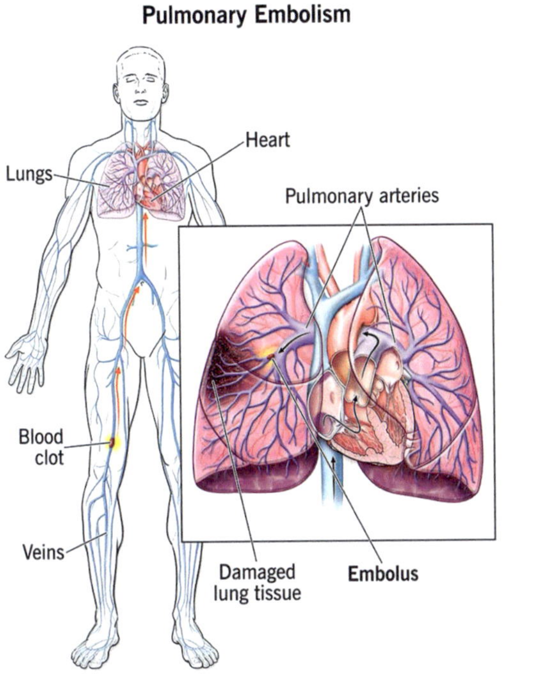

Figure 7.15. Pulmonary embolism illustration.

Source: https://my.clevelandclinic.org/-/scassets/images/org/health/articles/17400-pulmonary-embolism-illustration.ashx.

7.5.3. Chronic Obstructive Pulmonary Disease (COPD)

COPD is a significant and increasing public health problem, mainly because it leads to lasting breathing difficulties and airflow obstruction. The main cause is being exposed to irritants for a long time, such as tobacco smoke, air pollution, and risks at work. As the disease progresses, the airways become inflamed and damaged, which can result in significant changes in the lungs' blood circulation. This leads to a lack of oxygen in the lungs, which causes the blood vessels there to relax. This can, in turn, lead to pulmonary hypertension. COPD management should focus on stopping smoking, using medications, and changing daily habits, since these actions can help a lot in relieving symptoms and improving a patient's life. Therefore, understanding how COPD affects the lungs' blood circulation is crucial for designing more effective treatments and helping people with the disease manage their condition. The diagnostic landscape for COPD has expanded beyond traditional spirometry, which often overlooks small airway dysfunction (SAD). Recent studies have highlighted the utility of the impulse oscillometry system (IOS), which offers a more nuanced understanding of airway dynamics and resistance. IOS can detect small airway changes that other methods may not, which helps doctors respond earlier and monitor for any worsening of the disease. In this context, IOS metrics, including R5 – R20, are important because they can help distinguish between COPD and healthy individuals and predict the disease's outcome. Combining IOS information with clinical evaluations enables doctors to more accurately predict when COPD exacerbations may occur, which helps manage patients and reduces lung damage. As a result, it is now crucial to enhance the diagnostic tools used by doctors. Also, the fact that COPD is linked to oral health proves the strong relationship between body systems and the need for comprehensive patient care. It is now being discovered that changes in the oral microbiome may have a significant impact on lung health, particularly for individuals with COPD. For example, periodontitis can result in a higher number of specific pathogens in the mouth, which can harm the mouth and also cause breathing problems. Research suggests a strong link between periodontal disease measures and lung function, including FEV1 and FEV1/FVC, which may make oral health treatments beneficial for individuals with COPD. So, looking after oral health well is an important way to prevent complications, and it can also benefit overall lung health, which stresses the importance of teamwork in handling chronic lung diseases like COPD.

7.6. Diagnostic Techniques

To look into pulmonary circulation, doctors must use accurate tools to spot both structural and functional issues in the cardiovascular system. Imaging modalities such as echocardiography, computed tomography (CT), and MRI have emerged as pivotal tools in the evaluation of pulmonary vascular conditions. Echocardiography enables the real-time observation of the heart and allows for the visualization of the right heart chambers and pulmonary arteries without the need for invasive procedures, thereby facilitating the early detection of pulmonary hypertension. Besides, CT pulmonary angiography allows for detailed pictures of blood vessels, which help find any blockages or abnormalities that might influence pulmonary circulation. These approaches allow clinicians to confirm diagnoses and plan treatments which shows why they should be part of regular cardiovascular exams. Along with imaging, invasive procedures are still important for a comprehensive understanding of how pulmonary circulation works. Right heart catheterization is the most effective method for measuring pulmonary artery pressure and assessing a patient's response to medication. For diagnosing pulmonary hypertension, this technique is crucial because it provides clear measurements that aid in determining treatment options. Additionally, the use of diagnostic biomarker testing, which helps identify related diseases at a molecular level, has been noted. Examining blood samples for signs of endothelial dysfunction or inflammation can provide valuable insights into the health of the pulmonary vessels. All of these methods, when combined, enhance traditional imaging, which improves diagnosis and facilitates more effective patient management. Improvements in nanotechnology are leading to new methods for diagnosing pulmonary circulation. Nanomedicine introduces new methods that utilize nanotechnology to create more precise and sensitive diagnostic imaging agents. For example, using lipid-based systems can allow contrast agents to be delivered to the lungs which improves the contrast seen in lung imaging. It helps address the solubility issue common in regular imaging agents, potentially allowing for quick and precise imaging of the lungs and blood vessels. By harnessing the capabilities of nanomaterials, researchers aim to refine the diagnostic process, leading to more effective disease management. This ultimately caters to the unique physiological challenges presented by the pulmonary circulation and its associated pathologies, as outlined in Danaei et al. (2018) and Patra et al. (2018).

7.6.1. Imaging Methods: X-Rays and CT Scans

Evaluating lung circulation is much easier with the help of X-rays and CT scans which allow doctors to find problems related to lung health. X-rays help doctors see the structures inside the chest which allows them to spot problems like infiltrates, masses or fluid buildup that might affect the pulmonary vessels. Because it is non-invasive, this technique is beneficial in emergencies since results are available quickly. Along with regular clinical checks, X-rays can be used for initial screening; however, their interpretation may be limited by structures that overlap and by findings that are not easily visible. Alternatively, CT scans provide clearer images and an increased ability to detect changes in the lungs, which is very useful for evaluating pulmonary circulation. Using this method, doctors can see detailed cross-sectional images of the thorax, which helps them assess the lungs and the blood vessels that keep blood flowing. Notably, advancements in CT technology, such as dual-energy CT (DECT), have optimized material differentiation and reduced radiation exposure, thereby improving image quality and diagnostic accuracy. Because of DECT, fewer full-angle projections are needed, which improves the visibility of blood vessels and areas affected by diseases such as pulmonary embolism or pulmonary hypertension, key causes of problems in the pulmonary circulation.

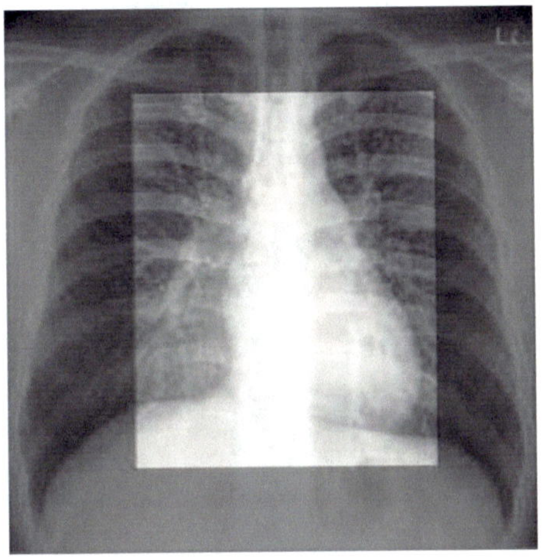

Figure 7.16. Chest X-ray.

Source: https://encrypted-tbn0.gstatic.com/images?q=tbn:ANd9GcR-uU4NcyiC24d0QxUrV58RvI9mqnLTA2oYjg&s.

The integration of artificial intelligence (AI) into imaging methods such as X-rays and CT scans further enhances diagnostic capabilities in pulmonary assessments. AI algorithms have been shown in recent studies to be effective at detecting lung nodules on chest X-rays, which may indicate lung cancer, and are therefore considered important for studying the pulmonary system. AI tools can also support radiologists by making it easier to identify and group lung nodules, which improves the accuracy of diagnosis. Even so, just because AI tools do well in research settings does not guarantee they are reliable in real-world situations. As imaging technology evolves and AI becomes more integrated, these methods exemplify a dynamic approach to enhancing diagnostic workflows, ultimately improving patient outcomes in lung health and related circulatory conditions (Figure 7.16).

7.6.2. Pulmonary Function Tests

Pulmonary function tests (PFTs) are essential tools for assessing various aspects of lung health and function, playing a critical role in diagnosing and monitoring pulmonary diseases. PFTs help doctors by measuring lung volume, the speed of airflow, and how well gas is exchanged, which reveals information about breathing and blood circulation in the lungs. These tests are particularly significant in evaluating conditions such as COPD, asthma, and interstitial lung disease (ILD), where abnormalities in pulmonary function can indicate the severity of the underlying pathology. PFTs can also be used to measure a patient's condition at the beginning, and these results can be followed over time to guide the proper treatment and care for each patient. Right ventricular function should be understood by looking at the results of PFT tests in pulmonary circulation. Right ventricular (RV) performance often reflects the health of pulmonary circulation, as it is responsible for pumping blood into the pulmonary arteries. Suppose someone has mitral regurgitation for a long time. In that case, the right ventricle may be affected by increased pressure and extra blood which is caused by higher pressures in the pulmonary arteries. The changes in the right ventricles can be measured by combining PFTs and echocardiography. By identifying how pulmonary dysfunction translates to changes in RV performance, clinicians can better predict patient outcomes and the need for more invasive diagnostic procedures or treatments, thereby enhancing the overall understanding of the interdependence between respiratory and cardiovascular systems (Maheut et al., 2024). Furthermore, the integration of cardiopulmonary exercise testing (CPX) into clinical practice extends the utility of pulmonary function assessments. CPX tests both lung function and the heart's reaction to exercise, providing a comprehensive picture of both systems. This test measures oxygen uptake and ventilation, providing information on how effectively patients can perform gas exchange and the health of their lungs. If something unusual is found during CPX, it can be linked to certain pulmonary or cardiac diseases, which helps doctors diagnose more accurately. Moreover, the ability of CPX to account for multiple medical issues faced by patients enhances its relevance in real-world settings, making it a vital component of both diagnostic and therapeutic strategies for managing pulmonary circulation disorders (Figure 7.17).

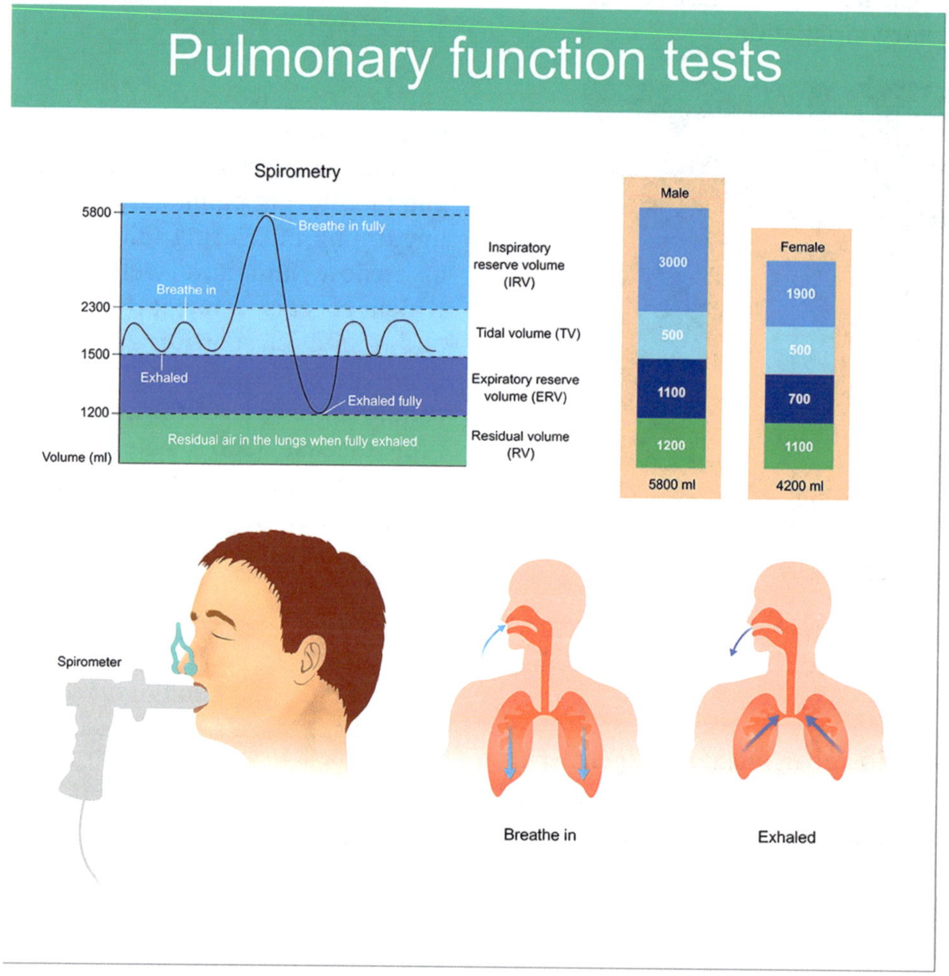

Figure 7.17. Pulmonary function tests (PFTs).

Source: https://www.aurorahealthcare.org/-/media/Project/Health-System-Enterprise/AuroraHealthCareOrg/aurorahealthcare/images/services/heart-vascular/services-treatments/testing-diagnosis/pulmonary-function-tests.webp?h=1200&iar=0&w=1200&rev=fde3e41270bf4491a18b930634a2bec8&hash=4A66C67C3F1AF5339DB579B8506E9FE1.

7.6.3. Blood Tests and Biomarkers

Examining blood tests and biomarkers is crucial for understanding the intricacies of pulmonary circulation in patients with complex heart conditions. Biomarkers give clues to clinicians about the underlying causes of a disease. For example, a rise in angiogenesis-related proteins may indicate that the endothelium is not functioning properly, which can lead to problems in the lungs. In a study concerning patients with Fontan physiology, elevations in angiopoietin-2 (Ang-2) were noted, particularly among those with a history of arrhythmias. These findings underscore the importance of monitoring specific biomarkers, which can provide clinicians with valuable insights into potential complications that may arise in pulmonary conditions, thereby enhancing patient management and informing therapeutic strategies (Aboulhosn et al., 2019). Besides congenital heart diseases, biomarkers may be helpful in other areas of pulmonary medicine. Using blood tests and identifying biomarkers can help monitor inflammation in pulmonary vascular diseases. For example, recent investigations into amniotic fluid embolism have highlighted the role of the immune and inflammatory responses, suggesting that specific serum markers may be implicated in the condition's pathophysiology (Busardo' et al.). Using blood-based tests in conjunction with other methods can enhance the ability to predict outcomes and provide prompt assistance to individuals with lung problems. Routinely using these tests in clinical practice could change the way pulmonary circulatory problems are managed. Basically, blood tests and biomarkers play a key role in monitoring and treating pulmonary circulation disorders. Besides identifying current heart problems, biomarkers help predict risks, allowing doctors to take action early. Higher levels of Ang-2 suggest a risk for arrhythmias and help predict them, and studies on other diseases confirm their importance in general pulmonary assessments. As a result, ongoing research on biomarkers is expected to enhance the understanding of pulmonary circulation and improve patient care through personalized medicine. This integration of blood tests and biomarker analysis holds significant potential for advancing clinical outcomes in pulmonary health (Figure 7.18).

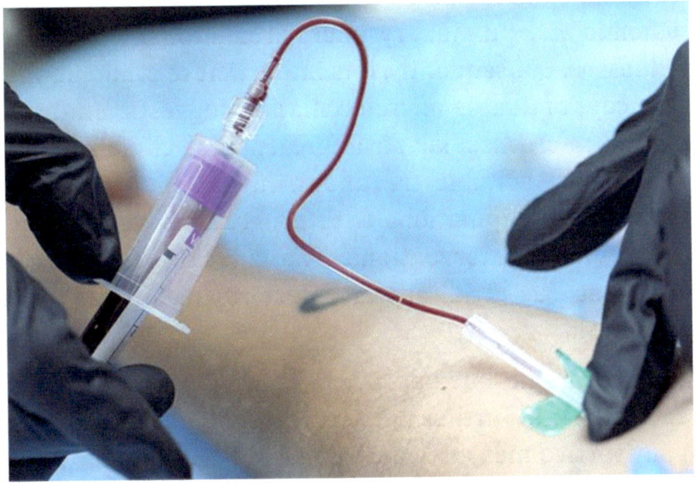

Figure 7.18. Venipuncture for blood collection.

Source: https://uwnewsroom-prod-backend.parallelpublicworks.com/sites/default/files/styles/wide/public/2024-12/Blood%20draw%20cbc%20ojas%20de%20hojalata%20GettyImages-2169206675.jpg?itok=uQenXIna.

SUMMARY

The mechanism of action of pulmonary circulation and its effects on health are a significant topic. This system, which transports deoxygenated blood to the lungs for reoxygenation and then returns it to the heart, is crucial for many bodily functions. A clear understanding of pulmonary circulation helps guide clinical actions, especially in distinguishing between asthma and COPD. Recent studies emphasize that while BDR may serve as a key marker, its efficacy as a diagnostic tool remains inconsistent across various patient groups, indicating a need for more precise identification methods within the realm of pulmonary medicine (Aggarwal and Aggarwal, 2024). Also, the treatment of pulmonary complications such as postoperative chylothorax points to the value of a multidisciplinary approach to lung health. Using pleural effusion triglyceride levels as a new indicator has dramatically improved the way surgery is planned and managed after the procedure.

This predictive capability enhances clinical decision-making, enabling healthcare professionals to tailor interventions effectively and improve patient outcomes, thereby highlighting the interconnectedness of various pulmonary conditions and their eventual outcomes (Ji et al., 2024). With ongoing research in pulmonary circulation, it is clear that new studies are crucial for enhancing clinical treatments. Studying BDR definitions and understanding how they work will clarify COPD diagnostics and treatment methods. Additionally, utilizing new prognostic indicators can help surgeons achieve better outcomes and provide prompt care for patients with chylothorax. Because of these advancements, it is important for healthcare professionals to keep learning and changing their practices in pulmonary circulation management to benefit patients and gain a better grasp of respiratory health issues.

Pulmonary circulation helps support many cardiovascular functions and is essential for overall macrocirculation. It is essential to distinguish between systemic circulation and pulmonary circulation, as they operate differently and have distinct structures. Macrovascular understanding requires comprehending both systemic and pulmonary microcirculations, which play a major role in the development of critical illnesses. Consequently, it is important to study pulmonary microcirculation in greater detail, as the concept of double microcirculation suggests. Understanding the differences in blood flow regulation and microvascular structure enables clinicians to provide patients with pulmonary dysfunction the most suitable treatment. In the clinical management of pulmonary conditions, especially in pediatric populations with progressive pulmonary hypertension (PH), it is crucial to adopt evidence-based interventions. The current guidelines point out that various approaches are important, such as atrial septal defect repair, making a pulmonary-to-systemic shunt, and lung transplantation.

They are used when patients do not improve with drugs, which shows that treatment plans should be tailored to each patient. Furthermore, extracorporeal membrane oxygenation (ECMO) is recognized as a vital supportive measure in cases where traditional therapies are unsuccessful. This evidence-based focus aims to optimize patient outcomes by refining treatment methodologies based on specific patient profiles and evolving clinical knowledge (Ryan et al.). In short, the comprehensive view of pulmonary circulation encompasses both its normal functions and its medical implications. As time passes, applying the knowledge gained from critical reviews and guidelines is essential to deliver more effective care to patients. Having a strong understanding of double microcirculation supports the use of various treatments and increases the likelihood of predicting outcomes in critically ill patients. By paying attention to the specific characteristics of systemic and pulmonary microcirculation, doctors can develop therapies tailored to each patient's needs. Additionally, ongoing studies on progressive lung diseases help us gain a deeper understanding, which in turn can improve patient care and health outcomes, demonstrating that pulmonary circulation is a complex system that requires careful management.

CLOSER LOOK

EXTRACORPOREAL MEMBRANE OXYGENATION (ECMO)

ECMO is a life-support technique in which a machine outside the body takes over the work of the heart and lungs, allowing them to rest and recover. It is used for patients with life-threatening heart or lung conditions when conventional treatments fail. ECMO involves drawing blood from the body, oxygenating it in a machine, and then returning it to the body (Figure 7.19).

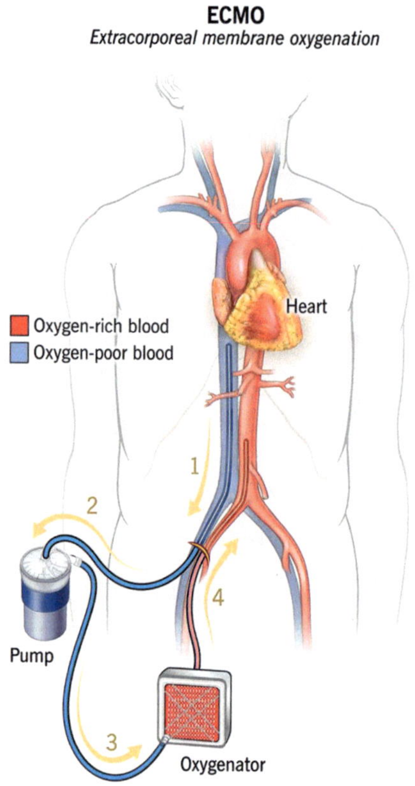

Figure 7.19. Extracorporeal membrane oxygenation.

Source: https://my.clevelandclinic.org/-/scassets/images/org/health/articles/21722-ecmo-illustration.

How It Works?

- **Cannulation:** Two cannulas are inserted into the patient's arteries or veins, usually in the neck or groin, to draw blood into the ECMO circuit.
- **Blood Flow:** The ECMO machine pumps the blood through a membrane oxygenator, which adds oxygen and removes carbon dioxide.

- **Return to the Body:** The oxygenated blood is then returned to the patient through the other cannula.

When It's Used?

- **Severe Acute Respiratory Distress Syndrome (ARDS):** A condition where the lungs are severely damaged, making it difficult to breathe.
- **Cardiac Arrest or Cardiogenic Shock:** When the heart stops beating or is unable to pump blood effectively.
- **Other Conditions:** COVID-19, severe infections, and other conditions that severely impair heart or lung function.

Benefits

- **Provides a Bridge:** ECMO allows patients to recover from their underlying condition while their heart and lungs rest.
- **Improved Survival:** ECMO has been shown to improve survival rates in some instances, particularly for severe ARDS and cardiac arrest.

Risks and Complications

- **Bleeding:** Due to the need for anticoagulation to prevent blood clots in the ECMO circuit.
- **Infections:** The ECMO circuit can be a source of infection.
- **Organ Damage:** ECMO can sometimes lead to organ damage, especially to the kidneys.
- **Other complications, including neurological issues, blood clots, and other serious issues,** are also possible.

REFERENCES

1. Aggarwal, A., & Agarwal, R. (2024). Bronchodilator responsiveness in chronic obstructive pulmonary disease: Prevalence, significance, and clinical implications. *Current Opinion in Pulmonary Medicine.* https://www.semanticscholar.org/paper/7e86cbae748525cf6d2bbf784cf4a0a6c5415962 (accessed on 31st May 2025).
2. Alba, G. A., Samokhin, A., Wang, R., Zhang, Y. Y., Wertheim, B. M., Arons, E., Greenfield, E., et al. (2021). NEDD9 is a novel and modifiable mediator of platelet-endothelial adhesion in the pulmonary circulation. *American Journal of Respiratory and Critical Care Medicine.* https://www.semanticscholar.org/paper/b461e0d34b9dcd1e4da78cce325e00d26e40068e (accessed on 31st May 2025).
3. Anastasiou, V., Alexandrou, M., Kamperidis, V., Daios, S., Tsilonis, K., Theodorakopoulou, M., Moysidis, D., et al. (2023). Changes on right ventricular dimensions, function, and pulmonary circulation loading according to the degree of interdialytic weight gain in maintenance hemodialysis patients. *Journal of Hypertension*, *41*(Suppl. 1), e54, e55. https://www.semanticscholar.org/paper/adf3e7c93f64bcc235e2f27087422759c9fece27 (accessed on 31st May 2025).
4. Arena, R., & Sietsema, K. (2011). Cardiopulmonary exercise testing in the clinical evaluation of patients with heart and lung disease. *Circulation*, *123*, 668–680. https://www.semanticscholar.org/paper/331b5aecf16f6f387a617e894637efca21d51bfa (accessed on 31st May 2025).
5. Arzamasov, K., Vasilev, Y., Zelenova, M., Pestrenin, L., Busygina, Y., Bobrovskaya, T., Chetverikov, S., et al. (2024). Independent evaluation of the accuracy of 5 artificial intelligence software for detecting lung nodules on chest X-rays. *Quantitative Imaging in Medicine and Surgery*, *14*, 5288–5303. https://www.semanticscholar.org/paper/3a1152462881f4da2497c8d705ef2dd8016f7aa2 (accessed on 31st May 2025).
6. Auckburally, A., & Nyman, G. (2017). *Review of Hypoxemia in the Anaesthetized Horse: Predisposing Factors, Consequences and Management.* Elsevier BV. https://core.ac.uk/download/46558350.pdf (accessed on 31st May 2025).
7. Bailey, M., Durst, L., Cajigas, H., Kane, G., Krowka, M., Kushwaha, S. S., McCully, R., et al. (2024). Using PAH-SYMPACT to assess quality of life in patients with pulmonary hypertension associated with chronic lung disease. *Pulmonary Circulation.* https://www.semanticscholar.org/paper/fb5d7a067674a01b36991d57d45f0582d27ca0a9 (accessed on 31st May 2025).
8. Burrowes, K. S., Clark, A. R., Geier, E. T., Kang, et al. (2018). *In Silico Modeling of Oxygen-Enhanced MRI of Specific Ventilation.* eScholarship, University of California. https://core.ac.uk/download/323065291.pdf (accessed on 31st May 2025).
9. Busardò, F. P., Fineschi, V., Frati, P., Zaami, et al. (2015). Amniotic fluid embolism pathophysiology suggests the new diagnostic armamentarium: β-tryptase and complement fractions C3-C4 are the indispensable working tools. *Int. J. Mol. Sci.* MDPI AG. https://core.ac.uk/download/54249007.pdf (accessed on 31st May 2025).
10. Cash, M., Giambra, B., Stone, L., Magness, M., Luebbe, K., Moore, S., Moore, R., et al. (2025). Hank the Heart and animation-based education for pulmonary hypertension. *Pulmonary Circulation.* https://www.semanticscholar.org/paper/2d408a8a427830c6cb47716990957e11e969e9ae (accessed on 31st May 2025).

11. Charalampopoulos, A., Connolly, S. B., Davies, R. J., Gibbs, et al. (2014). Response to pulmonary arterial hypertension drug therapies in patients with pulmonary arterial hypertension and cardiovascular risk factors. University of Chicago Press. *Pulm. Circ.* https://core.ac.uk/download/76996385.pdf (accessed on 31st May 2025).

12. Cheyne, W. S., Harper, M., Gelinas, J., Sasso, J., & Eves, N. (2020). Mechanical cardiopulmonary interactions during exercise in health and disease. *Journal of Applied Physiology*, *128*. https://www.semanticscholar.org/paper/18b674aaf0534ccc445ff5eb9235cf3fe5e8e47a (accessed on 31st May 2025).

13. Coleman, R. D., Cohen, S. P., Eghtesady, P., Grady, R. M., Morales, D. L. S., Hayes, D., Ruminjo, J. K., et al. (2025). Summary for clinicians: Clinical practice guideline on interventional strategies for children with progressive pulmonary hypertension despite optimal therapy. *Annals of the American Thoracic Society*. https://www.semanticscholar.org/paper/561c6dff128a15d4f3491578351cefbb9bd5922a (accessed on 31st May 2025).

14. Danaei, M., Dehghankhold, M., Ataei, S., Hasanzadeh, D. F., Javanmard, R., Dokhani, A., Khorasani, S., et al. (2018). Impact of particle size and polydispersity index on the clinical applications of lipidic nanocarrier systems. *Pharmaceutics*, *10*, 57. https://doi.org/10.3390/pharmaceutics10020057 (accessed on 31st May 2025).

15. Danduran, M. J., Dixon, J. E., & Rao, R. P. (2012). Near infrared spectroscopy describes physiologic payback associated with excess postexercise oxygen consumption in healthy controls and children with complex congenital heart disease. *Pediatric Cardiology*. e-Publications@Marquette. https://core.ac.uk/download/213086415.pdf (accessed on 31st May 2025).

16. Dickson, K. J., Hess, E., Powers, J. V., Wallace-Robinson, et al. (2025). Publications of the Space Physiology and Countermeasures Program, Cardiopulmonary Discipline: 1980–1990. https://core.ac.uk/download/pdf/42809290.pdf (accessed on 31st May 2025).

17. Ding, X., Cheng, Z., & Qian, Q. (2017). Intravenous fluids and acute kidney injury. *Blood Purification*, *43*, 163–172. https://doi.org/10.1159/000452702 (accessed on 31st May 2025).

18. Elmaghawry, M., Thiene, G., Zampieri, F., Zanatta, et al. (2015). *Andreas Vesalius: Celebrating 500 Years of Dissecting Nature*. Hamad bin Khalifa University Press (HBKU Press). https://core.ac.uk/download/53526658.pdf (accessed on 31st May 2025).

19. Finney, S. J. (2014). *Extracorporeal Support for Patients with Acute Respiratory Distress Syndrome*. European Respiratory Society (ERS). https://core.ac.uk/download/77004032.pdf (accessed on 31st May 2025).

20. Fletcher, E. S. (2016). *Organ Specific Vascular Response to Fibrosis Affects Breast Cancer Metastatic Organotropism*. DigitalCommons@TMC. https://core.ac.uk/download/80296557.pdf (accessed on 31st May 2025).

21. Goetz, A. E., & Kuebler, W. M. (2002). *The Marginated Pool*. S. Karger AG. https://core.ac.uk/download/16432675.pdf (accessed on 31st May 2025).

22. Harvey, J. (2017). *Incidence and Predictors of Premature Ventricular Complexes Following Catheter Ablation for Atrial Fibrillation*. https://open.bu.edu/bitstream/2144/23785/5/Harvey_bu_0017N_12743.pdf (accessed on 31st May 2025).

23. Heydari, K., Johnson, C., Cooper, I. D., Hersi, K., Tanba, C., Sun, J., Solomon, M. A., et al. (2025). Flow cytometric determination of circulating progenitor cells in patients with

pulmonary arterial hypertension: A systematic review. *Pulmonary Circulation*. https://www.semanticscholar.org/paper/33ce533439f7a7019f36ee3302342b74c88023f0 (accessed on 31st May 2025).

24. Huang, Y., Zhang, X., Wang, J., Bao, W., Lv, C., Zhang, Y., Tian, X., et al. (2025). Role of impulse oscillometry in chronic obstructive pulmonary disease and asthma-chronic obstructive pulmonary disease overlap. *Clinical and Translational Allergy*. https://www.semanticscholar.org/paper/f568d23c36c004ca316b9b834cb77f911f853fa6 (accessed on 31st May 2025).

25. Itoh, H., Ichiba, S., Obata, H., Futami, M., Okahara, S., Kawabata, T., Nguyen, T. B., et al. (2024). Pulsatile right ventricle to pulmonary artery extracorporeal membrane oxygenation in pigs. *Tạp chí Phẫu Thuật Tim Mạch Và Lồng Ngực Việt Nam*. https://www.semanticscholar.org/paper/abb9fa5efdfa099a4c5014b1aa65bead769465d2 (accessed on 31st May 2025).

26. Ji, H., Wang, Z., Xu, C., Yu, X., & Huang, H. (2024). Prognostic significance of pleural fluid triglyceride levels based on a low-fat diet management strategy in patients with chylothorax following pulmonary resection. *Journal of Cardiothoracic Surgery*. https://www.semanticscholar.org/paper/0690b5c62c8f8d6345c407963052a209c4a5652c (accessed on 31st May 2025).

27. Kitsiou, A., Caforio, A. L. P., Porta-Sanchez, A., Vahanian, A., Iung, B., Carrera, C., Szymanski, C., et al. (2013). *ESC Core Curriculum for the General Cardiologist*. Oxford University Press (OUP). https://core.ac.uk/download/55756305.pdf (accessed on 31st May 2025).

28. Liu, J., Xiao, Q., Xiao, J., Niu, C., Li, Y., Zhang, X., Zhou, Z., et al. (2022). Wnt/β-catenin signaling: Function, biological mechanisms, and therapeutic opportunities. *Signal Transduction and Targeted Therapy*. https://doi.org/10.1038/s41392-021-00762-6 (accessed on 31st May 2025).

29. Maheut, R., Trousselle, L., Eggenspieler, F., Pace, N., Filippetti, L., Fraix, A., Popovic, B., et al. (2024). Echocardiographic assessment of the right heart pulmonary circulation unit in mitral regurgitation due to mitral valve prolapse. *European Heart Journal*. https://www.semanticscholar.org/paper/52c3dd214ddb5a5b3ace67f7766dc78177976aaf (accessed on 31st May 2025).

30. Mahmood, R., Shaik, T., Kaur, I. P., Gupta, V., Shaik, A., Anamika, F., Garg, N., et al. (2024). Cardiovascular challenges beyond Earth: Investigating the impact of space travel on astronauts' cardiovascular health. *Cardiology in Review*. https://www.semanticscholar.org/paper/5b77cf12933237a41dbe8d740a4a02630df916de (accessed on 31st May 2025).

31. Männer, J. (2024). The functional significance of cardiac looping: Comparative embryology, anatomy, and physiology of the looped design of vertebrate hearts. *Journal of Cardiovascular Development and Disease*. https://www.semanticscholar.org/paper/f81b4e760a36767c905093690cc89889a2f58c47 (accessed on 31st May 2025).

32. Mithradas, N., Sudhakar, U., Shanmugapriya, K., Jeddy, N., & Ram, S. (2024). The oral-lung microbiome dysbiosis: Unravelling its role in implications for chronic obstructive pulmonary disease (COPD) pathogenesis. *Journal of Oral and Maxillofacial Pathology: JOMFP*, *28*, 619–625. https://www.semanticscholar.org/paper/e42edbf85871b2dbd0ee1947b679b1c45765ff0b (accessed on 31st May 2025).

33. Murtada, S. I., Ramachandra, A., & Humphrey, J. (2023). Ex vivo biomechanical characterization of umbilical vessels: Possible shunts in congenital heart palliation. *Journal of Biomechanics*. bioRxiv. https://www.semanticscholar.org/paper/d01737d0dfef4da11bf08cd0150f84845649267e (accessed on 31st May 2025).

34. N/A. (2025). *Prognosis of the State of Health of a Person Under Spaceflight Conditions.* https://core.ac.uk/download/pdf/42875329.pdf (accessed on 31st May 2025).

35. Neidenbach, R., Freilinger, S., Stöcker, F., Ewert, P., Nagdyman, N., Oberhoffer-Fritz, R., Pieper, L., et al. (2023). Clinical aspects and targeted inspiratory muscle training in children and adolescents with Fontan circulation: A randomized controlled trial. *Cardiovascular Diagnosis and Therapy, 13*, 11–24. https://www.semanticscholar.org/paper/64d181939eb9281580787463c7e52a54591e5e00 (accessed on 31st May 2025).

36. Pagnamenta, A., Azzola, A., Beghetti, M., Lador, F., & On Behalf of the Swiss Society of Pulmonary Hypertension. (2017). Invasive hemodynamic evaluation of the pulmonary circulation in pulmonary hypertension. *Swiss Medical Weekly, 2017*, w14445. https://www.semanticscholar.org/paper/02cb26dc16288e85efc1a73867c3a978bf3c7d78 (accessed on 31st May 2025).

37. Patra, J. K., Das, G., Fraceto, L. F., Campos, E. V. R., Rodriguez-Torres, M. del P., Acosta-Torres, L. S., Díaz-Torres, L. A., et al. (2018). Nano based drug delivery systems: Recent developments and future prospects. *Journal of Nanobiotechnology*. https://doi.org/10.1186/s12951-018-0392-8 (accessed on 31st May 2025).

38. Plunkett, M. J., Paton, J. F., & Fisher, J. P. (2024). Autonomic control of the pulmonary circulation: Implications for pulmonary hypertension. *Experimental Physiology, 109*, 42–57. https://www.semanticscholar.org/paper/ccf36ee5ea8956ab93b1657ccd4f4f4f13becc3c (accessed on 31st May 2025).

39. Ponikowski, P., Voors, A. A., Anker, S. D., Bueno, H., Cleland, J. G. F., Coats, A. J. S., Falk, V., et al. (2016). 2016 ESC guidelines for the diagnosis and treatment of acute and chronic heart failure. *European Heart Journal, 37*, 2129–2200. https://doi.org/10.1093/eurheartj/ehw128 (accessed on 31st May 2025).

40. Ren, J., Zhang, W., Wang, Y., Liang, N., Wang, L., Cai, A., Wang, S., et al. (2024). A dual-energy CT reconstruction method based on anchor network from dual quarter scans. *Journal of X-ray Science and Technology*. https://www.semanticscholar.org/paper/dfe2d5e3f68bd9a66bd70c4bd193255dc8fdb774 (accessed on 31st May 2025).

41. Scheffers, L., Helbing, W., Utens, E., Dieleman, G., Dulfer, K., Noske, J., Van Den, B. E. A., et al. (2022). Study protocol of the exercise study: Unraveling limitations for physical activity in children with chronic diseases in order to target them with tailored interventions—A randomized cross over trial. *Frontiers in Pediatrics*. https://www.semanticscholar.org/paper/e336e106bc38057ff68fea4d356fc6279a04a54c (accessed on 31st May 2025).

42. Sheahan, T. P., Sims, A., Leist, S. R., Schäfer, A., Won, J. J., Brown, A. J., Montgomery, S. A., et al. (2020). Comparative therapeutic efficacy of remdesivir and combination lopinavir, ritonavir, and interferon beta against MERS-CoV. *Nature Communications*. https://doi.org/10.1038/s41467-019-13940-6 (accessed on 31st May 2025).

43. Shirali, A. S., Lluri, G., Guihard, P. J., Conrad, M. B., Kim, H., Pawlikowska, L., Boström, K. I., Iruela-Arispe, M. L., & Aboulhosn, J. A. (2019). Angiopoietin-2 predicts morbidity in adults with Fontan physiology. *Scientific Reports, 9*(1). https://doi.org/10.1038/s41598-019-54776-wAbraham, A. S., Bahl, D., Clague, V. A., Cotton, et al. (2020). Presyncope is associated with intensive care unit admission in emergency department patients with acute pulmonary embolism. *West J. Emerg. Med.* eScholarship, University of California. https://core.ac.uk/download/305124092.pdf (accessed on 31st May 2025).

44. Shoemaker, J., & Gros, R. (2024). A century of exercise physiology: Key concepts in neural control of the circulation. *European Journal of Applied Physiology*. https://www.semanticscholar.org/paper/510d4ff457dd6ed40b461a60dc043af1f1423154 (accessed on 31st May 2025).

45. Singer, M., Deutschman, C. S., Seymour, C. W., Shankar-Hari, M., Annane, D., Bauer, M., Bellomo, R., et al. (2016). The Third International Consensus Definitions for Sepsis and Septic Shock (Sepsis-3). *JAMA, 315*, 801. https://doi.org/10.1001/jama.2016.0287 (accessed on 31st May 2025).

46. Soni, M., Joshi, P., Patel, S. C., Shreya, D., Zamora, D. I., Patel, G. S., Grossmann, I., et al. (2021). Persistent pulmonary hypertension: A look into the future therapy. *Cureus*. https://www.semanticscholar.org/paper/b456b3b552bcf253915287a083458286c2e2f45d (accessed on 31st May 2025).

47. Sun, I., & Lee, K. (2013). Cyclophosphamide dose: How much is needed to win the war against paraquat poisoning? *The Korean Journal of Internal Medicine, 28*, 410–412. https://www.semanticscholar.org/paper/6ec54caab407653bb14e39ca3242eb4191fa8dc7 (accessed on 31st May 2025).

48. Tomarchio, E., Momigliano, F., Giosa, L., Collins, P., Barrett, N., & Camporota, L. (2024). The intricate physiology of Veno-venous extracorporeal membrane oxygenation: An overview for clinicians. *Perfusion, 39*(Suppl. 1), 49S–65S. https://www.semanticscholar.org/paper/d085f37dd2e0d56b3cc123b2feab488ac3b35d74 (accessed on 31st May 2025).

49. Uzkan, S., Korkmaz, M. F., & Altın, H. (2025). *Congenital Corrected Transposition of the Great Arteries (ccTGA): An Incidental Case Report*. Pediatric Academic Case Reports. https://www.semanticscholar.org/paper/2e19e98704b95210bb753b4440e33ca542310b81 (accessed on 31st May 2025).

50. Van de, B. A., Claessen, G., Salaets, T., & Gewillig, M. (2022). Late Fontan circulatory failure: What drives systemic venous congestion and low cardiac output in adult Fontan patients? *Frontiers in Cardiovascular Medicine*. https://www.semanticscholar.org/paper/4c89c179ca3b9ed4dfcd2c4a0fe1a5cc3cbe614e (accessed on 31st May 2025).

51. Wang, G., Deng, Q., Wang, J., Zhang, Q., Lian, H., & Wang, X. (2025). Systemic and pulmonary microcirculation, double microcirculation: From basic concepts to treatment key points. *Journal of Intensive Care Medicine, 2025*, 8850666251321786. https://www.semanticscholar.org/paper/61dea9a1b9fe69f5f325c4975cd65e3a075b9561 (accessed on 31st May 2025).

52. Wichmann, D. (2020). Autopsy findings and venous thromboembolism in patients with COVID-19. *Annals of Internal Medicine, 173*, 1030. https://doi.org/10.7326/l20-1206 (accessed on 31st May 2025).

53. Zaky, A. F., Froelich, M., Meers, B., Sturdivant, A. B., Densmore, R., Subramaniam, A., Carter, T., et al. (2021). Noninvasive assessment of right ventricle function and pulmonary artery pressure using transthoracic echocardiography in women with pre-eclampsia: An exploratory study. *Cureus*. https://www.semanticscholar.org/paper/347c9c39da14bc27b1f53ad03f60695e0969dd02 (accessed on 31st May 2025).

54. Zheng, D., Liwinski, T., & Elinav, E. (2020). Interaction between microbiota and immunity in health and disease. *Cell Research, 30*, 492–506. https://doi.org/10.1038/s41422-020-0332-7 (accessed on 31st May 2025).

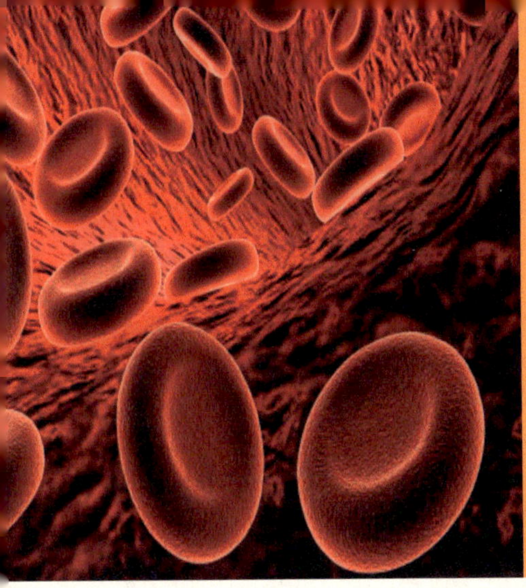

Chapter 8
OXYGEN TRANSPORT

Contents

Introduction

The survival of aerobic organisms depends on the important process of oxygen transport. Oxygen is delivered through this mechanism from the respiratory surfaces to various parts of the body, allowing cells to produce energy. The complexity of this process is exemplified by the role of hemoglobin, a protein found in red blood cells (RBCs), which binds to oxygen molecules in the lungs and releases them in tissues where they are needed. It is responsible for delivering oxygen efficiently and also helps control blood pH and remove carbon dioxide, illustrating the numerous roles respiratory physiology plays. Understanding these processes is crucial for recognizing how oxygen transport varies with different needs and conditions. In addition to its biological significance, oxygen transport has profound implications in clinical settings, particularly in the diagnosis and treatment of respiratory and cardiovascular diseases (CVDs). For instance, conditions such as chronic obstructive pulmonary disease (COPD) or anemia severely impair the body's oxygen-carrying capacity, leading to hypoxemia and a host of related symptoms. Clinicians often assess oxygen saturation levels using pulse oximetry and arterial blood gases (ABGs), which provide insight into the efficacy of oxygen transport in patients. In addition, new medical technologies have led to therapies that help improve oxygen delivery, for example, supplemental oxygen and erythropoietin-stimulating agents. Understanding oxygen transport helps explain normal body functions and also guides the treatment of diseases that affect oxygen supply. Studying how oxygen is transported enables scientists to discover ways to enhance energy production through new biotechnologies. For example, microbial solar cells (MSCs) have garnered attention as a means of converting solar energy into usable electrochemical forms through the use of photosynthetic and electrochemically active microorganisms. It demonstrates a new approach to energy systems by combining biology and energy efficiency. Exploring these new areas can show how to make energy more sustainable and offer ideas for making oxygen delivery systems better in various uses, such as in hospitals and for cleaning up the environment. Ultimately, the continued research into oxygen transport is pivotal, as it not only addresses fundamental biological inquiries but also contributes to advancements in health technology and sustainable practices (Buisman et al., 2010; Kaag et al., 2009).

Definition of Oxygen Transport

Oxygen transport helps move oxygen from outside the body to every cell. Oxygen is mainly carried in the body by hemoglobin in the RBCs through the circulatory system. Oxygen transport is more involved than simply moving it through the body.

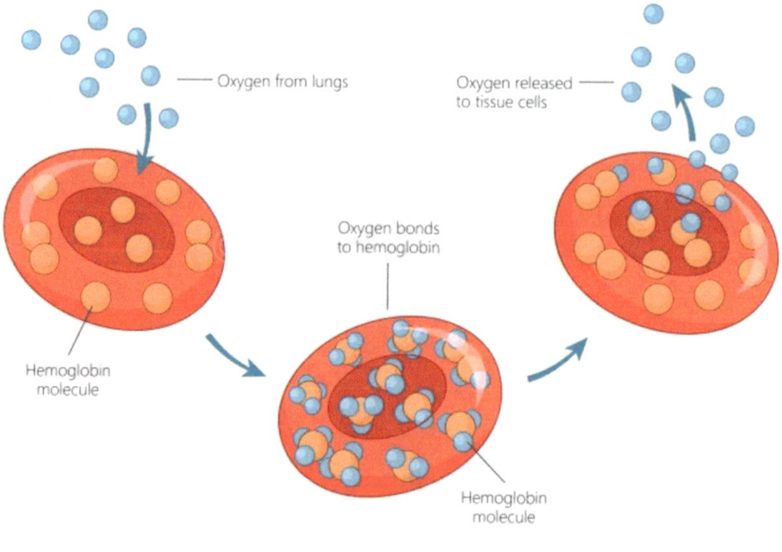

Figure 8.1. Transport of oxygen in the blood.

Source: https://thumbs.dreamstime.com/b/oxygen-transport-blood-structure-diagram-oxygen-transport-blood-showing-red-blood-cells-hemoglobin-molecules-oxygen-369026701.jpg.

Many things, like pH and carbon dioxide levels, can influence how hemoglobin binds to oxygen, which in turn changes the protein's saturation. It is important because it guarantees that tissues receive the oxygen they need. Understanding these factors is crucial to comprehend how oxygen moves from the lung alveoli to the rest of the body, which is essential for overall health. The way oxygen moves through the microcirculation is more complicated than in the macrocirculation. Both diffusion and convection are used as oxygen is released from the RBCs into nearby tissues. It has been shown that the axial convective flux is important, but its effect on delivering oxygen to the radial direction is much less than that of the diffusive flux. Most of the latter occurs where RBCs and capillary walls are in close proximity, making diffusion seem more important for oxygen supply to tissues.

The intricate balance between these mechanisms underscores the importance of microvascular architecture and blood flow dynamics in optimizing oxygen availability for cellular respiration and metabolic functions (Zhang, 2025). Additionally, the manner in which oxygen is transported affects the function of mitochondria within cells. Mitochondria are responsible for utilizing oxygen to produce adenosine triphosphate (ATP), which is essential for various cellular processes. Good oxygen transport and utilization help maintain normal, everyday mitochondrial function and cellular balance. However, disruptions in oxygen supply, such as those occurring during traumatic brain injury (TBI), can lead to mitochondrial dysfunction, further exacerbating the issue of insufficient ATP production.

This discordance between oxygen transport, mitochondrial efficiency, and cellular energy demands underscores the need to comprehend the mechanisms of oxygen delivery, not only to sustain energy metabolism but also to maintain vital physiological functions (Carteri, 2025) (Figure 8.1).

Importance of Oxygen in Biological Systems

Oxygen is vital for life because it is essential for many metabolic activities, not just breathing. During cellular respiration, oxygen is necessary for accepting electrons and facilitating the conversion of glucose into ATP, a form of usable energy. It primarily occurs in mitochondria, facilitated by a series of biochemical reactions known as the electron transport chain. Oxidative phosphorylation enables oxygen to facilitate the cell's production of ATP, a crucial energy source. Oxygen is also needed for the formation of important cellular molecules such as lipids and nucleotides, which are key for cellular structure and function. Cells cannot work correctly if there is not enough oxygen, showing how important oxygen is for life and energy production. Oxygen's significance is also profoundly illustrated by the roles of heme and coenzyme Q (CoQ) in the transport and utilization of oxygen in living organisms. Heme, which is part of hemoglobin, facilitates the binding and unbinding of oxygen, allowing it to be carried from the lungs to other parts of the body. It helps the body utilize oxygen and also enables cells to respond quickly to changes in oxygen supply. Moreover, the transport of heme itself, as indicated by research on bacterial cytochrome c biogenesis pathways, is crucial since heme needs to be tightly regulated due to its potential cytotoxicity (Alicia et al., 2025). The way oxygen is transported and heme functions show how complicated biological systems are and how they depend on oxygen for different functions. Apart from heme, CoQ is important for oxygen-dependent metabolism since it transports electrons across cell membranes. CoQ's hydrophobic structure enables it to reside within the mitochondrial membrane, thereby facilitating its function as a crucial component of the electron transport chain (Wang et al., 2024). It helps produce ATP and also maintains the balance of oxidation and reduction within cells. Because oxygen can perform many functions, it is clear that it is essential for the body in multiple ways, not just for biochemistry. Hence, the importance of oxygen in life is evident in the way it is transported and utilized by heme and CoQ in biological systems.

8.1. The Role of Hemoglobin

Hemoglobin helps move oxygen from the lungs to all parts of the body. This iron-rich protein, located in red blood cells (RBCs), binds to oxygen in the lungs and releases it in tissues requiring energy for metabolic processes. The ability of hemoglobin to bind oxygen is influenced by pH, temperature, and the presence of carbon dioxide in the blood. Thanks to these changes, hemoglobin can respond to the body's changing oxygen needs and make sure oxygen delivery is adequate for metabolism. The importance of hemoglobin's oxygen-binding capabilities is underscored by studies demonstrating how environmental factors, such as exposure to ozone, can affect its functionality and, consequently, overall oxygen transport efficiency (Zinchuk et al., 2023). Problems with hemoglobin can significantly impact how oxygen is transported in the body, leading to various health issues. For instance, conditions such as idiopathic pulmonary arterial hypertension (IPAH) are characterized by changes in hemoglobin's biochemical and biophysical properties, resulting in a diminished capacity for oxygen binding. Scientists have found that the shape of hemoglobin differs in IPAH patients compared to healthy individuals using Raman spectroscopy. Due to these changes, oxygen delivery is impaired, and thus it is clear to see how hemoglobin structure, oxygen transport, and disease states are related. Such findings are crucial for understanding how pathologies may disrupt the finely tuned mechanisms of oxygen transport, implicating hemoglobin not only as a vital oxygen transporter but also as a potential biomarker for assessing related health conditions (Allakhverdiev et al., 2023). The ways hemoglobin responds to different stimuli are proof of its importance in carrying oxygen. If oxygen levels are low, such as in high altitudes, hemoglobin adjusts its structure to better hold on to oxygen and carry it through the blood. Being able to adapt allows aerobic metabolism to continue in different conditions. Furthermore, external factors such as pollutants—including ozone—can influence hemoglobin's oxygen transport efficiency, suggesting that environmental considerations are increasingly relevant in discussions surrounding respiratory health and overall well-being (Zinchuk et al., 2023). Knowing the many roles of hemoglobin highlights how oxygen is transported and also how environmental or health problems can disrupt this important function.

8.1.1. Structure of Hemoglobin

The structure of hemoglobin, which is vital for oxygen transport, is special because it has four subunits: two alpha and two beta chains. A heme group is found in every subunit and is necessary for oxygen binding, as it contains an iron atom and a porphyrin ring. As a result of being a tetramer, hemoglobin can cooperatively bind oxygen, so the binding of oxygen to one group makes it easier for the others to bind as well. Because of this feature, hemoglobin can absorb oxygen in the lungs and deliver it to tissues that need it most. The way amino acids are arranged in the subunits significantly affects the stability and functioning of hemoglobin, enabling it to work effectively in various body conditions. Additional analysis of hemoglobin proves that its shape is responsible for transporting oxygen and also affects its reactions to various body conditions. For example, when pH changes, the structure of hemoglobin is altered, which affects how strongly it binds to oxygen. It is called the Bohr effect, and it occurs when increased carbon dioxide and a lower pH in tissues cause hemoglobin to release oxygen more easily. Research suggests that hemoglobin can also adopt different structural states, including the relaxed (R) and tense (T) states, depending on the oxygen saturation levels. It is essential for the blood to be able to adapt quickly, especially in environments where oxygen consumption fluctuates significantly. This adaptability is also mirrored in other hemoglobin-like proteins, such as dehaloperoxidase (DHP) found in marine species like Amphitrite ornata, which demonstrates similar functional versatility by alternating between peroxidase and peroxygenase activities (Fehr et al., 2017). Additionally, the way hemoglobin interacts with various metabolites can significantly impact its ability to carry oxygen when health issues arise. For example, in states of hyperglycemia, conformational changes in the hemoglobin molecule may lead to a decreased affinity for oxygen, manifesting in a higher ratio of deoxyhemoglobin and methemoglobin (Bourdon et al., 2017). These changes are also linked to alterations in the erythrocyte membrane, such as increased glycosylation of proteins, which can reduce the oxygen transport ability. Changes in metabolism can alter the shape of red blood cells, making it clearer how the hemoglobin structure relates to its function. Understanding these complex interactions within the context of health and disease underscores the importance of hemoglobin's structural integrity in its role as the primary oxygen carrier in the bloodstream (Figure 8.2).

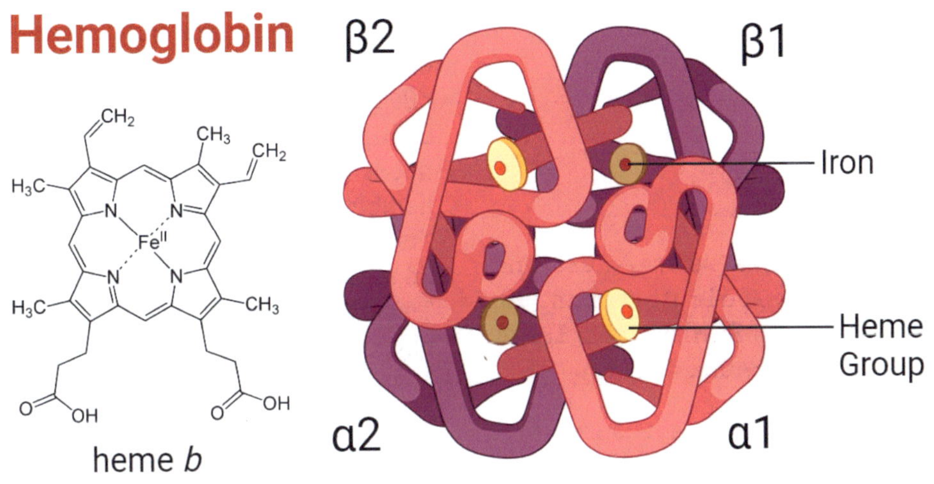

Figure 8.2. Structure of hemoglobin.

Source: https://microbenotes.com/wp-content/uploads/2023/08/Structure-of-Hemoglobin.jpeg.

8.1.2. Mechanism of Oxygen Binding

Oxygen is transported in the body mainly because hemoglobin can bind to oxygen in the blood. Because hemoglobin has four chains, each with a heme group, it can change its shape and bind or release oxygen. When oxygen molecules bind to the iron atom within the heme group, there is an alteration in the hemoglobin structure from the tense (T) state to the relaxed (R) state. The change in hemoglobin causes it to become more attracted to oxygen molecules, a phenomenon known as cooperative binding. Thus, when the lungs have more oxygen, the hemoglobin can accept more oxygen, which is then delivered efficiently to tissues that need it for metabolism. It is essential to understand the factors that affect oxygen binding to comprehend the role of hemoglobin in oxygen transport. The amount of oxygen hemoglobin can hold is influenced by pH, carbon dioxide, and temperature, as demonstrated by the Bohr effect. For instance, increased carbon dioxide and decreased pH (increased acidity) can lead to a shift in the hemoglobin equilibrium toward the release of oxygen, which is particularly advantageous in metabolically active tissues. On the other hand, in the lungs, where the pH is higher and carbon dioxide levels are lower, hemoglobin is more attracted to oxygen, which facilitates its absorption.

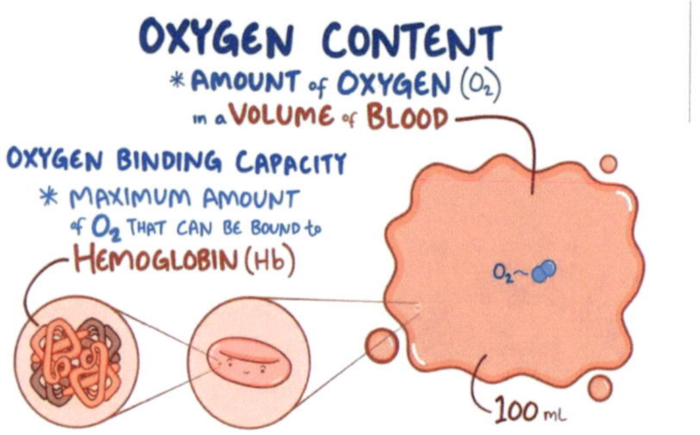

Figure 8.3. Oxygen binding.

Source: https://www.osmosis.org/_next/image?url=https%3A%2F%2Fd16qt3wv6xm098.cloudfront.net%2FFCHiIJo3RHitVr2zhL_1rngEQouIAVRd%2F_.jpg&w=3840&q=75.

This method of adjustment ensures that the body can always supply oxygen in the correct amounts based on its needs. Modern biochemistry has revealed the molecular basis for oxygen binding, which is similar to findings in other biological areas. Exploring the effects of toxins on cells has revealed similarities in the way substances are transported within cells. Microcystin-LR is taken up into plant cells by active protein-mediated processes, just as oxygen is transported by hemoglobin. The way the heme group in hemoglobin interacts with biogenic stabilizers illustrates the complexity of controlling the movement and binding of gases. This comparative analysis further enriches our understanding of oxygen transport mechanisms and their physiological roles, illustrating the fundamental importance of molecular dynamics in biological systems (Li et al., 2025; Wai et al., 2025) (Figure 8.3).

8.1.3. Factors Affecting Hemoglobin's Affinity for Oxygen

Many physiological and biochemical factors can change the affinity of hemoglobin for oxygen. A critical determinant is the concentration of carbon dioxide (CO_2) in the blood, which governs the Bohr effect. As CO_2 levels go up, hemoglobin's attraction to oxygen decreases, which helps oxygen be released in parts of the body where it is used. Additionally, the presence of lactic acid and hydrogen ions (H^+) further lowers hemoglobin's affinity through competitive inhibition, thereby ensuring efficient oxygen delivery where it is most needed. It demonstrates that metabolism can change oxygen transport to meet different needs. Furthermore, the structural changes in hemoglobin—leading to a more relaxed (R) state that binds oxygen more tightly—contrast with its tense (T) state, which readily releases oxygen. This explains the accuracy of our body in moving oxygen and adjusting to different conditions. Temperature has a significant influence on how hemoglobin binds to oxygen. When the body temperature rises, such as during exercise or a fever, hemoglobin becomes less able to hold oxygen, so it releases oxygen in areas where it is needed most. This effect is significant during exercise, as it allows tissues to get more oxygen to meet their increased needs. Alternatively, lower temperatures can increase the ability of hemoglobin to hold onto oxygen, which is seen during hypothermia. The way these shifts are balanced is significant for efficient oxygen movement and delivery in the body. According to models of erythropoiesis, as suggested by recent studies, the feedback regulation of RBC production is also intricately tied to temperature-induced changes in hemoglobins oxygenation, expanding our understanding of systemic responses to environmental changes and physical demands (Leonard, 2025). Additionally, the physiological process of erythrocyte formation significantly impacts how hemoglobin transports oxygen. Research indicates that patients with cardiovascular diseases (CVDs) often display altered erythrocyte morphology and membrane lipid composition, which can disrupt normal oxygen transport dynamics.

When the microviscosity of erythrocyte membranes changes, it leads to difficulties in how hemoglobin binds and releases oxygen. Antiaggregants and beta-blockers, which are standard treatments, have not been very successful in improving hemoglobin function. For this reason, new treatment methods should also take into account hemoglobin's ability to transport oxygen, especially for individuals with heart problems. The integration of innovative diagnostic techniques, such as laser interference microscopy and Raman spectroscopy, may prove crucial in identifying and addressing erythrocyte dysfunctions at an early stage, thereby fostering better clinical outcomes in oxygen transport management (Gromova et al., 2016).

8.2. Oxygen Transport in the Blood

Oxygen is carried to all parts of the body by hemoglobin in RBCs, which is necessary for life. Hemoglobin, which is made of four subunits, easily attaches to oxygen in the lungs, where oxygen levels are very high. As soon as one oxygen molecule binds, hemoglobin becomes more likely to bind more oxygen molecules. With this, hemoglobin can collect a good amount of oxygen as it moves through the pulmonary capillaries. The oxygen is released in the tissues, where the pressure of oxygen is lower, which demonstrates how oxygen is dissociated. The adaptation guarantees that tissues get the oxygen they need, depending on their metabolism, which is necessary for all cells to function correctly. Additionally, oxygen transport is significantly influenced by pH, temperature, and carbon dioxide levels. The Bohr effect shows that more carbon dioxide and lower pH encourage the release of oxygen from hemoglobin, which matters a lot when exercising hard or dealing with illness.

This regulation helps ensure that muscles actively working during exercise receive the oxygen they need at the right moment. In the same way, temperature influences how hemoglobin connects with oxygen, so that higher temperatures cause hemoglobin to release oxygen more easily. They highlight how the circulatory and respiratory systems cooperate to ensure the body receives enough oxygen, demonstrating the various ways oxygen is transported throughout the body. Additionally, recent advances in understanding how hypoxia affects oxygen transport have opened up new avenues for research, primarily related to chronic diseases.

The adaptation of tissues under hypoxic conditions involves a myriad of cellular responses, including the potential activation of hypoxia-inducible factors (HIFs), which regulate the expression of genes involved in angiogenesis and erythropoiesis. In diseases such as chronic obstructive pulmonary disease (COPD) and pulmonary hypertension, the adaptation mechanisms can become maladaptive, leading to further complications. Therefore, understanding how these processes occur at the molecular level is crucial for discovering new treatments and therapies. Such insights underscore the importance of maintaining adequate oxygen transport, as disruptions in this process can lead to significant pathophysiological states, ultimately shaping future research endeavors in both pathology and treatment modalities (Figure 8.4).

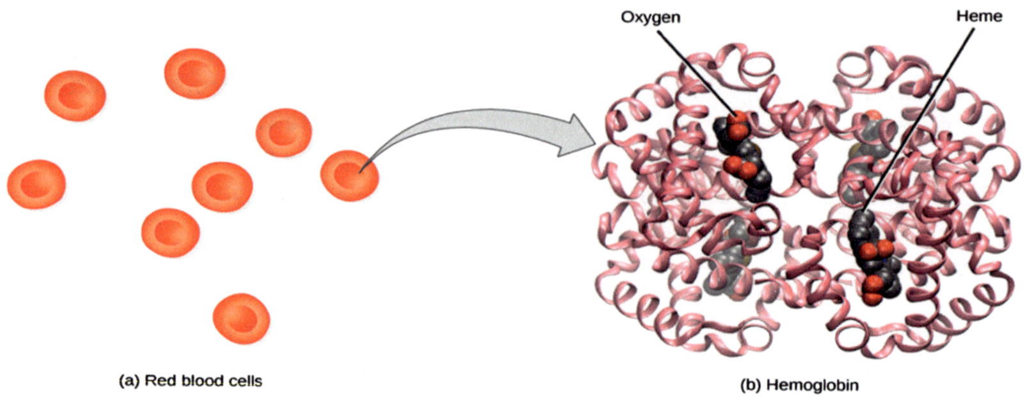

Figure 8.4. The protein inside (a) red blood cells that carries oxygen to cells and carbon dioxide to the lungs is (b) hemoglobin. Hemoglobin is made up of four symmetrical subunits and four heme groups. Iron associated with the heme binds oxygen. It is the iron in hemoglobin that gives blood its red color.

Source: https://s3-us-west-2.amazonaws.com/courses-images/wp-content/uploads/sites/1223/2017/02/08195831/Figure_39_04_01-1024x432.jpg.

8.2.1. Oxygen Saturation Levels

Oxygen saturation levels indicate how well the respiratory system is functioning and the overall health of the body, by showing the percentage of hemoglobin sites in the blood that are filled with oxygen. Proper cellular metabolism depends on having enough oxygen which is delivered by blood to different tissues. In most healthy adults, oxygen saturation typically ranges from 95% to 100%. When oxygen levels are below this point, people may feel tired, have trouble breathing normally, and find it hard to exercise, which can greatly impact their quality of life. Therefore, checking oxygen saturation is very important, particularly for individuals with respiratory illnesses, as ensuring sufficient oxygen is a primary goal in their treatment and clinical evaluation. The protein hemoglobin, which binds oxygen in RBCs, relies on oxygen transport for its proper function. Conditions in the environment, the efficiency of hemoglobin in binding to oxygen, and health problems such as anemia or lung diseases can all impact oxygen saturation. In hospitals, pulse oximetry is a non-invasive method for measuring oxygen levels in the blood, which helps identify hypoxemia sooner. If someone is pregnant or has a chronic illness, keeping an eye on their oxygen saturation makes it possible to react quickly. The physiological adaptations during pregnancy, for example, create an increased demand for oxygen, thereby necessitating vigilant monitoring to ensure both maternal and fetal health during this critical period (Liang et al., 2020). The relationship between oxygen saturation levels and health is also influenced by changes in the body's physiology. If oxygen levels in the body become low, it can cause erythropoietin to be released, which helps make more RBCs to transport oxygen. Conditions such as high-altitude exposure also induce changes in oxygen saturation, prompting the body to adjust to lower oxygen environments by increasing breathing rate and RBC production (Locatelli et al., 2017). They demonstrate the importance of monitoring oxygen saturation levels in both medical testing and understanding human body functions in various settings. As research continues, enhancing our understanding of factors affecting oxygen transport and saturation remains essential for improving health outcomes across diverse populations (Figure 8.5).

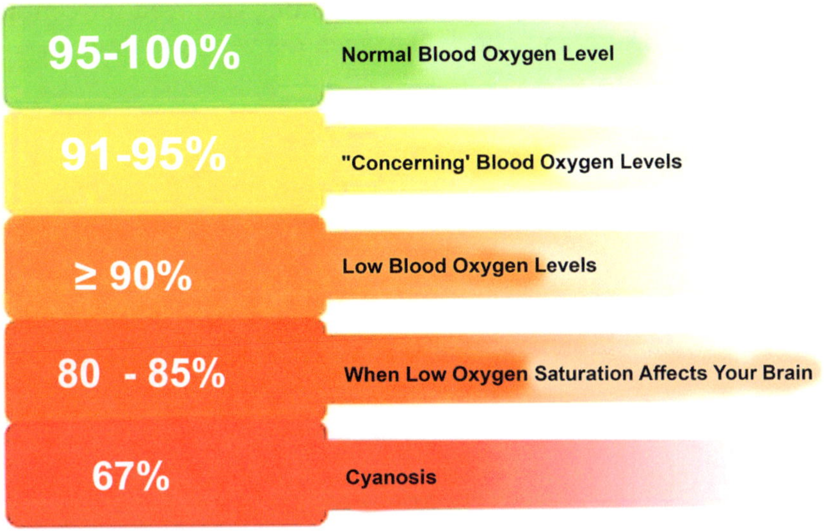

Figure 8.5. Oxygen saturation levels.

https://cdn.prod.website-files.com/65056ba428fdd5501ff0ef16/66a3d674277ddb50a133a834_66217c213d188cadfa38d50e_51020214218pulse-oximeter-readings-chart-gen.png.

8.2.2. Role of Red Blood Cells (RBCs)

RBCs, or erythrocytes, play a crucial role in the biological process of oxygen transport, which is essential for sustaining cellular metabolism throughout the human body. Due to the fact that RBCs are biconcave and do not have a nucleus, they can have a large surface area for gas exchange. This design helps the lungs take in oxygen efficiently and also makes them more flexible, allowing them to fit through the smallest capillaries. Additionally, hemoglobin in RBCs is essential for transferring oxygen from the lungs or gills to the body tissues that utilize it in aerobic respiration. Through this intricate system, RBCs significantly contribute to maintaining optimal physiological function, providing the necessary resources to support complex metabolic processes essential for survival (Singh et al., 2024). RBCs are also key to the body's system for controlling oxygen supply and use. Hemoglobin can change its shape, which helps it bind to more oxygen in various situations. It is important because the level of hemoglobin saturation depends on pH, temperature, and carbon dioxide, which is known as the Bohr effect. A rise in carbon dioxide in active tissues causes hemoglobin to bind less strongly to oxygen, allowing oxygen to be released where it is most needed. This dynamic relationship between RBCs and their environment exemplifies the sophisticated adaptations that have evolved to optimize oxygen delivery, demonstrating the versatility and importance of these cells in maintaining homeostasis within the body (Lamichhane et al., 2024). Maintaining healthy RBCs is crucial to prevent hematological problems that can impair the body's ability to transport oxygen. Conditions such as anemia, thalassemia, and sickle cell disease (SCD) directly impact the production, structure, and function of RBCs, leading to diminished oxygen-carrying capacity. A lack of functional RBCs in anemia means there is insufficient oxygen for the tissues, which can lead to fatigue and pale skin. However, when someone has SCD, the RBCs are shaped differently, which blocks blood flow, leads to pain crises, and shortens their lifespan. Understanding the medical implications related to RBC functionality underscores their significance within the broader context of oxygen transport, highlighting the need for continual research into therapies that enhance RBC health and effective oxygen delivery (Singh et al., 2024) (Figure 8.6).

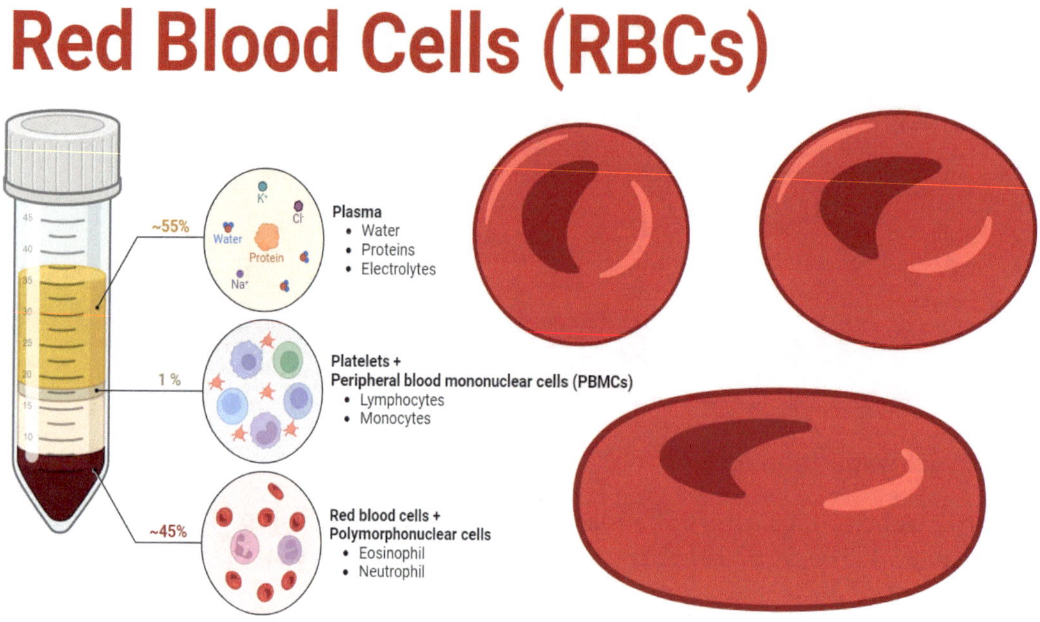

Figure 8.6. Red blood cells (RBCs).

Source: https://microbenotes.com/wp-content/uploads/2024/04/Red-Blood-Cells-RBCs.jpeg.

8.2.3. Transport Dynamics in the Circulatory System

Understanding the transport dynamics in the circulatory system is crucial for understanding how oxygen is effectively delivered to tissues and organs. RBCs are key to this process, since they carry oxygen attached to hemoglobin and also affect the movement of oxygen molecules. The movement of blood and the tissues around it makes a complex area where diffusion takes place. The latest simulations reveal that RBCs can influence how quickly small molecules, such as oxygen, diffuse. In particular, when RBCs use tank-treading motion, they cause flows that help reduce the movement of nearby particles. This highlights the intricacies of diffusion in biological systems, suggesting that cellular motion fundamentally impacts how efficiently oxygen is transported to where it is needed most in the body (Nix, 2025). The production of energy within the circulatory system is also an important factor in understanding oxygen transport. Earlier, it was believed that ATP synthesis provided the energy for cardiac contractions; however, recent studies reveal a different picture for multicellular organisms. Heart muscle cells do not have unlimited ATP, which limits the use of this method. Replacing this viewpoint highlights that the circulatory system uses both ATP and extracellular Fenton reactions working together to produce energy. The model proposes that cellular energy helps the heart maintain its regular contractions, which improves the delivery of oxygen to all parts of the body. The interplay of these energy systems contributes to the overall efficiency of the circulatory system, underscoring the complexity of biological energy dynamics (Wang et al., 2025).

In addition, how much energy each cell has and how the circulatory system works together are important for both health and disease. Oxygen transport in the body helps explain several biological functions, such as tumor formation and overall health. Combining individual cellular energy with a central circulatory system explains many different conditions in the body. For instance, pulse diagnosis in traditional Chinese medicine (TCM) relies on understanding these vascular dynamics to evaluate systemic health. By examining how holistic energy influences individual cellular function, researchers can gain a deeper understanding of how disruptions in these processes may lead to health issues, thereby illuminating new pathways for both diagnosis and treatment (Wang et al., 2025).

8.3. The Process of Oxygen Delivery

The process of oxygen delivery is a vital component of the human respiratory and circulatory systems, relying heavily on the role of RBC. RBCs do not have organelles because they are highly specialized to carry out gas exchange. They transport oxygen to all parts of the body and help eliminate carbon dioxide, a waste product of metabolism. RBCs can adjust their shape to fit through the many types of blood vessels, including the very narrow capillaries. Because of this ability, oxygen can reach every tissue, supporting cellular respiration and metabolism – vital processes which are needed for maintaining homeostasis. Furthermore, the lifespan of RBCs, averaging 120 days, allows them to continually engage with numerous cell types, facilitating significant physiological interactions required for health and disease management (Pretini et al., 2019). The environment RBCs are in strongly affects their structure and function, which in turn impacts how efficiently oxygen is delivered. Endothelial cells, platelets, and immune cells all interact to keep the blood in a balanced state. At this stage, RBCs help transport gases and also affect hemostasis and thrombosis, which are essential for managing injuries. RBC membrane components, like proteins and ion channels, are important for these interactions. They also interact with the immune system by combating pathogens to prevent infections.

As such, understanding these interactions and how RBCs adapt to physiological challenges is essential for comprehending the complexities of oxygen transport and the overall functioning of the cardiovascular system (Pretini et al., 2019). Recent advancements in scientific research have highlighted the significance of reactive oxygen and nitrogen species (RONS) in therapeutic applications, particularly in the treatment of various diseases. New ways to produce RONS, such as with cold atmospheric pressure plasma jets, offer a different method for increasing oxygen delivery. Because of this, RONS can enter cells and help oxygen reach them by influencing various cellular activities and the healing process. Their ability to make RONS at specific depths and interact with tissues shows that these jets can be used in many ways to help with oxygen problems in diseases. It could be helpful in treating tumors below the skin as well as for improving oxygen delivery to tissues that are not getting enough. Thus, exploring novel treatments that leverage RONS generation could significantly impact the field of oxygen transport and its application in medical therapies (Figure 8.7).

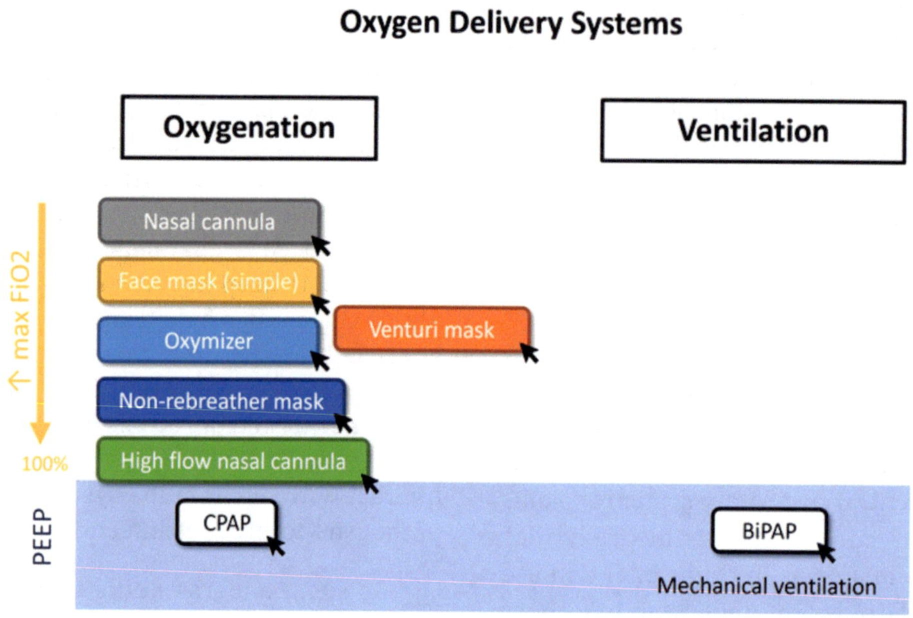

Figure 8.7. Oxygen delivery systems.

Source: https://teachim.org/wp-content/uploads/2021/10/Oxygen-delivery-scaled.jpg.

8.3.1. Oxygen Release at the Tissue Level

The release of oxygen at the tissue level is a crucial aspect of the oxygen transport system, facilitating the delivery of this essential gas to metabolically active cells. The main way oxygen is transported in the blood is by hemoglobin which picks up oxygen in the lungs and brings it to tissues where it is used for aerobic metabolism. Several factors affect the efficiency of oxygen release, including pH levels and the amount of carbon dioxide, which are involved in the Bohr effect. As a result of tissues using glucose and releasing carbon dioxide and hydrogen ions, the pH of the blood goes down, which promotes oxygen release from hemoglobin. Due to this relationship, it is evident that local metabolic needs play a role in controlling oxygen transport and that the body can adapt to various situations. New studies have shown how adipokines can affect the amount of oxygen available to tissues. Asprosin, a recently discovered compound, helps regulate the body's oxygen transport, particularly in individuals with excess body weight and insulin resistance. A rise in asprosin in the body is linked to changes in the oxyhemoglobin dissociation curve, which suggests the body is adjusting to problems with oxygen delivery. Higher levels of nitrogen monoxide and lower levels of hydrogen sulfide, which are important for blood flow and oxygen release, are part of these changes. By affecting the bioenergetic status of tissues, asprosin exemplifies how metabolic conditions can directly influence the efficiency of oxygen transport and availability, offering a new perspective on the complexities of oxygen release at the cellular level (Zinchuk et al., 2024). Moreover, the intricate relationship between oxygen release and the formation of reactive oxygen species (ROS) highlights the importance of cellular conditions in oxygen transport. Ischemia-reperfusion injury (IRI) represents a significant challenge, as the sudden restoration of oxygen can lead to excessive ROS production, causing tissue damage and inflammation. Using ROS-responsive nanoparticles to deliver medicine is a novel approach to mitigating these adverse effects. Empagliflozin, which is often prescribed for type 2 diabetes, has demonstrated the ability to protect against IRI by affecting pathways that create ROS. Using EMPA-loaded nanomicelles helps deliver the drug to the needed areas in the ischemic tissues. Such advances underscore the need for a comprehensive understanding of how tissue conditions affect oxygen transport and release (Cheng et al., 2024).

8.3.2. Role of Myoglobin in Muscle Tissues

Myoglobin, which is mostly found in muscles, helps carry and store oxygen. Myoglobin allows oxygen to be absorbed from the blood and then released inside muscle cells, mainly when the body needs more energy. During strenuous exercise, when muscles require more oxygen than the blood can supply, this function is crucial. The structure of myoglobin enables it to tightly bind oxygen, allowing it to store oxygen until it is used in the mitochondria. Moreover, studies on myoglobin saturation during activities such as diving illustrate its capacity to adapt to varying oxygen availability, highlighting its importance not only in sustaining muscle function but also in supporting the overall metabolic flexibility of muscle tissues in different environments (Ponganis et al., 2024). It has been found that myoglobins do more than just move oxygen around. Recent studies have shown that myoglobin is involved in lipid transport and several metabolic reactions in muscle cells. For example, it is involved in the way lactate and pyruvate interact, which are important during anaerobic conditions. Myoglobin has also been identified as a modulator of nitric oxide (NO) pools, suggesting its involvement in signaling pathways that regulate muscle metabolism. Because myoglobin has multiple functions, it is crucial for muscle physiology, particularly in regulating changes in oxygen and energy utilization. By acting as an oxygen sensor, myoglobin can influence intracellular processes that determine how effectively muscles utilize energy substrates during activity (Adepu et al., 2024). The evolution of myoglobin in different species over time highlights its importance in muscle tissue. For example, the myoglobin saturation in diving mammals, such as the emperor penguin, demonstrates their adaptation to underwater environments. When diving, these animals exhibit different mechanisms by which myoglobin loses oxygen, reflecting their methods of utilizing oxygen. Specific patterns limit the amount of oxygen that can reach the muscles, leading to myoglobin depletion, but others maintain steady oxygen flow by regulating blood flow. These results indicate that myoglobin is essential for all living things to store oxygen and can also adapt to the specific demands of each organism. Consequently, understanding myoglobin's role in diverse contexts enhances our comprehension of muscle oxygen transport mechanisms and metabolic regulation (Ponganis et al., 2024) (Figure 8.8).

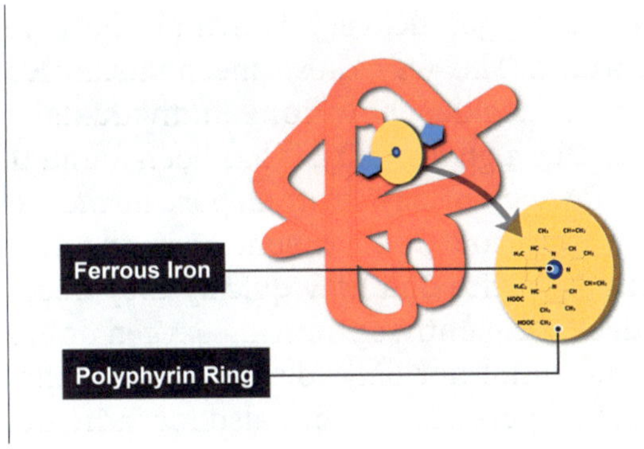

Figure 8.8. Myoglobin.

Source: https://www.getbodysmart.com/wp-content/uploads/2017/09/Globin-Polyphyrin-Ring-1024x732.png.

8.3.3. Impact of Exercise on Oxygen Delivery

The relationship between exercise and oxygen delivery is multifaceted, significantly influencing physical performance and overall health. When you exercise, your muscles use more oxygen to maintain their function. The need for more oxygen triggers changes in the body to enhance oxygen delivery. The main adaptations include increased blood pumping by the heart and a more efficient blood supply to the muscles. As you work out harder, your heart rate and stroke volume go up, which improves blood delivery to the active tissues. Exercise also stimulates the growth of small blood vessels in muscles, which helps oxygen reach the cells more easily. These adaptations not only support improved athletic performance but also contribute to long-term health benefits, particularly in populations engaging in regular physical activity as recommended by the new WHO guidelines (Richie et al., 2023). Oxygen transport is also essential for how muscles metabolize energy. It shows that when the body's critical power is reached, it can no longer control its metabolism, which depends on oxygen supply and use. The use of oxygen by muscles is affected by both convective and diffusive oxygen delivery, which are both very important. The way these mechanisms work together decides how long individuals can exercise at high intensity. It has been found that the efficiency of oxygen transport in the body affects both how well someone performs during intense exercise and how quickly they become tired. Consequently, optimizing oxygen delivery becomes vital not only for athletes seeking to maximize performance but also for individuals involved in rehabilitation or exercise programs aimed at improving health outcomes (Richie et al., 2023). Exercise regularly helps deliver oxygen more effectively and also benefits the heart, which is crucial for oxygen transport. The WHO recommends engaging in regular physical activity to strengthen the heart, which in turn helps the body deliver more oxygen. Engaging in 150 to 300 minutes of moderate aerobic exercise weekly significantly enhances the body's oxygen transport and utilization. Additionally, when people remain seated for extended periods, their hearts do not function as efficiently, resulting in reduced oxygen delivery to the muscles and decreased strength during exercise. If people reduce the time spent sitting and engage in aerobic and muscle-strengthening exercises, they can improve the efficiency of their heart and lungs. This holistic approach to physical activity highlights the importance of regular exercise in promoting a more robust oxygen delivery system, which supports both athletic performance and health maintenance in diverse populations (Bull et al., 2020) (Figure 8.9).

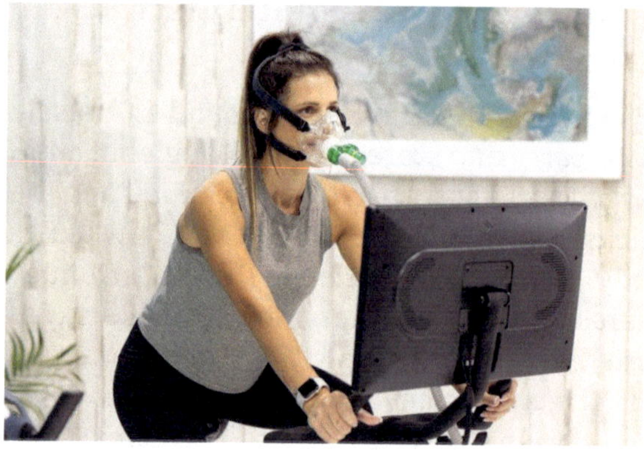

Figure 8.9. Cardiopulmonary exercise testing (CPET) during stationary cycling.

Source: https://www.onethousandroads.com/cdn/shop/articles/573dcb9d6567ac78753a6a9c53c64802.jpg?v=1672593783.

8.4. Regulation of Oxygen Transport

There are many biochemical and physiological systems in place to ensure the body receives enough oxygen to its tissues. The regulation of oxygen transport in RBCs primarily depends on hemoglobin, which adjusts its structure to optimize binding and release of oxygen according to the environment. Hemoglobin's ability to release oxygen is affected by pH, carbon dioxide, and temperature, which allows more oxygen to be released in tissues that are active in metabolism. Further supporting the dynamic nature of oxygen transport is the influence of 2,3-bisphosphoglycerate, which can modulate hemoglobin affinity in response to various physiological demands, highlighting the complexity of oxygen delivery systems in living organisms. This is supported by cellular metabolic processes that influence oxygen transport efficiency (Deborah et al., 2016).

Besides hemoglobin, several signaling pathways that oversee blood vessels are also important in oxygen transport. Nitric oxide, produced by endothelial cells, helps relax blood vessels and increase blood flow to tissues that need oxygen. During times when oxygen demand is high such as during exercise or injury, this mechanism makes sure blood flows more quickly to the affected areas. There are complex feedback systems that monitor oxygen levels in tissues and initiate pathways to provide sufficient oxygen when needed. Such regulation is vital for sustaining cellular respiration and energy production, underlining the physiological significance of the orchestrated regulation of oxygen transport (Şükrü et al., 2014). Furthermore, the way oxygen is transported changes in different health and disease states, demonstrating the body's ability to maintain stability. When oxygen is scarce, such as at high altitudes or with chronic lung diseases, the body increases the number of RBCs, raises hemoglobin, and improves oxygen transport proteins. They help the body get enough oxygen to the tissues and also make it easier to use oxygen when supplies are low. Additionally, factors such as illness and nutrition can influence how oxygen is transported, highlighting the need for comprehensive healthcare that considers the entire picture. This multifaceted regulation reflects the complexity and vital importance of maintaining efficient oxygen transport, which supports life (Deborah et al., 2016).

8.4.1. Role of the Respiratory System

The respiratory system plays a crucial role in transporting oxygen, serving as the primary gateway through which oxygen enters the body. Inhalation starts by air entering through the nose or mouth, then moving down the trachea into the bronchi, which lead to the lungs. Air in the alveoli contains oxygen which diffuses into the blood, where it is quickly attached to hemoglobin in RBCs. Hemoglobin moves oxygen to different parts of the body and also helps control the amount of carbon dioxide in the blood. It is essentialcrucial for this process to be efficient, as oxygen is essential for cells to produce energy. If the respiratory system is not functioning properly, the entire metabolic system of the body would be affected, highlighting the importance of maintaining balance. After oxygen enters the blood, it is delivered to tissues and organs by the careful cooperation between the respiratory and circulatory systems. Oxygen-rich blood in the arteries supplies cells with oxygen, which the mitochondria need for their function. In the electron transport chain (a primary process of cellular respiration), oxygen is used by mitochondria to create ATP, the key energy source for cells. A byproduct of cellular respiration is carbon dioxide, which the body must get rid of. The respiratory system facilitates both breathing in air and breathing out carbon dioxide, allowing metabolic activities to continue normally. The fact that they occur together indicates how the respiratory system is involved in energy use and balance within the body. In addition to its primary role in respiration, the respiratory system also plays a crucial role in defending the body and regulating several vital processes. For example, mucous membranes and tiny hairs in the respiratory tract help by catching and removing harmful substances and germs, making infection less likely. Additionally, the respiratory system helps maintain the correct blood pH by regulating the amounts of carbon dioxide and oxygen.

As noted in respiratory research, disturbances in respiratory function can lead to significant metabolic consequences, affecting systems such as mitochondrial activity (Povea-Cabello et al., 2024). Furthermore, emerging studies have shown that changes in respiratory function correlate with pathological conditions like prostate cancer, where metabolic alterations occur in mitochondrial respiration (Zhang et al., 2022). Overall, the respiratory system is vital not only for oxygen transport but also for maintaining overall health and metabolic efficiency in the body (Figure 8.10).

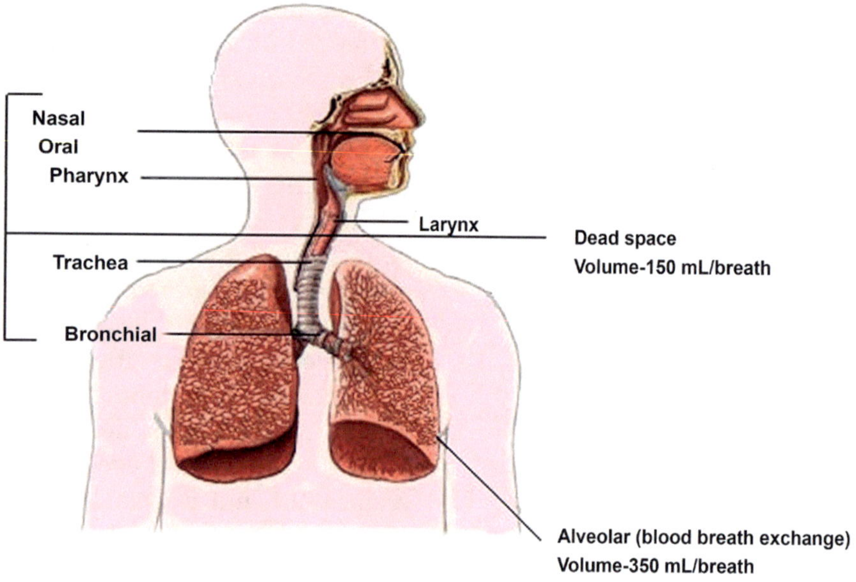

Figure 8.10. Respiratory system and its relation to breath.

Source: https://www.researchgate.net/publication/272158440/figure/fig9/AS:668864123781139@1536481042802/Respiratory-system-and-its-relation-to-breath-Adapted-with-permission-from-15.jpg.

8.4.2. Influence of pH and Carbon Dioxide Levels

The effect of pH levels on oxygen transport is crucial in physiology and biochemistry. Changes in pH may influence the way hemoglobin binds to oxygen. In acidic conditions, the Bohr effect occurs, causing hemoglobin to bind less oxygen. When we exercise intensely, this biochemical response helps by removing lactic acid and carbon dioxide, which makes the area around the muscle more acidic. So, having oxygen in these conditions supports efficient cellular respiration and increases energy production. It is essential to understand these dynamics for both treating lung diseases and improving athletic performance. Exploring the relationship between pH and oxygen reveals that maintaining a suitable pH level is essential for the body's metabolism. Oxygen transport is significantly influenced by carbon dioxide levels, which affect both the body and the environment during breathing. Elevated carbon dioxide concentration can lead to the formation of carbonic acid (H_2CO_3), lowering the pH of the blood. So, the Bohr effect is strengthened as the lower pH encourages hemoglobin to release oxygen. The bicarbonate buffer system helps maintain the balance of carbon dioxide and oxygen in the blood as well as keeps blood pH within a healthy range. Hypercapnia, a common occurrence in various respiratory disorders, increases carbon dioxide levels and can lead to respiratory acidosis, thereby making it more challenging to deliver oxygen to the tissues. Because carbon dioxide levels affect the way oxygen is transported, it is clear that balancing respiratory gases is crucial for maintaining good health and protecting the environment. Moreover, studying the interaction between pH and carbon dioxide in various environments, particularly in relation to climate change and the environment, is crucial. Rising carbon dioxide levels worldwide because of human actions cause changes in pH in natural water bodies, which may influence aquatic life and their ability to get oxygen. Due to these changes, marine organisms may exhibit altered breathing patterns and shifts in the types of species present. Studying the outcomes of pH and carbon dioxide changes is necessary to understand how ecosystems react to climate change and to develop methods to mitigate negative effects. When all these ideas are brought together, they guide conservation efforts and help create policies to maintain a sustainable balance in ecosystems, thereby supporting global environmental initiatives.

8.4.3. Adaptations to High Altitude

Adaptations to high altitude represent a remarkable intersection of evolutionary biology and physiology, particularly in relation to oxygen transport mechanisms. At high altitudes, there is less oxygen, which causes severe difficulties for organisms trying to use aerobic metabolism. The adaptations observed in species such as deer mice (*Peromyscus maniculatus*) elucidate how natural selection acts on physiological traits that enhance oxygen transport under hypoxic conditions. They have increased their affinity for hemoglobin to obtain more oxygen, which enables them to live in areas that are too high for many other animals. The intricate changes in the oxygen transport cascade demonstrate how adaptation can effectively counteract environmental stressors, ensuring survival and metabolic efficiency even in extreme settings (Harter et al., 2024). In addition, ongoing hypoxia leads the body to change in ways that help it get more oxygen. A change that occurs is higher hemoglobin levels, which can be strongly affected by genes. Studies have shown that genes such as Endothelial PAS Domain Protein 1 (EPAS1) play a crucial role in mediating these adaptations. Differences in the EPAS1 gene have been related to how Tibetans and Andeans adjust to living at high altitudes. While some groups have more hemoglobin, others, for example, Tibetans, can use oxygen efficiently with normal hemoglobin, showing how different groups adapt in different ways. This genetic basis for physiological responses underscores the complexity of adaptation to high altitude and its implications for oxygen transport systems (Moya, 2022). Examining high-altitude adaptations reveals how species have evolved and may also lead to new approaches for managing human health issues. Learning about how deer mice manage oxygen transport in low-oxygen environments can help identify new treatments for people with COPD or sleep apnea. Studies on how RBCs change and signal under hypoxia may discover new ways to improve oxygen delivery in humans. Studies of people living at high altitudes have shown that their cardiovascular and respiratory systems adapt, which may lead to new medical developments. By examining these natural adaptations, we can glean valuable insights from evolution and potentially apply these lessons in clinical settings to enhance oxygen transport in patients facing similar challenges (Harter et al., 2024).

8.5. Advances in Oxygen Transport Research

Recent innovations in oxygen transport research have focused on the development of advanced membrane technologies that enhance the efficiency of oxygen delivery systems. One potential area is the use of membrane separation in conjunction with chemical reactions in oxygen transport dual-functional membrane reactors. Due to this method, people are interested in how it can boost efficiency and also help the environment by using less energy and reducing its environmental impact. Although there have been many positive changes, there is still a significant gap in reviews that cover all the advances in dual-functional membrane reactors for oxygen transport. Addressing this gap is essential for understanding how to optimize membrane performance and unlock the full potential of these advanced systems in industrial applications (Chen et al., 2023).

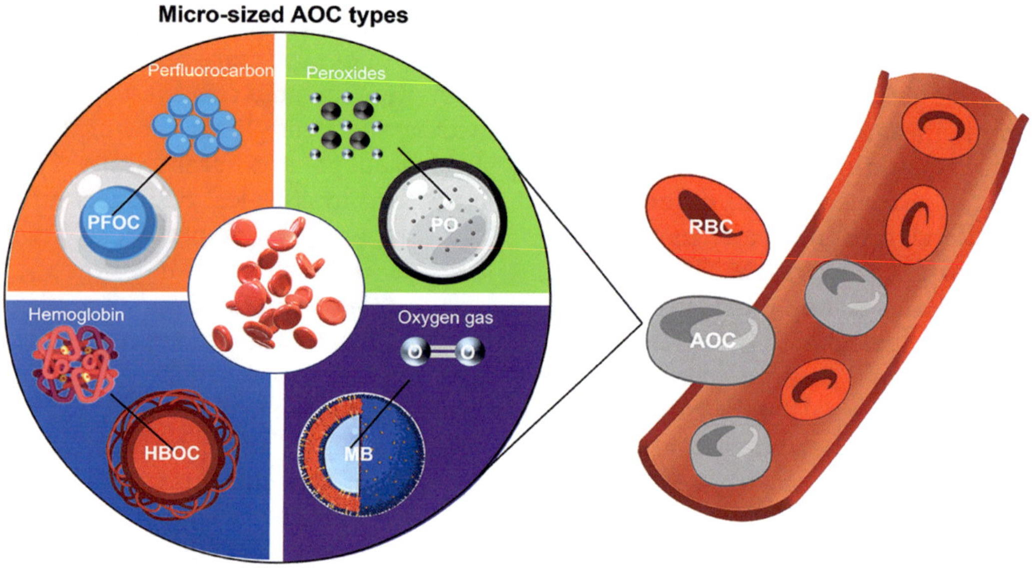

Figure 8.11. Recent advances in micro-sized oxygen carriers inspired by red blood cells.

Source: https://www.tandfonline.com/cms/asset/35571d20-a0e0-4020-a709-ceeb69e89e66/tsta_a_2223050_uf0001_oc.jpg.

The mechanisms by which oxygen is carried in RBCs are now a primary subject of study. Earlier, RBCs were thought to primarily carry oxygen, but it is now known that they play a more significant role in controlling metabolism. Omics technologies have shown that the RBC proteome and metabolomes are more complex than expected, suggesting RBCs participate in many body functions besides oxygen delivery. Additionally, studies over time have highlighted changes in RBCs that occur during storage in blood banks, prompting concerns about whether these alterations affect their performance during transfusions. Insights from these investigations are crucial for improving blood storage methods and transfusion practices, ultimately supporting better patient outcomes (Angelo et al., 2023). There are many issues and challenges in the future that could shape further research on oxygen transport. It is critical to find new materials for oxygen transport membranes to improve their performance and durability. Also, enhancing membrane engineering and reactor design can help make reactors more efficient, which could bring about significant changes in both industry and medicine. Experts are urged to investigate new ways reactions can occur and new applications for dual-functional membrane reactors, which combine chemistry, biology, and engineering. As investigations continue, the integration of cutting-edge technologies is poised to reshape our understanding and application of oxygen transport processes, thereby contributing to more sustainable and practical solutions (Chen et al., 2023) (Figure 8.11).

8.5.1. Innovations in Medical Treatments

Innovations in medical treatments have significantly enhanced the understanding and management of oxygen transport within the human body. Targeted therapies and personalized medicine are enabling improvements in oxygen delivery, particularly for individuals with respiratory and cardiovascular diseases. For instance, the invention of monoclonal antibodies has provided new approaches to addressing diseases that damage the lungs by targeting specific inflammatory pathways. They help the body take in more oxygen and, at the same time, reduce the common side effects of traditional therapies. These discoveries underscore the importance of understanding how oxygen is transported, which in turn helps create more effective treatment methods that lead to improved patient outcomes. As we learn more through research, these inventions may improve the lives of people with conditions caused by oxygen shortages. The use of technology in medicine has transformed various aspects of oxygen transport, primarily due to digital health solutions. Wearable devices and telemedicine enable the real-time monitoring of patients' oxygen levels and vital signs, allowing for swift action to be taken if necessary. They can inform healthcare providers about important changes, allowing them to quickly adapt the treatment. Additionally, the information gathered from these devices can be used in broader studies to understand trends in oxygenation and the effectiveness of various treatment methods across populations. They allow patients to look after themselves and also make sure healthcare resources are used wisely which is a significant change in how oxygen transport problems are handled. The evolution of healthcare means that strong leadership in clinical settings is more necessary for using innovative treatments. Many different health service providers using various leadership styles now indicate that the approach to oxygen transport problems is changing, which affects how patients are cared for. Working together with private companies has encouraged public services to reevaluate medical treatments and adopt new leadership methods to enhance the delivery of services. Because everyone collaborates, new treatment ideas are shared, with a focus on improving oxygen transport for different patient groups. Notably, such interorganizational synergies are likely to fuel ongoing research and development that are essential for addressing complex medical challenges in oxygen transport and related health outcomes (N/A, 2017; Siriwardena et al., 2006).

8.5.2. Use of Artificial Blood Substitutes

Due to the increased demand for effective oxygen transport in medicine, numerous new artificial blood substitutes have been developed. They are designed to perform the important tasks of human blood, mainly by providing oxygen and replacing blood volume. Among the most prominent types of artificial blood substitutes are perfluorocarbons and hemoglobin-based oxygen carriers (HBOCs), which offer specific mechanisms to enhance oxygen transport within the bloodstream. In particular, HBOCs are designed to resemble natural red blood cells, allowing them to deliver oxygen to body tissues more efficiently than regular blood products. It is essential during surgery or when there is significant bleeding, as fast and effective oxygen delivery may be needed to save a person's life. Due to their unique characteristics, they can supply oxygen in a manner that helps overcome the issues associated with blood transfusions in humans. Additionally, these artificial substitutes help address the primary difficulties associated with collecting and storing blood traditionally. Blood transfusions are required to go through strict matching and can only be kept for a short time, which makes them hard to use in emergencies. Artificial blood substitutes, particularly HBOCs, are designed to maintain stability over a wider range of temperatures and exhibit longer shelf life than human blood, making them more accessible and consistently available in medical settings (Ager et al., 2009). Being able to store blood for an extended period is highly beneficial in remote or resource-poor areas where traditional blood banking is not feasible. Since these substitutes are pathogen-free, they help prevent infections that can be transmitted by transfusion which is a significant safety issue in patient care. Although artificial blood substitutes show considerable promise, further research is necessary to ensure they are both safe and effective for use in clinics. The development of microscopic robots, for example, indicates new frontiers in oxygen transfer, as these nanorobots could assume roles akin to erythrocytes by utilizing ambient oxygen for localized delivery (Ager et al., 2009). The addition of such technology could enhance the capabilities of artificial substitutes, particularly in tissues with numerous blood vessels, where rapid oxygenation is required. Still, before they are used widely in medicine, ethical questions, strict laws, and detailed clinical trials must be dealt with. Ultimately, as these developments progress, artificial blood substitutes may play a transformative role in oxygen transport, significantly impacting medical procedures and emergency care protocols (Figure 8.12).

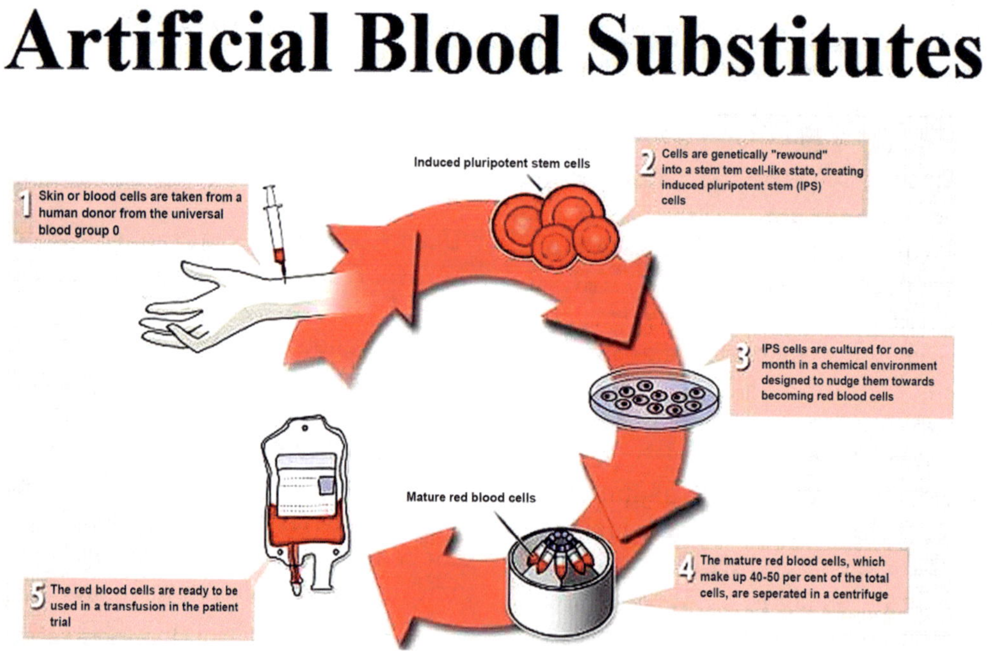

Figure 8.12. Artificial blood substitutes.

Source: https://cdn.open-pr.com/T/2/T220765814_g.jpg.

8.5.3. Future Directions in Oxygen Transport Studies

As the field of oxygen transport studies continues to evolve, researchers are increasingly recognizing the significance of molecular and catalytic advancements in optimizing oxygen delivery systems. The integration of oxygen vacancy (OV) engineering into catalyst design presents a promising avenue for enhancing oxygen transport dynamics. It has been demonstrated recently that controlling the number of oxygen vacancies in catalysts enables scientists to make reactions more efficient and easier to control. Using this method, reactants are activated better, and the movement of electrons is increased, which is important for efficient chemical reactions. As a result, using catalysts with engineered OVs brings about a significant change toward more sustainable ways to move oxygen in systems, dealing with energy efficiency and environmental issues at the same time. These advancements mark a pivotal step forward in optimizing oxygen transport mechanisms, which may ultimately lead to broader applications in various industrial and medical fields (Wang et al., 2025). Additionally, research on oxygen transport is becoming increasingly linked to new approaches in personalized medicine and therapy. As researchers strive to enhance oxygen delivery in hospitals, particularly for patients with compromised lungs or metabolic disorders, the development of targeted therapies will be crucial. New types of antidiabetic drugs, such as glucagon-like peptide-1 receptor agonists and sodium-glucose co-transporters, are being studied for how they help manage metabolism and improve oxygen transport. Because of this research, it is clear that more research is needed to see how these drugs help tissues receive oxygen, which is important for personalized care. Future studies should focus on elucidating the pathways involved and identifying patient-specific factors that influence oxygen transport, paving the way for tailored interventions that improve patient outcomes (Chatzianagnostou et al., 2024). In the future, it will be crucial for various experts to collaborate to advance studies on oxygen transport. Merging biophysics, materials science, and biological research can create new ways to study how oxygen is transported. Joining real-time imaging methods with advanced materials engineering may help design new oxygen carriers or delivery systems that are more efficient and meet the demands of living organisms. Nanotechnology also holds promise for the design of oxygen nanocarriers, highlighting the potential in this area of research. Working together across these fields can lead to significant discoveries about oxygen and its movement, which can be applied to develop better treatments for various diseases. Focusing on research that combines different fields strengthens the science of oxygen transport and also ensures that new technologies are used to solve urgent global health problems.

SUMMARY

Several biological and physical mechanisms interact to form the processes of oxygen transport. One important point is to find and study materials that allow oxygen to pass through easily, whether in biological membranes or in new synthetic forms. It has been found that improving these materials can enhance the delivery of oxygen to cells, which benefits many applications, particularly in biomedical fields. Through the analysis of materials like Bombyx mori silk fibroin (BMSF), which exhibits potential but limited real-world applications, it becomes clear that further studies are needed to elucidate their true capabilities and limitations when it comes to oxygen permeability, as highlighted by the existing literature on BMSF's shortcomings in contact lens application (Chirilă, 2021).

Additionally, studies have demonstrated that understanding how oxygen is transported in the body is crucial. For example, understanding how synapses function under oxygen stress underscores the importance of focusing on key physical properties, such as the location and thickness of transport barriers. Using models to simulate these properties can help us understand how oxygen transport is affected by things like temperature and current, which leads to the creation of better materials. By employing advanced modeling approaches and validating them through experimentation, researchers can deepen their understanding of the transport mechanisms of oxygen, thereby contributing significantly to both scientific and practical advancements in the field (Athena et al., 2023). By combining biology and materials science, there are now more opportunities for new oxygen transport technologies. Examining various types of materials, including those derived from living organisms and those synthesized in laboratories, is crucial for advancing applications in wound healing and respiratory devices. While some issues are still unclear such as the exact oxygen permeability of BMSF and the detailed study of conductive filaments in synapses, the existing research forms a solid base for further studies. By addressing these issues, we can benefit from new oxygen transport solutions that could transform healthcare and improve patients' lives, highlighting the importance of collaboration across different fields.

Several complex mechanisms are required to transport oxygen throughout the body and maintain a proper balance of cells. Oxygen is bound to hemoglobin in RBCs in the lungs, which is how the process of transport begins. Because of its structure, hemoglobin can easily grab oxygen molecules, and the more oxygen it grabs, the stronger its attraction to oxygen becomes. It is important to make sure tissues get the oxygen they need under different conditions, such as when exercising or at high altitudes. The dissociation of oxygen from hemoglobin is influenced by factors such as pH and carbon dioxide levels, emphasizing the dynamic relationship between oxygen transport and cellular metabolism (Grady et al., 2011).

As a result, it is evident why hemoglobin is crucial for transporting oxygen to all parts of the human body. At the same time as hemoglobin, myoglobin in muscle tissues is important for storing and releasing oxygen. Myoglobin holds on to oxygen more tightly than hemoglobin which allows it to save oxygen for the muscles when they need it. This function becomes particularly important during anaerobic exercise, as the supply of oxygen can be limited. In addition, things like altitude, temperature and pH influence how hemoglobin and myoglobin function which can change the efficiency of oxygen transport. Such adaptability is crucial for sustaining aerobic metabolism and ensuring that tissues receive sufficient oxygen, particularly during periods of increased energy expenditure (Neet et al., 2008). So, the way hemoglobin and myoglobin work together demonstrates how the body carefully regulates oxygen levels. Additionally, the regulation of oxygen transport is also influenced by various physiological and pathological conditions. An example is that anemia or carbon monoxide poisoning can reduce oxygen delivery, illustrating the importance of hemoglobin functioning properly. Additionally, studies on methods to increase hemoglobin or utilize erythropoietin to enhance RBCs in patients underscore the importance of oxygen transport in medical care. Understanding the details of hemoglobin and myoglobin influences can inform strategies to enhance sports performance or manage ongoing respiratory conditions. Therefore, the synthesis of knowledge surrounding oxygen transport mechanisms provides valuable insights into both normal physiology and potential clinical applications, illustrating its pivotal role in sustaining life (Grady et al., 2011; Neet et al., 2008).

CLOSER LOOK

HYPOXIA-INDUCIBLE FACTOR (HIF)

HIFs are proteins that respond when there is insufficient oxygen in the cell, a condition known as hypoxia. Pseudohypoxia may occur when there is a deficiency of thiamine, which is addressed. Both hypoxia and pseudohypoxia lead to impairment of ATP production by the mitochondria (Figure 8.13).

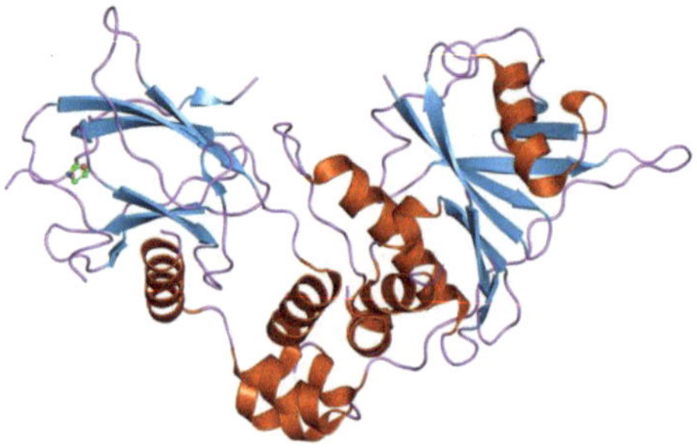

Figure 8.13. Structural representation of hypoxia-inducible factor (HIF).

Source: https://upload.wikimedia.org/wikipedia/commons/9/90/PDB_1lm8_EBI.jpg.

Structure

Oxygen-breathing species express the highly conserved transcriptional complex HIF-1, which is a heterodimer composed of an alpha and a beta subunit, the latter being a constitutively-expressed aryl hydrocarbon receptor nuclear translocator (ARNT). HIF-1 belongs to the PER-ARNT-SIM (PAS) subfamily of the basic helix-loop-helix (bHLH) family of transcription factors. Alpha and beta subunits are similar in shape, and they share these domains:

- N-terminus – a bHLH domain for DNA binding.
- Central region – Per-ARNT-Sim (PAS) domain, which facilitates heterodimerization.
- C-terminus – recruits transcriptional coregulatory proteins.

Function

HIF1α in hematopoietic stem cells means the cells remain inactive and use little energy, which helps them remain powerful for a long time during the organism's life.

HIF signaling causes the effects of hypoxia, which occurs when there is insufficient oxygen in the cell. Hypoxia often keeps cells from differentiating. Hypoxia causes the embryo and tumors to produce new blood vessels, which is important for the vascular system. Because there is not enough oxygen in wounds, keratinocytes can migrate to the area and help the epithelium regenerate. Because of these findings, controlling HIF-1 is considered a promising way to treat wounds.

In general, HIFs play a vital role in development. Mammals will not live past birth if HIF-1 genes are absent. HIF-1 allows chondrocytes to live when there is not much oxygen in the bones' growth plates. The regulation of human metabolism greatly depends on HIF.

Mechanism

Hydroxylation of the alpha subunits of HIF by HIF prolyl-hydroxylases makes them targets for the VHL E3 ubiquitin ligase, which attaches a ubiquitin tag for their rapid breakdown by the proteasome. This occurs only in normoxic conditions. Since oxygen is required for the work of HIF prolyl-hydroxylase, it is inhibited when there is insufficient oxygen.

If there are mutations in the SDHB or SDHD genes, the build-up of succinate stops HIF prolyl-hydroxylase from working, which keeps HIF-1α stable. This is termed pseudohypoxia.

With low oxygen levels, HIF-1 stabilizes and switches on many genes that help cells survive. These include glycolysis enzymes, which allow ATP synthesis in an oxygen-independent manner, and vascular endothelial growth factor (VEGF), which promotes angiogenesis. HIF-1 acts by binding to hypoxia-responsive elements (HREs) in promoters that contain the sequence 5'-RCGTG-3' (where R is a purine, either A or G). Evidence suggests that hypoxia can alter the methylation of histones and impact chromatin.

It has been shown that muscle A kinase–anchoring protein (mAKAP) organizes E3 ubiquitin ligases, affecting the stability and positioning of HIF-1 inside its action site in the nucleus. Depletion of mAKAP or disruption of its targeting to the perinuclear (in cardiomyocytes) region altered the stability of HIF-1 and transcriptional activation of genes associated with hypoxia. Thus, "compartmentalization" of oxygen-sensitive signaling components may influence the hypoxic response.

There is much more known about how HIF1 is regulated at the molecular level under hypoxia than about how NF-κB affects HIF1 regulation under normal oxygen levels. Still, HIF-1α can be stabilized in normal oxygen levels by a mechanism that is not yet known. It has been demonstrated that nuclear factor κB (NF-κB) is a direct modulator of HIF-1α expression under normal oxygen pressure. Small interfering RNA (siRNA) studies for individual NF-κB members revealed differential effects on HIF-1α mRNA levels, indicating that NF-κB can regulate basal HIF-1α expression. Finally, it was demonstrated that when endogenous NF-κB is induced by tumor necrosis factor α (TNF-α) treatment, HIF-1α levels also change in an NF-κB-dependent manner. HIF-1 and HIF-2 have different physiological roles. HIF-2 regulates erythropoietin production in adult life.

REFERENCES

1. Adepu, K. K., Anishkin, A., Adams, S. H., & Chintapalli, S. V. (2024). A versatile delivery vehicle for cellular oxygen and fuels, or metabolic sensor? - A review and perspective on the functions of myoglobin. *Physiological Reviews, 104*(4), 1611–1642. https://doi.org/10.1152/physrev.00031.2023Ager, A., Andrianantoandro, E., Arbuckle, D., Bailey, A., Baker, M., Bao, G., et al. (2009). *Chemical Power for Microscopic Robots in Capillaries.* https://arxiv.org/abs/0906.5022 (accessed on 31st May 2025).
2. Allakhverdiev, E. S., Rezukhina, E. A., Slatinskaya, O., Rodnenkov, O., Maksimov, G., & Martynyuk, T. (2023). Possibility of evaluation of oxygen transport function in PAH patients on effective selexipag-based therapy. *Eurasian Heart Journal.* https://www.semanticscholar.org/paper/c3c06f34665cf397e3677592970973f9fb79de87 (accessed on 31st May 2025).
3. Ankrah, A., Glaudemans, A., Sathekge, M., & Klein, H. (2016). Imaging latent tuberculosis infection with radiolabeled nitroimidazoles. *Clinical and Translational Imaging, 4*, 157–159. https://www.semanticscholar.org/paper/2a5270918dfaeacd66e8fb8975739924633b14e7 (accessed on 31st May 2025).
4. Athena, F. F., & Vogel, E. M. (2023). Describing the analog resistance change of HfOx-based neuromorphic synapses using a compact series trap-assisted tunneling and Ohmic conduction model. *Applied Physics Letters.* https://www.semanticscholar.org/paper/5d0e1b4acc7e4558e91083bf47e2c7423803e351 (accessed on 31st May 2025).
5. Azmat, J., Waseem, M., Dar, Y. F., Ambreen, S., Shafqat, H., & Yousaf, Z. (2024). Role of hemoglobin and its impact on human health: A narrative review. *Insights—Journal of Health and Rehabilitation.* https://www.semanticscholar.org/paper/84e57bd0920f704689f74fec6ee32929d1a7ac46 (accessed on 31st May 2025).
6. Bourdon, J. C., Gromova, N. V., Grunyushkin, I. P., Klenova, et al. (2017). Physical and chemical processes and the morphofunctional characteristics of human erythrocytes in hyperglycemia. *Front. Physiol.* https://core.ac.uk/download/141567522.pdf (accessed on 31st May 2025).
7. Brindha, D. P., Krishna, V. R., & Romauld, S. I. (2017). *A Review on Artificial Blood: A Source We Need.* https://core.ac.uk/download/477853072.pdf (accessed on 31st May 2025).
8. Buisman, C. J. N., Hamelers, H. V. M., Helder, M., Steinbusch, et al. (2010). *Microbial Solar Cells: Applying Photosynthetic and Electrochemically Active Organisms.* https://core.ac.uk/download/30436016.pdf (accessed on 31st May 2025).
9. Bull, F., Al-Ansari, S. S., Biddle, S., Borodulin, K., Buman, M. P., Cardon, G., Carty, C., et al. (2020). World Health Organization 2020 guidelines on physical activity and sedentary behavior. *British Journal of Sports Medicine, 54*, 1451–1462. https://doi.org/10.1136/bjsports-2020-102955 (accessed on 31st May 2025).
10. Carteri, R. (2025). Mitochondria as a therapeutic target: Focusing on traumatic brain injury. *Journal of Integrative Neuroscience, 24*(1), 25292. https://www.semanticscholar.org/paper/7542140cbc6e3207fb126c6dbc9369cb24e08eba (accessed on 31st May 2025).
11. Chatzianagnostou, K., Gaggini, M., Florentin, A. S., Simonini, L., & Vassalle, C. (2024). New molecules in type 2 diabetes: Advancements, challenges and future directions. *International Journal of Molecular Sciences, 25.* https://www.semanticscholar.org/paper/a324411af6ff54aae428b5276a9466c10ae60cc2 (accessed on 31st May 2025).

12. Chen, G., Widenmeyer, M., Yu, X., Han, N., Tan, X., Homm, G., Liu, S., et al. (2023). Perspectives on achievements and challenges of oxygen transport dual-functional membrane reactors. *Journal of the American Ceramic Society, 107,* 1490–1504. https://doi.org/10.1111/jace.19411 (accessed on 31st May 2025).

13. Cheng, J., Zhang, X., Zheng, Q., Shi, S., & Wang, J. (2024). Empagliflozin-loaded nanomicelles responsive to reactive oxygen species for renal ischemia/reperfusion injury protection. *Open Chemistry, 22.* https://www.semanticscholar.org/paper/ffc682eb3f092cd7ea1e4b40f2a0456b1ba14af1 (accessed on 31st May 2025).

14. Chirilă, T. (2021). Oxygen permeability of silk fibroin hydrogels and their use as materials for contact lenses: A purposeful analysis. *Gels, 7.* https://www.semanticscholar.org/paper/cc2bbc3aa02fc2400645c823e937a7302b5ce9d1 (accessed on 31st May 2025).

15. D'Alessandro, A., Anastasiadi, A. T., Tzounakas, V. L., Nemkov, T., Reisz, J. A., Kriebardis, A. G., Zimring, J. C., et al. (2023). Red blood cell metabolism *in vivo* and *in vitro. Metabolites, 13,* 793. https://doi.org/10.3390/metabo13070793 (accessed on 31st May 2025).

16. Dehghani, M., Ghazi, S. F., & Kazemzadeh, Y. (2024). Interfacial tension and wettability alteration during hydrogen and carbon dioxide storage in depleted gas reservoirs. *Scientific Reports, 14.* https://www.semanticscholar.org/paper/6176f76cf17c2988fad748544d504e98fe0ca63c (accessed on 31st May 2025).

17. Fehr, T. (2017). *A pH Dependent Switch in DHP Oxidation Mechanism.* https://core.ac.uk/download/158970007.pdf (accessed on 31st May 2025).

18. Ghimire, B., Szili, E. J., Lamichhane, P., Short, R. D., Lim, J. S., Attri, P., Masur, K., et al. (2019). The role of UV photolysis and molecular transport in the generation of reactive species in a tissue model with a cold atmospheric pressure plasma jet. *Applied Physics Letters, 114.* https://doi.org/10.1063/1.5086522 (accessed on 31st May 2025).

19. Goberdhan, D. C. I., Wilson, C., & Harris, A. L. (2016). Amino acid sensing by mTORC1: Intracellular transporters mark the spot. *Cell Metabolism, 23,* 580–589. https://doi.org/10.1016/j.cmet.2016.03.013 (accessed on 31st May 2025).

20. Goulding, R. P., & Marwood, S. (2023). Interaction of factors determining critical power. *Sports Medicine, 53,* 595–613. https://doi.org/10.1007/s40279-022-01805-w (accessed on 31st May 2025).

21. Grady, C., Daigger, G., Love, N., & Filipe, C. (2011). *Biological Wastewater Treatment.* https://www.semanticscholar.org/paper/9f74aab3fed3459fecbdc8046d61da743ab0703e (accessed on 31st May 2025).

22. Gromova, N. V., Imarova, O. G., Martynova, M. I., Revin, et al. (2016). Role of membrane lipids in the regulation of erythrocytic oxygen-transport function in cardiovascular diseases. *BioMed Research International.* https://core.ac.uk/download/228177833.pdf (accessed on 31st May 2025).

23. Güleç, Ş., Anderson, G. J., & Collins, J. F. (2014). Mechanistic and regulatory aspects of intestinal iron absorption. *AJP Gastrointestinal and Liver Physiology, 307,* G397–G409. https://doi.org/10.1152/ajpgi.00348.2013 (accessed on 31st May 2025).

24. Harter, T., & Scott, G. R. (2024). Linking red blood cell functional phenotypes to environmental tolerance in high-altitude adapted deer mice. *Physiology.* https://www.semanticscholar.org/paper/fc8c5d0a7ec7488cc5141f0e1a1d0f3024620897 (accessed on 31st May 2025).

25. Kaag, N. H. B. M., Karman, C. C., & Tamis, J. E. (2009). *Feasibility Studies in Relation to the IMO Ballast Water Convention.* https://core.ac.uk/download/pdf/29252094.pdf (accessed on 31st May 2025).

26. Kreiman, A. N., Garner, S. E., Carroll, S. C., & Sutherland, M. C. (2025). Biochemical mapping reveals a conserved heme transport mechanism via CcmCD in System I bacterial cytochrome c biogenesis. *mBio.* https://www.semanticscholar.org/paper/5e8d5d4c0defc1f26622d1ae814bd76a7fb683bd (accessed on 31st May 2025).

27. Lamichhane, S., Carreto Guevara, E., Fescenko, I., Liou, S. H., Lai, R. Y., & Laraoui, A. (2024). Magnetic relaxometry of methemoglobin by widefield nitrogen-vacancy microscopy. *Applied Physics Letters.* https://www.semanticscholar.org/paper/7cf1d1ede03461e3bb7820087ca5fee9e660a20a (accessed on 31st May 2025).

28. Lazic, D., Grujić, V., & Cvetković, D. (2023). Results of using sustainable aviation fuel in transport aircraft on different flight levels and their influence on carbon-dioxide CO_2 emissions. *Scientific Journal of Silesian University of Technology. Series Transport.* https://www.semanticscholar.org/paper/af0ac36c529c736daeeb44d5675a972b3cd54bfb (accessed on 31st May 2025).

29. Leonard, J. I. (2025). A systems analysis of the erythropoietic responses to weightlessness. Volume 2: Description of the model of erythropoiesis regulation. Part A: Model for regulation of erythropoiesis. Part B: Detailed description of the model for regulation of erythropoiesis. https://core.ac.uk/download/pdf/42844719.pdf (accessed on 31st May 2025).

30. Li, Y. W., Zheng, Q. J., Zheng, N. J., Meng, J. Z., Liu, B. L., Liu, X., Zhao, H. M., et al. (2025). Novel insights into microcystin-LR uptake, accumulation, and toxicity mechanisms in lettuce (*Lactuca sativa* L.) using a protoplast model. *Journal of Agricultural and Food Chemistry.* https://www.semanticscholar.org/paper/72b7e79ad11ed618ccc62bbaf649d60d0ffa3af1 (accessed on 31st May 2025)

31. Liang, H., & Acharya, G. (2020). Novel coronavirus disease (COVID-19) in pregnancy: What clinical recommendations to follow? *Acta Obstetricia et Gynecologica Scandinavica, 99,* 439–442. https://doi.org/10.1111/aogs.13836 (accessed on 31st May 2025).

32. Locatelli, F., Fishbane, S., Block, G. A., & Macdougall, I. C. (2017). Targeting hypoxia-inducible factors for the treatment of anemia in chronic kidney disease patients. *American Journal of Nephrology, 45,* 187–199. https://doi.org/10.1159/000455166 (accessed on 31st May 2025).

33. Moya, E. (2022). EPAS1/HIF-2α: A key regulator for chronic hypoxia across species. *The Journal of Physiology, 600.* https://www.semanticscholar.org/paper/7fd9ea325220ad378a8733cf9ccd827fe2c4be68 (accessed on 31st May 2025).

34. N/A. (2017). *Outlook Magazine, Spring 2017.* https://core.ac.uk/download/212868995.pdf (accessed on 31st May 2025).

35. Neet, K., & Thinakaran, G. (2008). Thematic minireview series on the molecular basis of Alzheimer disease. *Journal of Biological Chemistry, 283,* 29613–29614. https://www.semanticscholar.org/paper/08210c13fa19a6f599a99ffad86082e244d5cc3b (accessed on 31st May 2025).

36. Nix, S. (2025). Transport characteristics of small molecules diffusing near deforming blood cells. *Computation.* https://www.semanticscholar.org/paper/b8c4150554e940db9ebeffade2587b610707924f (accessed on 31st May 2025).

37. Ponganis, P., Williams, C. L., & Kendall-Bar, J. M. (2024). Blood oxygen transport and depletion in diving emperor penguins. *The Journal of Experimental Biology, 227*. https://www.semanticscholar.org/paper/a1763b31e3401303b198dfb13c3a281cc88da611 (accessed on 31st May 2025).

38. Povea-Cabello, S., Brischigliaro, M., & Fernández-Vizarra, E. (2024). Emerging mechanisms in the redox regulation of mitochondrial cytochrome c oxidase assembly and function. *Biochemical Society Transactions*. https://www.semanticscholar.org/paper/9d60b5100601098b04e896aafd513dc06f417a60 (accessed on 31st May 2025).

39. Pretini, V., Koenen, M. H., Kaestner, L., Fens, M. H. A. M., Schiffelers, R. M., Bartels, M., & Van Wijk, R. (2019). Red blood cells: Chasing interactions. *Frontiers in Physiology, 10*. https://doi.org/10.3389/fphys.2019.00945 (accessed on 31st May 2025).

40. Singh, A., Maurya, N., Saxena, R., & Saxena, S. (2024). An overview of red blood cell properties and functions. *Journal of International Research in Medical and Pharmaceutical Sciences*. https://www.semanticscholar.org/paper/1dbe43da39e789b1cb096e3126e11a7eff6856de (accessed on 31st May 2025).

41. Siriwardena, A. N. (2006). *Releasing the Potential of Health Services: Translating Clinical Leadership into Healthcare Quality Improvement*. https://core.ac.uk/download/52745.pdf (accessed on 31st May 2025).

42. Tokodi, N., Latkowska, E., Klimczak, B., Kłodawska, K., Malec, P., Willis, A., Kokociński, M., et al. (2025). Toward understanding the mechanisms of *Raphidiopsis raciborskii* response to chill/light stress. *Journal of Phycology*. https://www.semanticscholar.org/paper/d6ff6e888a0eceb7e4eb57bf0e86c6926ad53fc9 (accessed on 31st May 2025).

43. Wai, P. P., Yamaguchi, H., Hitachi, K., Tsuchida, K., & Komatsu, S. (2025). Morphological and proteomic analyses to reveal salt-tolerant mechanisms in soybean seedlings treated with titanium-oxide nanoparticles. *Oxygen*. https://www.semanticscholar.org/paper/2a964b4aa2a9f82e4384a44ec144f078e3b674c7 (accessed on 31st May 2025).

44. Wang, D., Zhou, J., Sun, X., & Niu, X. (2025). The essence of nature can be the simplest (3) holistic energy: Extracellular Fenton reactions of all cells. *Chemistry & Biodiversity*. https://www.semanticscholar.org/paper/17068e6effffa2431a7038aa283c275d59d49785 (accessed on 31st May 2025).

45. Wang, Y., Lilienfeldt, N., & Hekimi, S. (2024). Understanding coenzyme Q. *Physiological Reviews, 104*, 1533–1610. https://www.semanticscholar.org/paper/75af8bf88a826823e04ab4b0ec772e03481478c2 (accessed on 31st May 2025)

46. Wang, Z., Lin, S., Wang, L., Qian, J., He, M., Lu, B. H., & Wang, Y. (2025). Oxygen vacancy engineering for enhancing catalytic performance in CO_2 hydrogenation: Recent advances and future directions. *ChemCatChem*. https://www.semanticscholar.org/paper/aed53063cd5db941f537943ee318f9fb626b3612 (accessed on 31st May 2025)

47. Zafar, S., Raza, A. A., Lakhair, J. A., Murad, S., Fatah, A., & Fatima, E. (2023). Dried fruit and Aspaghola: New approaches in treating lipid metabolism. *Journal of Clinical Research and Case Studies*. https://www.semanticscholar.org/paper/9bc7624c52522b28e8912fb4e8eec01d51af02f6 (accessed on 31st May 2025).

48. Zhang, A., Gupte, A., Chatterjee, S., Li, S., Ayala, A., Miles, B., & Hamilton, D. (2022). Enhanced succinate oxidation with mitochondrial complex II reactive oxygen species generation in human

prostate cancer. *International Journal of Molecular Sciences, 23.* https://www.semanticscholar.org/paper/5f5fca8cbe50d450866392fd8fe9b8126c9225f2 (accessed on 31st May 2025).

49. Zhang, J. (2025). Convection effect of plasma flow on oxygen transport in capillaries: An in-depth numerical investigation. *Microcirculation, 32.* https://www.semanticscholar.org/paper/b48f6d1c8a95f4083dfe384ae1e89ed85704affd (accessed on 31st May 2025).

50. Zinchuk, V. V., & Al-Jebur, J. S. O. (2024). Oxygen-dependent aspects of the action of Asprosyn. *Rossijskij Fiziologičeskij Žurnal im. I. M. Sečenova.* https://www.semanticscholar.org/paper/f21a4c1a79e11f8443f98a9fd994bc76fcf352ca (accessed on 31st May 2025).

51. Zinchuk, V., & Biletskaya, E. (2023). Effect of ozone on oxygen transport and pro-oxidant–antioxidant balance of red blood cell suspension. *Acta Chimica Slovenica.* https://www.semanticscholar.org/paper/60aef47ac34b1bf03d404f63183aed7201b5810c (accessed on 31st May 2025).

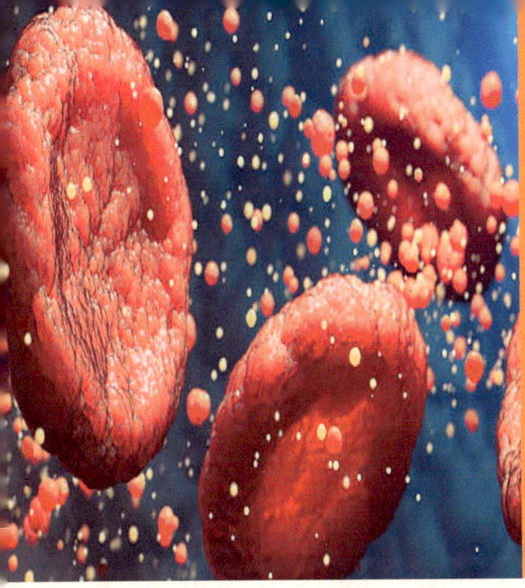

Chapter 9

CARBON DIOXIDE TRANSPORT IN THE BLOOD

Contents

Introduction

The transport of carbon dioxide (CO_2) in the blood is a crucial physiological process that is integral to maintaining homeostasis within the human body. Cells release CO_2 while processing nutrients, and this gas must be removed to keep it from becoming dangerous. This dynamic process includes various mechanisms of transport, primarily through bicarbonate ions in the plasma, dissolved CO_2, and the binding of CO_2 to hemoglobin in red blood cells (RBCs). By understanding these pathways, we can observe both the primary functions of the respiratory system and how metabolism influences it. The ability of the body to maintain appropriate levels of CO_2 is essential, as deviations can lead to respiratory acidosis or alkalosis, which can have profound effects on physiological function and ultimately systemic health (Pöschl et al., 2015). In addition to its importance for respiration, transporting CO_2 highlights issues related to public health and the environment. Due to climate change and poor air quality in cities, the relationship between CO_2 levels and human health is a significant concern. An increase in carbon dioxide can exacerbate respiratory diseases and impact the overall health of individuals. For this reason, it is important to have effective carbon management, and this means learning more about how CO_2 is transported in blood. As highlighted by recent research, the biogeochemical cycling of carbon compounds is inextricably linked to Earth's health, urging an investigative approach that encompasses both physiological and environmental science (Pöschl et al., 2015). The exploration of carbon dioxide transport mechanisms also yields insights into treatment approaches for various respiratory conditions, such as chronic obstructive pulmonary disease (COPD) and asthma. In the past, attention in respiratory physiology was primarily focused on airflow and lung function, which often overlooked the details of CO_2. Knowing how CO_2 transport changes in diseases can give a clearer view of pulmonary physiology. For example, reduced ability to transport CO_2 in the blood may result in actions that further harm breathing. By elucidating these mechanisms, researchers can better address the needs of patients and contribute to the advancement of clinical strategies that enhance respiratory health (Wouters, 2008).

Definition of Carbon Dioxide Transport

The transport of carbon dioxide (CO_2) in the blood is a critical physiological process essential for maintaining acid-base balance and facilitating respiration. Carbon dioxide, which is produced during cellular respiration, moves in the bloodstream mainly by dissolving in the plasma, forming bicarbonate ions, or binding to hemoglobin. Approximately 7% of CO_2 is transported in its dissolved form, while 70% is converted into bicarbonate ions through a reaction catalyzed by the enzyme carbonic anhydrase (CA). Most of this conversion happens in RBCs and it is needed because bicarbonate helps control the pH level in blood. The remaining bicarbonate (23%) is bound to hemoglobin, forming carbamino compounds that facilitate the transport of CO_2 from the body to the lungs for exhalation. Knowing about these mechanisms is important for recognizing how the body effectively controls CO_2 levels. CO_2 transport is important not only for removing waste; it also supports breathing and helps maintain the body's balance. For example, the bicarbonate buffering system helps maintain the pH of blood within a narrow range, which is essential for normal cell and enzyme function. This regulation occurs through a dynamic equilibrium between CO_2, bicarbonate ions, and carbonic acid (H_2CO_3) in the blood. Additionally, when CO_2 transport is altered, it can have a significant impact on the body; for example, hypercapnia, characterized by an increase in CO_2, can lead to respiratory acidosis. Hypocapnia which means there is less CO_2 in the blood, may cause respiratory alkalosis. Both conditions highlight the role of CO_2 transport in helping metabolic processes continue without being disrupted, which shows how the body carefully balances its functions in response to different needs. In addition to supporting normal body functions, removing CO_2 is crucial in diseases and the environment. For example, conditions that impair respiratory function, such as chronic obstructive pulmonary disease (COPD) or pneumonia, can hinder the effective transport of carbon dioxide, leading to significant health complications. Additionally, understanding how CO_2 moves through the atmosphere is crucial for addressing the broader issues resulting from higher CO_2 levels caused by human activities. When CO_2 builds up in the body, it can harm various parts of the body, so a comprehensive approach is needed to assess and treat the effects on health. Research and initiatives aimed at addressing the global carbon budget are crucial in mitigating the effects of climate change on human health, highlighting the interconnectedness of carbon dioxide transport in both biological and environmental contexts (Livingston et al., 2020; Saunois et al., 2020) (Figure 9.1).

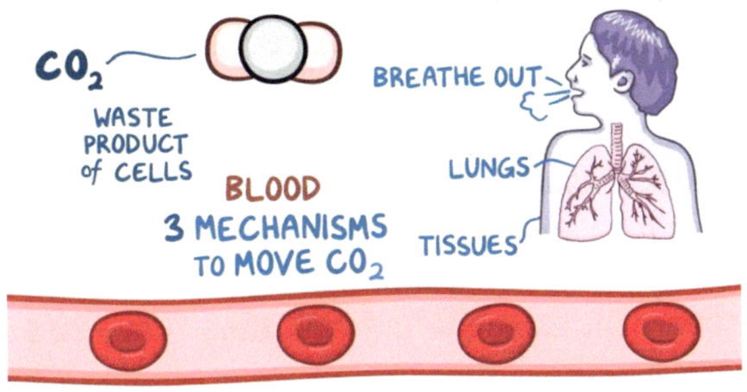

Figure 9.1. Carbon dioxide transport.

Source: https://d16qt3wv6xm098.cloudfront.net/UDvojzodRvWVHUKwvPv0h2CyS86LEX4B/_.jpg.

Importance of Carbon Dioxide in the Body

Carbon dioxide in the body is not only excreted; it is important for a range of life-sustaining processes. Most of the CO_2 produced in the body comes from cellular respiration, which takes place in the mitochondria. CO_2 is produced as a result of energy metabolism, which involves breaking down glucose and other substances to produce ATP. Furthermore, CO_2 exists in equilibrium with bicarbonate (HCO_3^-), facilitating the maintenance of acid-base balance, which is crucial in regulating pH levels in blood and tissues. This buffering system is vital, as deviations from normal pH can disrupt homeostasis and impair various enzyme functions necessary for metabolic processes (Rad, 2022). CO_2 is constantly generated and transported throughout the body, highlighting its importance for cellular activities and overall health. In addition to its basic functions, CO_2 is involved in important pathways that regulate various physiological responses. A rise in CO_2 may lead to increased production of peroxynitrite, which in turn affects the pathways that regulate redox signaling. CO_2 reacts with peroxides in the body, which helps control oxidative stress inside cells. This interaction is noteworthy, as CO_2 not only participates in generating reactive species but also influences gene expression related to redox metabolism and inflammatory responses (Rad, 2022). These functions of CO_2 highlight its role in cellular balance and its potential contribution to disease when its levels are not properly regulated. Knowing that CO_2 plays a role in metabolism and participates in cell signaling is crucial for understanding its role in both health and disease. Also, the body relies on CO_2 transport in the blood to maintain its balanced state. CO_2 is mainly transported in the body as dissolved CO_2, bicarbonate ions, and carbamino compounds, which illustrates the complexity of gas exchange and pH control. The enzyme CA allows CO_2 to be quickly changed into bicarbonate in RBCs, which helps it reach the lungs for exhalation. Maintaining the balance between CO_2 and HCO_3 is necessary to keep acid-base homeostasis. Increased CO_2 in tissues leads to vasodilation, which enhances the flow of blood and oxygen to areas that require more energy. It demonstrates that CO_2 plays a crucial role in waste removal, as well as in the proper functioning of all the body's systems.

9.1. The Role of Carbon Dioxide in Metabolism

The biochemical processes underlying metabolism are intricately linked to the levels and roles of carbon dioxide in the body. Cellular respiration releases CO_2, mainly because of the oxidative decarboxylation reactions that happen in the mitochondria. They include the conversion of metabolic intermediates such as pyruvate, isocitrate, and α-ketoglutarate, which produce CO_2 and reduce NAD+ to NADH, which is then used to make ATP in the electron transport chain. Furthermore, CO_2 exists dynamically within the bicarbonate (HCO_3^-) buffer system, essential for maintaining acid-base balance in the body. This equilibrium helps neutralize excess acids produced during metabolism, underscoring the critical role of CO_2 as both a waste product and a regulator of metabolic processes, ensuring that cellular functions proceed optimally in various physiological contexts (Rad, 2022). New research suggests that CO_2 can act as a messenger molecule, influencing redox reactions and gene expression in metabolic pathways. New studies have revealed that CO_2 and peroxides interact and change the way oxidative stress, signaling, and inflammation occur in mammalian cells. CO_2 increases the activity of peroxides, which can affect important oxidative processes, such as changes to proteins, including thiol oxidation and tyrosine nitration. These modifications have significant implications for cellular functions and mechanisms of damage control, indicating that CO_2 is not merely a metabolic byproduct but an active participant in cellular signaling cascades (Rad, 2022). Because CO_2 is involved in numerous processes, it plays a crucial role in energy production and cellular regulation. Besides its role in metabolism, CO_2 is important for lymphatic function and homeostasis. Keeping CO_2 levels under control helps the blood and lymphatic vessels communicate, which is necessary for the body to maintain a balance of nutrients, waste, and the immune system. Researchers are now investigating the relationship between lymphatic vessel function and carbon dioxide metabolism. Although the mechanisms by which lymph vessels grow are better understood, the impact of CO_2 on these processes remains unclear. This emerging area of study exemplifies how CO_2 not only facilitates metabolic reactions but also drives physiological functions across interconnected biological systems, highlighting its importance beyond metabolism alone (Figure 9.2).

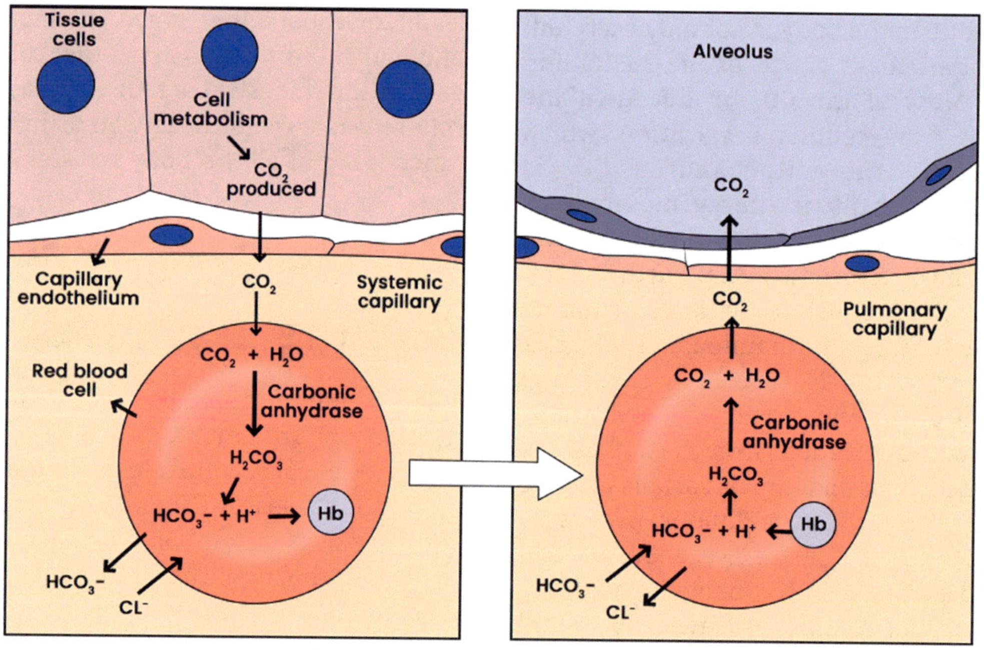

Figure 9.2. Transport of carbon dioxide in the blood.

Source: https://media.geeksforgeeks.org/wp-content/uploads/20240606102206/Transport-of-Carbon-Dioxide-in-the-Blood.png.

9.1.1. Production of Carbon Dioxide During Cellular Respiration

The production of carbon dioxide (CO_2) during cellular respiration is a fundamental biochemical process that occurs in both prokaryotic and eukaryotic cells. Cellular respiration consists of glycolysis, the Krebs cycle, and oxidative phosphorylation, culminating in the conversion of energy from nutrients into adenosine triphosphate (ATP). The process involves oxidizing organic compounds, which results in the release of CO_2. In aerobic respiration, the mitochondria use the pyruvate dehydrogenase complex to change pyruvate, which is from glucose, into CO_2. CO_2 that collects in the body affects the body's acid-base balance, which influences the pH of tissues and blood. This, in turn, helps control metabolic processes and cellular activities. The Krebs cycle, a part of cellular respiration, causes intermediates such as isocitrate and α-ketoglutarate to release more CO_2 through decarboxylation. They also play a role in creating important electron carriers called NADH and $FADH_{2,}$ which have much energy. They are necessary for the next part of electron transport, where ATP is mainly produced. CO_2 is important because it interacts with energy metabolism, helping to control the rate of respiration and the way cells utilize various substances. Understanding this dynamic relationship is essential for grasping how CO_2 generation during cellular respiration links to broader metabolic and physiological processes, ultimately affecting the organism's health and homeostasis (Li et al., 2022). Additionally, the fact that CO_2 is formed during cellular respiration suggests its role as a primary regulator of redox biology within mammalian cells. The carbon dioxide/bicarbonate (CO_2/HCO_3^-) equilibrium plays a pivotal role in maintaining acid-base homeostasis. In this context, excess CO_2 reacts with water to form carbonic acid (H_2CO_3), which can dissociate into bicarbonate ions and hydrogen ions, thereby buffering pH levels in the blood and tissues. It is needs more energy, and CO_2 production increases. The influence of CO_2 extends beyond being a mere waste product; it actively modulates cellular processes, such as gene expression related to redox metabolism, oxidative stress responses, and inflammatory pathways (Rad, 2022). Understanding these intricate interactions elucidates how CO_2 production during cellular respiration is integral not only to energy metabolism but also to the regulation of vital physiological functions (Figure 9.3).

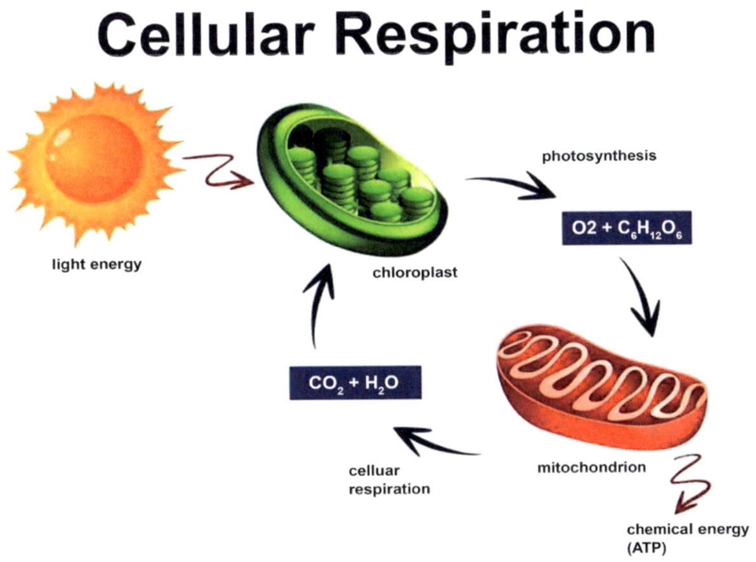

Figure 9.3. Understanding the process of cellular respiration.

Source: https://fatty15.com/cdn/shop/articles/Understanding_the_Process_of_Cellular_Respiration_1200x1200.png?v=1696520936.

9.1.2. Impact of Carbon Dioxide on Blood pH

An acute understanding of how CO_2 influences blood pH is essential to grasp its vital role in physiological processes. Within the bloodstream, CO_2 exists in dynamic equilibrium with bicarbonate (HCO_3^-) and H2CO3, which significantly affects blood pH levels. When CO_2 dissolves in water, it forms H_2CO_3, which can dissociate into bicarbonate and hydrogen ions (H^+). This reaction demonstrates that an increase in CO_2 in the blood causes the pH to drop, making the blood more acidic, a condition known as acidosis. Bicarbonate ions can also neutralize excess hydrogen ions in the bloodstream when CO2 is exhaled, thereby increasing the pH and making the environment more alkaline. So, balancing CO_2 levels is necessary to keep blood pH at the right level which helps the body function properly. The bicarbonate buffer system helps maintain the proper pH of blood as carbon dioxide levels change. Changes in CO_2 concentration cause a shift in the carbon dioxide-bicarbonate equilibrium, as determined by the Henderson-Hasselbalch equation. Rising CO_2 levels cause more H2CO3 to form, which moves the equilibrium to the side with more hydrogen ions and a lower pH, encouraging acidosis. When CO_2 decreases, the hydrogen ion concentration also decreases, which increases pH and may lead to metabolic alkalosis. Metabolic alkalosis is often observed in the clinic when bicarbonate levels are elevated, particularly when bicarbonate is gained or retained without a corresponding decrease in CO_2. It is further supported by research that, when COPD leads to chronic hypercapnia, it exacerbates acidosis and makes it significantly harder for the body to maintain its normal state, highlighting the close relationship between CO_2 levels and blood pH. The CO_2 regulation of blood pH also relies on the kidneys' function, highlighting the importance of adjusting to changes in CO_2 levels. Bicarbonate reabsorption and hydrogen ion excretion are ways in which the kidneys help maintain acid-base balance. If CO_2 levels are high, the kidneys try to lower acidosis by increasing the amount of bicarbonate they excrete. Additionally, if hypercapnia persists for an extended period, as can occur in certain metabolic disorders, the kidneys may increase ammonia production, which aids the body in eliminating excess hydrogen ions. If the body is exposed to a low pH for a prolonged period, it may develop mechanisms to manage the issue, which can eventually disrupt kidney function and affect the body's acid-base balance. As detailed in research, the intricate relationships between CO_2 metabolism and blood pH regulation highlight not only the physiological significance of CO_2 transport in the blood but also its impact on overall health and disease states, warranting further exploration of (Do et al., 2022; Rad Rí, 2022).

9.1.3. Relationship Between Carbon Dioxide and Oxygen Transport

The intricacies of gas exchange in human physiology hinge significantly on the relationship between carbon dioxide and oxygen transport within the bloodstream. Oxygen (O_2) is primarily transported by hemoglobin in RBCs, where it binds to iron-containing heme groups. Concurrently, carbon dioxide generated from cellular metabolism is released from tissues back to the lungs via three mechanisms: dissolution in plasma, conversion to bicarbonate, and binding to hemoglobin. Because of this system, oxygen is delivered to the tissues efficiently, and at the same time, CO_2 is eliminated. How these gases work together demonstrates the basic functions of the body and highlights that any upset in one can disrupt the other, showing how important it is for these gases to remain in balance. An interesting thing about CO_2 and O_2 is the Bohr effect, which means that more CO_2 in the blood makes hemoglobin less likely to hold onto oxygen. As tissues are more active, they produce more CO_2, which allows hemoglobin to release the O_2 it is carrying more easily. It is adjusted to meet local needs so that active tissues can always get enough oxygen. How these gases influence each other demonstrates how homeostasis happens and also explains how changes in their levels can indicate changes in tissue blood flow and breathing, making it clear why correct gas exchange is important for the body. Additionally, carbon dioxide transport is crucial in situations where individuals experience extreme conditions, such as astronauts. Studies have found that when blood flow is altered, as in microgravity, it can disrupt the standard mechanisms by which CO_2 and O_2 are transported. For instance, alterations in intracranial pressure associated with elevated CO_2 levels can lead to complications in brain perfusion and overall oxygen delivery (Sándor et al., 2023). Understanding how these systems are linked enhances our knowledge of physiology and also helps establish safety measures and health monitoring in hazardous situations. Enhanced techniques, such as diffuse optical flowmetry (DOF), can elucidate RBC dynamics, offering novel insights into the crucial interactions between oxygen and carbon dioxide transport within the human body (Kholiqov et al., 2020) (Figure 9.4).

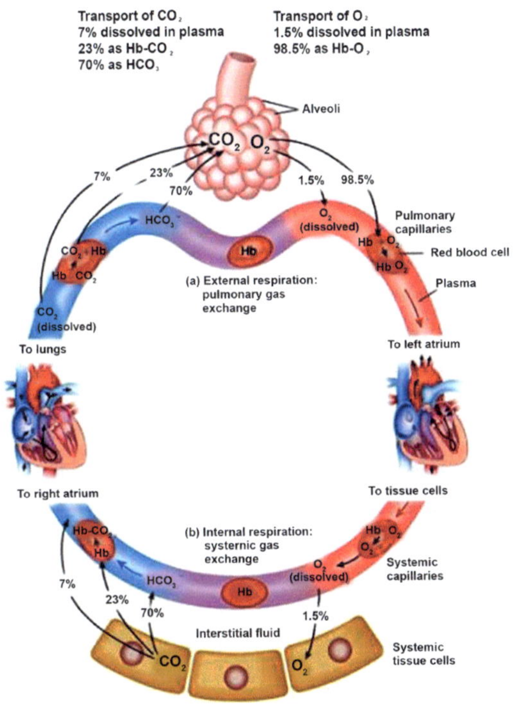

Figure 9.4. Transport of oxygen and carbon dioxide.

Source: https://slideplayer.com/slide/4157061/13/images/37/Transport+of+Oxygen+and+Carbo n+Dioxide.jpg.

9.2. Mechanisms of Carbon Dioxide Transport

The transport of carbon dioxide (CO_2) in the blood is a complex process that involves various mechanisms facilitated by RBCs. Besides transporting oxygen, RBCs are responsible for carrying away CO_2, which is a waste product of metabolism. Approximately 70% of CO_2 is transported in the form of bicarbonate (HCO_3^-), created via a reaction mediated by the enzyme carbonic anhydrase (CA) within RBCs. CO_2 is hydrated by this enzyme to become H_2CO_3, which rapidly separates into bicarbonate and hydrogen ions. By converting, the body helps maintain a proper acid-base balance in the blood and can easily move CO_2 from other tissues to the lungs. Moreover, the flexible structure of RBCs enables them to navigate through microcapillaries, ensuring effective gas exchange during their 120-day lifespan, while also interacting with various cell types (Pretini et al., 2019). Besides bicarbonate, hemoglobin transports about 23% of the carbon dioxide in the blood. As RBCs move through the body, CO_2 binds to different parts of the hemoglobin than oxygen, allowing them to carry both gases simultaneously. As a consequence, carbamino compounds form, which are necessary for hemoglobin to hold on to oxygen properly. Notably, the Bohr effect demonstrates that more CO_2 in the blood causes the pH to decrease which makes more oxygen available for tissues that need it the most. Their ability to carry out both roles is essential for both breathing and the overall balance of metabolic functions in different situations. Such intricate functions highlight the adaptive nature of RBCs in varying environmental scenarios (Pernow et al., 2019). RBCs play a crucial role in gas transport and also influence the functioning of blood vessels and the overall health of the body. Latest research indicates that RBCs are involved in signaling pathways that regulate blood vessel tone, particularly in the absence of oxygen, by releasing nitric oxide and ATP. This function of RBCs has been studied more because it affects cardiovascular health and disease. When RBCs aggregate and are exposed to increased oxidative stress, they can damage the endothelium, a condition often observed in diabetes mellitus. These problems in RBCs reduce CO_2 transport and also highlight the importance of RBCs in various cardiovascular functions. Therefore, understanding the multifaceted roles of RBCs in carbon dioxide transport opens pathways for novel therapeutic approaches in managing related cardiovascular disorders, emphasizing their importance beyond gas exchange (Pretini et al., 2019).

9.2.1. Dissolved Carbon Dioxide in Plasma

Dissolved carbon dioxide in plasma plays a crucial role in transporting CO_2 from tissues to the lungs. About 5–10% of carbon dioxide in the blood is dissolved and stays in balance with the bicarbonate and H_2CO_3 present in the surrounding fluid. Cell metabolism produces CO_2, which dissolves in the plasma. The level of dissolved CO_2 in blood depends on its partial pressure, which indicates the level of activity in the tissues. The amount of gas dissolved in a liquid is described by Henry's law, which shows that it is proportional to the gas's partial pressure. Thus, changes in metabolic rate will alter the dissolved carbon dioxide levels, which play a role in gas exchange in the respiratory system. Though dissolved carbon dioxide makes up only a small part of the total CO_2 transport, it is essential for the body. Carbon dioxide in the bloodstream helps maintain the body's acid-base balance, which is crucial for homeostasis. CO_2 dissolved in plasma plays a role in buffering, which impacts blood pH and the body's ability to regulate acid-base balance. An example is that when CO_2 dissolves, it forms H_2CO_3, which then breaks into bicarbonate and hydrogen ions. This change can cause the respiratory rate to increase, as the lungs remove both CO_2 and hydrogen ions, which helps maintain the blood pH stability. Such interactions exemplify the importance of bodily fluids, extracellular and intracellular buffers, as well as kidneys in regulating pH levels and serving the needs of metabolic processes – emphasizing the interconnectedness of various biological systems (White, 2025). The transport of dissolved carbon dioxide has consequences for clinical conditions, particularly for individuals in high-stress occupations, such as aviation. Increased physical demands can lead to elevated levels of dissolved CO_2, which may exacerbate cardiovascular challenges (Аралова et al., 2019). As a result, understanding how dissolved CO_2 is involved in carbon dioxide transport facilitates the early detection of problems in critical areas. Managing these levels effectively helps flight crews stay healthy, which in turn reduces the risk of accidents caused by stress. In other words, studying how carbon dioxide moves and is controlled in the blood is essential for ensuring that people can function well in conditions where their health and safety are most at risk.

9.2.2. Formation of Bicarbonate Ions

The formation of bicarbonate ions is a crucial biochemical process within the framework of carbon dioxide transport in the blood. The enzyme CA causes carbon dioxide to react with water when it enters the blood from tissues.

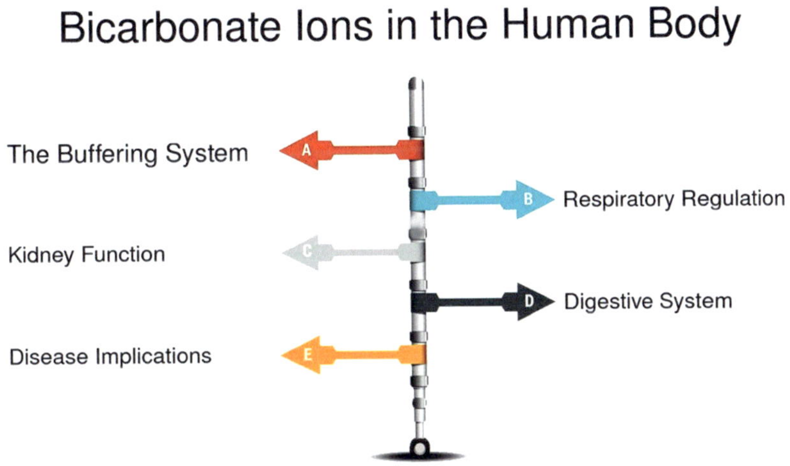

Figure 9.5. Bicarbonate ions in the human body.

Source: https://fastercapital.co/i/Bicarbonate-ions--The-Mighty-BICarbonate-Ions--Regulating-pH-Balance--Bicarbonate-Ions-in-the-Human-Body.webp.

This reaction transforms CO_2 and water (H_2O) into H_2CO_3, a transient compound that quickly dissociates into bicarbonate ions (HCO_3^-) and hydrogen ions (H^+). The role of this dissociation is crucial, as it helps maintain the blood pH within a narrow range, which is essential for cells to function correctly. The capacity of bicarbonate to neutralize acids is vital in conditions where carbon dioxide levels fluctuate, such as during intense physical activity or respiratory distress, emphasizing its role in acid-base homeostasis (Prado, 2024). Bicarbonate ions and CO_2 are in a dynamic balance that is essential to respiratory physiology. Bicarbonate ions usually act as the main way for carbon dioxide to be transported in the blood. Carbon dioxide is carried in the atmosphere primarily as carbonic acid. The remaining CO_2 is either dissolved directly in plasma (about 7%) or transported bound to hemoglobin as carbamino compounds. Bicarbonate ions help transport CO_2 and also facilitate its release from RBCs in the lungs, where it is converted back into CO_2 for exhalation. This reversible process underscores the interrelationship between bicarbonate formation and respiration, making bicarbonate a pivotal player in both gas exchange and acid-base balance (Baloğlu et al., 2021). As well as their role in the body, bicarbonate ions are significant in clinical situations and should be noted. Having abnormal bicarbonate levels may suggest that a person has metabolic acidosis or alkalosis. The diagnostic algorithms derived from blood gas analysis rely on measurements of bicarbonate and related variables to understand acid-base disturbances, as discussed in recent research that emphasizes a biochemical approach to diagnosing these conditions (Prado, 2024). The interplay between bicarbonate and acid-base balance highlights its significance not only in normal physiological processes but also in clinical settings, reinforcing its importance in the transport of carbon dioxide in the bloodstream and its broader health implications (Baloğlu et al., 2021) (Figure 9.5).

9.2.3. Binding to Hemoglobin and Other Proteins

The mode of which CO_2 and hemoglobin interact together dictates their importance in gas transport and the dramatic effect they have on the delivery of oxygen to different body parts. Hemoglobin mainly works with CO_2 in the RBCs by creating carbamate.

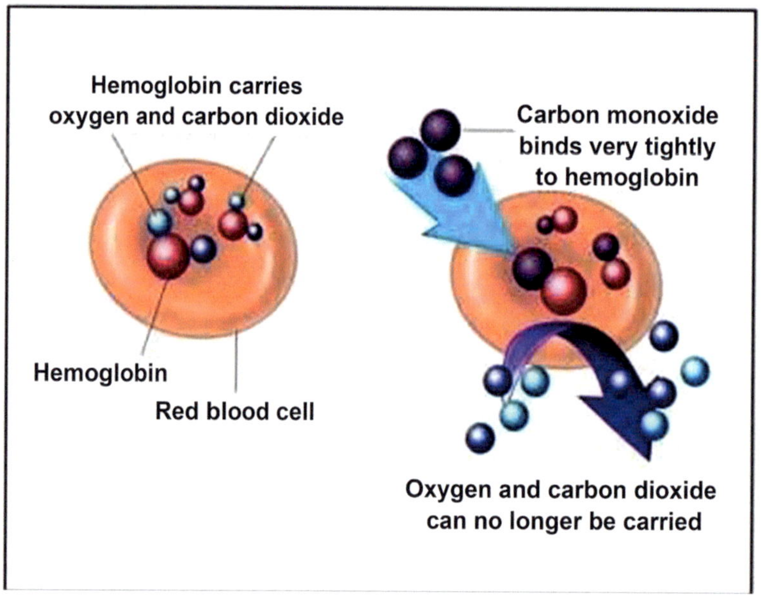

Figure 9.6. CO_2 binding to hemoglobin.

Source: https://www.researchgate.net/profile/Ekramul-Haque-Ehite/publication/344463481/figure/fig11/AS:942752053329925@1601781013087/b-CO-binding-to-Hemoglobin.jpg.

After CO_2 reaches the blood, it can attach to the amino termini of hemoglobin, which helps hemoglobin release more oxygen. This relationship is significant because, when metabolism is high, such as during intense exercise, more CO_2 leads hemoglobin to release oxygen to the tissues that require it. Additionally, this phenomenon illustrates that pH and temperature influence the ability of hemoglobin to transport oxygen and CO_2, which is crucial for its function in various parts of the body. Besides carrying O_2, hemoglobin is necessary for handling the harmful effects of too much CO_2. Elevated CO_2 concentrations in blood can lead to hypercapnia, resulting in a decrease in blood pH (acidosis). Some species, for example, the white seabass, have specialized cellular adaptations to mitigate these effects. Research reveals that these fish utilize sodium-proton exchangers (β-NHEs) to stabilize intracellular pH, thereby preserving hemoglobin's oxygen-binding capacity even under hypoxic or hypercapnic conditions. These adaptations have significant effects on the body, protecting against environmental changes and highlighting the crucial role of hemoglobins in evolution. As water bodies are increasingly affected by climate change, understanding these mechanisms may provide insight into how species can survive and adapt. Examining other protein interactions beyond hemoglobin enhances our understanding of CO_2 transport in the blood. Albumin and other proteins in the blood, besides hemoglobin, help carry CO_2 in its dissolved state, which is important for blood gas exchange. This transport route is especially needed when blood chemistry needs to be balanced and hemoglobin may not be able to do its job correctly. It is also the BBB's job to manage the movement of molecules such as CO_2, to avoid harmful effects on the brain and keep neurons working well. By studying these different pathways and their regulatory mechanisms, we can gain a comprehensive understanding of not only how CO_2 is transported but also how the body maintains homeostasis in response to varying loads of metabolic byproducts, highlighting the intricate balance required for optimal physiological functioning (Melanie et al., 2018) (Figure 9.6).

9.3. The Bicarbonate Buffer System

The bicarbonate buffer system plays a pivotal role in maintaining acid-base homeostasis in the human body, particularly in the context of carbon dioxide transport in the blood. Carbon dioxide, which is made by cellular respiration, moves into the blood and combines with water to form H_2CO_3 through a hydration reaction. This dynamic equilibrium between H_2CO_3, bicarbonate (HCO_3^-), and CO_2 is crucial for stabilizing blood pH levels. The bicarbonate ion acts as a weak base to neutralize excess hydrogen ions. Additionally, H2CO3 can release hydrogen ions when the pH increases, which helps maintain the body's stable conditions. The buffering ability is most important in places where the pH often changes, to maintain the proper function of enzymes and chemical pathways. Studying the bicarbonate buffer system also means looking at CAs which help quickly convert carbon dioxide into bicarbonate. They help the bicarbonate buffer system function more effectively, allowing blood pH to be regulated quickly. CAs help by facilitating the conversion of CO_2 into H2CO3 and vice versa, which is crucial for meeting metabolic needs, particularly during exercise when CO_2 levels increase. Additionally, bicarbonate's buffering role is crucial in acidosis, which results from an excessive number of hydrogen ions that can cause the pH to drop dangerously. Here, bicarbonate helps maintain acid-base balance and also signals cells to influence different cellular activities and metabolic pathways. The role of the bicarbonate buffer system and respiration demonstrates the importance of carbon dioxide transport in the blood. When CO_2 rises, it stimulates breathing centers in the brain, which makes us breathe more quickly and deeply to get rid of extra carbon dioxide. The influence of bicarbonate and carbon dioxide on pH is explained by the Henderson–Hasselbalch equation. Grasping this balance gives clues to situations such as respiratory failure or major metabolic problems, when the body's buffering ability is reduced. Thus, the bicarbonate buffer system is not merely a passive regulator; it actively engages in physiological processes, ensuring the stability of internal environments crucial for health, as evidenced by the profound implications of disturbances in blood pH levels on overall metabolic function (Li et al., 2022; Rad, 2022) (Figure 9.7).

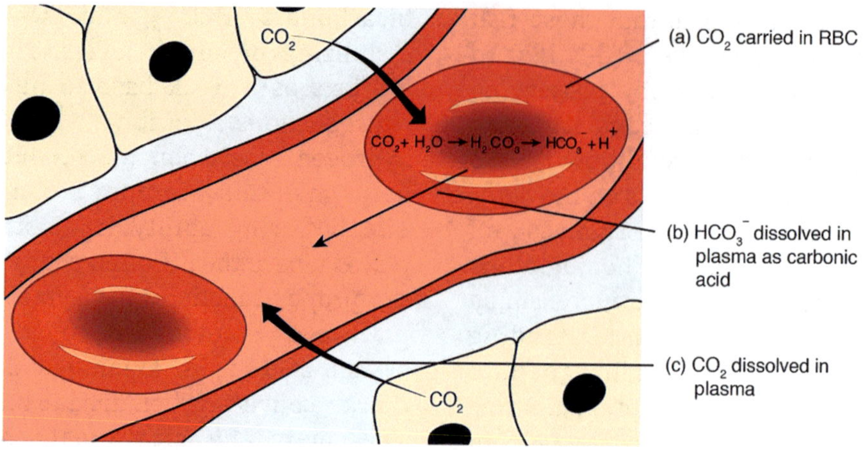

Figure 9.7. Carbon dioxide, a by-product of cellular respiration, is dissolved in the blood, where it is taken up by red blood cells and converted to carbonic acid by carbonic anhydrase. Most of the carbonic acid then dissociates to bicarbonate and hydrogen ions.

Source: https://upload.wikimedia.org/wikipedia/commons/thumb/9/98/2325_Carbon_Dioxide_Transport.jpg/1280px-2325_Carbon_Dioxide_Transport.jpg.

9.3.1. Function of Bicarbonate in Maintaining pH Balance

The function of bicarbonate in maintaining pH balance plays a significant role in the transport of carbon dioxide in the blood. Bicarbonate is important for blood pH because it responds to changes in hydrogen ions and helps keep the pH stable. Carbon dioxide that enters the blood is changed into H_2CO_3, which then dissociates into bicarbonate and hydrogen ions. This is necessary because a rise in hydrogen ions can cause acidosis, which makes the blood acidic and disrupts cellular functions. Because of bicarbonate, these excess acids are neutralized, preventing disruptions and keeping the body's pH at the right level for proper functions. Additionally, the level of bicarbonate in the blood is closely linked to the respiratory system, particularly when carbon dioxide levels fluctuate. For instance, in the studied case of sheep undergoing anesthesia, elevated arterial pH and bicarbonate concentration were observed despite controlled ventilation, indicating that the buffering capacity of bicarbonate was effectively maintaining acid-base balance during stress conditions (Grimm et al., 2021). This points out that the bicarbonate system adjusts to changes in breathing and metabolism. Additionally, when blood bicarbonate levels increase, it indicates that the body is effectively regulating carbon dioxide and preventing the complications of respiratory acidosis, underscoring the importance of this bicarbonate buffer system in transporting carbon dioxide. The importance of bicarbonate for maintaining pH is demonstrated in several physiological situations, for example, in marine amphipods such as *Orchestia gammarellus*. Studies have shown that amid environmental stresses such as immersion, significant increases in blood bicarbonate concentrations occur while pH remains stable (Spicer et al., 1987). This highlights that bicarbonate helps regulate pH and demonstrates how the body responds to various conditions. Maintaining bicarbonate levels is crucial for healthy bodily functions, so changes in bicarbonate balance can be detrimental to health. Understanding the role bicarbonate plays is important for grasping how carbon dioxide is transported and utilized in the body.

9.3.2. Role of Carbonic Anhydrase in Bicarbonate Formation

CA plays a pivotal role in the physiological process of bicarbonate formation, which is essential for the transport of carbon dioxide (CO_2) in the blood. This enzyme catalyzes the reversible reaction between CO_2 and water, producing bicarbonate (HCO_3^-) and protons (H^+) during its action. CO_2 being converted into bicarbonate is crucial for facilitating the efficient transfer of CO_2 from the rest of the body to the lungs. RBCs use CA to make sure carbon dioxide, which is produced as waste, is quickly changed into a more soluble form and carried by the blood. So, CA is key for maintaining acid-base balance and helping with gas exchange, which are both important parts of respiratory physiology. CA is important not only for making bicarbonate; it also affects the ability of blood to resist changes in pH. Most of the protons that form during the reaction are countered by hemoglobin, which plays a role in controlling blood pH. This is particularly important when CO_2 levels in the blood increase, as the body needs to respond quickly to prevent acidosis. Additionally, bicarbonate ions are transported in the blood as the primary form of CO_2, accounting for most of the CO_2 that is released from tissues to the lungs. In this manner, CA allows CO_2 to be transported and also plays a crucial role in maintaining the balance of acids and bases in the body, which is essential for proper cell function and metabolism. Studies have found that CAs are involved in several diseases, which proves their importance in the body. Many diseases, such as respiratory, metabolic, and neurological problems, are associated with abnormal amounts or activities of CA. In hypoxia, for example, some CA isoforms may be more active, which increases bicarbonate and leads to a change in blood pH. By explaining the part CA plays in these processes, researchers have designed new probes, such as FMRs-CA, to observe CA activity in living tissues. Such advancements enrich our understanding of the connection between abnormal CA function and disease states, thus highlighting the enzyme's critical role not only in bicarbonate formation but also in the larger context of carbon dioxide transport and its implications for human health (Hisar et al., 2003; Zhang et al., 2023) (Figure 9.8).

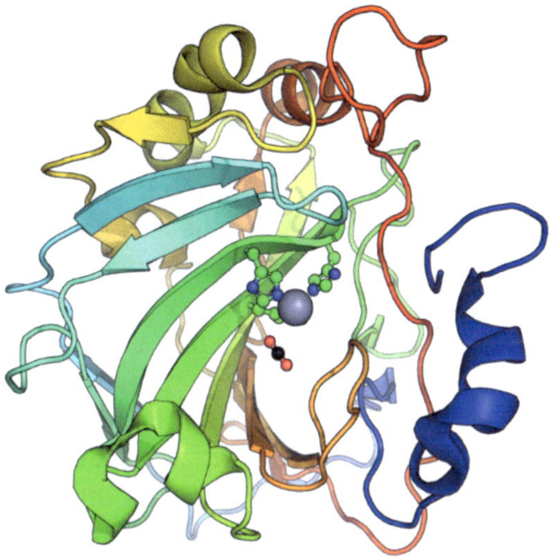

Figure 9.8. Human carbonic anhydrase II with bound Zinc and carbon dioxide.

Source: https://upload.wikimedia.org/wikipedia/commons/thumb/d/d2/Human_carbonic_anhydrase_II_PDB%3D6LUX.png/800px-Human_carbonic_anhydrase_II_PDB%3D6LUX.png.

9.3.3. Impact of the Bicarbonate System on Respiratory Function

The bicarbonate system is essential for balancing acidity and helping the body breathe efficiently by moving carbon dioxide. Carbon dioxide (CO_2), a byproduct of cellular metabolism, is primarily transported in the blood as bicarbonate (HCO_3^-). The process is carried out in erythrocytes by the enzyme CA, which helps turn CO_2 and water into H_2CO_3. H_2CO_3 then dissociates into bicarbonate and hydrogen ions, which buffer changes in blood pH. Having an effective buffering system is important for regulating blood pH and controlling breathing, which results in changes in ventilation as CO_2 levels rise or fall in the body. If this system did not exist, acid-base balance would be at risk, which could result in respiratory acidosis or alkalosis. When CO_2 levels are high, as in hypercapnia, the bicarbonate system responds by producing more hydrogen ions, which makes the blood more acidic. The body attempts to eliminate excess CO_2 through breathing when such conditions occur, which can alter respiratory drive and breathing patterns. Individuals with respiratory disorders may have a reduced ability to buffer metabolic changes, which increases the risk of serious metabolic complications. Because of these changes, the body must adapt which is seen in both standard and abnormal conditions. In people with metabolic or respiratory problems, the control of tumor pH can be affected which leads to more difficulties in transporting CO_2 and providing oxygen. Due to this interaction, the bicarbonate system is crucial for maintaining proper breathing in various bodily conditions. Also, the knowledge gained from bicarbonate and CO_2 management is helpful in other fields such as the exploration of space. Having high levels of carbon dioxide inside space suits can be very dangerous for astronauts. Existing research indicates that the way individuals react to hypercapnia varies, highlighting the importance of customized methods to manage CO_2 during spacewalks. If bicarbonate levels are well-controlled in these situations, it can prevent performance from dropping, highlighting the value of the bicarbonate system in various contexts. Ultimately, the bicarbonate system's integral role in respiratory function and carbon dioxide transport underscores the necessity for ongoing research to explore its implications across various physiological and environmental contexts, including the challenges posed by emerging technologies and exploration missions (Abercromby et al., Alarcon et al., 2011) (Figure 9.9).

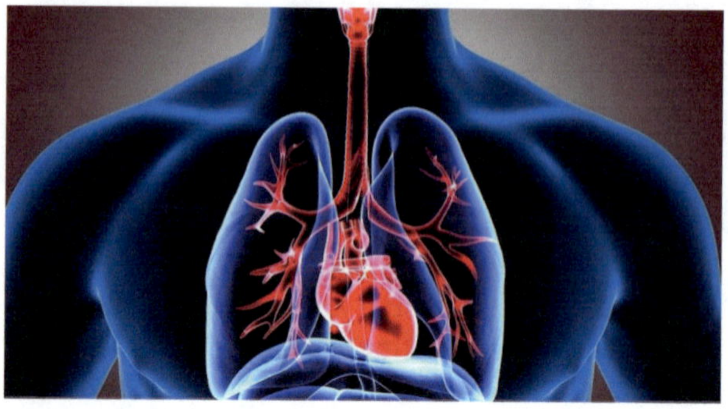

Figure 9.9. Anatomical illustration of the cardiopulmonary system.

Source: https://stgaccinwbsdevlrs01.blob.core.windows.net/newcorporatewbsite/blogs/october2023/detail-main-Respiratory-System.jpg.

9.4. Transport Pathways in the Circulatory System

Carbon dioxide and other substances are moved around the body by the human circulatory system. After oxygen is used during cellular respiration, the body produces carbon dioxide as waste, which must be carried back to the lungs for release. Most of this process occurs when the plasma carries carbon dioxide, attaches to hemoglobin, and changes into bicarbonate ions. Carbon dioxide is transported by dissolving in plasma, but this accounts for only a small fraction, usually 5–10%. Most of the time, carbon dioxide is attached to hemoglobin in RBCs or changed by the CA enzyme to bicarbonate ions, which carry carbon dioxide from body tissues to the lungs. Understanding these transport mechanisms is fundamental, particularly as they connect seamlessly to the metabolic processes occurring in tissues and their effect on overall organ homeostasis (Averell et al., 2015). Several factors influence how efficiently carbon dioxide is transported by blood, including its pH, temperature, and the concentrations of gases in the blood. Higher carbon dioxide and lower pH levels in working tissues, resulting from metabolism, facilitate the release of oxygen by hemoglobin, which supports better CO_2 capture. It demonstrates the detailed relationship between the movement of oxygen and carbon dioxide in the circulatory system. Fluctuating temperatures can also alter how hemoglobin binds to oxygen and carbon dioxide, which affects the efficiency of gas exchange. Such mechanisms illustrate the remarkable adaptability of the circulatory system in maintaining homeostasis, emphasizing the need for a comprehensive understanding of these pathways and their broader implications for health and disease (Özay et al., 2024). The structure of the heart and blood vessels is very helpful for moving carbon dioxide through the body. The right atrium collects blood from the systemic circulation, which contains a lot of carbon dioxide. The blood flows from the right ventricle to the pulmonary arteries, which carry it to the lungs for gas exchange. In the lungs, the blood gives off carbon dioxide into the alveoli which helps it to be exhaled. The way circulatory anatomy and transport routes are interconnected allows for more efficient gas exchange. Recognizing the importance of this anatomical and functional relationship is vital in modern biology, particularly in educational contexts where grasping the complexities of the circulatory system fosters a deeper appreciation for health sciences and metabolic processes (Averell et al., 2015).

9.4.1. Movement of Carbon Dioxide from Tissues to Blood

The movement of CO_2 from tissues to blood is an essential physiological process that ensures the removal of metabolic waste while maintaining acid-base homeostasis. Cells use nutrients, which create CO_2 that moves from the cytoplasm into the interstitial fluid and then into the blood. Because CO_2 is usually more concentrated in tissues than in the blood, the concentration gradient causes passive diffusion. CO_2 is mainly carried in the blood by being dissolved in plasma, attached to hemoglobin, and as HCO_3^-. The enzyme CA helps CO_2 change into bicarbonate by assisting the reaction between CO_2 and water, which produces H_2CO_3 that splits into bicarbonate and hydrogen ions, controlling pH. This illustrates the close relationship between cellular metabolism and respiration. In the context of gas exchange, the efficiency of CO_2 transport from tissues to blood is further enhanced by the Bohr effect, where increased levels of CO_2 and H+ ions result in hemoglobin releasing more oxygen (O_2) to tissues. The process is most important when the body is working hard, such as during exercise, because tissue CO_2 levels rise. ATP and other messenger molecules released by RBCs help regulate blood flow by dilating local blood vessels, which facilitates the supply of nutrients and the removal of CO_2. Critical research, such as that examining high-altitude animal adaptations, reveals that adaptations in RBC function can enhance both O_2 delivery and CO_2 transport under hypoxic conditions, emphasizing the importance of examining biochemical interactions in diverse environments (João et al., 2024). When CO_2 reaches the lungs, it is released into the atmosphere, completing the process of circulating it throughout the body. Gradients are formed by the way respiration works, allowing CO_2 to move from the blood, which has a higher concentration of it, to the alveoli for exhalation. It is very important to control this exchange, since CO_2 helps control blood pH and the rate at which we breathe. More CO_2 in the blood causes H_2CO_3 to rise, resulting in respiratory acidosis and prompting chemoreceptors to increase the breathing rate to eliminate CO_2. This tightly integrated system of CO_2 transport and regulation underscores its broader physiological implications, linking metabolic processes with respiratory responses that adapt to varying atmospheric and physiological conditions, providing insights valuable for future clinical applications (Harter et al., 2024) (Figure 9.10).

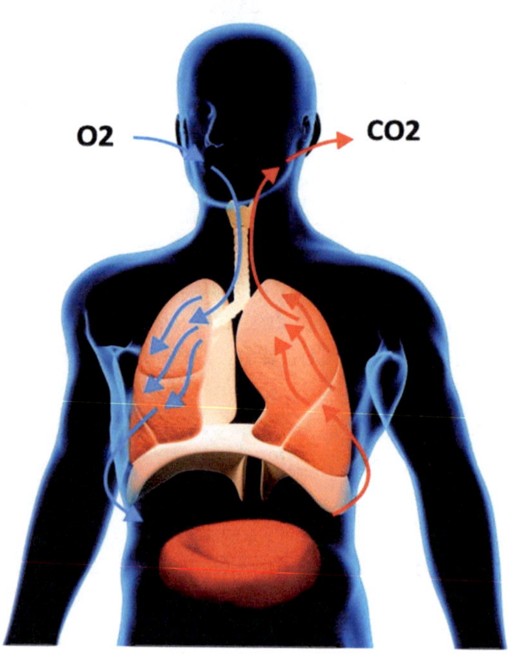

Figure 9.10. Physiological mechanism of carbon dioxide (CO_2) and oxygen (O_2) exchange in the human respiratory system.

Source: https://substackcdn.com/image/fetch/f_auto,q_auto:good,fl_progressive:steep/https%3A%2F%2Fsubstack-post-media.s3.amazonaws.com%2Fpublic%2Fimages%2F24ab47ff-a295-4c56-85c8-e8256d989315_696x628.png.

9.4.2. Transport From Blood to Lungs

The movement of CO_2 from the blood to the lungs is essential for proper gas exchange, which is necessary for the body to remain in balance. Dissolved gas in plasma, carbamino compounds, and bicarbonate ions are the main ways gas moves in the blood. The direct dissolving of CO_2 in blood plasma is possible, but it accounts for only a small portion of the total CO_2 transport. A big part of CO_2 is attached to hemoglobin as carbamino compounds, which happen when CO_2 and amino acids in hemoglobin react. Also, most of the CO_2 in blood is carried as bicarbonate ions, which is made possible by the enzyme CA in red blood cells. This demonstrates how the body maintains balance by regulating respiratory gases, which in turn affects its response to varying energy needs and environmental conditions. Blood in the systemic circulation gradually collects CO_2 from the tissues because of metabolism. As blood reaches the lungs, the primary task is to exchange gases. CO_2 can move from the blood into the alveoli due to the partial pressure gradient and it is expelled during exhalation. One important aspect is the connection between the composition of blood and the function of the lungs.

Changes in blood CO_2 can cause the body to adjust its breathing rate and depth, which is controlled by the body's chemoreceptors. Notably, end-tidal carbon dioxide ($ETCO_2$) values serve as vital indicators, reflecting both gas exchange efficiency and overall respiratory mechanics. It is crucial to understand this relationship to accurately diagnose and treat conditions such as respiratory failure or shock, which can significantly impact CO_2 transport. Assessing $ETCO_2$ is crucial in trauma or medical emergencies because it helps to understand the patient's condition. For example, a lower $ETCO_2$ value in intubated trauma patients often means the patient is in hemorrhagic shock, which highlights the need for constant monitoring during transport. Doctors can decide which treatments to give first, such as blood transfusions or increasing the patient's care, based on how the vital signs correlate. Therefore, being able to model and predict CO_2 transport helps us understand respiratory physiology and also supports better outcomes for patients in critical care. With robust models increasingly providing insights into gas exchange processes, as noted in the existing literature, they can also effectively guide treatment strategies, ultimately bridging the gap between theoretical knowledge and clinical practice (Bulger et al., 2021; Snapper et al., 2021) (Figure 9.11).

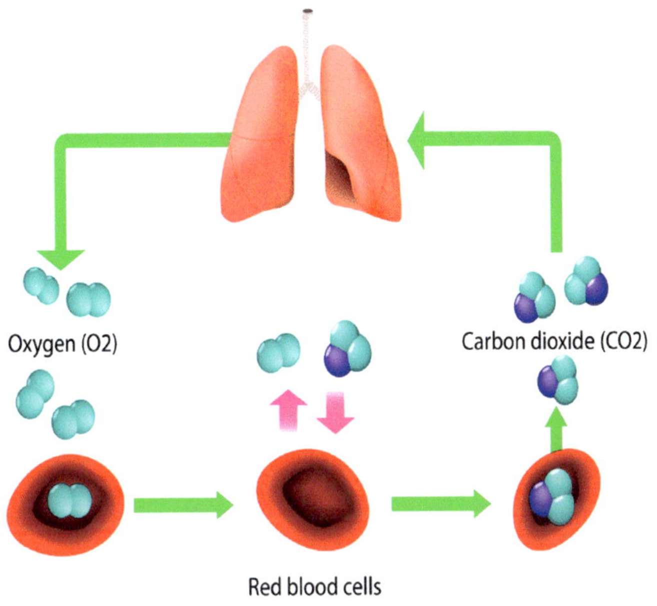

Figure 9.11. Transport of CO_2 from the blood to the lungs.

Source: https://www.respiratorytherapyzone.com/wp-content/uploads/2023/09/Transport-of-Oxygen-and-Carbon-Dioxide-in-Blood-Gas-Exchange-Illustration.png.

9.4.3. Role of the Pulmonary Capillaries in Gas Exchange

Pulmonary capillaries are essential for gas exchange, as they connect the alveoli with the blood in the body. They enable oxygen and carbon dioxide to diffuse, which is essential for maintaining homeostasis. As we breathe in, oxygen-rich air enters the alveoli, increasing the oxygen level there above that in the blood, which causes oxygen to diffuse from the alveoli into the blood. At the same time, CO_2 which is produced during metabolism, moves from the blood into the alveoli to be exhaled. The effectiveness of gas exchange depends on the condition and function of the pulmonary capillaries, which must be unblocked to allow gases to pass easily between the airspace and the blood. Any disturbance in the pulmonary capillary network can significantly impair gas exchange and lead to adverse outcomes for patients. Pulmonary hypertension and heart failure cause higher pressure, which can damage the endothelial cells in capillaries. Due to this injury, the alveolar-capillary membrane is damaged, making it more difficult for gases to pass through and thereby affecting lung function. Pressure-related damage can alter the structure and permeability of capillaries, making it harder for them to exchange gases properly. As cardiac dysfunction progresses, these structural changes can further contribute to decreased alveolar gas diffusion properties, leading to lower oxygen levels and higher carbon dioxide retention in the blood, a condition that has significant implications for overall respiratory and cardiovascular health, as described in the literature regarding chronic heart failure (Arena et al., 2015). In addition, pulmonary capillaries help manage the amount of fluid in the lung interstitium, not just passively exchange gases. Their role is highlighted in many health and disease states, where the balance of fluid entering and leaving the kidneys is very important. An increase in left atrial pressure due to heart issues can injure capillaries and disrupt fluid control, resulting in less efficient gas exchange. Clinical insights suggest that chronic conditions causing capillary remodeling not only impede the transport of gases but may also have prognostic implications for patients' overall health (Arena et al., 2015). Understanding these dynamics reinforces the importance of maintaining pulmonary capillary health as a critical component in the management of carbon dioxide transport and respiratory function in the clinical setting (Figure 9.12).

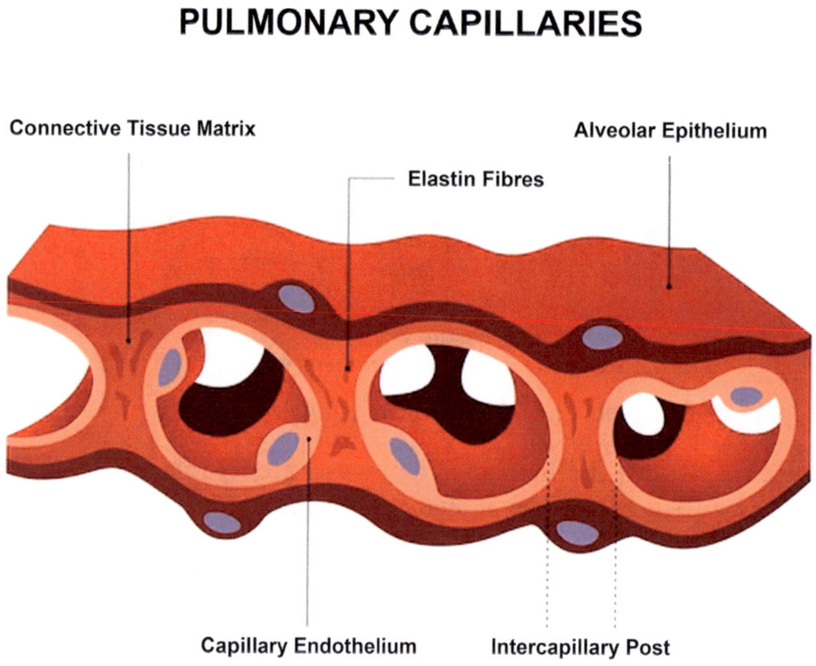

Figure 9.12. Pulmonary capillaries.

Source: https://img.freepik.com/premium-vector/diagram-pulmonary-capillaries-structure_278713-1571.jpg.

9.5. Factors Affecting Carbon Dioxide Transport

The transport of CO_2 in the blood is a complex process influenced by several physiological factors. The concentration difference between CO_2 in tissues and in the bloodstream is what drives the movement of CO_2 from tissues into the blood. As CO_2 levels increase in the blood, the transport capacity also escalates, primarily through the formation of bicarbonate ions (HCO_3^-) via the enzyme CA. It helps CO_2 and water be quickly turned into bicarbonate and hydrogen ions, which aids in keeping the body's acid-base balance. Consequently, the rate at which CO_2 is produced in tissues directly correlates with its transport capacity in the blood, illustrating how metabolic activity can influence gas exchange within the circulatory system, as highlighted by Marken (2020). Another significant factor affecting carbon dioxide transport is the partial pressure of oxygen (pO_2) in the blood. When oxygen levels increase, the Haldane effect explains that hemoglobin becomes less able to hold CO_2, due to the relationship between CO_2 transport and oxygen. When oxygen levels are high, such as in the lungs, hemoglobin gives up CO_2 more easily. In places far from the heart, where oxygen is used and CO_2 is created, the low pO_2 helps hemoglobin to carry CO_2 more effectively. As oxygen and carbon dioxide are exchanged efficiently, the body can easily respond to different physical conditions. Understanding these interactions is crucial for comprehending the dynamics of blood gases and their implications for respiratory physiology, as elaborated by Kelly (2004). The temperature and pH of the blood also play a significant role in how carbon dioxide is transported. When the body gets hot, such as during exercise or a fever, CO_2 becomes more soluble and moves more quickly into the blood. Similarly, the Bohr effect describes how a decrease in blood pH (resulting from an increase in hydrogen ion concentration, often due to lactic acid during strenuous activity) enhances the release of carbon dioxide from hemoglobin. It is necessary to help the body remove CO_2, mainly in tissues that are working hard. Thus, temperature and pH changes in the body help ensure that carbon dioxide is transported properly to maintain balance and meet energy needs. These factors underscore the complexity of the respiratory and circulatory systems working in tandem to ensure proper gas exchange and transport, as emphasized in the analyses of Kelly (2004) and Marken (2020).

9.5.1. Influence of Exercise on Carbon Dioxide Levels

The influence of exercise on carbon dioxide levels is a critical area of study within the broader context of respiratory and metabolic physiology. While exercising, the muscles need more energy, which causes metabolic processes to work harder and create more CO_2 as a byproduct of cellular respiration. As CO_2 levels rise, the body must breathe more efficiently to eliminate this gas and maintain balance. More intense exercises cause the body to produce more carbon dioxide which means more ventilation is required. When carbon dioxide levels increase in the blood, it can make the blood more acidic, a condition known as respiratory acidosis, which highlights the importance of making respiratory adjustments during and after exercise. In addition, exercise raises CO_2 levels and alters the way it is transported throughout the body. CO_2 moves in the blood by being dissolved in the plasma, as bicarbonate ions, and by binding to hemoglobin. Moving the muscles causes CO_2 to be converted into bicarbonate, making it easier for the lungs to remove CO_2 during exhalation. This change in the body is significant for maintaining acid-base balance when you exercise more. During prolonged exercise, improved CO_2 transport is crucial to prevent acid-base imbalances that could compromise muscle function and overall performance.

The relationship between how hard you exercise, how long you exercise and CO_2 transport points out the need for fine-tuned respiratory compensation to keep your body's metabolism in balance. The way exercise, carbon dioxide and metabolism interact stresses how fitness supports healthy breathing. Regular exercise is linked to better respiratory function, which allows the body to better handle changes in CO_2 levels. Even small amounts of exercise have been linked to better oxygen use and breathing which helps the body get rid of waste. Additionally, when people engage in regular exercise, their muscles and cardiovascular systems adapt, which helps them remove carbon dioxide more effectively. This physiological response to exercise is not only vital for athletic performance but also highlights the broader implications for health, particularly in older adults or those with respiratory conditions, underscoring the importance of exercise as a preventive and therapeutic measure in respiratory health management (Figure 9.13).

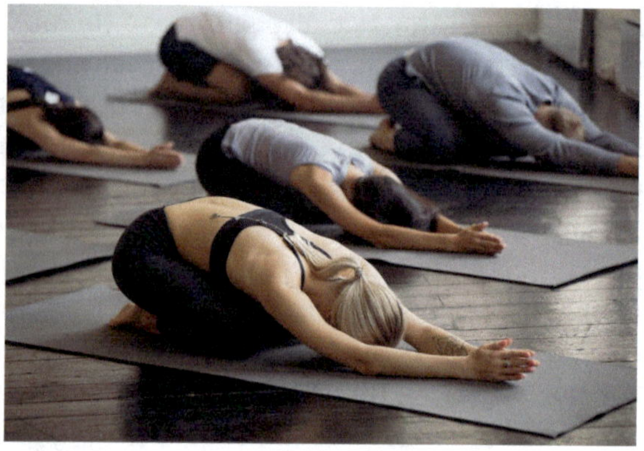

Figure 9.13. Yoga-based physical activity to enhance respiratory efficiency.

Source: https://media.rnztools.nz/rnz/image/upload/s--kHZkNB4r--/c_scale,f_auto,q_auto,w_1050/v1657739357/4O9RCY3_94827649_I_jpg?_a=BACCd2AD.

9.5.2. Effects of Altitude on Transport Efficiency

The transport efficiency of carbon dioxide in the bloodstream is significantly influenced by altitude, primarily due to alterations in atmospheric pressure and oxygen availability. Because there is less air pressure at higher altitudes, the oxygen pressure also decreases, which directly influences the body's breathing and heart functions. When oxygen levels drop, the body may raise its breathing and heart rates to try to maintain a stable oxygen level. By doing this, the body may actually reduce its ability to move carbon dioxide, since lower oxygen levels make it harder to remove carbon dioxide. As a result, adjustments in the body at altitude indicate that changes in carbon dioxide transport involve both changes in oxygen levels and the breathing adjustments typical for such environments. Additionally, hemoglobin plays a more complex role in transporting carbon dioxide as altitude increases. In most cases, hemoglobin binds both oxygen and carbon dioxide, facilitating the exchange of gases between the lungs and tissues. If altitude-induced hypoxia occurs, it can affect how hemoglobin binds to carbon dioxide, potentially reducing its ability to remove carbon dioxide from the body. When oxygen levels are low, hemoglobin tends to bind more oxygen and less carbon dioxide which can disturb systemic acid-base balance. Additionally, the Bohr effect influences this situation, as increased carbon dioxide in the blood can cause hemoglobin to release more oxygen; however, this may not fully compensate for the poorer oxygen transport at high altitudes, which can lead to problems maintaining bodily balance. The effect of altitude on moving carbon dioxide is also connected to the ways humans adapt to living at high altitudes for long periods. People who live at high altitudes gradually adapt, making changes such as producing more red blood cells and adjusting their breathing patterns. These changes are designed to help vehicles operate efficiently in low-pressure environments. However, how well these changes manage the effects of altitude on carbon dioxide transport is still being studied. Understanding these dynamics is crucial for developing strategies for individuals who travel to or live in high-altitude areas, particularly regarding how to manage respiratory and metabolic functions during periods of hypoxia (N/A, 2025).

9.5.3. Impact of Respiratory Diseases on Carbon Dioxide Transport

The relationship between respiratory diseases and the transport of carbon dioxide in the blood is intricate and critical to understanding pulmonary and cardiovascular function. Conditions such as interstitial lung disease (ILD) disrupt normal respiratory mechanics, leading to impaired gas exchange. In patients with fibrotic ILD, for instance, mean arterial blood gas (ABG) measurements reveal significant variations in carbon dioxide levels, as the condition can lead to chronic respiratory acidosis due to inadequate ventilation and impaired gas exchange. Abnormalities in carbon dioxide transport, characterized by an elevated partial pressure of carbon dioxide ($PaCO_2$), further exacerbate the disease process, complicating clinical outcomes by increasing the risk of respiratory distress and potential mortality. Such findings underscore the importance of closely monitoring and managing carbon dioxide levels in patients with compromised pulmonary function due to respiratory diseases (Mira et al., 2024). Carbon dioxide moves efficiently in the body due to several physiological processes, which can be affected by respiratory illnesses. Hemoglobin, which primarily transports oxygen, also facilitates the transport of carbon dioxide. If someone has COPD or severe asthma, their respiratory system does not work well, which affects gas exchange. When these diseases occur, carbon dioxide may not be released from tissues as it should, causing more carbon dioxide to accumulate in the blood. Consequently, elevated $PaCO_2$ levels can result in systemic effects, including altered blood pH due to respiratory acidosis, which further complicates the clinical management of these patients (Harter et al., 2024). The extent to which the lungs are affected and how carbon dioxide is transported are both crucial for guiding treatment and helping patients improve. Also, factors in the environment like air quality and altitude can make respiratory diseases have a more substantial effect on carbon dioxide transport. People in areas with high air pollution or low oxygen levels have to deal with additional problems. Such environmental problems can make existing lung diseases worse, which can cause more carbon dioxide and oxygen to be transported in the blood. As a result of reduced oxygen at high altitudes, the body increases the work of RBCs to help gas exchange. Still, the change in blood may not compensate for the reduced CO_2 transport that occurs in people with restrictive lung diseases. Thus, understanding these multifaceted interactions is crucial for developing comprehensive treatment approaches to mitigate the effects of respiratory diseases on carbon dioxide transport (Mira et al., 2024).

9.6. Clinical Implications of Carbon Dioxide Transport

The way carbon dioxide is transported in the body is important for the care of many respiratory and metabolic diseases. Since carbon dioxide is produced by cells, the body needs effective ways to transport it to maintain a stable acid-base balance. Pathologies such as COPD and respiratory distress syndrome (RDS) can disrupt normal CO_2 transport, leading to dangerous accumulations of carbon dioxide in the bloodstream, a condition known as hypercapnia. This situation significantly impacts how patients are cared for, particularly when making decisions about mechanical ventilation. An enhanced understanding of CO_2 transport dynamics can inform clinicians about optimal ventilation settings and the necessity for interventions such as extracorporeal carbon dioxide removal ($ECCO_2R$) to alleviate hypercapnic states (Zhuo et al., 2024). Therefore, managing these transport mechanisms is essential for better results in patients with respiratory problems. Besides affecting critical care, how carbon dioxide is transported also plays a role in treating conditions like anemia. The formation and removal of RBCs are affected by $CO_{2,}$ which is important for regulating the way hemoglobin binds to oxygen. When examining treatments that aid erythropoiesis, this relationship is particularly important, as it is being studied in greater detail through clinical research. Better RBC enucleation methods could increase the ability of blood to carry oxygen which would improve the delivery of oxygen to tissues. Studies on these processes offer possible ways to treat anemia, mainly for patients whose RBC production is affected. A robust understanding of the intricate balance between CO_2 transport and RBC development could lead to innovative interventions for patients suffering from anemia, further emphasizing the importance of CO_2 in clinical pathways related to blood function (Zhuo et al., 2024). New methods for removing carbon dioxide from the body also highlight the need for updated medical practices related to respiratory support. Technologies such as extracorporeal membrane oxygenation (ECMO) and $ECCO_2R$ serve as crucial forms of therapy for patients with severe respiratory failure, providing both oxygenation and CO_2 removal. $ECCO_2R$ has demonstrated potential for patients with hypercapnic respiratory failure, giving them a better option than standard mechanical ventilation. Because critical care is constantly evolving, it is essential to understand how CO_2 is transported in the body to utilize these advanced methods effectively. By refining our comprehension of carbon dioxide's role in pathophysiological contexts, healthcare providers can develop more targeted therapeutic approaches, thereby improving patient outcomes in settings of acute respiratory distress and enhancing overall management of respiratory conditions (Conrad, 2020).

9.6.1. Conditions Related to Impaired Carbon Dioxide Transport

Impaired carbon dioxide transport in the blood can lead to a variety of pathological conditions, significantly affecting respiratory function and homeostasis. Pulmonary embolism is a significant problem, since it happens when blood clots block the pulmonary arteries, making it much harder for gas exchange to occur. When this condition occurs, there is an increase in carbon dioxide in the blood, which leads to respiratory acidosis and a decrease in blood pH. If the body cannot eliminate enough CO_2, it may initiate a series of compensatory changes, such as faster and deeper breathing, to correct the problem. Because insufficient CO_2 transport can be dangerous, it is important to diagnose and manage pulmonary embolism quickly, since it can turn into serious complications or even death. COPD is another condition that happens when carbon dioxide is not transported well, and it is often linked to smoking and air pollution. COPD makes it difficult for air to leave the lungs properly, which slows down gas exchange and may result in too much carbon dioxide in the blood. People with this condition tend to experience shortness of breath and may exhibit symptoms of respiratory failure, as the body is unable to properly remove CO_2. Over time, the persistent buildup of CO_2 can stimulate the central nervous system (CNS) and the respiratory muscles, leading to hypoventilation and further exacerbating the condition. For COPD, doctors may prescribe bronchodilators and corticosteroids to help open the airways and improve gas exchange, which helps reduce the risks associated with impaired carbon dioxide transport. Working in specific jobs where people are exposed to toxins can seriously affect carbon dioxide transport and may cause acute breathing problems. Firefighters may encounter hazardous materials when fighting fires, which can impair the lungs' function and affect the transport of oxygen in the blood. Specific toxicants produced during combustion can disturb normal respiratory processes or cause chemical pneumonitis, which makes it hard for oxygen to be released and carbon dioxide to be taken in. Additionally, new approaches, such as respiratory challenge MRI, are being developed to gain a deeper understanding of the effects of carbon dioxide on brain function. By manipulating arterial gas concentrations, researchers can study profound changes in cerebral hemodynamics, yielding insights into the effects of impaired gas transport on cognition and overall brain health (Brown et al., 1990; Dani et al., 2016). Addressing the implications of toxic exposure is crucial for improving the safety and efficacy of interventions in both emergency and routine settings (Figure 9.14).

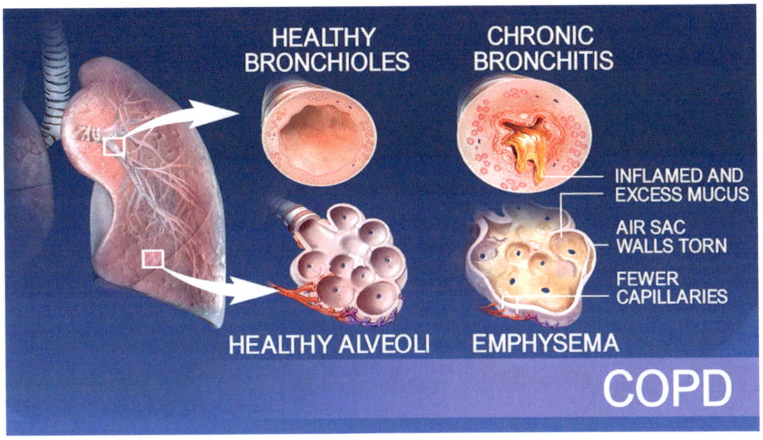

Figure 9.14. Lung disorder.

Source: https://regencyhealthcare.in/wp-content/uploads/2019/09/12_09_Sept.jpg.

9.6.2. Diagnostic Tests for Assessing Carbon Dioxide Levels

Diagnostic tests play a pivotal role in assessing carbon dioxide levels in the bloodstream, which is crucial for understanding the respiratory and metabolic states of patients. The primary test used for this purpose is the ABG analysis, which measures the partial pressure of carbon dioxide ($PaCO_2$), along with other vital parameters such as pH and oxygen levels. High $PaCO_2$ is generally a sign of hypoventilation or respiratory acidosis and low $PaCO_2$ may point to hyperventilation or metabolic alkalosis. Interpreting these values in conjunction with the rest of a patient's symptoms enables health practitioners to detect COPD and respiratory failure. Accurately checking carbon dioxide levels is crucial for both diagnosing patients and designing the most effective treatment plan for each individual. Along with ABG analysis, capnometry is a primary method for checking carbon dioxide levels, particularly in emergency and perioperative situations. They measure the amount of carbon dioxide in the air a patient exhales, providing instant information about their breathing. Because it is non-invasive, this method is suitable for monitoring patients under anesthesia or those who are short of breath, so that any hypercapnia or hypocapnia can be treated quickly. Advanced capnography equipment can create a waveform, called a capnogram, which helps visualize how breathing patterns change and allows for the detection of unusual breathing responses. Improvements in technology, including capnometry in clinical care, boost the accuracy of carbon dioxide measurements and highlight the significance of proper gas exchange. Lastly, the use of exhaled breath condensate (EBC) analysis is an emerging area of research in assessing carbon dioxide and other biomarkers associated with respiratory function. EBC is obtained by collecting moisture from the breath, which may enable the analysis of metabolic waste products, including carbon dioxide. However the sensitivity and specificity of EBC testing are still being studied. Currently, EBC is believed to provide insights into the lungs and the entire body; however, further research is necessary to establish standardized methods for collecting and analyzing samples. The ongoing exploration of EBC, alongside established methods such as ABG and capnometry, highlights the evolving landscape of diagnostic tests for assessing carbon dioxide levels and emphasizes the need for continued innovation in this critical area of respiratory medicine (N/A, 2025) (Figure 9.15).

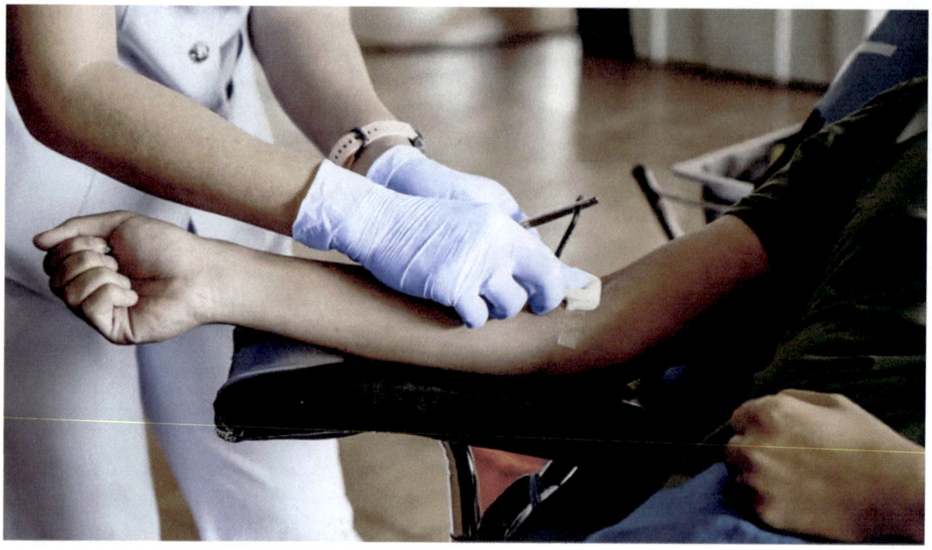

Figure 9.15. CO_2 blood test.

Source: https://media.post.rvohealth.io/wp-content/uploads/sites/3/2024/09/nurse-preparing-blood-test-1296x728-header-1024x575.jpg.

9.6.3. Treatment Options for Carbon Dioxide Retention

Addressing carbon dioxide retention is crucial in the management of respiratory illnesses, where ineffective gas exchange leads to elevated blood CO_2 levels. There are several ways to treat these conditions, each designed to improve lung function and facilitate sufficient gas exchange. In many cases, supplemental oxygen therapy is administered to help alleviate hypoxia, which also enhances the body's ability to remove carbon dioxide. When the blood has more oxygen, patients may breathe less and receive better oxygen and carbon dioxide exchange. It is essential for clinicians to monitor oxygen levels to prevent hypercapnia, which can occur when excessive oxygen reduces the need for deep breathing. Bronchodilators are often helpful for COPD patients since they help open the airways and improve airflow which reduces CO_2 in the body and improves their quality of life. If a patient has acute respiratory failure or high CO_2 levels, mechanical ventilation is often used as a significant treatment. It increases the pressure on inhalation, which improves the amount of air reaching the alveoli and facilitates the removal of carbon dioxide. Invasive or non-invasive ventilation (NIV) strategies may be employed depending on the specific clinical circumstances and the degree of respiratory compromise. NIV, such as bilevel positive airway pressure (BiPAP), has gained favor in managing chronic respiratory conditions, allowing increased comfort and compliance. The appropriate use of mechanical ventilation has been found to lower arterial CO_2 levels, which helps relieve the physical stress on patients with significant carbon dioxide retention. Importantly, careful management of ventilatory settings is necessary to avoid complications, such as barotrauma or ventilator-induced lung injury (VILI). Drugs play a crucial role in managing carbon dioxide retention, particularly for patients with pre-existing respiratory conditions. Corticosteroids are medications that can reduce inflammation in the airways, which improves the amount of air that can flow and the efficiency of gas exchange. Moreover, the development of controlled drug delivery systems has emerged as a potential advancement in pharmacotherapy, ensuring sustained release of therapeutic agents over specified periods (Adepu et al., 2021). These new inventions could help patients with chronic respiratory diseases get even better treatment results. Additionally, the use of bronchodilators in combination with other agents has been shown to more effectively reduce CO_2 retention. Importantly, ongoing evaluation of the treatment approach is crucial for adjusting strategies according to each patient's needs, ultimately improving the overall management of carbon dioxide retention and enhancing both respiratory function and patient quality of life (Saleh et al., 2020) (Figure 9.16).

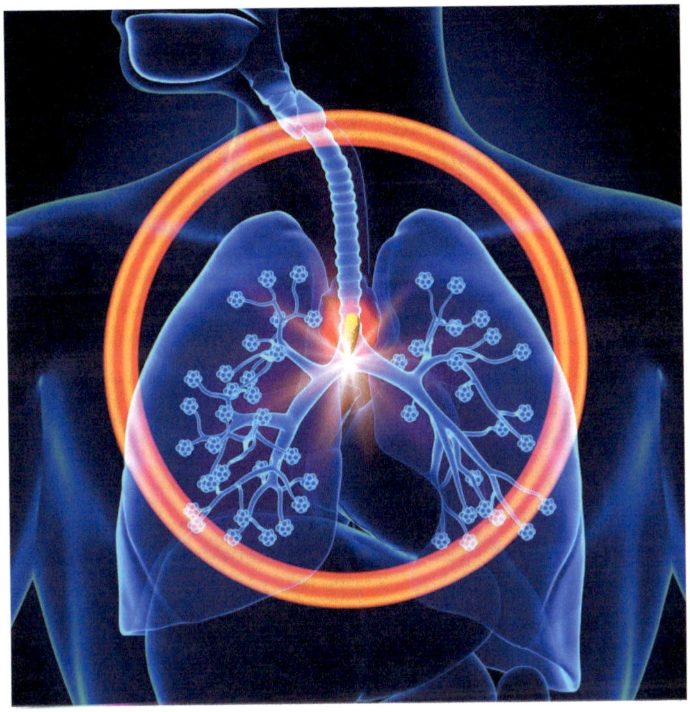

Figure 9.16. Hypercapnia.

Source: https://health.selfdecode.com/app/uploads/2018/08/bigstock-Lungs-Foreign-Object-inhaled-66734512-min.jpg.

SUMMARY

The movement of carbon dioxide in the blood is a crucial aspect of respiratory physiology that influences the body's oxygen utilization and overall metabolism. The fact that carbon dioxide is transported through dissolving, converting and binding to hemoglobin shows how complex this process is. Dissolved CO_2 in the blood helps maintain its pH, bicarbonate is important for gas exchange in tissues and lungs, and carbamino compounds increase hemoglobin's ability to carry oxygen. It highlights the role that effective transport of carbon dioxide plays in keeping the body's balance. The relationship between carbon dioxide transport and many other physiological functions is significant. When carbon dioxide levels change, the body's pH balance can be significantly affected, which influences its acid-base system. Bicarbonate's ability to buffer excess acid underlines the close link between breathing and metabolism. Any issue with carbon dioxide transport could lead to significant health problems, harming both the heart and lungs. That is why ongoing studies and education in this field are essential for enhancing medical knowledge and improving methods. The effects of carbon dioxide transport also affect public health and the environment, not just individuals. As studies continue, it becomes increasingly clear how human actions impact respiratory physiology. Relevant studies demonstrate these connections, such as the impact of increased atmospheric CO_2 on human health and the physiological adaptations required in various medical procedures, like laparoscopic surgeries, where CO_2 insufflation plays a critical role (Kim et al., 1992). This demonstrates that incorporating various fields of science is crucial for comprehending how carbon dioxide moves. An integrated understanding of these relations will be crucial for developing strategies that encompass not only individual health assessments but also global environmental health initiatives in the Anthropocene (Pöschl et al., 2015). CO_2 transport in the blood is necessary for keeping the body's balance and for effective breathing. Primarily, CO_2 is transported in three forms: dissolved in plasma, as bicarbonate ions (HCO_3^-), and bound to hemoglobin (Hb) as carbamino compounds. Around 7–10% of the CO_2 is found in plasma, and the other 70% is changed to bicarbonate by the action of CA. This change is necessary because it helps move CO_2 and also helps maintain blood pH levels under control. The last 20–23% of CO_2 combines with hemoglobin to make carbaminohemoglobin, which helps CO_2 be released at the lungs and O_2 be taken up at the tissues. It is essential to understand these mechanisms to comprehend how the body regulates carbon dioxide and adapts to varying needs. In addition to these transport mechanisms, CO_2 in the blood also plays a role in metabolic processes. Respiration relies on the feedback provided by the conversion of CO_2 and its effect on pH. If CO_2 rises, the blood becomes more acidic, which prompts the brain's respiratory centers to make us breathe faster and exchange more gas. When CO_2 levels are lower, respiratory rate slows down, which helps the body regulate how much oxygen is brought in and how much carbon dioxide is removed. Furthermore, recent studies have found that lactate affects CO_2 production in tissues and also functions as a signaling molecule in metabolic processes. The integration of these transport and regulatory mechanisms highlights the complexity of respiratory physiology and underscores the need for further research on their implications in health and disease (Li et al., 2022). A disturbance in the movement of carbon dioxide can cause significant health problems, such as respiratory acidosis or alkalosis, which highlights the need for homeostasis. If the balance between CO_2 production and elimination is disrupted, it can lead to both short-term and long-term health issues, particularly in individuals with respiratory difficulties, cardiovascular disease, or metabolic disorders. In urgent cases, doctors may use mechanical ventilation, and for chronic conditions, they may use drugs to help restore normal CO_2 levels. As we learn more about how CO_2 is transported, it becomes evident that this subject is crucial for both respiratory specialists and clinicians in other fields.

CLOSER LOOK

ENDOTHELIAL DYSFUNCTION

Endothelial dysfunction is a condition in which the endothelium, the inner lining of blood vessels, fails to function properly, resulting in reduced nitric oxide (NO) production and a shift toward vasoconstriction, inflammation, and clot formation. This dysfunction can contribute to various cardiovascular diseases (CVDs), including atherosclerosis and coronary artery disease (Figure 9.17).

- Endothelial dysfunction occurs when the endothelium's normal functions are impaired, such as reduced nitric oxide production.
- NO is a signaling molecule that helps relax blood vessels and prevent blood clots.
- When NO production is reduced, blood vessels may constrict more easily, and the risk of blood clots increases.
- Endothelial dysfunction is also associated with increased inflammation and a pro-thrombotic state.

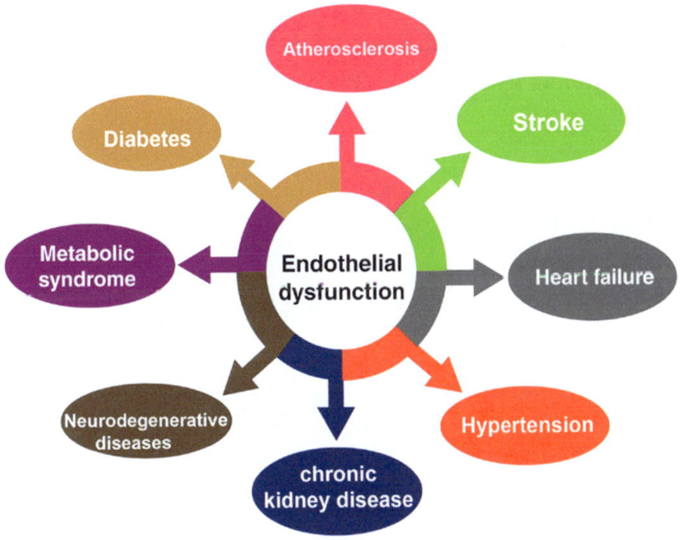

Figure 9.17. Endothelial dysfunction.

Source: https://onlinelibrary.wiley.com/cms/asset/de174742-262e-4c33-bca0-cbd5dd1d0d5a/mco2651-gra-0001-m.jpg?trick=1745187787632.

1. **Causes of Endothelial Dysfunction**

   Lifestyle Factors: Smoking, high blood pressure, high cholesterol, high blood sugar, and physical inactivity can all contribute to endothelial dysfunction.

- **Medical Conditions**: Conditions like diabetes, kidney disease, and heart disease can also damage the endothelium.

- **Infections**: Severe infections, such as sepsis, can also lead to endothelial dysfunction.

2. **Consequences of Endothelial Dysfunction**

- **Atherosclerosis**: Endothelial dysfunction is an early stage in the development of atherosclerosis, characterized by the accumulation of plaque in the arteries.
- **Coronary Artery Disease**: Endothelial dysfunction can contribute to coronary artery disease by making arteries less responsive to dilate.
- **Other Cardiovascular Diseases**: Endothelial dysfunction is also associated with hypertension, heart failure, and peripheral artery disease.

3. **Diagnosis and Treatment**

- **Endothelial Function Tests**: These tests assess the ability of blood vessels to dilate, a measure of endothelial function.
- **Biomarkers**: Certain blood tests can detect markers of endothelial dysfunction, such as cellular adhesion molecules.
- **Lifestyle Changes**: Adopting a healthy lifestyle, including regular exercise, a balanced diet, and avoiding smoking, can help improve endothelial function.
- **Medications**: Medications like ACE inhibitors, statins, and nitrates can also be used to treat endothelial dysfunction and reduce the risk of CVD.

REFERENCES

1. Abercromby, A. F. J., Bekdash, O. S., Conkin, J., Downs, et al. (2025). *Evidence-Based Approach to Establish Space Suit Carbon Dioxide Limits.* https://core.ac.uk/download/pdf/323104209.pdf (accessed on 31st May 2025).
2. Adepu, S., & Ramakrishna, S. (2021). Controlled Drug Delivery Systems: current status and future directions. *Molecules, 26*(19), 5905. https://doi.org/10.3390/molecules26195905Alarcon, M., Chambrey, R., Chegwidden, W., Cooper, G., Dadiani, M., Davenport, A., Gaffney, E. A., et al. (2011). *A Mathematical Model of Tumor and Blood pHe Regulation: The HCO_3^-/CO_2 Buffering System.* https://core.ac.uk/download/pdf/6185666.pdf (accessed on 31st May 2025).
3. Aralova, N. I., Klyuchko, O. M., Mashkin, V. I., & Mashkina, I. V., et al. (2019). Математические модели развития и компенсации гипоксических состояний при ишемической болезни сердца у лиц летного состава (mathematical models for development and compensation of hypoxic states during ischemic heart disease in flight crews' personnel). *Electronics and Control Systems.* https://core.ac.uk/download/286372200.pdf (accessed on 31st May 2025).
4. Arena, R., Guazzi, M., Lavie, C. J., & Phillips, S. A. (2015). *Endothelial Dysfunction and Lung Capillary Injury in Cardiovascular Diseases.* https://core.ac.uk/download/43367888.pdf (accessed on 31st May 2025).
5. Averell, P. M., Deguchi, H., Elias, D., Griffin, et al. (2015). *Arteriovenous Blood Metabolomics: A Readout of Intra-Tissue Metabostasis.* https://core.ac.uk/download/323066228.pdf (accessed on 31st May 2025).
6. Baloğlu, E., & Mairbäurl, H. (2021). In search of a sensor: How does CO_2 regulate alveolar ion transport? *American Journal of Respiratory Cell and Molecular Biology, 65*, 571–572. https://www.semanticscholar.org/paper/096daf98c4c6d6c73279eb23471b4607439c034d (accessed on 31st May 2025).
7. Baumgartner, H., De Backer, J., Babu-Narayan, S. V., Budts, W., Chessa, M., Diller, G. P., Lung, B., et al. (2020). 2020 ESC guidelines for the management of adult congenital heart disease. *European Heart Journal, 42*, 563–645. https://doi.org/10.1093/eurheartj/ehaa554 (accessed on 31st May 2025).
8. Brown, N. J. (1990). *Health Hazard Manual for Firefighters.* https://core.ac.uk/download/5122113.pdf (accessed on 31st May 2025).
9. Bulger, N., Harrington, B. K., Krieger, J. A., Latimer, A. J., Arbabi, S., Counts, C., Sayre, M., et al. (2021). Prehospital end-tidal carbon dioxide predicts hemorrhagic shock upon emergency department arrival. *Journal of Trauma and Acute Care Surgery, 91*, 457–464. https://www.semanticscholar.org/paper/e82ab1b4936908f8589d5fd4d60362d34042d684 (accessed on 31st May 2025).
10. Conrad, S. (2020). Extracorporeal carbon dioxide removal: From bench to bedside and back. *Critical Care Medicine.* https://www.semanticscholar.org/paper/1d6e69d4ec1c0fc9f0f413c2354f023bb496a206 (accessed on 31st May 2025).
11. Dani, K. A., Goutcher, C., Moreton, F. C., Muir, et al. (2016). *Respiratory Challenge MRI: Practical Aspects.* https://core.ac.uk/download/42371355.pdf (accessed on 31st May 2025).
12. Do, C., Vasquez, P. C., & Soleimani, M. (2022). Metabolic alkalosis pathogenesis, diagnosis, and treatment: Core curriculum 2022. *American Journal of Kidney Diseases, 80*, 536–551. https://doi.org/10.1053/j.ajkd.2021.12.016 (accessed on 31st May 2025).

13. Donaldson, M. A., Donohoe, K., Assayag, D., Durand, C., Fisher, J., Johannson, K. A., Kolb, M., et al. (2024). Characteristics of pulse oximetry and arterial blood gas in patients with fibrotic interstitial lung disease. *BMJ Open Respiratory Research, 11.* https://www.semanticscholar.org/paper/7ecd8d432e86ab339cb0c863bb2cc9b306bda984 (accessed on 31st May 2025).

14. Gaspary, J. F. P., Edgar, L., Lopes, L. F. D., Rosa, C. B., & Siluk, J. (2024). Translational insights into the hormetic potential of carbon dioxide: From physiological mechanisms to innovative adjunct therapeutic potential for cancer. *Frontiers in Physiology, 15.* https://www.semanticscholar.org/paper/fdb12a36e321f5afb93d2db18488492f2f751b71 (accessed on 31st May 2025).

15. Grimm, L., Humann-Ziehank, E., Zinne, N., Zardo, P., & Ganter, M. (2021). Analysis of pH and electrolytes in blood and ruminal fluid, including kidney function tests, in sheep undergoing long-term surgical procedures. *Acta Veterinaria Scandinavica, 63.* https://www.semanticscholar.org/paper/83410f774efb08ad44c480a6e39010e609e09aaf (accessed on 31st May 2025).

16. Harter, T. S., Clifford, A. M., & Tresguerres, M. (2021). Adrenergically induced translocation of red blood cell β-adrenergic sodium-proton exchangers has ecological relevance for hypoxic and hypercapnic white seabass. *AJP Regulatory Integrative and Comparative Physiology, 321*, R655–R671. https://doi.org/10.1152/ajpregu.00175.2021 (accessed on 31st May 2025).

17. Harter, T., & Scott, G. R. (2024). Linking red blood cell functional phenotypes to environmental tolerance in high-altitude adapted deer mice. *Physiology*. https://www.semanticscholar.org/paper/fc8c5d0a7ec7488cc5141f0e1a1d0f3024620897 (accessed on 31st May 2025).

18. Hisar, O., Hisar, Ş. A., Yanik, T., & Aras, M. (2003). Balık kan karbondioksitinin taşınması ve atılmasında karbonik anhidraz izoenzimlerinin fonksiyonları / The functions of carbonic anhydrase isozymes at fish blood carbon dioxide transport and excretion. *Journal of the Faculty of Agriculture, 34.* https://www.semanticscholar.org/paper/140e8a6cb6cebb0a6f0d1a28341acf0a429fcecb (accessed on 31st May 2025).

19. Kelly, L. (2004). *Essentials of Human Physiology for Pharmacy*. https://www.semanticscholar.org/paper/4219f4edcfbeb281dc54006ce947a2795fbfb510 (accessed on 31st May 2025).

20. Kholiqov, O., Zhou, W., Zhang, T., Le, D., & Srinivasan, V. (2020). Time-of-flight resolved light field fluctuations reveal deep human tissue physiology. *Nature Communications, 11.* https://www.semanticscholar.org/paper/8e9bf2bd52a87f49fa574a3d51ff0df542cf82e5 (accessed on 31st May 2025).

21. Kim, Y. I., Shur, M., Kim, H. S., Hong, S., Moon, S., & Chung, W. H. (1992). Change of hemodynamic parameters and plasma catecholamine level during laparoscopic cholecystectomy. *Korean Journal of Anesthesiology, 25*, 515–520. https://www.semanticscholar.org/paper/505c29fd31591b363d5aca1d73ea570f733e20ca (accessed on 31st May 2025).

22. Köse, E. Ö. (2024). *Biology Teacher Candidates Drawings About Circulatory System*. https://core.ac.uk/download/618266545.pdf (accessed on 31st May 2025).

23. Lee, H. W., Yu, P., & Simons, M. (2018). Recent advances in understanding lymphangiogenesis and metabolism. *F1000Research, 7*, 1114. https://doi.org/10.12688/f1000research.14803.1 (accessed on 31st May 2025).

24. Li, X., Yang, Y., Zhang, B., Lin, X., Fu, X., An, Y., Zou, Y., et al. (2022). Lactate metabolism in human health and disease. *Signal Transduction and Targeted Therapy, 7.* https://doi.org/10.1038/s41392-022-01151-3 (accessed on 31st May 2025).

25. Livingston, G., Huntley, J., Sommerlad, A., Ames, D., Ballard, C., Banerjee, S., Brayne, C., et al. (2020). Dementia prevention, intervention, and care: 2020 report of the Lancet Commission. *The Lancet, 396*, 413–446. https://doi.org/10.1016/s0140-6736(20)30367-6 (accessed on 31st May 2025).

26. Magor-Elliott, S. R., Fullerton, C. J., Richmond, G., Ritchie, G., & Robbins, P. (2021). A dynamic model of the body gas stores for carbon dioxide, oxygen, and inert gases that incorporates circulatory transport delays to and from the lung. *Journal of Applied Physiology, 130*, 1383–1397. https://www.semanticscholar.org/paper/1608537de240a76408d8455331404a78225 5a269 (accessed on 31st May 2025).

27. Marken, F. (2020). Future challenges in electrochemistry: Linking membrane-based solar energy conversion mechanisms to water harvesting. *Journal of Solid State Electrochemistry*. https://www.semanticscholar.org/paper/50273bb97002f7d090b54d70bf5873557cdeb52d (accessed on 31st May 2025).

28. N/A. (2025). *Aerospace Medicine and Biology: A Continuing Bibliography with Indexes (supplement 309)*. https://core.ac.uk/download/pdf/42832898.pdf (accessed on 31st May 2025).

29. Pernow, J., Mahdi, A., Yang, J., & Zhou, Z. (2019). Red blood cell dysfunction: A new player in cardiovascular disease. *Cardiovascular Research, 115*, 1596–1605. https://doi.org/10.1093/cvr/cvz156 (accessed on 31st May 2025).

30. Pöschl, U., & Shiraiwa, M. (2015). Multiphase chemistry at the atmosphere-biosphere interface influencing climate and public health in the Anthropocene. *Chemical Reviews, 115*(10), 4440–4475. https://www.semanticscholar.org/paper/8606070cc7b3f62d2e453547cb2117 e79c56689c (accessed on 31st May 2025).

31. Prado, A. N. (2024). Biochemical approach of acid-base disturbances: Diagnosis algorithm. *Revista Colombiana de Nefrología*. https://www.semanticscholar.org/paper/4b7206dad5e8a 4592a530b03a350b2455f3798e5 (accessed on 31st May 2025).

32. Pretini, V., Koenen, M. H., Kaestner, L., Fens, M. H. A. M., Schiffelers, R. M., Bartels, M., & Van, W. R. (2019). Red blood cells: Chasing interactions. *Frontiers in Physiology, 10*. https://doi.org/10.3389/fphys.2019.00945 (accessed on 31st May 2025).

33. Radí, R. (2022). Interplay of carbon dioxide and peroxide metabolism in mammalian cells. *Journal of Biological Chemistry, 298*, 102358. https://doi.org/10.1016/j.jbc.2022.102358 (accessed on 31st May 2025).

34. Saleh, I., Zouari, N., & Al-Ghouti, M. A. (2020). Removal of pesticides from water and wastewater: Chemical, physical and biological treatment approaches. *Environmental Technology & Innovation, 19*, 101026–101026. https://doi.org/10.1016/j.eti.2020.101026 (accessed on 31st May 2025).

35. Saunois, M., Stavert, A. R., Poulter, B., Bousquet, P., Canadell, J. G., Jackson, R. B., Raymond, P. A., et al. (2020). The global methane budget 2000–2017. *Earth System Science Data, 12*, 1561–1623. https://doi.org/10.5194/essd-12-1561-2020 (accessed on 31st May 2025).

36. Spicer, J., & Taylor, A. (1987). Carbon dioxide transport and acid-base regulation in the blood of the beach-hopper *Orchestia gammarellus* (Pallas) (Crustacea: Amphipoda). *Ophelia, 28*, 49–61. https://www.semanticscholar.org/paper/426739f0ad364709e1d38d1f6dee422d657 cf5fc (accessed on 31st May 2025).

37. Sweeney, M. D., Zhao, Z., Montagne, A., Nelson, A. R., & Zloković, B. V. (2018). Blood-brain barrier: From physiology to disease and back. *Physiological Reviews, 99*, 21–78. https://doi.org/10.1152/physrev.00050.2017 (accessed on 31st May 2025).

38. Szabó, S., Bodó, M., Nagy-Bozsóky, J., Pintér, I., Bagány, M., Kóra, S., & Dunai, P. (2023). Physiological challenges of space travel and ground-based simulation possibilities for monitoring brain circulatory changes: A rheoencephalography study. *Repüléstudományi Közlemények*. https://www.semanticscholar.org/paper/1359e450bd653e47292044fe171dbbc951a6b731 (accessed on 31st May 2025).

39. White, R. J. (2025). *Acid-Base Homeostasis in the Human System*. https://core.ac.uk/download/pdf/42869639.pdf (accessed on 31st May 2025).

40. Wouters, E. (2008). COPD: From an organ- to a disease-oriented approach. *COPD: Journal of Chronic Obstructive Pulmonary Disease, 5*, 73, 74. https://www.semanticscholar.org/paper/a7929f5bf5d81c2c8c871ded99d3c9f1cc72ff44 (accessed on 31st May 2025).

41. Zhang, F., Chen, F., Zhong, M., Shen, R., Zhao, Z., Wei, H., Zhang, B., et al. (2023). Imaging of carbonic anhydrase level in epilepsy with an environment-sensitive fluorescent probe. *Analytical Chemistry*. https://www.semanticscholar.org/paper/6b4cd1a6a869e0ea9a216bd1c75bb485d6dad906 (accessed on 31st May 2025).

42. Zhuo, Q., Zhang, Z., & Fang, X. (2024). New insights into the mechanisms of red blood cell enucleation: From basics to clinical applications. *EJHaem, 5*, 1301–1311. https://www.semanticscholar.org/paper/e5829f271c2eb0ae4596bfc98356fdefbb0c753a (accessed on 31st May 2025).

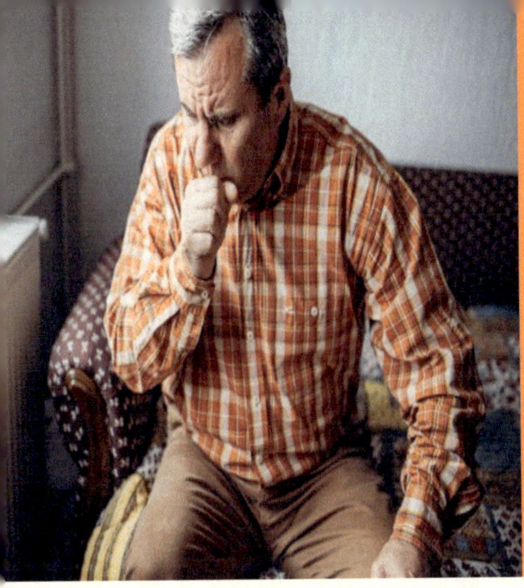

Chapter 10

REGULATION OF BREATHING

Contents

Introduction

Breathing is controlled by the body using both nerve and chemical signals. Essentially, this system enables organisms to adapt to various physical conditions and environmental changes, including altitude and atmospheric variations. An adequate supply of oxygen and the removal of carbon dioxide are both important for homeostasis and these are made possible by proper ventilation. Recently, new imaging and recording methods have helped us gain a deeper understanding of the brain circuits that control breathing, revealing how sleep apnea can disrupt normal breathing patterns. This research continues to demonstrate the importance of understanding these mechanisms in developing effective treatments for respiratory diseases that can significantly impact a person's health and daily life. Examining the systems that govern breathing in more detail reveals that sensory information and central circuits are involved. The brainstem, specifically the nucleus tractus solitarius (NTS), is critical for processing information related to blood gas levels and integrating sensory feedback to modulate ventilation accordingly. For instance, studies indicate that synaptic plasticity, particularly in response to hypoxia, can enhance the hypoxic ventilatory response (HVR), allowing for improved adaptation to lower oxygen environments. This demonstrates that the brain can adapt and highlights the importance of glutamate receptors in the NTS for regulating changes in breathing. Understanding these processes is vital, especially when considering their implications for various conditions that may alter normal breathing regulation, including those resulting from neurological events such as stroke (Calistri et al., 2017). Additionally, the complex ways breathing regulation is linked to other bodily functions can be observed when examining the effects of systemic changes. To illustrate, when someone becomes used to hypoxia, their body responds by altering breathing patterns, which also leads to lasting changes in the brain pathways involved in breathing. Even after returning to normal oxygen levels, the animals continued to hyperventilate, which suggests that these adaptations persist and raises doubts about how to treat people with related respiratory disorders. Studying these interactions enables researchers to understand the causes and broader effects of diseases that involve respiratory issues. Harnessing this knowledge is crucial for developing effective strategies to mitigate the impact of respiratory disorders on human health, thereby emphasizing the importance of ongoing research in this vital area (Carr et al., 2014).

Definition of Breathing Regulation

Breathing regulation is important because it constantly adjusts the body's breathing to keep the internal balance. This dynamic regulation is primarily managed by the central nervous system (CNS), particularly involving structures such as the brainstem, which integrates signals related to metabolic demand, emotional state, and environmental factors. The autonomic nervous system (ANS) plays a crucial role in regulating breathing patterns, allowing the body to adapt to physiological needs such as exercise or changes in atmospheric conditions. Breathing regulation is important because it supports gas exchange and also impacts the heart and immune systems, highlighting its significance for overall health. move. Additionally, breathing regulation utilizes several feedback mechanisms that extend from peripheral chemoreceptors to central processing areas. All of these elements cooperate to check the blood's levels of carbon dioxide, oxygen, and pH. For example, when CO_2 levels increase, receptors trigger the body to breathe more deeply, removing the excess CO_2 and maintaining balance. As a result, the body can respond to changes in its environment and within itself. There is a clear link between emotions and breathing, since stress can affect our breathing patterns, which may either help or worsen anxiety and similar problems. By learning about breathing regulation, we can see how its dysregulation can lead to various health problems, making it more important in clinical settings. Studies done recently suggest that controlling your breathing can have therapeutic effects on mental health issues. Slow, deep breathing helps increase the activity of the parasympathetic nervous system, resulting in lower stress and anxiety. They improve how well individuals notice and respond to their body's signals. Besides, scientists are now examining the link between the microbiota in the gut, the gut itself, and the brain to understand how breathing regulation is affected by gut health and mental state, since the microbiota and the CNS are closely involved in emotional and mental processes. Consequently, defining breathing regulation extends beyond basic respiratory mechanics; it integrates physiological, psychological, and environmental dimensions that are critical for health maintenance and therapeutic interventions in various clinical contexts (John et al., 2019; Camilla et al., 2022) (Figure 10.1).

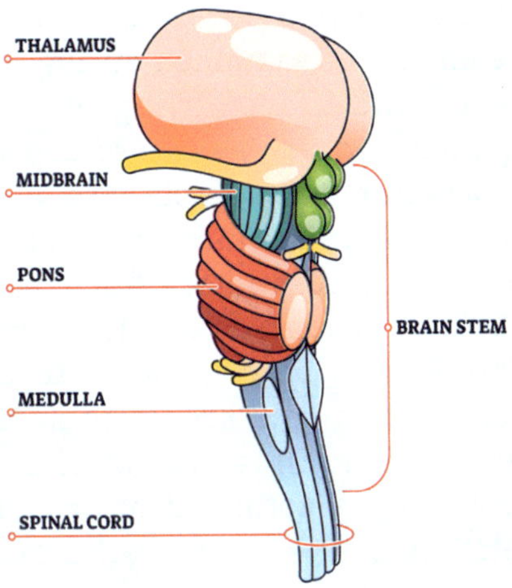

Figure 10.1. Brainstem regulation of breathing vector illustration.

Source: https://www.respiratorytherapyzone.com/wp-content/uploads/2022/04/Brainstem-Regulation-of-Breathing-Vector-Illustration.png.

Importance of Breathing Regulation in Human Physiology

Breathing regulation plays a crucial role in maintaining homeostasis within the human body. Besides helping gas exchange, the detailed workings of respiration also help maintain the right balance of carbon dioxide and oxygen in the body, which is necessary for proper cell function. The CNS and ANS work together to make sure breathing is adjusted as needed by the body. When someone exercises, their body needs to take in more oxygen and eliminate more carbon dioxide, which leads to faster and deeper breathing. Additionally, breathing is crucial for overall health because it impacts other vital physiological functions. If the breathing regulatory system is disrupted, it can lead to numerous health problems, underscoring the importance of understanding how these systems function and their impact on the body. Additionally, breathing regulation is not limited to gas exchange; it is also related to both our emotions and our thoughts. As an example, stress can change how we breathe, which can affect both our emotions and how well we think. Vocalization is explained in terms of the way voice production and respiratory control interact with the CNS and ANS. This demonstrates that the body must utilize its ventilation processes for both speaking and meeting its energy needs when under stress, highlighting the complexity of the relationship between respiration and human function. Understanding this interaction enables a more profound comprehension of how breathing regulation affects not only communication but also emotional and cognitive faculties, thereby highlighting its significance in human physiology (Puyvelde et al., 2018). New research suggests that the microbiota-gut-brain axis plays a crucial role in regulating breathing. The makeup of the microbiota can alter gut health as well as brain functions related to breathing and stress. The gut microbiome can influence the CNS which could change the way breathing is controlled under stress and other conditions. It means that taking care of your microbiome's health can support both your gut and your lungs. Thus, breathing regulation emerges as a multifaceted aspect of human physiology, intimately linked with various biological systems and influences, making it essential for both physical performance and mental well-being (John et al., 2019).

10.1. Neural Control of Breathing

The neural control of breathing is a complex process orchestrated by various brain structures, primarily the medulla oblongata and the pons. These regions are responsible for generating and regulating the rhythmic pattern of respiration through the integration of sensory feedback from chemoreceptors and mechanoreceptors dispersed throughout the respiratory system. Any changes in carbon dioxide and oxygen in the blood are detected by the medullary respiratory center, which then adjusts ventilation. This quick reaction is necessary to maintain homeostasis, whether the body is active or at rest. Disruptions to this neural control, particularly in individuals with chronic obstructive pulmonary disease (COPD), can lead to maladaptive breathing patterns and increased arterial carbon dioxide pressure, necessitating interventions like nocturnal NIV as a means to optimize respiratory function and enhance overall health outcomes (Alexandra et al., 2022).

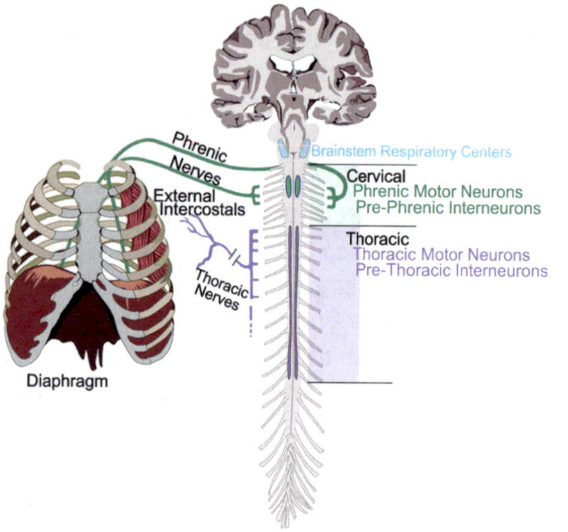

Figure 10.2. Central organization for the neural control of breathing.

Source: https://www.researchgate.net/profile/Ian-Malone/publication/353094269/figure/fig1/AS:1055352057520129@1628626946504/Central-organization-for-the-neural-control-of-breathing-Timing-and-coordination-of.png.

Additionally, understanding how sleep affects the brain's control of breathing can help us study how different states of consciousness alter respiration. During sleep, particularly rapid eye movement (REM) sleep, notable alterations occur in the neural command system, which can challenge the regulation of ventilation. COPD patients may experience significant changes in their arterial carbon dioxide levels, which can be dangerous for their health. Studying these interaction points out that ventilatory neural drive should be examined during sleep as well as when awake. Identifying the physiological adaptations linked to various sleep stages could inform therapeutic approaches that address the distinct challenges faced by individuals with compromised respiratory function (Alexandra et al., 2022). So, sleep and its effects on brain control should be considered together when understanding how breathing is regulated. A new approach in research involves combining neurobiology, breathing control, and emotional regulation to develop innovative treatments for patients. Precision medicine is highlighting the role of understanding the brain mechanisms that control breathing when someone is stressed. Studies in animals and humans enable researchers to understand the relationship between emotions and breathing patterns. This approach enables the development of mind-body therapies that utilize breathing techniques to support individuals with stress-related conditions, as they are both affordable and easily accessible. The main reason these therapies may help public health is that they are simple and can be used by people from different cultures. Ultimately, advancing our understanding of the neural control of breathing within this broader context may facilitate the refinement of clinical practices and improve outcomes for individuals facing respiratory and psychological challenges (Figure 10.2).

10.1.1. Role of the Brainstem in Respiratory Regulation

Breathing is primarily controlled by the brainstem, which serves as the primary center for regulating respiratory rhythms. The brainstem, which includes the midbrain, pons, and medulla oblongata, combines different neural messages to control respiration. The ventral respiratory group and the pre-Bötzinger complex, located in the medullary centers, help produce the primary rhythmic pattern of breathing. They obtain information from peripheral chemoreceptors located in the carotid body and other areas, which detect variations in blood oxygen and carbon dioxide levels. Thanks to their interaction, these receptors and the brainstem ensure that ventilation is appropriate for the body's metabolism, maintaining homeostasis during both rest and exercise. Recent studies have found that mitochondrial function in chemoreceptors and their connection with the brainstem play a crucial role in maintaining breathing under low-oxygen conditions. The hypoxic ventilatory response (HVR), a critical reflex for survival, is directly linked to the activation of glomus cells in the carotid body, which communicate with the brainstem respiratory centers. Research has shown that a change in mitochondrial complex I can disrupt respiratory function and lead to a weaker HVR response. Therefore, arterial chemoreceptors rely on mitochondrial NADH dehydrogenase to detect oxygen, thereby linking cellular respiration to the regulation of breathing by nerves. Understanding these mechanisms is vital, as they elucidate how the brainstem interprets and responds to fluctuating oxygen levels, ensuring that appropriate ventilatory adjustments are made in real-time (Jim et al., 2023). When novel pathogens cause respiratory complications, it highlights the brainstem's susceptibility to problems. For instance, severe cases of COVID-19 have revealed the neurotropic nature of SARS-CoV-2, which can directly impact the central nervous system (CNS), including brainstem nuclei responsible for regulating breathing. These patients often have difficulty breathing, which is related to acute changes in their blood gases, as the virus can significantly harm their lungs. It demonstrates the close link between the brainstem and respiratory events when the body is affected by systemic disease. It also suggests that harm to the respiratory centers in the brainstem may make it difficult for patients to recover and could mean they require ventilation for a more extended period. Consequently, comprehending the brain stem's role in respiratory regulation is vital, particularly when considering the implications of viral infections on the respiratory system as a whole (Baig, 2020) (Figure 10.3).

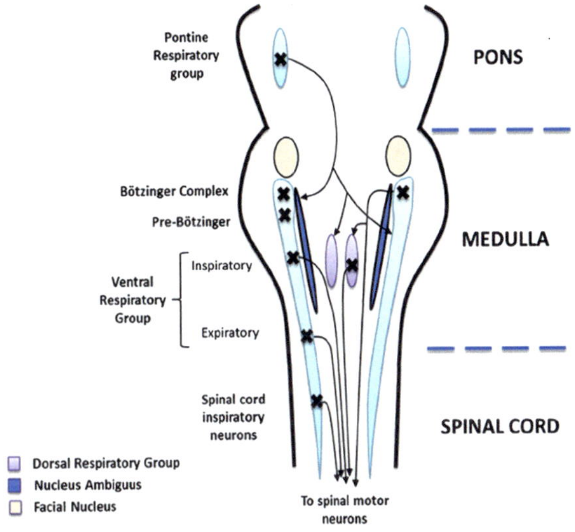

Figure 10.3. Brainstem centers contributing to the control of respiratory drive.

Source: https://www.researchgate.net/profile/Mudiaga-Sowho-2/publication/264312906/figure/fig1/AS:295827403755520@1447542157159/Brainstem-centers-contributing-to-the-control-of-respiratory-drive-Adapted-from-Horner.png.

10.1.2. Influence of the Cerebral Cortex on Breathing Patterns

The cerebral cortex plays a pivotal role in modulating breathing patterns, reflecting its complex interaction with the lower brain centers responsible for autonomic regulation. Usually, the brainstem handles the automatic parts of breathing, but the cortex can also shape these patterns by our thoughts and feelings. When people sing or talk, they often adjust the rate and depth of their breathing. This cognitive influence suggests that the cortex can influence respiratory actions beyond the usual physical responses. It has been found that activating brain regions responsible for voluntary movement can cause significant changes in ventilation, showing the role of the cerebral cortex in managing both thought processes and breathing. By knowing this relationship, we can understand how our feelings and thoughts can change our breathing which is important for breathing regulation in the human body. Importantly, the interaction between the cerebral cortex and respiratory centers also encompasses responses to events occurring around us. Because of the cortex, we can respond to changes in carbon dioxide or oxygen saturation and initiate deeper or faster breathing if necessary. Studies using functional magnetic resonance imaging (fMRI) have shown that areas within the parietal cortex and cingulate cortex become active during periods of hypoxia and hypercapnia, revealing a neural network that coordinates these responses. This suggests that humans can adapt to new environmental conditions by utilizing higher brain functions. This means the cerebral cortex helps with both automatic and purposeful changes in breathing which are both important for keeping the body stable. Additionally, the way the cerebral cortex influences breathing is closely tied to our overall sense of consciousness and body awareness. Studies have shown that synchronizing brain waves during breathing is crucial for maintaining a coherent mind. The cerebral cortex is involved in combining information from the senses and emotions, which affects how individuals perceive their breathing. As the mind and body are connected, being aware of breathing can actually alter how we breathe, demonstrating that the mind and body are closely linked. For example, treating anxiety disorders may include breathing exercises that demonstrate the usefulness of understanding how the cortex affects breathing. Ultimately, recognizing the cerebral cortex's contributions to both voluntary and involuntary breathing regulation reveals its integral role in the comprehensive regulation of breathing, demonstrating the complexity of the interactions between consciousness and physiological function (Figure 10.4).

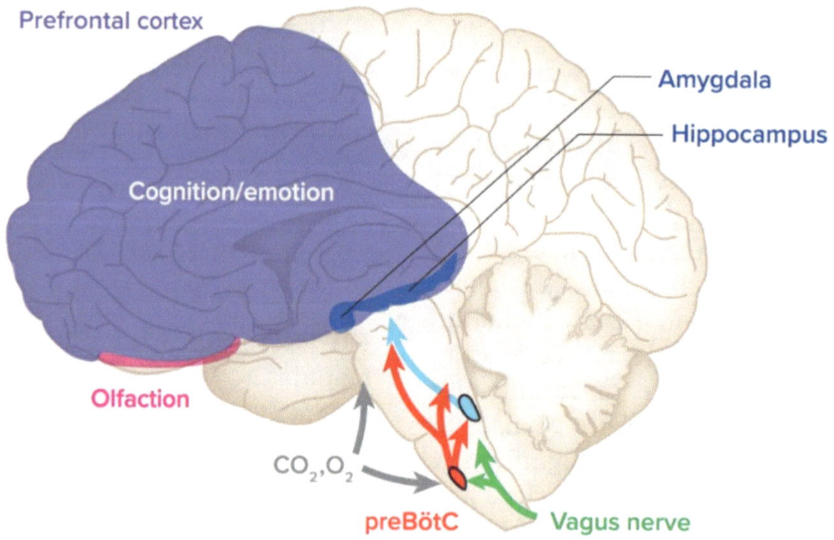

Figure 10.4. How breathing influences the brain.

Source: https://th-thumbnailer.cdn-si-edu.com/Im5gNORqvfV863oQ_RjtshV8yK4=/fit-in/1072x0/filters:focal(625x455:626x456)/https://tf-cmsv2-smithsonianmag-media.s3.amazonaws.com/filer_public/8b/44/8b44a730-eaa8-433f-bc2e-be763785e3be/g-breathing-influences-brain-alt.png.

10.1.3. Feedback Mechanisms From Chemoreceptors

The intricate regulation of breathing is significantly influenced by feedback mechanisms originating from chemoreceptors. Most of these sensory cells are found in the carotid and aortic bodies, and they monitor changes in carbon dioxide, oxygen, and pH in the blood. If carbon dioxide rises or oxygen drops, chemoreceptors alert the CNS, mainly the medulla oblongata, which then starts breathing to restore balance. It is essential because changes in gas levels may result in metabolic problems that disrupt the whole body. Understanding the roles of these chemoreceptors not only illustrates the complexity of respiratory regulation but also highlights their relevance in potential pathophysiological conditions, especially those related to respiratory irregularities and associated disorders that complicate respiratory drive, as discussed in Barnes et al. (2014). Additionally, when you exercise, your body requires more oxygen and must regulate the amount of carbon dioxide. These receptors play a crucial role in bringing sensory information under the control of breathing. As exercise causes more metabolism, chemoreceptors notice the increase in carbon dioxide and the decrease in oxygen which leads to an autonomic response that makes breathing faster and deeper. It ensures that the muscles have enough oxygen and that waste products are removed. The ability of chemoreceptors to integrate various physiological signals demonstrates the remarkable adaptability of the respiratory system under varying demands, affirming their crucial function in maintaining metabolic homeostasis, particularly during strenuous activities, as outlined in Crisafulli et al. (2014). The way chemoreceptors work with the CNS shows that feedback is essential for regulating breathing. These chemoreceptors send information about gas levels in the blood and also regulate heart function, indicating that they are involved in numerous body functions. For example, when we feel inspired, chemoreceptors may cause changes in heart rate and blood pressure, allowing the entire system to support breathing. Inspiration causes a slight hyperpolarization, and expiration leads to depolarization, as demonstrated in recent studies, revealing the intricate control of respiratory drive. This ongoing communication between chemoreceptors and the respiratory centers enables real-time adjustments that are vital for sustaining life and managing the body's responses to internal and external stimuli, thereby advancing our understanding of respiratory physiology and its clinical implications, as discussed in Barnes et al. (2014) (Figure 10.5).

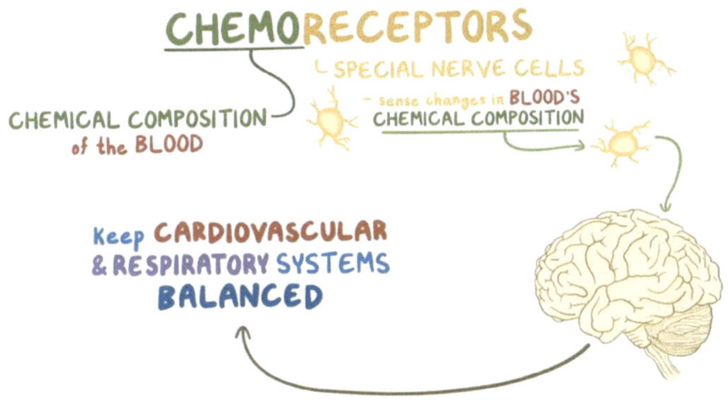

Figure 10.5. Chemoreceptors.

Source: https://d16qt3wv6xm098.cloudfront.net/MiQJCuUrSru6vyer7hT63SssQcukFioC/_.jpg.

10.2. Chemical Regulation of Breathing

The chemical regulation of breathing is a complex interplay of various physiological mechanisms that respond to changes in blood chemistry. The central part of this regulation is chemoreceptors, which are present in the carotid and aortic bodies and also in the CNS. These receptors detect fluctuations in carbon dioxide (CO_2), oxygen (O_2), and pH levels in the blood, effectively serving as sensors that relay vital information to the respiratory centers in the brainstem. When CO_2 levels increase and hypercapnia occurs, the chemoreceptors stimulate the body to breathe faster and deeper, thereby removing excess CO_2, which helps maintain a balanced blood pH and keep the body stable. It is particularly important during physical activity, as the body requires more oxygen and produces more CO_2.

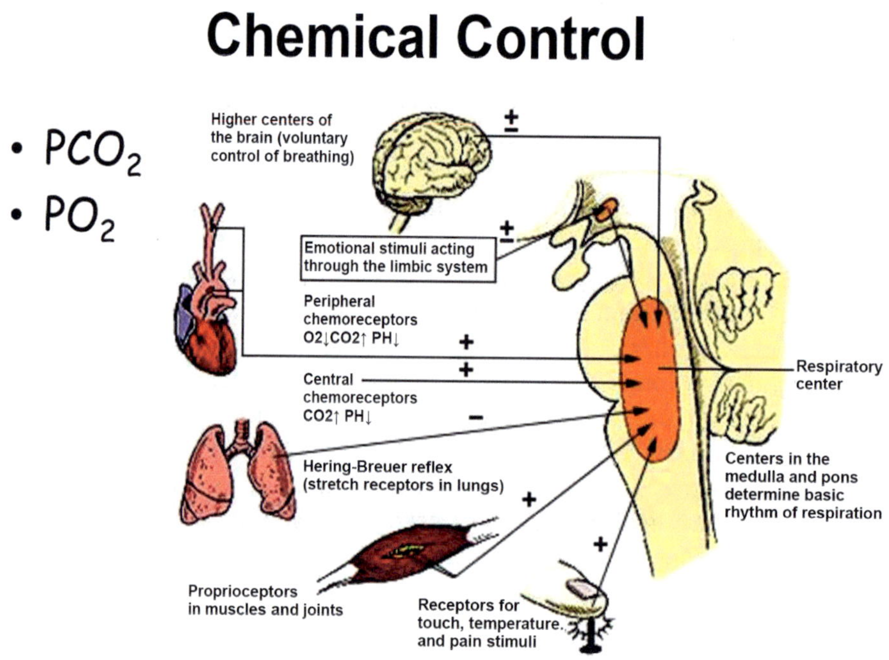

Figure 10.6. Chemical control.

Source: https://image.slideserve.com/764250/chemical-control-l.jpg.

The brain is crucial in regulating the numerous details of chemical balance and respiratory responses. The medulla oblongata and pons work together to receive signals from both peripheral and central chemoreceptors, which help the body respond appropriately to changes in blood gas levels. In addition, new research has pointed out that the way the brain is connected can strongly affect breathing control, especially in patients with sleep apnea after a stroke. Research indicates that enhanced thalamic connectivity in these individuals could influence networks responsible for both arousal and breathing control, as noted in findings showing increased functional coupling with brain regions involved in breathing modulation during sleep (Calistri et al., 2017). It means that problems with normal nerve pathways can seriously reduce breathing efficiency and lead to health issues.

Chemical processes that regulate breathing are also linked to sleep-related breathing disorders, which can impact the quality of life. When people have sleep apnea, the chemoreceptors may not respond appropriately to changes in oxygen and carbon dioxide, which is caused by the disruption of neural signals. It highlights the need to carefully investigate the effects of pathological changes on respiratory regulation. When patients exhibit excessive connectivity between sensory processing regions and areas involved in modulating respiratory patterns, it becomes clear that understanding these alterations may pave the way for targeted therapeutic interventions (Calistri et al., 2017). Thus, the study of chemical regulation is not only a matter of elucidating fundamental biological processes but is also crucial for developing strategies to mitigate the adverse effects of related respiratory ailments (Figure 10.6).

10.2.1. Role of Carbon Dioxide and Oxygen Levels

The regulation of breathing is intricately linked to the levels of carbon dioxide (CO_2) and oxygen (O2) in the bloodstream. The CNS, particularly the brainstem, plays a pivotal role in monitoring these gas levels. In the brainstem and peripheral arteries, chemoreceptors detect changes in the levels of CO_2 and O_2. If CO_2 levels rise, blood pH falls, prompting the body to increase its breathing rate and depth to remove the excess CO_2 and maintain balance. If oxygen levels are low, the body automatically increases breathing to obtain more oxygen, demonstrating that O_2 supply is a top priority. Having both gases watched by this system emphasizes their role in helping the body meet its metabolic needs. Rising CO_2 levels may also cause the airways to narrow because of their effect on airway hyperreactivity. Certain situations, such as anesthesia, clearly demonstrate how changes in CO_2 levels can lead to bronchospasm. In a real case, a patient who started bronchospasm after intubation was found to have low end-tidal $CO_{2,}$ which pointed to ineffective ventilation. It proves that not having enough oxygen and too much CO_2 in the air can quickly cause severe breathing problems, so quick action is necessary. In some cases, drugs are used to help alleviate both bronchospasm and CO_2 retention, emphasizing the importance of managing airways and gas exchange together in clinical practice. The need for vigilance in monitoring these levels cannot be overstated, particularly in anesthetic settings where the potential for life-threatening complications exists (Dewachter et al., 2011). In addition, managing carbon dioxide and oxygen levels is important in both hospitals and when exploring diseases of the respiratory system, such as asthma. Changes in these gases can make breathing more difficult and worsen breathing problems. Treatment of these conditions relies on administering oxygen and bronchodilators. Asthma symptoms are often managed by boosting oxygen levels and avoiding carbon dioxide accumulation, as occurs in COPD. To design the treatment, clinicians should understand how oxygen saturation, carbon dioxide levels, and respiratory rate interact with each other. Thus, the regulation of breathing, heavily influenced by these gas levels, is integral to maintaining respiratory health and addressing pathological states (Charles et al., 2019).

10.2.2. Importance of pH Balance in Blood

The significance of pH balance in blood cannot be overstated, particularly in the context of respiratory regulation. The ideal blood pH for human health is very narrow, ranging from 7.35 to 7.45, and this is very important for proper body function. Acidemia or alkalosis, which happen when the pH is outside the normal range, can cause problems for cells and organs. It is the respiratory system that ensures the blood has the right amount of CO_2. As CO_2 dissolves in blood, it forms carbonic acid (H_2CO_3), thus lowering pH. Therefore, good ventilation is necessary to maintain homeostasis; when the breathing rate increases, it helps eliminate CO_2 and raise blood pH, illustrating the strong link between respiration and acid-base balance. Additionally, the respiratory system plays a crucial role in maintaining the optimal acidity level in the blood, which supports the body's overall health and metabolism. Acidic byproducts are produced by metabolism, and they should be quickly buffered and removed from the body.

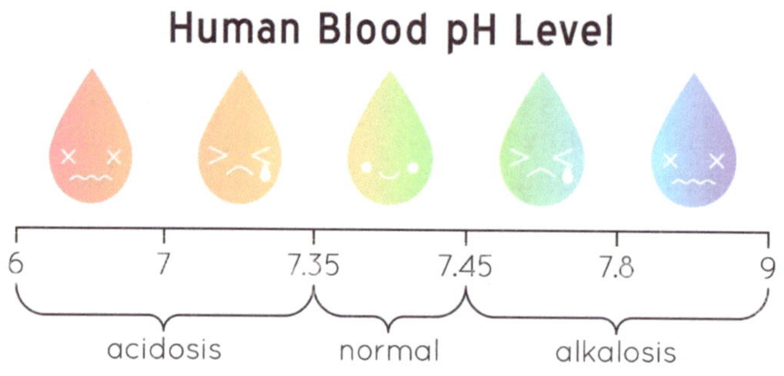

Figure 10.7. Human blood pH level.

Source: https://thumbs.dreamstime.com/z/human-blood-ph-scale-vector-diagram-acidic-to-normal-alkaline-rainbow-laboratory-paper-indicator-chemistry-science-concept-221278700.jpg.

The lungs ensure the body stays balanced by expelling CO_2, which directly affects the H_2CO_3 level in the blood. The way the respiratory system controls hydrogen ions and bicarbonate stresses the importance of respiration in maintaining acid-base balance. If the body needs more energy, such as during exercise, it increases its respiratory rate to ensure there is enough oxygen and to maintain a balanced pH. The ability of the respiratory system to adjust demonstrates the importance of a well-functioning regulatory system for life. Not maintaining the proper pH can cause problems for the nervous and muscular systems. If blood pH is outside the normal range, the nervous system may exhibit symptoms such as confusion, fatigue, or muscle twitches, which occur because neurons and muscle fibers are more or less excitable. Enzymes responsible for metabolism may not function properly when blood pH is abnormal which reduces energy and causes problems with function. Disruptions in neural activity can lead to issues with cognitive functions, illustrating the relationship between gas exchange and pH balance. In conclusion, the interdependence of the respiratory system and acid-base homeostasis is vital for maintaining not only physical health but also neurological integrity, thus demonstrating the essential nature of pH balance in blood in the broader context of respiratory regulation (Figure 10.7).

10.2.3. Interaction Between Respiratory and Metabolic Processes

The regulation of breathing is intricately linked to metabolic processes, reflecting a dynamic interaction that is essential for maintaining homeostasis. Oxygen is needed, and carbon dioxide is produced in cells as a result of metabolic activity. For example, while exercising, oxygen consumption increases as your muscles burn nutrients to generate energy. Due to the increased metabolism, the respiratory system works harder to maintain oxygen levels and remove more carbon dioxide. This relationship demonstrates that the body must adjust breathing to meet its energy needs and it shows that the two systems work together to allow the body to use oxygen and produce energy efficiently. The CNS is significant in connecting the respiratory and metabolic systems. There are respiratory centers in the brainstem that receive input from peripheral chemoreceptors, which are sensitive to changes in oxygen and carbon dioxide levels in the blood. The feedback loop is necessary because it guides the respiratory centers to adjust breathing in the correct manner. If metabolic activity causes more carbon dioxide to be produced, the respiratory centers increase breathing rate and depth to restore blood gas levels to normal. This system is not only responsive; it also anticipates needs, adjusting metabolism based on the bodyis activity and the environment, so that needs are met ahead of time. Therefore, the CNS helps control breathing and ties together the processes of respiration and metabolism. Additionally, disturbances in the interaction between these two systems can lead to significant changes in the body. Problems such as metabolic disorders, lung diseases, or exposure to harmful substances can impair the respiratory system's ability and, consequently, the body's metabolic efficiency. For instance, individuals exposed to pollutants such as polycyclic aromatic hydrocarbons (PAHs) may experience compromised lung function, which in turn affects oxygen delivery and carbon dioxide removal, resulting in altered metabolic states. Researchers are now discovering that the gut and its microbes play a role in both breathing and metabolism, which adds to the understanding of how these processes are controlled. Understanding these interconnections is crucial for developing therapeutic strategies that optimize respiratory and metabolic health, underscoring the need for a comprehensive approach in the study of respiratory regulation (Figure 10.8).

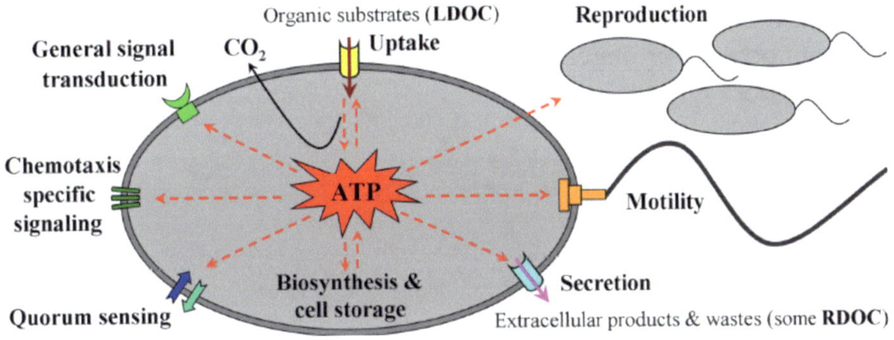

Figure 10.8. Schematic of metabolic energy transduction by microbial respiration and certain MCP-related cellular processes.

Source: https://www.researchgate.net/profile/Hongyue-Dang/publication/274684649/figure/fig1/AS:294851158528000@1447309402307/Schematic-of-metabolic-energy-transduction-by-microbial-respiration-and-certain.png.

10.3. Respiratory Reflexes

The intricate network of respiratory reflexes plays a crucial role in regulating breathing, ensuring that the body adapts effectively to varying physiological demands. The central command mechanism is central to the system because it starts and controls breathing when you are active. The higher brain centers monitor the body's need for oxygen and the need to eliminate carbon dioxide, which influences this reflex. As you engage in dynamic exercise, your body makes adjustments one after another to maintain oxygen and acid-base balance. This orchestration of respiratory reflexes exemplifies the body's ability to dynamically respond to both internal and external stimuli, thereby supporting metabolic activity during heightened physical demands and ensuring homeostasis remains intact through effective regulation of arterial blood pressure and ventilation (Crisafulli et al., 2014). Changes in blood chemistry are detected by the chemoreflex, which then controls the rate of breathing. In this reflex, the main central chemoreceptors are located in the medulla oblongata, which react to changes in carbon dioxide. The peripheral chemoreceptors, situated in the carotid and aortic bodies, are sensitive to both oxygen and carbon dioxide. When the body is active, these receptors stimulate the breathing centers, causing them to breathe faster and deeper, which facilitates gas exchange. The way these chemoreceptors interact suggests that metabolic signals can influence breathing control. Recent findings suggest that venous chemoreceptors may play a more significant role in regulating breathing and metabolism, which could be useful for understanding this process. Indeed, evidence suggests that these receptors may serve as significant sensors in managing the respiratory response to changing metabolic states (Parkes et al., 2017). It is also important that these reflexes are integrated, as they both respond to sudden physiological changes and help explain a range of health problems. If the body is in a diseased state, these reflexes might not function properly, which can result in problems such as being unable to exercise well or gas exchange troubles in those with respiratory problems. Knowing how the brain reacts and adapts reflexes during emergencies can help manage conditions that affect breathing. Also, scientists are still researching the ways in which respiratory reflexes work, and this is helping to adjust existing theories. This evolving knowledge base underscores the complexity of the regulatory processes involved in breathing, highlighting their relevance in both healthy and diseased states, and reflecting the importance of ongoing research in this area (Crisafulli et al., 2014; Parkes et al., 2017) (Figure 10.9).

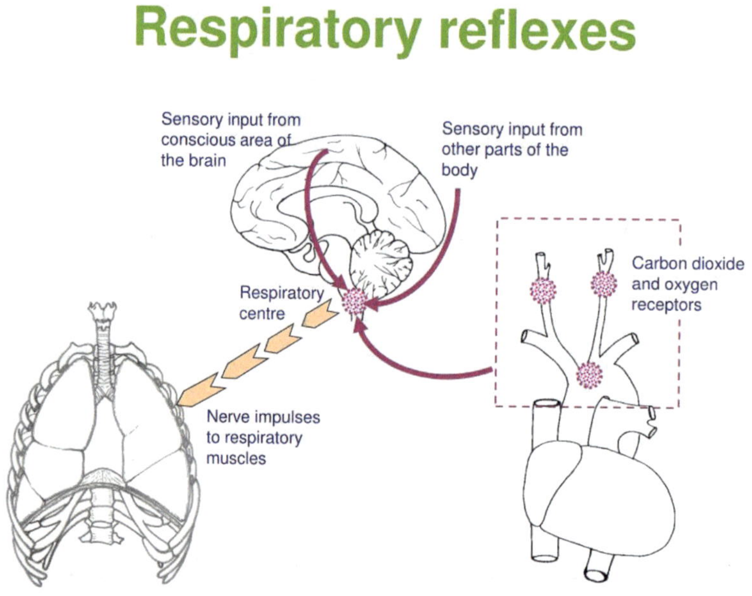

Figure 10.9. Respiratory reflexes.

Source: https://image2.slideserve.com/4059553/respiratory-reflexes1-l.jpg.

10.3.1. Overview of Protective Reflexes (E.g., Coughing, Sneezing)

Protective reflexes, such as coughing and sneezing, play a critical role in maintaining respiratory health by safeguarding the airways from various irritants and pathogens. Coughing is the main way the airway is defended and it is mainly set off by nociceptive stimuli.

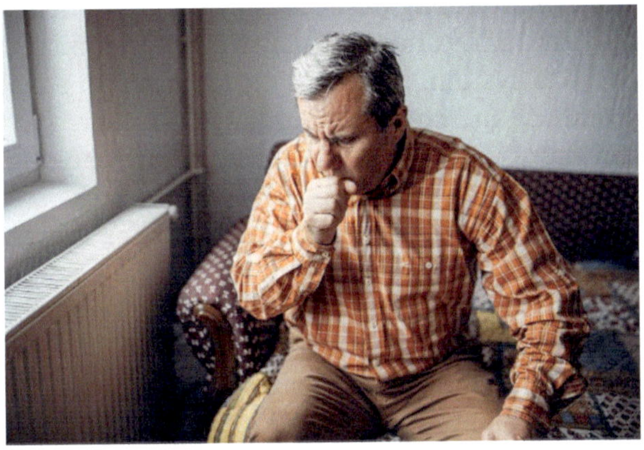

Figure 10.10. Coughing.

Source: https://www.hackensackmeridianhealth.org/-/media/project/hmh/hmh/public/healthu/healthu-images/education-stories/2023/03/2023-03-08.jpg?h=533&iar=0&w=800&hash=B007A4CF834C987BB5D7EEC71E56A6EA.

The process involves a complex interaction of neural pathways, particularly those found in the caudal ventral respiratory group (cVRG) of the brainstem. The region helps coordinate the exhalation needed to produce a strong cough. Korpáš and Tomori pointed out that this reflex calls for muscle contractions, and cVRG neurons coordinate the sequence of breathing in and out. Such precise neural coordination ensures that coughs are effective in clearing the airways, illustrating the central role of this reflex in respiratory regulation (Bongianni et al., 2020). Sneezing, which is less often studied than coughing, is also a valuable reflex that supports respiratory health. When irritants reach the nasal passages, it causes a reflex that makes air and particles leave the body through the nose and mouth. The mechanism begins when sensory fibers detect irritation; this information is relayed to the brain, which activates the appropriate motor pathways (Figure 10.10).

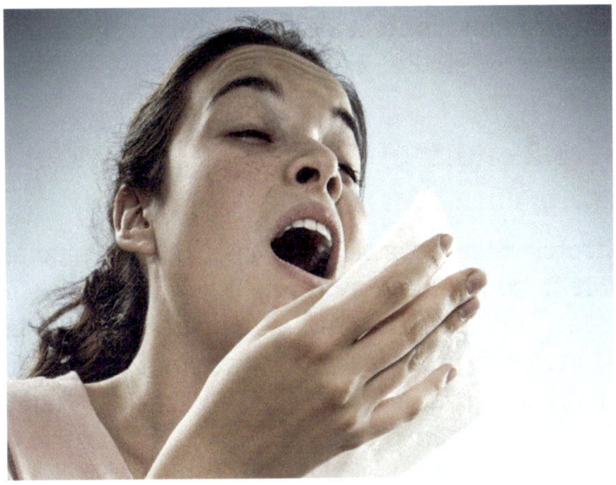

Figure 10.11. Sneezing.

Source: https://media-cldnry.s-nbcnews.com/image/upload/streams/2013/April/130423/6C7058857-tdy-130418-sneezing-stock-1.jpg.

Sneezing, like coughing, depends on several respiratory events, including inhaling deeply and then expelling air forcefully. The reflex helps clear irritants, such as pollen, dust, or pathogens, and also helps control airflow and pressure in the sinuses. Sneezing helps remove irritants from the air, which is crucial for maintaining the respiratory system's health and balance. Coughing and sneezing are examples of how the human body adapts to its environment, demonstrating that these behaviors are regulated by evolution. It has been found through research that the cough reflex which comes in mechanosensory and chemosensory forms, may have evolved to help people survive a variety of dangers to the lungs. Aδ. Aδ fibers trigger the mechanosensory reflex to prevent swallowing dangerous things, and the chemosensory cough, which is relayed by unmyelinated C fibers, helps protect against infectious agents and irritants. As people evolved, these reflexes became increasingly important for maintaining lung health in the face of air pollution and diseases. The synchronization of these protective reflexes underscores the intricate neuromuscular networks involved, ultimately highlighting their significance in the broader context of respiratory regulation (Brooks et al., 2011) (Figure 10.11).

10.3.2. Role of Stretch Receptors in Lung Function

Stretch receptors in the lungs play a crucial role in controlling breathing and maintaining a steady breathing rhythm as our needs change. Stretch receptors located in the smooth muscle of the airways and lungs play a crucial role in detecting when the lungs expand or contract. They give sensory information to the CNS, which helps control the rate and depth of breathing. When the lungs enlarge, stretch receptors send messages through afferent pathways to the brainstem, mainly the medulla oblongata and pons, which then control the diaphragm and intercostal muscles. This reflex prevents the lungs from being overstretched and injured, which helps the breathing pattern stay efficient. This coordination highlights how neural control in respiration functions and emphasizes the role of these receptors in maintaining stable breathing during various activities. Stretch receptors are important because they enable reflexes that help the airway narrow and prepare the body for environmental changes. Together with pulmonary stretch receptors, the Hering-Breuer reflex stops further inspiration when the lungs are fully inflated. It enables the body to intake the optimal amount of oxygen and eliminate the correct amount of carbon dioxide, thereby maintaining respiratory stability. Under certain situations, such as when exercising intensely or going to high altitudes, these receptors become more sensitive to maintain efficient gas exchange. The brain uses the information from stretch receptors to respond to outside changes, which improves how the lungs work and makes them more efficient. Therefore, the way these sensors interact is crucial for maintaining the respiratory system's well-regulation and enabling it to respond as needed to changes in the body and the environment. Moreover, stretch receptors have been implicated in influencing autonomic nervous system (ANS) activities, particularly related to stress responses and emotional regulation. Research suggests that altering breathing patterns may influence heart rate variability and the balance of the autonomic nervous system. For example, focusing on slow breathing and noticing your lungs fill and empty can increase parasympathetic activity, making you feel calm and reducing stress, which is a sign of good mental health. Research has shown that controlled breathing helps people engage their stretch receptors, which not only supports the lungs but also calms the nervous system, making individuals feel more emotionally stable. This connection between stretch receptor function and psychophysiological outcomes underscores the significance of understanding lung mechanics beyond basic respiratory physiology, particularly in therapeutic contexts that leverage breathing techniques for health benefits, thereby highlighting the multifaceted role of stretch receptors in lung function (Donald, 2022; Zaccaro et al., 2018).

10.3.3. Impact of Reflexes on Breathing Efficiency

Reflexes play a crucial role in ensuring efficient breathing during the body's various stages. These reflexes, for example, the cough reflex and the sneeze reflex, are important for keeping the airways open and facilitating gas exchange. For example, when irritants are present in the airway, the cough reflex is triggered, causing one to quickly expel air to clear the obstruction. It works to protect the airways in the moment and also helps breathing work better by making sure the airways are not blocked. Additionally, the coordination of breathing and swallowing demonstrates the close relationship between reflexes and regulating breathing, as the body adjusts its breathing to avoid aspiration and maintain a stable state. It is necessary to look at the role of the nervous system when studying the effect of reflexes on breathing. Studies have found that the CNS manages reflexes that help respiratory movements work together with swallowing.

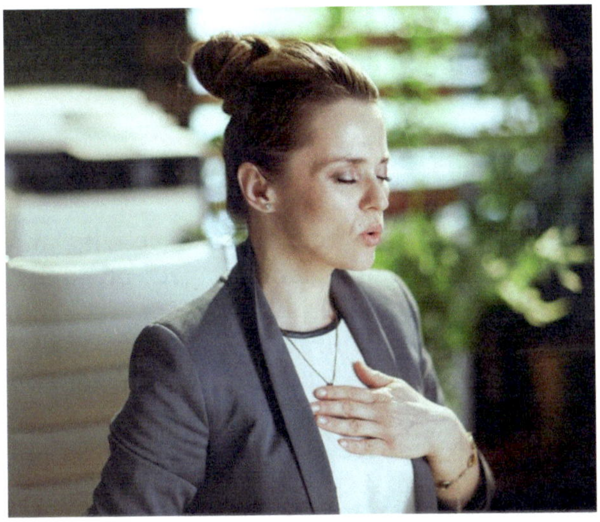

Figure 10.12. Practicing controlled breathing for stress management and respiratory regulation.

Source: https://media.licdn.com/dms/image/v2/D4D12AQEPWk7ekRJeLg/article-cover_image-shrink_720_1280/article-cover_image-shrink_720_1280/0/1711451382018?e=2147483647&v=beta&t=j2Q0ldRFuFQLaWJqP1CDw6bHyg9_PaOW_GQEKjJa1OU.

Studies of opioid effects on the respiratory system point out that there are reflex pathways that control both breathing and swallowing. It was discovered in a study of the upper aerodigestive tract that opioid use can reduce the airway's natural reflexes, which may cause patients to develop aspiration pneumonia. These findings underscore the complexity of neural interactions and their direct impact on both the efficiency of breathing and the integrity of airway protection mechanisms, as highlighted in Frazure et al. (2023). Additionally, the central and peripheral components of reflex actions can be influenced by factors such as age, gender, and various health conditions. It has been found that the responses to opioids may be quite different for males and females, which may influence the way respiratory reflexes work. The observations made in studies examining these variations illustrate that females may be more susceptible to opioid-induced respiratory depression, as found in Frazure et al. (2023). Due to the fact that breathing efficiency changes differently, there is a higher risk of respiratory problems. Understanding how these reflexive adaptations operate within the regulatory framework of breathing not only provides insight into the mechanics of respiration but also emphasizes the clinical importance of addressing how reflex actions contribute to respiratory health and the potential consequences of their disruption, as stated in (Figure 10.12).

10.4. Factors Affecting Breathing Regulation

A myriad of factors, both physiological and environmental influences breathing regulation. A key feature is the impact of metabolic processes on respiratory function. Conditions such as obesity and metabolic disorders can severely affect breathing patterns, with obstructive sleep apnea (OSA) being a prime example. Studies show that OSA is prevalent among individuals with obesity, impacting not only sleep quality but also contributing to the development of further complications such as cardiovascular diseases (CVDs) and diabetes. This bidirectional relationship between OSA and metabolic conditions underscores the importance of understanding the physiological mechanisms underlying breathing regulation, as interventions targeting these factors could improve overall health outcomes in affected populations (Arble et al., 2018). For this reason, examining these areas is crucial for designing effective strategies to manage both respiratory diseases and their associated health consequences. Besides metabolic reasons, psychological factors play a significant role in controlling breathing. When someone is stressed or anxious, they might change their breathing pattern and end up hyperventilating or breathing shallowly. These changes not only disrupt normal gas exchange but can also cause numerous other physiological changes that affect how the heart beats and how the body is regulated. It has been found through recent studies that pranayamic breathing encourages the body to use the parasympathetic system which can help manage stress-related changes.

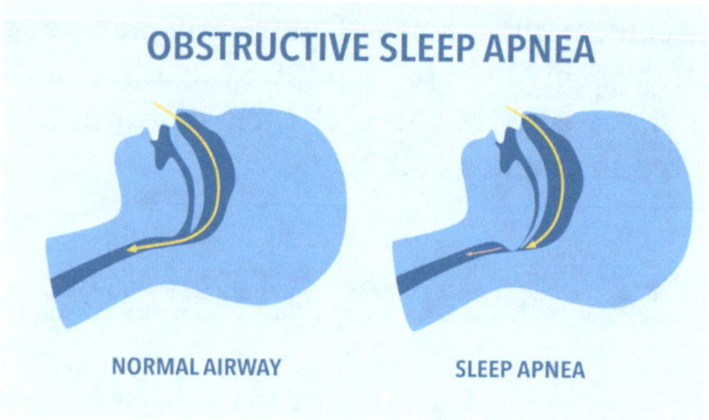

Figure 10.13. Obstructive sleep apnea (OSA).

Source: https://www.beaconhospital.com.my/wp-content/uploads/2024/07/Obstructive-Sleep-Apnea-scaled.webp.

This transition toward a more relaxed state is characterized by reduced heart rate and blood pressure, reflecting a shift in the ANSs balance (Austin et al., 2006). If we understand how emotions affect breathing, we can explore various ways to reduce anxiety and enhance lung health. Additionally, external factors in the environment also impact breathing regulation. Air quality, temperature, and altitude have a significant impact on respiratory patterns. Airway resistance can increase if someone is exposed to pollutants or allergens, which complicates the process of breathing. Those at high altitudes may also notice a change in their breathing rate because there is less oxygen available. The body needs to adjust the rate of breathing to maintain normal oxygen levels. Focusing on these environmental factors when planning treatments may boost the success of respiratory treatments. Therefore, recognizing the multifaceted influences on breathing regulation, including metabolic, psychological, and environmental factors, is essential for fostering a comprehensive understanding of respiratory health within the broader context of human physiology (Figure 10.13).

10.4.1. Influence of Physical Activity on Breathing

The interplay between physical activity and breathing is a fundamental aspect of human physiology that significantly impacts the regulation of respiratory function. Being physically active requires more oxygen, so breathing patterns must be adjusted. When you run or cycle, your breathing rate and the amount of air you take in go up to help your body take in more oxygen and release more carbon dioxide. Many neural and hormonal signals are involved in this dynamic process to maintain the body's balance. As a result, regular physical activity improves the function of your lungs and increases their capacity over time. When respiratory mechanics improve through training, both athletes and non-athletes can better control their breathing during intense activities, which supports improved performance and stamina. In addition to the physical changes brought about by exercise, the impact of exercise on breathing control is also substantial. Being physically active usually boosts your mood, which can improve your breathing. For example, meditation and yoga are practices that focus on breathing exercises, which help individuals relax and reduce stress. When these practices are combined with exercise, they lead to a harmonious functioning of the heart and lungs, which is beneficial for both the mind and body. In addition, using breathing exercises while exercising can reduce stress and make people more aware of themselves which supports a balanced ANS. When exercise and mindful breathing are combined, the positive effects include increased mental and emotional strength, promoting a balanced approach to overall health. It is crucial to regulate your breathing when exercising, as stress and anxiety can negatively impact your breathing. Many studies now show that stress can cause people to breathe in a shallow and rapid manner, which can worsen their anxiety and discomfort. When you use structured breathing during your workout, it can help you avoid these negative effects and support a state that promotes good recovery and relaxation. According to recent research, incorporating meditation and focused breathing into regular training routines can help mitigate the effects of stress on the body, suggesting that these practices should be included in daily training regimens. Ultimately, recognizing the profound influence of physical activity on breathing regulation not only enhances athletic performance but also promotes mental health, establishing a foundational connection vital to overall well-being (Barnes et al., 2015, 2016).

10.4.2. Effects of Altitude on Respiratory Function

The impact of altitude on respiratory function is a critical area of study, particularly in the context of human adaptation to lower atmospheric pressure and reduced oxygen availability. At higher altitudes, the barometric pressure drops, causing the oxygen partial pressure to be lower. When there is less oxygen, the body may increase its breathing rate to try to get more oxygen. At higher altitudes, the body must work harder to breathe, which can lead to changes in the volume of air inhaled and exhaled, as well as the rate of breathing. These adaptations are essential for maintaining adequate oxygen delivery to tissues, a process that becomes increasingly challenging as elevations surpass 2,500 meters. Beyond this threshold, individuals may begin experiencing symptoms indicative of acute mountain sickness and other high-altitude illnesses (Jean-Richalet, 2020). Additionally, research indicates that altitude can impact both the body's ability to exchange gases and the overall functioning of the respiratory system. For instance, not everyone can adjust well to high altitudes; some individuals may feel weaker and experience lower oxygen levels during exercise. When hypoxia occurs at high altitudes, the carotid chemoreceptors are activated, and this causes a person to hyperventilate to maintain their blood oxygen levels. Still, how many of these responses a person has depends on their own background, genes, and physical condition. The complex interplay between these factors highlights the need for comprehensive research to determine the precise effects of high altitude on respiratory physiology and the potential for interventions aimed at alleviating hypoxia-related complications (Gali et al., 2015). It is important to look at how altitude affects breathing, as this can have significant health effects, especially for people involved in sports and expeditions. Athletes who train at high altitudes often use hypoxic environments to improve their endurance and body changes, but there is still much discussion about which types of training are best such as normobaric or hypobaric conditions. Recent studies on the effects of stress and performance have found that different types of hypoxic environments can result in varying changes in breathing and oxygen use. Understanding these effects can inform training practices and health strategies to mitigate altitude-related risks while optimizing respiratory function in extreme environments (Jean-Richalet, 2020).

10.4.3. Impact of Environmental Factors (E.g., Pollution, Allergens)

Environmental factors, such as pollution and allergens, play a significant role in regulating breathing, particularly in terms of their impact on respiratory health. Many cities are filled with pollutants such as particulate matter, nitrogen dioxide, and ozone, which have been associated with both short-term and long-term breathing problems. Breathing in these pollutants can cause inflammation and worsen problems such as asthma and COPD. Children and the elderly are especially at risk because their lungs might respond more strongly to these stresses. The high prevalence of respiratory ailments in urban areas, such as the South Bronx, where residents face elevated pollution levels alongside poor housing conditions, demonstrates the urgent need to address these interconnected environmental issues and their impact on public health Allergens from pollen, mold, and pests exacerbate the problem of respiratory health. Such organic triggers may start an allergic response, causing symptoms that make it hard to breathe normally. For example, people in low-income neighborhoods with poor housing are more likely to be affected by allergens found in their homes, such as mold and cockroach droppings. In the South Bronx, the presence of numerous cockroaches in homes is common due to poor housing conditions, which in turn leads to an increase in asthma exacerbations. Moreover, external allergens such as pollen contribute to seasonal asthma peaks, intensifying the burden on respiratory health during specific times of the year. Therefore, it is crucial to investigate how these allergens impact breathing to inform more effective public health policies. More generally, environmental influences play a role in creating health policies to address breathing problems. Awareness of the relationship between allergens and pollution and their impact on disease burdens highlights the need for specific public policies. Because Africa faces multiple health issues simultaneously, it is crucial to address allergies and general diseases concurrently to enhance public health. Awareness of environmental triggers for breathing issues enables policymakers to initiate programs that address health problems now and improve the environment for the future. This multifaceted strategy can enhance the quality of life for vulnerable populations by reducing exposure to detrimental environmental factors while promoting health equity across communities (Figure 10.14).

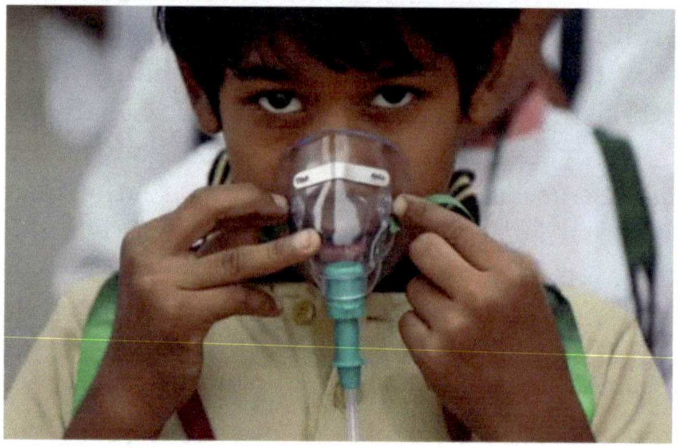

Figure 10.14. Child using an oxygen mask in response to air pollution exposure.

Source: https://ichef.bbci.co.uk/news/480/cpsprodpb/FFC5/production/_98677456_gettyimages-475812358.jpg.webp.

10.5. Disorders Related to Breathing Regulation

Problems with breathing regulation encompass various conditions that impair a person's ability to breathe correctly. Sleep apnea, COPD, and emphysema are examples of how breathing patterns can be changed. Sleep apnea is characterized by frequent pauses in breathing during sleep, which disrupts sleep and reduces the amount of oxygen in the blood. It leads to poor sleep and makes people feel exhausted and less able to think during the day. COPD and emphysema, however, damage the airways and airflow, so patients often feel out of breath when doing normal activities. All these disorders highlight the importance of correct breathing in maintaining health and well-being. Another important point is that disorders of breathing regulation can significantly impact a person's emotional and psychological state. Studies have shown that controlling breathing can significantly influence one's emotions, indicating a close link between the body and the mind. Those with chronic respiratory conditions tend to feel more anxious and depressed, which may make their symptoms worse and affect their compliance with treatment. Insomnia is particularly relevant in this context; it is prevalent among older adults and can lead to chronic sleep difficulties, further complicating the management of respiratory disorders (Estrine et al., 2003). Recognizing how these conditions can recur underscores the importance of adopting an approach that addresses both breathing and mental health issues. Additionally, recent developments in imaging technology have highlighted the CNS's role in controlling breathing and disorders associated with it. Experiments using functional neuroimaging have identified brain areas that regulate breathing and emotions. For instance, increased activity in areas such as the amygdala and striatum has been observed when individuals engage in tasks that modulate cardiovascular arousal, suggesting a connection between emotional states and physiological responses, including heart rate and breathing (Asmundson et al., 2015). The results suggest that biofeedback could be used to help individuals regulate their breathing and improve their emotional well-being, which may be particularly beneficial for those with breathing regulation disorders. As breathing disorders involve the brain, body, and feelings – managing them is not simple.

10.5.1. Overview of Common Respiratory Disorders (E.g., Asthma, COPD)

Asthma and COPD are two prevalent respiratory disorders that significantly impact the regulation of breathing. The primary symptoms of asthma include wheezing, difficulty breathing, a tight chest, and coughing, as the airways become inflamed and narrow. The symptoms may change in severity and can be triggered by environmental factors such as allergens, smoke, and pollution. Unlike asthma, COPD encompasses several lung diseases, including emphysema and chronic bronchitis, that impede airflow and impact breathing. Mainly, this is caused by years of exposure to dangerous particles, mainly from smoking. Both disorders present unique challenges in treatment and management, often requiring a combination of pharmacological interventions, lifestyle modifications, and pulmonary rehabilitation (PR) to improve respiratory function and enhance patient quality of life. It is crucial to understand the causes of these respiratory disorders to develop more effective treatment methods. When asthma is not treated, the airways become hyperreactive and undergo inflammation which results in airway remodeling. In addition, asthma attacks or exacerbations can become very serious and require prompt medical attention. The decline in lung function caused by COPD over time emphasizes the importance of early detection and treatment. Patients usually have exacerbations, and their symptoms tend to get worse when they are exposed to infections or changes in the environment. The clinical management of both conditions emphasizes the importance of personalized treatment plans, which may incorporate inhaled corticosteroids (ICSs) for asthma and bronchodilators for COPD, with the goal of maximizing lung function and minimizing symptoms. Also, using rehabilitation and holistic methods like yoga and pranayama has become popular for managing these disorders. Studies have found that breathing exercises can help people with asthma and COPD by improving lung function and reducing their symptoms, showing the importance of controlling breathing. It is known that diaphragmatic breathing and alternate nostril breathing can help people relax and enhance their breathing efficiency. If these exercises are performed regularly, they can significantly help individuals with chronic conditions that reduce lung capacity. Consequently, integrating such practices into conventional treatment regimens presents a promising avenue for enhancing patient outcomes and promoting overall well-being in individuals with respiratory disorders, particularly in light of current healthcare challenges (Dhaniwala et al., 2020; Donald, 2022).

10.5.2. Impact of Neurological Conditions on Breathing

Neurological conditions can significantly disrupt the complex mechanisms that regulate breathing, often resulting in severe respiratory complications. The control of breathing is managed by neural pathways that go from the brainstem to the respiratory muscles. In conditions such as amyotrophic lateral sclerosis (ALS), multiple sclerosis (MS), and spinal cord injuries, the efficacy of these neural connections can be compromised. As an example, ALS damages motor neurons, which might result in muscle weakness or paralysis, making it hard for the diaphragm to function correctly and breathe normally. Additionally, when someone has a stroke, it can disrupt the parts of the brainstem that control breathing, making it harder to maintain oxygen and carbon dioxide levels. Since neurological problems and breathing issues are often linked, it is essential to employ comprehensive assessment and treatment plans for these patients. Neurological problems can influence breathing by changing the control and strength of respiration. Neurological issues often result in abnormal chemoreception, which means the brain does not respond effectively to changes in carbon dioxide and oxygen levels. Sometimes, those with severe brain injuries do not respond well to increased carbon dioxide, which can cause respiratory acidosis and have effects throughout the body. Also, diseases such as Parkinson's disease can cause problems with how the body regulates breathing, which can make it more challenging to manage respiration. Proper monitoring and the right treatments are necessary to fix these autonomic problems and improve breathing, since neurological health and lung function are closely linked. The mental effects of neurological disorders can affect how well the lungs function. Many patients feel anxious and stressed, which can make their breathing problems worse. strong. Individuals with long-term neurological conditions are more susceptible to respiratory infections due to their weakened coughing and airway defense mechanisms. Mental stress can make breathing more difficult, since anxiety can cause people to breathe less deeply or panic, which reduces the amount of air they take in. Working on both the brain and mental aspects is important for improving respiratory health. Approaches in therapy should be based on this dual perspective to help patients achieve better outcomes and a better quality of life. Proper management strategies are crucial for avoiding complications associated with respiratory function in conjunction with neurological conditions, underscoring the need for interdisciplinary care models in clinical practice (Figure 10.15).

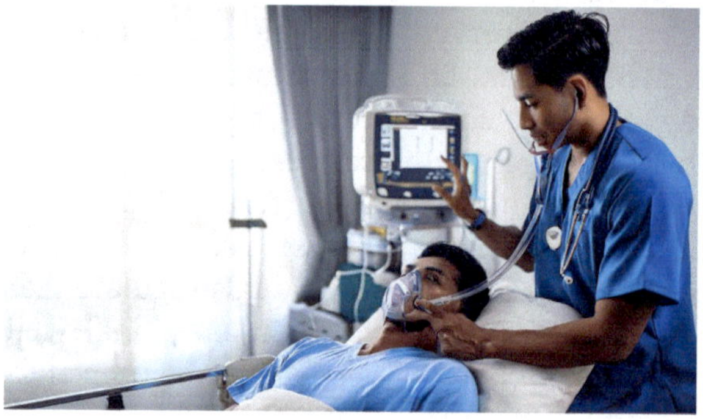

Figure 10.15. Nurse adjusting patients breathing apparatus monitoring their oxygen.

Source: https://citineurocentre.com/wp-content/uploads/2025/04/nurse-adjusting-patients-breathing-apparatus-monitoring-their-oxygen-1024x585.jpg.

10.5.3. Treatment Options and Management Strategies

The regulation of breathing encompasses various treatment options and management strategies that are critical for individuals suffering from respiratory conditions. Among the most common treatments are bronchodilators and corticosteroids, which help ease symptoms and reduce inflammation in the airways. They are used in asthma and COPD to improve breathing and raise the quality of life for patients. Additionally, PR methods are important because they encompass exercise, nutrition advice, and education on how to manage the disease. By using a holistic approach, health professionals can design these solutions to fit each patient, which improves their breathing and enables them to participate in more daily activities. Besides medicine and therapy, making specific lifestyle changes is crucial for controlling breathing. Smoking cessation and avoidance of pollutants are commonly recommended to patients, as they can exacerbate breathing problems. Additionally, incorporating physical activity into a daily routine helps strengthen the lungs and makes them more resilient to disease. What you eat is important, since a diet high in antioxidants can decrease inflammation and support your lung health. It is important to use psychological support and learn stress management, because anxiety might make it harder for the lungs to work correctly. When they recognize the relationship between these factors, healthcare providers can design plans that handle both the physical and mental health issues of respiratory patients. Utilizing advanced technologies to manage breathing is becoming a growing field. Using telemedicine and remote monitoring has helped patients adhere to their treatment plans and receive assistance promptly when needed. With telehealth, doctors can monitor patients in real-time and change treatments as needed. Additionally, these devices can help monitor a person's vital signs and breathing, which can inform personalized treatment plans. Using these approaches, established treatments can be made more effective, allowing patients to receive the care they need as their needs change. As scientists continue to discover more, these technologies are likely to continue shaping how respiratory health is managed, ultimately benefiting patients and improving their lives.

SUMMARY

It is essential to emphasize that respiration is regulated by both the body's internal systems and external influences. Breathing is not only controlled by the body automatically; it also depends on feedback systems responding to changes in the environment, metabolism, and health. It makes it possible to recognize the difficulties that some populations, such as preterm and low birth weight infants, experience. Their trouble breathing can result in various health problems, as research indicates that their lungs are not fully developed. Thus, the importance of specialized care becomes evident, as understanding risk factors enables healthcare professionals to tailor interventions to improve neonatal outcomes (Ap, 2024). Nasal breathing and its effect on metabolism point to the broader role respiratory physiology plays in overall health. A growing body of research, as shown in recent studies, reveals that nasal breathing can have a significant impact on metabolic rate, which might impact how much energy the body uses and how it regulates metabolism. Once the metabolic profiles of the subjects changed after nasal surgery, it was clear that the efficiency of breathing can affect more than just oxygen exchange in the body. This finding reinforces the importance of understanding the nuances of breathing regulation, as it has implications for both individual health and the effectiveness of medical interventions (Alves et al., 2024). All in all, the regulation of breathing involves several key components that are essential for both breathing and metabolism. Looking at at-risk populations such as premature infants and understanding how nasal breathing affects metabolism proves that a thorough approach to respiratory care is necessary. Researchers can continue to explore the importance of respiratory regulation for health and disease management, which will aid in the development of successful clinical treatments. Taking this approach helps us see the big picture of respiratory function, which proves the need to keep researching to benefit patients from all walks of life.

When we study how breathing is regulated, we discover several important mechanisms that describe the interaction between the body and the nervous system, enabling steady breathing. The regulation of breathing mainly depends on the ANS and the brainstem, especially the medulla oblongata and pons. These brain areas send messages to the diaphragm and intercostal muscles, which help with breathing in and breathing out. The medulla and peripheral arteries have chemoreceptors that sense changes in CO_2, O_2, and pH in the blood, and these adjust the breathing rate to maintain proper gas exchange. The way signals between neurons and chemicals are connected is crucial for matching respiration to the body's energy needs, illustrating the complexity of respiratory regulation. Pulmonary reflexes are also essential in regulating breathing because they provide immediate responses to changes in the lungs and their chemical composition. As an illustration, the Hering-Breuer reflex stops the lungs from overinflating by blocking signals for inhalation when stretch receptors in the airways sense that the lungs are too full. In addition, receptors in the lungs and airways can trigger coughing or sneezing to help remove any blockages that may be obstructing the airways. It emphasizes that the body can defend the respiratory system and ensure efficient gas exchange at the same time. They demonstrate how the nervous system and the body's mechanics work together to control breathing in response to your actions and the body's needs. The topic of regulating breathing examines how environmental factors and personal differences can impact breathing. Factors such as altitude, temperature, and environmental pollution can significantly alter breathing habits and the body's adjustment process.

CLOSER LOOK

HYPOXIC VENTILATORY RESPONSE (HVR)

The HVR is a physiological reflex that increases breathing rate and depth in response to low oxygen levels, primarily triggered by carotid body chemoreceptors. It is a crucial adaptation for the body to maintain adequate oxygen intake during hypoxia. The HVR is not a single, uniform response but rather a complex interplay of mechanisms that can change over time, depending on the duration and intensity of hypoxic exposure.

1. **Activation:** The HVR is initiated when peripheral chemoreceptors, primarily located in the carotid bodies, detect a decrease in arterial oxygen partial pressure (PaO_2).
2. **Mechanisms:** The response involves a cascade of events, including:

- Increased central respiratory drive, leading to faster and deeper breaths.
- Activation of the respiratory muscles, which can include the accessory muscles of respiration.
- Changes in the rate and depth of breathing to improve gas exchange in the lungs.

3. **Time Domains:** The HVR can be categorized into different time domains:

- **Acute Hypoxic Response**: The initial, rapid increase in ventilation triggered by low oxygen.
- **Hypoxic Ventilatory Decline (HVD)**: A gradual decrease in the ventilatory response after initial exposure to hypoxia.
- **Ventilatory Acclimatization to Hypoxia (VAH)**: Long-term adjustments in breathing patterns in response to chronic hypoxia, often seen during altitude acclimatization.

4. **Factors Affecting HVR**

- **Altitude**: HVR is significantly elevated at high altitude compared to sea level.
- **Individual Differences**: There are substantial differences in HVR sensitivity among individuals, influenced by factors such as genetics and fitness levels.
- **Age**: HVR can be altered during critical periods, such as infancy, when environmental factors can cause long-term changes in the respiratory system.

5. **Clinical Relevance:** The HVR is a key factor in understanding conditions related to hypoxia, including:

- **Altitude Sickness**: The HVR is a crucial factor in how the body adapts to high altitudes, but excessive HVR can contribute to altitude sickness.
- **Sleep Apnea**: Changes in HVR during sleep can contribute to the respiratory instability seen in OSA.
- **Exercise and Physical Activity**: HVR plays a role in how the body regulates breathing during exercise, and blunted HVR can limit exercise performance.

REFERENCES

1. Abdel-Shafy, H. I., & Mansour, M. S. (2015). A review on polycyclic aromatic hydrocarbons: Source, environmental impact, effect on human health and remediation. *Egyptian Journal of Petroleum, 25*(1), 107–123. https://doi.org/10.1016/j.ejpe.2015.03.011Ackland, D., Akopyan, G., Banzett, R., Bertrand, D., Bianchi, A., Brannan, J., Cavanna, A., et al. (2010). *Sub-Cortical and Brainstem Sites Associated with Chemo-Stimulated Increases in Ventilation in Humans.* https://core.ac.uk/download/10507.pdf (accessed on 31st May 2025).
2. Adams, R., Araujo, L., Araujo, J., Asmah, R., Breman, W., Brugman, H., Butler, M., et al. (2010). *Allergic Disorders in Africa and Africans: Is it Primarily a Priority?* https://core.ac.uk/download/pdf/18410775.pdf (accessed on 31st May 2025).
3. Alves de, S. F., Correia, J. T., Ferreira, M., Rios, M., Magalhães, M., & Santos, M. (2024). Nasal breathing: A neglected factor in metabolic regulation? *European Archives of Oto-Rhino-Laryngology, 282*, 869–879. https://www.semanticscholar.org/paper/adcfa50f510af01c398e1e0e4419d3f9c68a17be (accessed on 31st May 2025).
4. Ap, E. (2024). Risk factors and complications in premature and low birth weight newborns. *Trends in Nursing and Health Care Research*. https://www.semanticscholar.org/paper/a264c08bc8192072889e0f886ad61fdd32a68141 (accessed on 31st May 2025).
5. Arble, D. M., & Framnes, S. N. (2018). *The Bidirectional Relationship Between Obstructive Sleep Apnea and Metabolic Disease.* https://core.ac.uk/download/213087655.pdf (accessed on 31st May 2025).
6. Asmundson, G. J. G., Beacher, F. D. C., Beauregard, M., Beck, A. T., Beck, J. G., Beer, J. S., Bonn, M., et al. (2015). *Neuroanatomical Substrates for the Volitional Regulation of Heart Rate.* https://core.ac.uk/download/30611430.pdf (accessed on 31st May 2025).
7. Austin, D., Benson, H., Bhargava, R., Bhattacharya, R., Bijlani, R., Brown, K., Busek, P., et al. (2006). Physiology of long pranayamic breathing: Neural respiratory elements may provide a mechanism that explains how slow deep breathing shifts the autonomic nervous system. *Med. Hypotheses.* https://core.ac.uk/download/131210060.pdf (accessed on 31st May 2025).
8. Baig, A. M. (2020). Computing the effects of SARS-CoV-2 on respiration regulatory mechanisms in COVID-19. *ACS Chemical Neuroscience, 11*, 2416–2421. https://doi.org/10.1021/acschemneuro.0c00349 (accessed on 31st May 2025).
9. Barnes, V. A., Cearley, S. M., Jensen, M., Ravinder, S., et al. (2016). *Meditation Experiences, Self, and Boundaries of Consciousness.* https://core.ac.uk/download/131210053.pdf (accessed on 31st May 2025).
10. Barnes, V. A., Cearley, S. M., Junca, S., Ravinder, S., et al. (2017). The dynamic role of breathing and cellular membrane potentials in the experience of consciousness. World Journal of Neuroscience. https://core.ac.uk/download/131210584.pdf (accessed on 31st May 2025).
11. Barnes, V. A., Crawford, M. W., Harden, K., Ravinder, S., et al. (2014). *Widespread Depolarization During Expiration: A Source of Respiratory Drive?* https://core.ac.uk/download/131210052.pdf (accessed on 31st May 2025).
12. Barnes, V. A., Crawford, M. W., Harden, K., Ravinder, S., et al. (2015). *Self-Regulation of Breathing as a Primary Treatment for Anxiety*. https://core.ac.uk/download/131210063.pdf (accessed on 31st May 2025).

13. Bongianni, F., Cinelli, E., Iovino, L., Mutolo, D., et al. (2020). Essential role of the cVRG in the generation of both the expiratory and inspiratory components of the cough reflex. *Physiol. Res.* https://core.ac.uk/download/326839841.pdf (accessed on 31st May 2025).

14. Brooks, S. M. (2011). *Perspective on the Human Cough Reflex.* https://core.ac.uk/download/pdf/8655062.pdf (accessed on 31st May 2025).

15. Calistri, V., Caramia, F., De Lena, C., Di Mascio, M., et al. (2017). Resting state functional thalamic connectivity abnormalities in patients with post-stroke sleep apnea: A pilot case-control study. https://core.ac.uk/download/98345696.pdf (accessed on 31st May 2025).

16. Camacho-Ordonez, N., Ramirez, N., Posadas-Cantera, S., Caballero-Oyteza, A., Fliegauf, M., Zhao, F., Guarini, M., et al. (2022). *Integrated Multi-Omics Analyses of NFKB1 Patients B Cells Points Towards an up Regulation of NF-κB Network Inhibitors.* bioRxiv. https://www.semanticscholar.org/paper/6ed7876cdbfe3a9e7b5599934971ed530ecd9cd5 (accessed on 31st May 2025).

17. Carr, J. A., Nguyen, J., Pamenter, M. E., Powell, F. L., et al. (2014). The effect of combined glutamate receptor blockade in the NTS on the hypoxic ventilatory response in awake rats differs from the effect of individual glutamate receptor blockade. *Physiol. Rep.* https://core.ac.uk/download/323066789.pdf (accessed on 31st May 2025).

18. Coté, C. J., & Wilson, S. (2019). Guidelines for monitoring and management of pediatric patients before, during, and after sedation for diagnostic and therapeutic procedures. *Pediatrics, 143.* https://doi.org/10.1542/peds.2019-1000 (accessed on 31st May 2025).

19. Crisafulli, A., Marongiu, E., Nobrega, A. C. L., O'Leary, D. S., et al. (2014). Neural regulation of cardiovascular response to exercise: Role of central command and peripheral afferents. *Biomed. Res. Int.* https://core.ac.uk/download/pdf/54599119.pdf (accessed on 31st May 2025).

20. Cryan, J. F., O'Riordan, K. J., Cowan, C. S. M., Sandhu, K. V., Bastiaanssen, T. F. S., Boehme, M., Codagnone, M. G., et al. (2019). The microbiota-gut-brain axis. *Physiological Reviews, 99,* 1877–2013. https://doi.org/10.1152/physrev.00018.2018 (accessed on 31st May 2025).

21. Dewachter, P., Mouton-Faivre, C., Emala, C. W., Béloucif, S., & Riou, B. (2011). Case scenario: Bronchospasm during anesthetic induction. *Anesthesiology, 114,* 1200–1210. https://doi.org/10.1097/aln.0b013e3182172cd3 (accessed on 31st May 2025).

22. Dhaniwala, N. K. S., Dasari, V., & Dhaniwala, M. N. (2020). Pranayama and breathing exercises – Types and its role in disease prevention & rehabilitation. *Journal of Evolution of Medical and Dental Sciences, 9,* 3325–3330. https://doi.org/10.14260/jemds/2020/730 (accessed on 31st May 2025).

23. Estrine, J., & O'Brien, N. (2003). *Sleep, Health, and Aging.* https://core.ac.uk/download/71356671.pdf (accessed on 31st May 2025).

24. Frazure, M. L. (2023). *Swallow, Breathing and Survival: Sex-Specific Effects of Opioids.* https://core.ac.uk/download/588595902.pdf (accessed on 31st May 2025).

25. Galiè, N., Humbert, M., Vachiéry, J. L., Gibbs, S., Lang, I., Torbicki, A., Simonneau, G., et al. (2015). 2015 ESC/ERS guidelines for the diagnosis and treatment of pulmonary hypertension. *European Heart Journal, 37,* 67–119. https://doi.org/10.1093/eurheartj/ehv317 (accessed on 31st May 2025).

26. Ingber, D. E. (2022). Human organs-on-chips for disease modelling, drug development and personalized medicine. *Nature Reviews Genetics, 23,* 467–491. https://doi.org/10.1038/s41576-022-00466-9 (accessed on 31st May 2025).

27. Jiménez-Gómez, B., Ortega-Sáenz, P., Gao, L., González-Rodríguez, P., García-Flores, P., Chandel, N. S., & López-Barneo, J. (2023). Transgenic NADH dehydrogenase restores oxygen regulation of breathing in mitochondrial complex I-deficient mice. *Nature Communications, 14.* https://doi.org/10.1038/s41467-023-36894-2 (accessed on 31st May 2025).

28. Khalsa, S. S., Adolphs, R., Cameron, O. G., Critchley, H., Davenport, P. W., Feinstein, J. S., Feusner, J. D., et al. (2017). Interoception and mental health: A roadmap. *Biological Psychiatry: Cognitive Neuroscience and Neuroimaging, 3,* 501–513. https://doi.org/10.1016/j.bpsc.2017.12.004 (accessed on 31st May 2025).

29. Lavretsky, H., & Feldman, J. (2021). Precision medicine for breath-focused mind-body therapies for stress and anxiety: Are we ready yet? *Global Advances in Health and Medicine, 10.* https://www.semanticscholar.org/paper/fe68d6246f1655f2542ab1ecd0320d0a3b758d9e (accessed on 31st May 2025).

30. Machhi, J., Herskovitz, J., Senan, A. M., Dutta, D., Nath, B., Oleynikov, M., Blomberg, W. R., et al. (2020). The natural history, pathobiology, and clinical manifestations of SARS-CoV-2 infections. *Journal of Neuroimmune Pharmacology, 15,* 359–386. https://doi.org/10.1007/s11481-020-09944-5 (accessed on 31st May 2025).

31. McCartney, A. M., Phillips, D., James, M., Chan, O., Neder, J., de-Torres, J., Domnik, N., et al. (2022). Ventilatory neural drive in chronically hypercapnic patients with COPD: Effects of sleep and nocturnal noninvasive ventilation. *European Respiratory Review, 31.* https://www.semanticscholar.org/paper/26c0da1bf2dd448b23297ecc28c67cf2a4de4b81 (accessed on 31st May 2025).

32. N/A. (2011). *South Bronx Residents Solution on Greening Our Hood.* https://core.ac.uk/download/71361702.pdf (accessed on 31st May 2025).

33. N/A. (2025). *Aerospace Medicine and Biology: A Continuing Bibliography with Indexes, Supplement 125.* https://core.ac.uk/download/pdf/42897953.pdf (accessed on 31st May 2025).

34. Nord, C. L., & Garfinkel, S. N. (2022). Interoceptive pathways to understand and treat mental health conditions. *Trends in Cognitive Sciences, 26,* 499–513. https://doi.org/10.1016/j.tics.2022.03.004 (accessed on 31st May 2025).

35. Parkes, M. (2017). *Reappraisal of Systemic Venous Chemoreceptors—Might Venous Chemoreceptors Have Been Controlling Breathing all the Time?* https://core.ac.uk/download/267302079.pdf (accessed on 31st May 2025).

36. Percie Du, S. N., Ahluwalia, A., Alam, S., Avey, M. T., Baker, M., Browne, W. J., Clark, A., et al. (2020). Reporting animal research: Explanation and elaboration for the ARRIVE guidelines 2.0. *PLoS Biology, 18,* e3000411–e3000411. https://doi.org/10.1371/journal.pbio.3000411 (accessed on 31st May 2025).

37. Richalet, J.-P. (2020). CrossTalk opposing view: Barometric pressure, independent of, is not the forgotten parameter in altitude physiology and mountain medicine. *The Journal of Physiology, 598,* 897–899. https://doi.org/10.1113/jp279160 (accessed on 31st May 2025).

38. Sokolov, A. (2022). Issues of the improvement of the legal regulation of the academic titles. *European Proceedings of Social and Behavioral Sciences.* https://www.semanticscholar.org/paper/b0d3271c38c00aaf8de8131ff36bf8b986489760 (accessed on 31st May 2025).

39. Svanström, M., Heimersson, S., Peters, G., Peters, G., Harder, R., I'Ons, D., Finnson, A., et al. (2017). Life cycle assessment of sludge management with phosphorus utilization and improved hygienization in Sweden. *Water Science and Technology: A Journal of the International Association on Water Pollution Research*, *75*(9, 10), 2013–2024. https://www.semanticscholar.org/paper/4b2016dda0ef64bc141634ddeea2bb9ca592ad89 (accessed on 31st May 2025).

40. Van Puyvelde, M., Neyt, X., McGlone, F., & Pattyn, N. (2018). Voice stress analysis: A new framework for voice and effort in human performance. *Frontiers in Psychology*, *9*. https://doi.org/10.3389/fpsyg.2018.01994 (accessed on 31st May 2025).

41. Wassey, S. A., Shafeeq, S., Butt, J. A., Jamil, A. (2022). Remediation of polychlorinated biphenyls (PCBs) through bio and phytoremediation in the environment: A review study. *International Journal of Economic and Environmental Geology*. https://www.semanticscholar.org/paper/73635a8560c2da92aa55b34a9bf1c8ce45e7caa7 (accessed on 31st May 2025).

42. Zaccaro, A., Piarulli, A., Laurino, M., Garbella, E., Menicucci, D., Neri, B., & Gemignani, A. (2018). How breath-control can change your life: A systematic review on psycho-physiological correlates of slow breathing. *Frontiers in Human Neuroscience*, *12*. https://doi.org/10.3389/fnhum.2018.00353 (accessed on 31st May 2025).

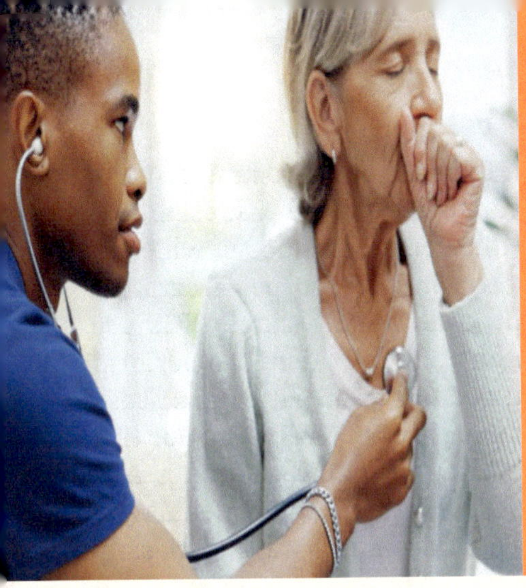

Chapter 11

PULMONARY FUNCTION TESTS (PFTS)

Contents

Introduction

Pulmonary function tests (PFTs) serve as an essential tool in assessing and managing respiratory diseases, providing critical data on lung capacity and airflow. Spirometry, lung volume measurement, and assessing diffusion capacity are some of the methods these tests use. Spirometry enables doctors to assess a patient's ability to breathe in and out, allowing them to identify any obstructions or restrictions in lung function. The results gleaned from these tests are pivotal in diagnosing conditions such as asthma, chronic obstructive pulmonary disease (COPD), and interstitial lung diseases (ILDs). In addition, PFTs are crucial for monitoring the progression of a disease and determining if treatment is effective, making them essential in medical care. Therefore, it is crucial for healthcare providers to understand how to accurately interpret these tests to deliver the best possible respiratory care. Experts in pulmonary medicine have recently emphasized the importance of rethinking the standard interpretation of PFT results. Current American Thoracic Society (ATS) standards recommend race and ethnicity-specific reference equations, a practice that is increasingly scrutinized for its potential to perpetuate health disparities. Some argue that using racial categories in PFT interpretation does not reveal the main social reasons for health such as environmental and economic factors. In turn, the ATS organized a workshop in 2021 and proposed the use of race-neutral average reference equations. This shift aims to ensure that pulmonary function interpretation is fairer which can lead to a new review of how PFTs affect medical and insurance decisions. Therefore, a discussion about PFT interpretation is now necessary and crucial for promoting health equity. Additionally, utilizing PFTs in clinical practice necessitates understanding their impact on patient health and the broader community. For children and adults with conditions like sickle cell disease (SCD), the uncertainty surrounding screening and management approaches can lead to significant variability in health outcomes. As PFTs help provide indicators of how the heart and lungs are working in these patients, their correct use can lead to more effective prevention and management. It is essential that healthcare providers understand how to utilize PFT to manage diseases and monitor changes in cardiopulmonary conditions effectively. Learning new skills in interpreting PFTs helps providers, which leads to improved care and quality of life for people with chronic lung diseases. The intense focus on education and research demonstrates the importance of PFTs in comprehensive healthcare.

Definition of Pulmonary Function Tests

PFTs are essential for evaluating the health and function of the lungs and respiratory system. Most of these tests are designed to measure lung volumes, capacities, airflow, and gas exchange, giving a complete view of how the lungs are functioning. By checking lung function, PFTs can help find out if someone has asthma, COPD, or a restrictive lung disease. The information from these assessments helps create a differential diagnosis, which is necessary for choosing the proper treatment for each patient. Additionally, since PFTs are non-invasive, healthcare providers can perform them multiple times to track a patient's disease progression or the effects of treatment. For this reason, PFTs are key in medical settings and play a significant role in managing patients with lung diseases. There are many ways to classify PFTs and each type has its own benefits and uses. Spirometry is commonly used because it measures the volume of air exhaled and the rate at which it is exhaled, which can signal problems such as obstructive or restrictive lung diseases. Tests like measuring lung volumes and diffusion capacity play a significant role in learning about the lungs' structure and function. Though spirometry can provide many details, a complete evaluation often includes several tests to see the lungs from all angles. Using different approaches helps doctors identify complex lung problems early, allowing them to be managed quickly. The advancement of pulmonary medicine leads to the use of new tools and methods in PFTs which helps improve both diagnosis and outcomes for patients. In recent times, PFTs are recognized as crucial for both diagnosis and the management of health conditions. For example, during the COVID-19 pandemic, assessing pulmonary function has become very important. A comprehensive PFT assessment can reveal how COVID-19 has impacted a person's lungs, which helps guide their medical care and rehabilitation. Additionally, understanding the correlation between pulmonary function and overall health outcomes has gained significant attention, particularly as studies highlight risk factors such as chronic comorbidities that may exacerbate respiratory conditions (Annemarie et al., 2020). Furthermore, as healthcare systems focus on evidence-based practice, PFT results contribute to developing protocols and guidelines that improve patient care, emphasizing the test's importance in lung health management and public health initiatives (Matthew et al., 2021) (Figure 11.1).

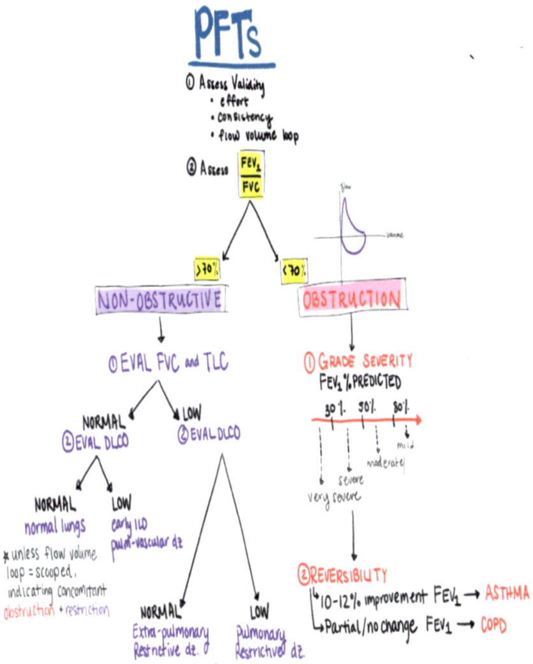

Figure 11.1. Pulmonary function tests.

Source: https://i0.wp.com/clinicalproblemsolving.com/wp-content/uploads/2019/12/PFTs.png?resize=1164%2C854&ssl=1.

Importance of PFTs in Respiratory Health

The significance of PFTs in maintaining respiratory health cannot be overstated, as they serve as critical diagnostic tools for assessing lung function and identifying underlying conditions. Spirometry and lung volume tests (PFTs) give important information about ailments including asthma, COPD, and restrictive lung disease. By measuring key parameters, such as forced vital capacity (FVC) and forced expiratory volume in one second (FEV1), healthcare providers can tailor management plans to patients' specific needs. Additionally, PFTs are crucial for monitoring the progression of the disease and assessing the effectiveness of treatment. As evidenced by recent studies, including findings related to the impact of smoking on respiratory health among healthcare workers, PFTs are fundamental to early diagnosis and timely intervention, ultimately improving patient outcomes and quality of life (Hasan et al., 2024). Because respiratory health assessment is constantly evolving, the use of technology in PFTs has benefited both patients and healthcare providers. Traditional spirometry is effective, but it has some drawbacks, particularly during health crises like COVID-19. The arrival of wearable devices has made it possible to monitor breathing continuously which has improved how reliable and accessible lung function data is. They rely on modern sensors and learning algorithms to detect even minor changes in lung function, providing reliable feedback. The implications of such technological advancements highlight the need for healthcare systems to embrace innovative methodologies while ensuring validation and calibration protocols are strictly adhered to Bernardo et al. (2024). As respiratory health becomes increasingly important, the strong connection between PFTs and new technologies can greatly benefit patient care. Additionally, PFTs have a positive impact on public health, helping to reduce the incidence of respiratory diseases in communities. Studying lung function trends in the population can guide efforts to reduce lung disease and change health policies. For example, studies showing that smoking causes lung problems prove the need for smoking cessation programs, mainly among healthcare workers. Providing caregivers with access to PFT data enables healthcare systems to deliver personalized care tailored to various patient groups. When more people are tested regularly, it becomes easier to spot changes in respiratory health, which encourages taking early action for public health. This comprehensive view of respiratory health, supported by PFTs, allows for more effective resource allocation, ultimately reducing healthcare costs associated with advanced disease management (Hasan et al., 2024).

11.1. Types of Pulmonary Function Tests

Various types of PFTs are employed to evaluate lung function, guiding the diagnosis and management of respiratory diseases. A standard test is spirometry, which measures the amount and speed of air entering and exiting the lungs. The test gives important details by checking FVC and FEV1. With these measurements, doctors can detect asthma and COPD. Additionally, the findings help track the progression of the disease and assess the effectiveness of treatment. Its widespread use in hospitals and clinics demonstrates the importance of spirometry in respiratory medicine and in helping patients. Plethysmography is a more advanced PFT that measures the air pressure within a chamber to determine the lung volumes. This provides an in-depth analysis of total lung capacity (TLC) and residual volume (RV), essential for diagnosing restrictive lung diseases. An added advantage of this procedure is its ability to determine functional residual capacity (FRC) without relying on gas dilution techniques. For patients diagnosed with interstitial lung disease (ILD), as highlighted in a study analyzing ILD management, plethysmography is often complemented by exercise oximetry to assess oxygen saturation during physical activity. These integrated assessments are crucial for developing tailored treatment plans and improving patient outcomes, making plethysmography an indispensable tool in respiratory diagnostics (Fenech et al., 2012). Diffusing capacity testing, specifically the diffusing capacity of the lungs for carbon monoxide (DLCO), serves as another critical component of PFTs. It checks how well gases move from the air in the lungs into the blood, which reflects the health of the alveolar-capillary membrane. When it comes to COPD and pulmonary fibrosis, the DLCO can identify changes that are not detected by regular spirometry. Moreover, a recent study demonstrated the potential of high-resolution computed tomography (HRCT) in correlating DLCO with emphysema severity, emphasizing the importance of integrating imaging and PFT data for comprehensive assessment and management of pulmonary conditions (Carl et al., 2018). So, PFTs, which use different methods, are necessary for correctly diagnosing, monitoring, and managing respiratory diseases.

11.1.1. Spirometry

The evaluation of PFTs relies greatly on spirometry, which gives important information about lung function by measuring both lung volume and airflow rates. The test measures FVC and FEV1, which indicate how well the lungs can expel air. The FEV1/FVC ratio is critical, as it helps distinguish between obstructive and restrictive lung diseases. Due to the rise in e-cigarette use and its possible health effects, studies have found some concerning trends. A recent study found that young adults who smoke e-cigarettes have less FEV1 and FVC than those who do not, which suggests their lungs are not working as well. This underscores the necessity of spirometry in both clinical settings and public health discussions regarding emerging respiratory risks (Digambiro et al., 2025). In addition to detecting lung problems, spirometry is essential for the regular monitoring of individuals with lung conditions. COPD and asthma are managed best when lung function is regularly checked to adjust the treatment plan. Doctors use spirometry to measure the extent of disease, check how the patient responds to treatment, and decide on changes to medications. Additionally, new technology in spirometry has made it easier to use and more reliable, allowing it to be utilized in many outpatient and community clinics. The incorporation of additional functional tests, such as body plethysmography and multiple breath washout (MBW), further enriches the understanding of complex pulmonary pathophysiology. However, while spirometry remains a foundational technique, it is essential to recognize its limitations and the need for comprehensive assessments of lung function (Short et al., 2024). As respiratory health is evolving, it is more crucial than ever to incorporate spirometry into regular pulmonary function testing. It helps not only by identifying diseases, but also by revealing how lungs behave in different patient groups. Recent studies of e-cigarette users show that spirometry can detect early signs of airway obstruction in individuals who seem healthy. Additionally, emerging techniques like MBWShX are being recognized for their sensitivity in detecting specific pathophysiological features, such as trapped air, which are crucial for monitoring diseases like cystic fibrosis (CF). Due to these changes, respiratory functions are being evaluated in a new way, integrating various testing methods. Consequently, spirometry remains an indispensable instrument in respiratory medicine, enhancing both clinical outcomes and public health initiatives (Digambiro et al., 2025; Short et al., 2024) (Figure 11.2).

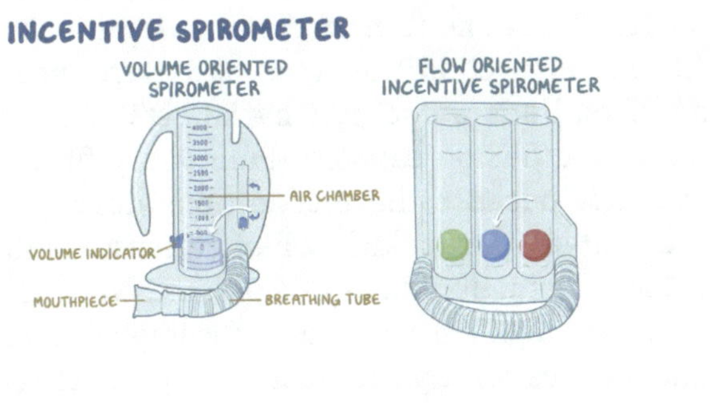

Figure 11.2. Incentive spirometer.

Source: https://www.osmosis.org/_next/image?url=https%3A%2F%2Fd16qt3wv6xm098.cloudfront.net%2F4MqDcdkRSSm4CmSBfO5ZIvjdTv61n-Hu%2F_.jpg&w=3840&q=75.

11.1.2. Lung Volume Measurement

Lung volume measurement is a crucial component of PFTs, providing valuable information about the lungs and any changes associated with disease. Spirometry, plethysmography, and gas dilution methods are often used to measure lung volumes because each has its own benefits. One example is spirometry, which is easy to use and accurate for measuring FVC and FEV1. Still, it may not be able to measure particular changes in lung volume in people with restrictive lung diseases. Plethysmography, unlike spirometry, measures the total volume of gas in the thorax, providing a more accurate representation of lung compliance. Therefore, these various techniques play a significant role in understanding lung function and directing patient care. Lung volume measurements are clinically important because they can predict different lung conditions. In patients with ILD, TLC measured by PFTs can indicate the severity of lung damage and the effectiveness of treatment. According to studies, KL-6 and IL-18 have been investigated as biomarkers for ILD; however, they may not always align with the results from standard volumetric measurements. In reality, the initial FVC measurements are important signs of how the disease will progress and the risk of death in patients with systemic sclerosis-related ILD. Integrating volumetric and biomarker assessments allows clinicians to sort patients better and decide on the best treatment. By understanding these correlations, we can better comprehend how lung volume mechanics impact the final outcomes for patients. Recent advancements in imaging, such as three-dimensional computed tomography (3D-CT), have revolutionized lung volume measurement by providing detailed visualizations of pulmonary structures. In particular, 3D-CT reconstruction enables the accurate assessment of total lung volume (TLV), which can significantly aid in pre- and post-operative evaluations, which can be carefully monitored using advanced imaging methods. Research indicates that severe scoliosis can lead to a decrease in lung volume, which can be closely observed using these methods. Evidence suggests that with appropriate interventions, such as halo-pelvic traction (HPT), there can be substantial increases in TLV following treatment. This demonstrates that combining novel imaging methods with standard PFTs enables a more comprehensive understanding of the lungs' workings and changes in various medical scenarios. Collectively, these methodologies highlight the essential role of lung volume measurement in navigating the complexities of pulmonary function testing and its implications for patient care (Figure 11.3).

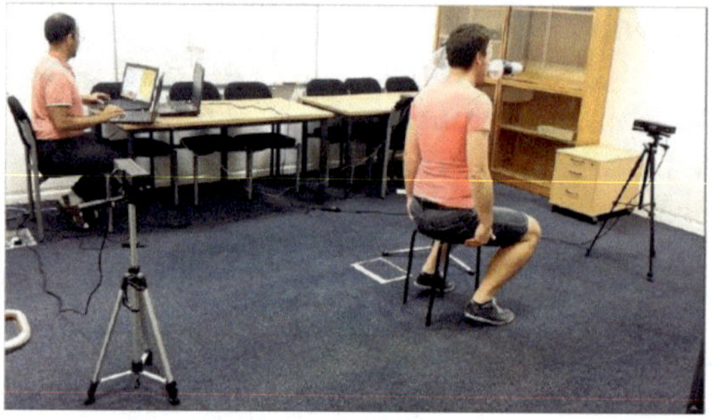

Figure 11.3. Measurement setup with two Kinect v2 cameras facing each other. The subject sits on a chair without a backrest and breathes through a reference spirometer.

Source: https://www.mdpi.com/sensors/sensors-22-09680/article_deploy/html/images/sensors-22-09680-g003.png.

11.1.3. Diffusion Capacity Tests

Diffusion capacity tests are important for evaluating pulmonary function, particularly in assessing how easily gases exchange between the alveoli and the blood. They mainly assess how well the lungs can exchange gases, such as oxygen and carbon dioxide, which is necessary for proper blood oxygenation. The most common method for assessing diffusion capacity is the carbon monoxide diffusion capacity (DLCO) test. Abnormal DLCO in patients with ILD or other lung diseases suggests impaired gas exchange and may direct the doctor's treatment plan. Finding the diffusion capacity helps healthcare providers understand the patient's condition and adjust treatment plans, highlighting the importance of this test among PFTs. Understanding what affects alveolar-capillary gas exchange is crucial for accurately interpreting diffusion capacity. Pulmonary fibrosis and emphysema can cause a decrease in diffusion capacity because these conditions destroy or thicken the alveoli. Diffusion capacity tests can aid in diagnosis, particularly when patients exhibit general respiratory symptoms. In a study examining the diagnostic journey of patients with ILD, only 15% underwent PFTs prior to referral to specialized care, highlighting an area for improvement in patient management (Adegunsoye et al., 2019). Adding diffusion capacity tests to regular check-ups allows both primary care doctors and specialists to make more accurate diagnoses and help patients by treating them sooner. Additionally, diffusion capacity tests play a role in predicting how a patient's condition may progress. Changes in DLCO over time suggest whether the disease is worsening or improving due to therapy, helping clinicians decide on further steps. For example, a longitudinal analysis of patients with ILD revealed that each year of diagnostic delay was associated with an increased percentage of fibrosis on chest CT, emphasizing the need for timely intervention

(Adegunsoye et al., 2019). Additionally, understanding pleural stress in the lungs can help predict surgical outcomes and any potential complications that may impact lung function after surgery. As part of the comprehensive evaluation provided by PFTs, diffusion capacity may ultimately guide interventions that can impact both immediate clinical management and long-term patient health trajectories (Figure 11.4).

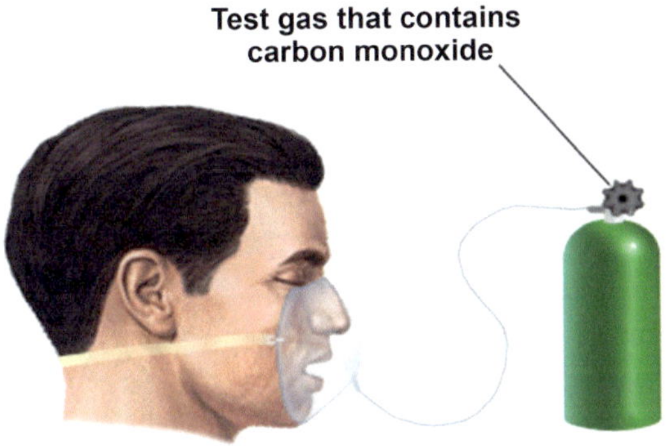

Figure 11.4. Lung diffusion testing.

Source: https://ssl.adam.com/graphics/images/en/9598.jpg.

11.2. Indications for Pulmonary Function Tests

The assessment of pulmonary function through PFTs is critical for diagnosing a variety of respiratory conditions. PFTs are ordered in many situations, such as when patients have a chronic cough, difficulty breathing, or wheezing that cannot be explained. They are used to prove if there is lung obstruction or restriction, as well as to measure the degree of lung impairment. Before undergoing thoracic or upper abdominal surgery, patients should undergo PFTs to assess their lung function and reduce the risk of postoperative complications. Incorporating such tests into clinical practice helps clinicians develop more effective management and treatment strategies for each patient. PFTs are essential for monitoring the progress of patients with existing respiratory illnesses. Regularly checking for asthma, COPD, and ILD is necessary to monitor the disease and determine if the treatment is effective. Repeated PFTs help clinicians assess the effectiveness of treatments, enabling them to make informed adjustments to the patient's therapy. Additionally, individuals with neuromuscular diseases or obesity hypoventilation syndrome may benefit from periodic PFTs to monitor their respiratory mechanics over time. Regularly checking lung function with PFTs is important for managing chronic diseases, which helps patients live better and improve their well-being. Recent changes in medical education have placed more emphasis on how to interpret and utilize PFTs in clinical practice. Teaching medical students the BORG model and similar frameworks helps these students to interpret test results and use these strategies in their clinical work. It enhances knowledge of the physiology underlying PFTs and clarifies their proper application in clinical settings. As elucidated in scholarly discussions, focused workshops help bridge the knowledge gap among trainees, enabling them to navigate complex cases involving pulmonary assessments more proficiently (Ryan et al., 2023). The evolving landscape highlights the importance of training in PFT utilization, ensuring that future clinicians are proficient in leveraging these tests to enhance patient care (Ethan et al., 2024).

11.2.1. Diagnosis of Respiratory Diseases

A diagnosis for respiratory diseases usually involves using several methods, including PFTs. PFTs help assess the lungs by measuring airflow and lung volumes, which can show if someone has obstructive or restrictive lung diseases. Respiratory tests, for example, spirometry, are often used to check how the lungs work and find problems like asthma, COPD, or pulmonary fibrosis. The findings from these tests help determine the severity of the disease and may guide doctors to conduct additional tests, such as scans or blood work, to confirm the diagnosis. Respiratory diseases are often diagnosed with the help of imaging techniques, which often add to the results of PFTs. HRCT has emerged as a crucial tool for identifying ILDs, particularly idiopathic pulmonary fibrosis (IPF). The proper understanding of HRCT images requires close cooperation between pulmonologists and radiologists, ensuring that the context of the patient's condition is taken into account. The partnership is important because not every radiology pattern is an absolute sign of a specific disease. If the initial results are not conclusive, holding a multidisciplinary meeting can improve diagnosis by including various medical opinions which helps understand the patient's breathing problem better. Along with imaging and functional tests, incorporating clinical information significantly enhances the diagnosis of respiratory diseases. A patient's history of possible exposure to toxins or allergens helps explain the test results and supports a thorough evaluation of the case. This way of thinking can be particularly useful when regular diagnostic methods are insufficient. For instance, in the investigation of conditions like fibrotic lung disease, a retrospective review of patient records can reveal patterns relevant to diagnosis and treatment, as illustrated by the prevalence of ILD in various populations (Fenech et al., 2012). Thus, ongoing evaluations of clinical, radiological, and laboratory data are crucial for refining a patient's diagnosis and ensuring the efficacy of their individualized treatment plan (Chung et al., 2018) (Figure 11.5).

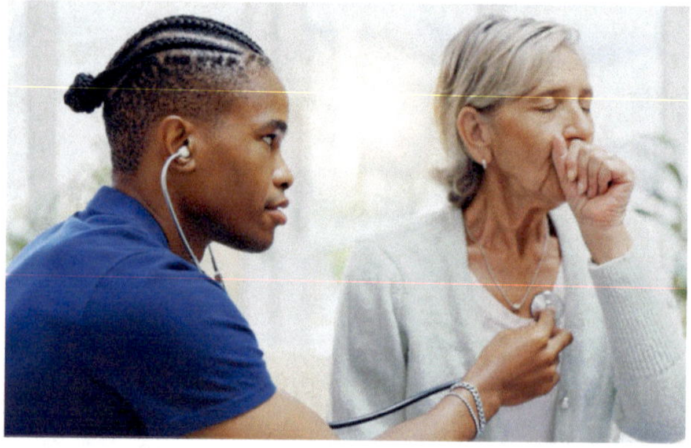

Figure 11.5. Clinical evaluation of respiratory symptoms during diagnostic assessment.

Source: https://thenativeantigencompany.com/wp-content/uploads/2025/02/iStock-1830136396_coughing-female-patient-with-male-doctor-in-blue-scrubs-1080x675.jpg.

11.2.2. Monitoring Disease Progression

Monitoring how a respiratory disease is depends mainly on using PFTs. These tests provide critical insights into lung function, typically measuring parameters such as forced expiratory volume (FEV1) and FVC. Routine assessments enable healthcare providers to detect any changes in lung function, allowing them to adjust treatment plans as needed. A significant part of this process is to know the patient's usual function and notice any changes that might suggest the disease is worsening. Clinicians should always perform PFTs in the same way, as changes in technique or patient effort can lead to incorrect results. Therefore, having standard practices and ensuring patients follow them can improve the accuracy of results, which is crucial for understanding how COPD and pulmonary sarcoidosis develop. When COPD is involved, PFTs are especially important because the link between smoking and the disease is so close. It has been found that early detection of COPD relies heavily on checking lung function, mainly in populations where many people have a history of smoking.

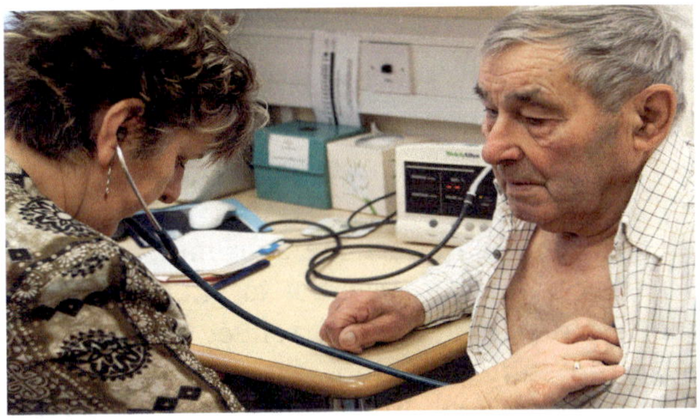

Figure 11.6. Lung examination for monitoring disease progression.

Source: https://www.pulsetoday.co.uk/wp-content/uploads/2020/11/p30_Lung_examination_SPL_1200x800px.jpg.

Lately, studies have found that using biological markers along with PFTs can help predict early-stage COPD more accurately, which may result in better treatment outcomes. For example, the GOLD 2022–2024 guidelines now pay closer attention to biological causes that may be more strongly linked to disease progression than the usual clinical signs and symptoms. It emphasizes the importance of developing more effective monitoring methods that can link simple evaluations with detailed bio-signals, revealing lung function changes in patients. Moreover, the exploration of complementary monitoring tools, such as cardiopulmonary exercise testing (CPET), can augment the efficacy of conventional PFTs in gauging disease progression. PFTs only provide a brief assessment of lung function, but CPET enables doctors to measure exercise capacity and heart response, providing more specific information. It has been found that CPET is especially useful for staging diseases and comparing with signs of inflammation seen in imaging in sarcoidosis. With this approach, PFTs and CPET provide more detailed information about the disease, enabling healthcare providers to customize care based on individual assessments. As the landscape of pulmonary disease management evolves, incorporating these diverse methodologies into routine clinical practice could significantly improve monitoring outcomes and ultimately patient care (Figure 11.6).

11.2.3. Preoperative Assessment

Preoperative assessment is a critical component of surgical planning, particularly for patients presenting with respiratory concerns. Spirometry and other lung function tests can help identify patients who are more likely to experience postoperative complications. A thorough preoperative assessment enables healthcare providers to tailor the anesthetic and surgical methods to each patient's specific needs. From the results of PFTs, FEV1 and FVC supply important information about lung capacity and the way air moves through the lungs. These factors can help decide if a patient needs preoperative treatments like bronchodilators or physiotherapy which can significantly reduce the risk of complications during and after surgery, mainly for those with lung diseases or weak respiratory function. It is well known that preoperative PFTs help predict surgical outcomes because they are strongly related to lung function. Research has shown that patients undergoing procedures such as rheumatic mitral valve surgery exhibit notable declines in FEV1 and FVC, corresponding to increased cardiac risk, which emphasizes the importance of these measures in risk stratification (Harneet et al., 2024). This change in vital signs could suggest there is not enough lung reserve, which might result in more complications during surgery if not addressed. Studies also show that PFT results are linked to more serious postoperative events such as needing extra ventilation and developing significant complications. By carrying out preoperative assessments that include PFTs, medical staff can be more prepared and help reduce risks for patients during surgery. When surgeons are performing corrective spinal surgery on people with major thoracic deformities, the importance of PFTs increases. For instance, the implementation of HPT prior to surgery has demonstrated improvements in pulmonary function metrics, indicating a direct relationship between structural spinal corrections and enhancements in lung capacity (Zhou et al., 2023). The significant rise in TLV and lung capacity after preoperative interventions demonstrates that incorporating thorough pulmonary evaluations into preoperative routines is crucial. This multifaceted approach not only prepares the patient's respiratory status for surgery but also contributes to more favorable long-term outcomes, reinforcing the critical role of preoperative PFTs in optimizing patient care and expanding the therapeutic options available to surgical teams (Figure 11.7).

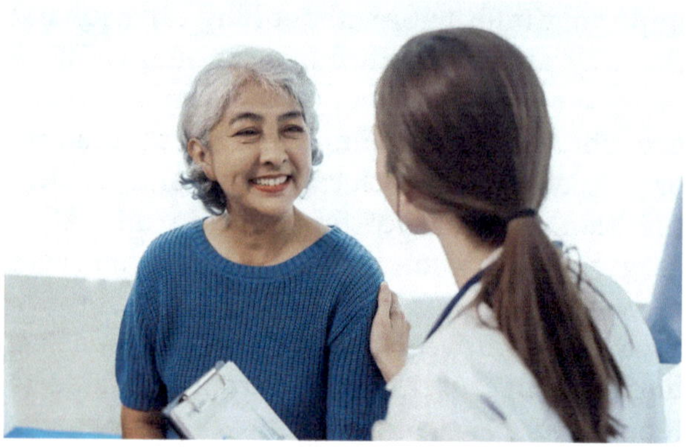

Figure 11.7. Preoperative consultation focused on patient-centered care.

Source: https://sa1s3optim.patientpop.com/filters:format(webp)/assets/production/practices/377012814fbb4323f1bc0008126ef1d839c9f69f/images/2710485.jpeg.

11.3. Procedure of Pulmonary Function Tests

The procedure of PFTs is pivotal in evaluating respiratory function and diagnosing various pulmonary conditions. Typically, the first step is to review the patient's medical history and explain the tests that will be performed. Clinicians ensure that patients understand the importance of the assessments and how accurate results can inform their treatment. Patients are often advised not to use bronchodilators for a certain period before the test, as these medications can affect the spirometry results. This precaution is essential to guarantee that the test results accurately reflect the patient's baseline lung function, thereby improving the reliability of subsequent interpretations (Vahanian et al., 2021). While being tested, patients undergo a series of measurements that assess various lung functions. The most common part of spirometry is for the patient to take a deep breath and then blow as hard as possible into a device called a spirometer. The FVC and FEV1 parameters are measured with this instrument, and these are key for diagnosing asthma and COPD. If the initial results are concerning, other tests, such as lung volume and diffusion capacity, may be performed. They check the lungs' ability as well as the efficiency of gas exchange between the air and blood. By incorporating these multifaceted assessments, clinicians can pinpoint abnormalities and tailor treatment plans effectively (Douglas et al., 2014). Once the procedure is complete, the PFT results are reviewed in conjunction with other medical information to assess the patient's lung health. Clinicians review the results to identify patterns that may indicate restrictive or obstructive airway diseases, which helps them better understand the patient's condition. It is important to interpret the results, since they can change depending on the patient's age, gender, height, and ethnicity so that changes may be needed for an accurate assessment. After the tests, healthcare providers will discuss the results with the patient and explain the necessary next steps, whether that involves treatment or additional tests. The comprehensive nature of PFTs plays a crucial role in respiratory medicine, influencing clinical decisions and enhancing patient outcomes through precise diagnoses and targeted therapies (Vahanian et al., 2021).

11.3.1. Preparation for the Tests

The preparation for PFTs is a crucial step that can significantly affect the accuracy of the results. Most patients are instructed to refrain from taking bronchodilators or other respiratory medications for a specified period before the test, typically between 4 and 12 hours. Not using the bronchodilator ensures that the lungs' normal function is not changed, and the results are accurate. Patients are also advised to refrain from vigorous exercise and smoking for at least one day before the test, as these activities can temporarily alter lung function. Educating patients about these preparations not only enhances the validity of the test outcomes but also promotes an understanding of their own respiratory health by encouraging them to consider behaviors that impact lung function (Dent et al., 2008). It is just as important to be psychologically ready for PFTs. Being anxious about testing can change your breathing, which can cause the results to be incorrect. Therefore, medical staff should clearly explain what the tests involve, what the patient can expect to feel, and what each part of the test aims to achieve. Being open and transparent can help people relax and team up, which results in better measurements of lung capacity and function. For example, knowing how to perform spirometry, which requires deep breathing, is very important. By demystifying the procedure, health professionals can increase patients' confidence and compliance, ultimately enhancing the diagnostic potential of the tests (Abrazado et al., 2014). Dietary rules are also a significant part of preparing for PFTs. It is generally recommended that patients avoid eating large meals before testing, as this can cause their abdomen to expand and reduce the movement of the diaphragm, potentially affecting lung function, healthcare locations advise against using caffeine or stimulants, as these can lead to unusual breathing patterns. Healthcare providers should always give detailed instructions about all of these points before any test. Clinicians who focus on both the physical and emotional aspects of preparation help the testing process go smoothly and provide accurate results for pulmonary health. Consequently, a well-prepared patient is likely to yield results that accurately reflect their true pulmonary function, facilitating the development of appropriate clinical interventions and management strategies (Dent et al., 2008) (Figure 11.8).

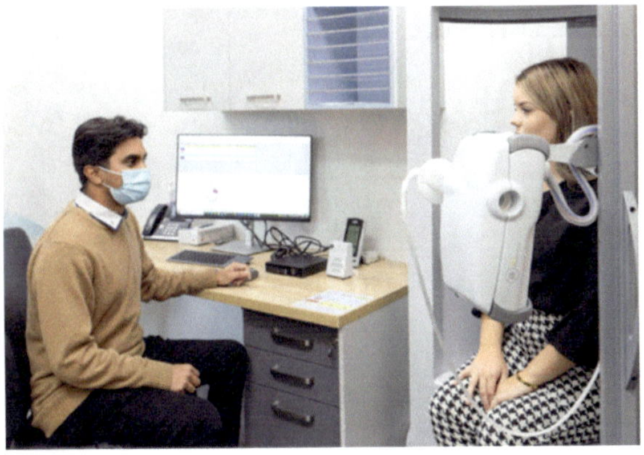

Figure 11.8. Preparing for pulmonary function testing.

Source: https://sydwestresp.com.au/wp-content/uploads/2022/07/consultation.jpg.

11.3.2. Step-by-Step Process of Conducting PFTs

Conducting PFTs involves a systematic approach to assess lung function and diagnose respiratory conditions accurately. The first step is to get the patient ready, which involves asking about their past health and examining them physically. It is essential for clinicians to know about any health problems, possible drug interactions or earlier lung conditions. It is usual for patients to be told to avoid bronchodilators, smoking, and strenuous exercise before the test, since these can alter the results. Clearly informing patients about what to do helps reduce their anxiety and increases their likelihood of following the instructions, which in turn improves the accuracy of the test results. Getting accurate data on a patient's lung function depends on proper preparation. Once the preliminary evaluations are complete, the actual testing process can begin. Tests conducted in this phase include spirometry, which measures lung volume, diffusion capacity tests, and bronchial provocation tests. Spirometry is usually performed first, as it measures the amount of air inhaled and exhaled by the patient, providing results such as FVC and FEV1. All these tests are conducted by qualified personnel using properly calibrated tools to ensure accuracy. Other tests might use inhaled agents to cause the airways to narrow or overinflate which is necessary for finding out if a person has asthma or COPD. Reviewing all the test results provides a comprehensive overview of lung function. The final part of PFTs involves analyzing and interpreting the data, which enables doctors to make informed decisions. The results are verified against established values for age, gender, race, and height. Clinicians compare the observed values with what is predicted to determine if a patient may have restrictive or obstructive lung disease. Additionally, recent advancements in PFT methodologies, such as airspace dimension assessment (AiDA), showcase promising implications for enhanced diagnostic precision. They can help find changes in the lungs that are not easily seen with traditional techniques. Consequently, rigorous evaluation of PFT results can identify lung impairments and guide treatment strategies more effectively, as evidenced in populations with unique health challenges, such as those with spina bifida (Cheng et al., 2014; Sj Pögren et al., 2023) (Figure 11.9).

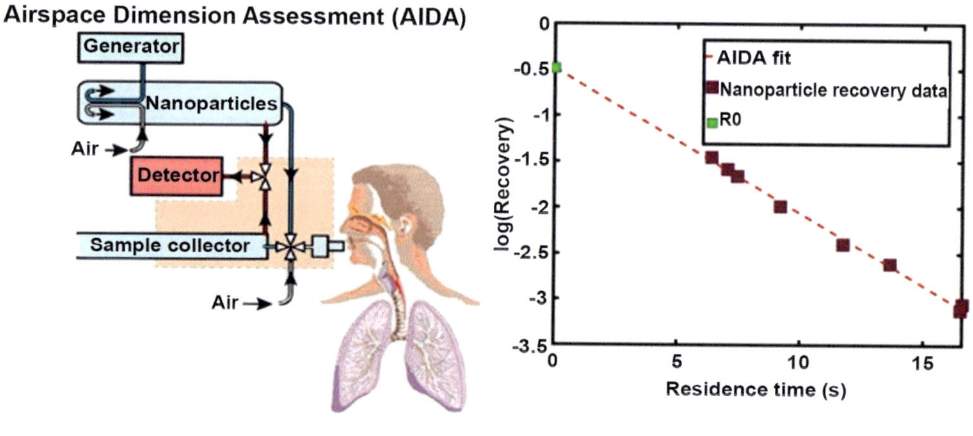

Figure 11.9. (Left) Schematic illustration of the AiDA method. The aerosol particles from the distal airspaces were sampled to obtain the distal airspace radius rAiDA and the zero-second recovery R0. (Right) Representative recovery data as a function of residence time in the lungs and AiDA fit obtained for one volunteer.

Source: https://www.researchgate.net/publication/349596061/figure/fig4/AS:995346113130520@1614320414861/Left-Schematic-illustration-of-the-AiDA-method-The-aerosol-particles-from-the-distal.png.

11.3.3. Safety and Comfort Measures During Testing

In the realm of PFTs, ensuring patient safety and comfort is paramount. At the beginning, healthcare providers provide a thorough explanation of the procedures, what the patient can expect to feel, and any potential discomfort. Being open about the process helps patients feel less anxious and get ready for what will happen. Temperature and noise in the room should be managed to help maintain a calm environment. All staff members should be adequately trained to address patient concerns and provide support during testing.

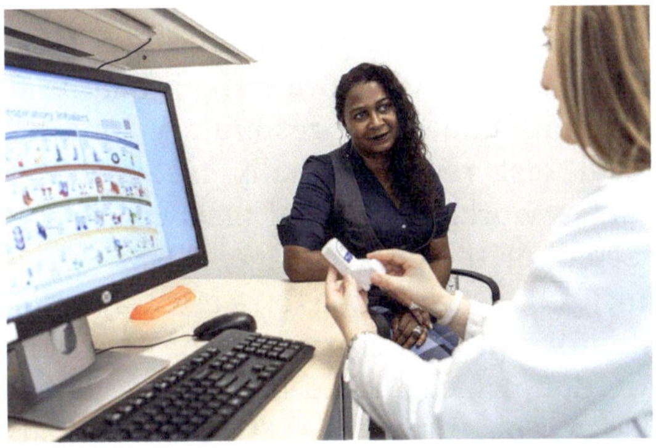

Figure 11.10. Patient-centered education and support in pulmonary function testing (PFT).

Source: https://my.clevelandclinic.org/-/scassets/images/org/care-pages/respiratory/respiratory-therapy-feature.jpg?w=640&q=75.

All of these efforts improve how patients feel and could also help ensure test results are more accurate by reducing the effects of anxiety on their breathing. Furthermore, following infection control guidelines has become increasingly important, especially in the wake of the COVID-19 pandemic. According to guidelines set forth by authorities such as the Thoracic Society of Australia and New Zealand, safety measures should be adapted based on local transmission rates and environmental factors (Borg et al., 2022). This includes the use of personal protective equipment (PPE) for healthcare workers, as well as maintaining appropriate distancing during tests when feasible. Additionally, ensuring that equipment is sanitized both before and after testing helps prevent cross-contamination and reassures patients that they are safe. If healthcare providers prioritize these protective strategies, patients will feel more comfortable undergoing important tests without worrying about infection. Besides the physical steps taken, more people are noticing the role of emotional well-being in how patients perform during PFTs. When tests cause discomfort, it may lead to physiological changes that could change the test results, especially in various populations. Research indicates that the removal of race correction in PFTs could contribute to more equitable assessments and treatment recommendations, particularly for African American individuals who have historically been subject to biased evaluations (Sidra et al., 2023). Emotional support is essential in healthcare; therefore, healthcare providers can help patients relax or teach them about the significance of the tests. By addressing both the physical and emotional factors, the potential for achieving accurate and meaningful pulmonary function results is significantly enhanced (Figure 11.10).

11.4. Interpretation of Pulmonary Function Test Results

The interpretation of PFT results is a critical aspect of diagnosing and managing various respiratory conditions. Doctors can distinguish between obstructive and restrictive lung diseases by examining the FVC, FEV1, and the FEV1/FVC ratio. In asthma and COPD, it is common to see a decrease in FEV1, but a normal FVC, which is indicative of an obstructive pattern. Conversely, when breathing patterns are restricted, both FEV1 and FVC decrease at the same time, which is often a sign of ILD or pulmonary fibrosis.

With this detailed understanding, healthcare providers can design treatments that fit each patient, which greatly helps patients. Their effectiveness is enhanced when their outcomes are aligned with what is observed in patients and on imaging. For instance, a chest computed tomography (CT) scan may reveal interstitial changes in patients with diminished lung function; thus, incorporating diagnostic imaging can provide valuable context for interpreting PFT results.

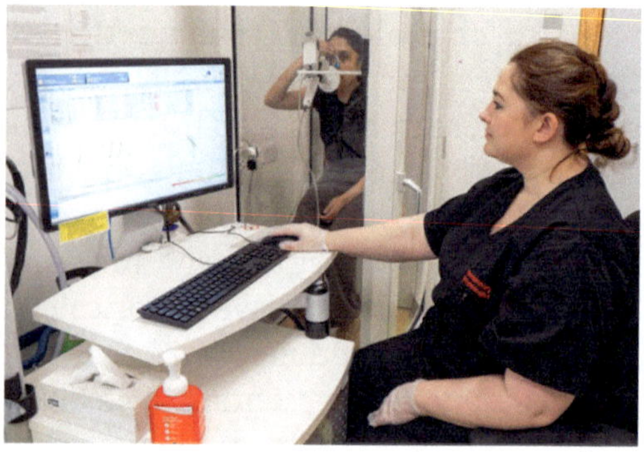

Figure 11.11. Interpreting pulmonary function test results.

Source: https://emedia1.nhs.wales/CAVUhb/cache/file/06AF67EE-2091-47A1-A2E46C5A630276BD.jpeg.

Evidence suggests that detecting ILD features on chest CT scans helps prompt pulmonologists to be consulted, highlighting the importance of using different tests to manage complex lung diseases. A retrospective analysis indicated that a significant percentage of patients experienced diagnostic delays due in part to inadequate reporting of ILD features on PFTs, highlighting the need for comprehensive assessment strategies to avoid missing critical diagnoses like ILD (Adegunsoye et al., 2019). Additionally, monitoring lung function over time can help identify any changes in lung disease, allowing for early treatment. Regular PFTs are helpful for patients with ILD to assess the effects of their treatment and monitor changes in their lung function. The results from PFTs should be considered in conjunction with age and any other existing health issues, as these factors can impact lung function. For example, a study conducted in Malta highlighted that worsening lung function correlated with advancing age among patients with ILD, suggesting a potentially critical relationship between demographic factors and pulmonary function (Fenech et al., 2012). Establishing such associations clarifies the interpretation of PFT results and reinforces the necessity for individualized care plans based on comprehensive data analysis (Figure 11.11).

11.4.1. Normal vs. Abnormal Results

The interpretation of PFTs is essential in determining whether a patient's results fall within the normal range or indicate abnormalities that may signify underlying respiratory conditions. Typical test results usually mean that the lungs are working well and their values are as expected for the person's age, height, sex, and ethnicity. Unusual findings on a test may indicate ventilatory problems, such as obstruction or restriction, which should be further examined and may require treatment. This differentiation is accomplished through a systematic approach outlined by recognized guidelines, such as those of the ERS/ATS, which compare individual results against established norms to identify deviations that may help diagnose specific respiratory diseases and manage treatment effectively (Barkous et al., 2024). PFT results may not be typical and can take various forms, so they need to be carefully sorted to find out the nature of the impairment. Obstructive pulmonary patterns seen in spirometry testing usually point to asthma or COPD. This occurs when the FEV1 is less than the FVC, which helps doctors assess the health of the lungs. Another example, such as pulmonary fibrosis, is characterized by small volumes for all measures, including FVC. The examination of these patterns is crucial, as it directly influences clinical decision-making and the urgency of follow-up actions, including potential bronchodilator testing or additional imaging (Chaithanya et al., 2024). The role of various factors in PFT is crucial because they influence the interpretation of normal and abnormal results. Age, sex, BMI, and past medical history can all significantly impact how the lungs function. According to the study, people recovering from COVID-19 often had more restrictive patterns in their PFTs, which highlights the links between past health problems and current lung function. Noticing these correlations highlights the importance of following up with patients over time and developing personalized plans for them in clinical care. Thus, distinguishing between normal and abnormal PFT results is not merely a technical exercise; it becomes a critical component in understanding patient health trajectories and tailoring appropriate therapeutic strategies (Chaithanya et al., 2024) (Figure 11.12).

	Lung perfusion	
Variable	Normal (n = 32)	Abnormal (n = 18)
FEV_1 (% of pred.)	83.38 ± 16.35	81.93 ± 16.67
FVC (% of pred.)	80.64 ± 15.93	79.64 ± 16.70
FEV_1/FVC (%)	88.41 ± 10.72	87.37 ± 8.70
DLco (% of pred.)	86.23 ± 15.85	85.41 ± 14.80
TLC (% of pred.)	95.13 ± 15.07	84.7 ± 11.79
SaO_2 (%)	96.90 ± 2.56	96.74 ± 2.62
6MWD (m)	603 ± 101	597 ± 76

Figure 11.12. Pulmonary function test results in the two groups of subjects.

Source: https://www.researchgate.net/profile/Eliezer-Klainman/publication/23311345/figure/tbl1/AS:601693494452263@1520466316911/Pulmonary-function-test-results-in-the-two-groups-of-sub-jects.png.

11.4.2. Common Patterns in PFT Results

PFTs are vital diagnostic tools that assess lung capacity and functionality, revealing common patterns indicative of various respiratory conditions. The FEV1 is a key factor measured in PFTs, and it may decrease significantly in people who have obstructive lung diseases, such as COPD and asthma. Emphysema, a type of COPD, can cause FEV1 to drop significantly, which is related to changes in the structure of the lungs. Due to emphysematous changes, the residual volume increases and the FVC decreases, making the patient's condition more difficult to treat. By recognizing these patterns, clinicians can classify the severity of lung conditions and plan the treatment, which is why patients with possible lung issues should have PFTs regularly. Additionally, the diffusion capacity of the lungs for carbon monoxide (DLCO) serves as another critical component of PFT results, often highlighting the presence of underlying pathologies. A drop in DLCO is mainly linked to pulmonary vascular diseases and ILD. It can suggest the presence of pulmonary fibrosis or emphysema. Research has shown that a significant decrease in DLCO can accompany both high attenuation volume (HAV) and low attenuation volume (LAV) in PFT results, providing insights into the fibrotic changes in the lung parenchyma and their impact on lung functionality (Doellinger et al., 2019). It demonstrates that both interstitial and emphysematous diseases can lower diffusion capacity, which can make the patient's condition more complex. Additionally, HRCT scans can be used to highlight emphysematous areas in patients with COPD, thereby enhancing the accuracy of PFT results analysis. Studies have demonstrated that automated methods for quantifying emphysema from HRCT can provide a robust correlation with traditional PFT measurements, such as FEV1 and DLCO (Carl et al., 2018). They are expected to decrease disagreements between doctors and help with more precise emphysema diagnoses. As PFTs remain a cornerstone in evaluating pulmonary health, integrating imaging data can enhance the interpretation of lung function, ultimately improving patient outcomes through tailored management strategies (Figure 11.13).

Respiratory Patterns in Common Diseases

	Asthma	Emphysema	Interstitial Lung Disease	Muscle Weakness
FVC	Normal or ↓	↓	↓	↓
$FEV_{1.0}$	↓	↓	↓	↓
$FEV_{1.0}/FVC$	↓	↓	Normal	Normal
TLC	Normal or ↑	↑	↓	↓
DLCO	Normal	↓	↓	Normal

Figure 11.13. Respiratory patterns in common diseases.

Source: https://hospitalmedicaldirector.com/wp-content/uploads/2021/12/Respiratory-patterns-in-common-diseases.jpg.

11.4.3. Role of Healthcare Professionals in Interpretation

The interpretation of PFTs plays a crucial role in the diagnostic process for various respiratory conditions. Interpreting the results of PFT tests is mainly the job of respiratory therapists and pulmonologists. Due to their expertise, they can identify the finer points in the data to inform further medical actions. They should be able to conduct the tests and also identify the signs that indicate diseases such as asthma or COPD. When healthcare professionals combine the data from PFTs with patients' clinical information, they can ensure that the diagnoses are accurate and tailored to each patient. This integrative approach enhances the effectiveness of treatment plans, which is vital given that many patients with COPD remain undiagnosed, as highlighted by recent findings in the field (Ching-Lin et al., 2023). Besides caring for patients, healthcare professionals are responsible for teaching patients about PFTs. Educating patients is essential to help them cooperate and understand the tests, which in turn affects the accuracy of the results. Educating patients properly helps them feel less anxious about what will happen and encourages them to take an active role in their healthcare. It is also important for healthcare professionals to ensure that test results are well understood, especially when discussing chronic lung diseases. Discussing a patient's PFT results with them encourages their active involvement in their treatment, which can lead to improved health outcomes. Therefore, the roles of educators and interpreters highlight the many responsibilities that healthcare professionals have in PFTs. Additionally, new technology in healthcare has enabled professionals to utilize advanced tools when interpreting PFTs. Advanced analytic techniques, including artificial intelligence (AI), are now being integrated into the interpretation process, enabling more precise readings and improved identification of subtle abnormalities in pulmonary function (Gali et al., 2023). Still, while technology is invaluable, medical interpretation relies heavily on the skills of people. Such advanced results should be understood by healthcare professionals, who can utilize their experience and knowledge of the patient. Respiratory care improves when technology and professional expertise are combined. As healthcare systems continue to adapt to technological innovations, the importance of skilled professionals in interpreting PFTs will only grow, reinforcing the essential nature of their roles in healthcare (Figure 11.14).

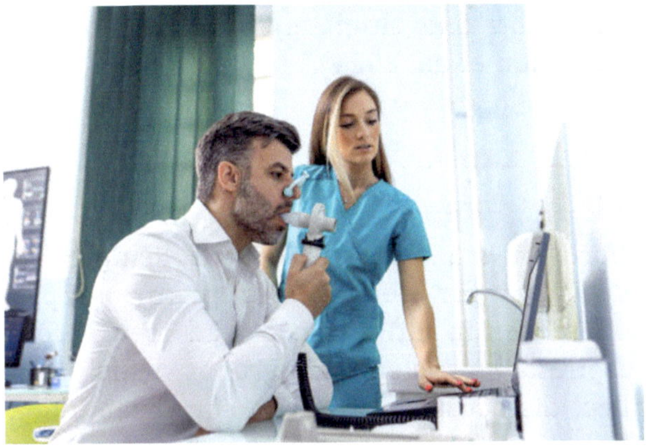

Figure 11.14. Healthcare professional overseeing pulmonary function testing and result interpretation.

Source: https://media.istockphoto.com/id/1497786387/photo/adult-man-testing-breathing-function-by-spirometry-having-health-problem-diagnosis-of.jpg?s=612x612&w=0&k=20&c=v5wHFGdCIaPOqlHM_6UpeF1OcB-lXDaiD6vd-VM2blw=.

11.5. Limitations of Pulmonary Function Tests

The limitations of PFTs are significant and can impact clinical decision-making. A primary concern is that patients must understand and follow the test instructions, as using the wrong technique can lead to incorrect results. Following the detailed instructions for spirometry and body plethysmography can be hard for people who are very ill or have mental impairments. Additionally, since these tests require a significant amount of time, healthcare providers may not consider other, faster methods to assess patients. Additionally, measuring surface topography has become a valuable addition to standard PFTs. Research indicates that these non-invasive scans can effectively correlate with vital pulmonary parameters in patients with idiopathic scoliosis, suggesting their potential to improve assessment accuracy while accommodating patient limitations (Jessica et al., 2024). Traditional PFTs have difficulty assessing every aspect of lung function, particularly in certain patient groups. For instance, in people with ankylosing spondylitis, the usual PFT tests may not reflect the complete impact on breathing, because the spine's deformities typically cause a restrictive lung disease. This highlights the need for advanced scanners, such as CT scans, to provide a clearer picture of lung volumes and their function. Studies have demonstrated a superior accuracy of CT-based lung volume measurements over conventional PFTs, highlighting that PFTs alone may fall short in delivering a complete assessment of the respiratory status in specific patient groups (Zhou et al., 2024).

While there have been many improvements, pulmonary diagnostics still struggles with making tests standard and limiting differences between testing centers. For example, the calibration and testing methods used for equipment may vary significantly from one facility to another, resulting in inconsistent outcomes for patients. In some cases, such as those with neuromuscular disorders or individuals with significantly different body sizes, the results may not accurately reflect their lung function. Using surface topography or CT lung volume measurements opens up new avenues to address these gaps and provides a more comprehensive view of lung health. As the medical field strives to improve the use of PFTs, it is essential to acknowledge their limitations and employ a combination of methods for pulmonary assessment.

11.5.1. Factors Affecting Test Accuracy

Several factors can significantly impact the accuracy of PFTs, ultimately affecting diagnosis and treatment decisions. Age, gender, and BMI are important factors in the patient's physiology, and they can affect the values of FVC and FEV1. As people age, their lung function often declines, which can make it more challenging for PFT tests to yield accurate results in older patients. Also, research has found that variations in BMI may help prevent or increase the risk of sarcopenia, which is linked to lung function problems in COPD patients. Accurate interpretation of these tests thus demands an understanding of how individual characteristics influence overall performance and results (Yang et al., 2025). The results of PFTs depend a lot on environmental and behavioral factors. Smoking, exposure to pollutants, and pre-existing lung conditions may affect the results, making it difficult to interpret how well the lungs are functioning. In these settings, testing must be done according to the rules and patients should be given clear instructions and reassured to avoid making the tests unreliable. Any difference in how the test is done may cause the results to be inaccurate. Additionally, it is crucial that spirometry equipment is well-calibrated, as any issues with the device or incorrect use can lead to incorrect test results and inaccurate assessments. Awareness and control of these factors are paramount to ensuring the reliability of PFT outcomes (Zhou et al., 2024). How the PFT is performed plays a significant role in how accurate the results are. The way selection is done, the criteria used for diagnosis, and the exact protocols can have a significant impact on how pulmonary function is understood. As an illustration, a study found that CT lung volume results are generally more accurate than those from traditional PFTs. Additionally, conducting PFTs on a wide range of patients can lead to variations in the results, which makes it more challenging to establish clear reference values. For this reason, it is necessary to use the same methods and regularly check how well diagnostic tools work in various clinical settings. These considerations are crucial in addressing the challenges inherent to achieving accurate PFT results and ultimately enhancing patient care (Zhou et al., 2024).

11.5.2. Limitations in Specific Populations

There are many restrictions on using PFTs, especially for certain groups of people. Differences in altitude can lead to different respiratory problems for groups, which may affect the accuracy of PFTs. It has been found through research that living at high altitudes can lower the risk of COPD for those at high risk. According to this study, altitude may play a role in influencing lung function and the way diseases appear, which means that interpreting PFTs the same way everywhere might not be right. The demographic and environmental factors, including ethnicity and exposure to biomass fuel, can further complicate the assessment and diagnosis of pulmonary diseases in these populations, necessitating specialized reference values that account for geographical and socioeconomic differences (Wen et al., 2025). People with connective tissue diseases can also make it difficult for PFT results to be accurate. When ILDs are linked to these conditions, PFTs may not fully reflect the level of lung damage or the progression of the disease. As shown in the analysis of KL-6 levels among patients with connective tissue disease-related ILDs, there exists a significant inverse correlation between biomarkers and pulmonary function (Álvarez et al., 2024). Therefore, simply using common PFT results might miss important changes in lung function, especially during the diagnosis or monitoring of disease in these patients. Because these diseases are complex, clinicians should use both biomarkers and regular lung function tests to get a better idea of the patient's breathing problems. Besides, PFTs can be limited when used with people who have low health literacy or come from different cultures. Patients who come from different backgrounds may not fully understand how to do PFTs, which can cause them to do poorly and misunderstand their test results. Additionally, beliefs and practices regarding health and sickness, as well as the accessibility of healthcare, can impact the accuracy of these tests. The results of PFTs can be wrong if the patient's culture is not adequately considered. For this reason, healthcare providers should employ strategies informed by culture and explore various methods to assess patients, ensuring they are diagnosed and treated properly. As a result, healthcare systems can effectively address the challenges of lung disease for all groups of people.

11.5.3. Misinterpretation of Results

Misinterpretation of results in PFTs poses significant challenges in accurately diagnosing and managing respiratory conditions. The way lung function data is interpreted can differ significantly if clinicians do not consider age, gender, and possible comorbidities. These variables significantly influence parameters such as FVC and Diffusion Capacity (DLCO), which, if not contextualized, could mislead healthcare providers. For example, many studies have found that people with long COVID have lung function problems without any noticeable symptoms, since many of them complained about breathing issues even when their lung tests were routine. This underscores the necessity for clinicians to contextualize PFT outcomes within a comprehensive clinical assessment to mitigate potential misinterpretations and ensure that patients receive appropriate treatment strategies (Lehmann et al., 2022). Also, problems in testing or the way experiments are performed can lead to misinterpretation. If PFTs are not performed according to the established guidelines, the results may be incorrect and misinterpreted by clinicians. For example, if the air is polluted during testing or the patient does not cooperate sufficiently, the results of spirometry may be affected. The study found that lung function tests did not always consider lung conditions and the effects of surgery on patients, which shows how important it is to use the proper methods. Ensuring that methodology aligns with clinical standards not only enhances the validity of PFT outcomes but also minimizes the risk of misdiagnosis or mistreatment stemming from flawed interpretations (Choi et al., 2021). Incorrect interpretation of PFT results may result in doctors making wrong choices about a patient's care. A wrong diagnosis might lead to unnecessary treatments and missing out on the right therapy for genuine respiratory problems. During COVID-19, patients with reduced FVC and TLCO might be wrongly diagnosed with COPD, not taking into account their recent viral infection. Since there are many different views, it is essential for clinicians to adopt an integrative approach to patient care that considers all the contextual factors influencing lung function. Thus, fostering clinician education on the importance of comprehensive data interpretation may hold the key to improving clinical outcomes and reducing the likelihood of errors resulting from misinterpretation of PFTs (Lehmann et al., 2022) (Figure 11.15).

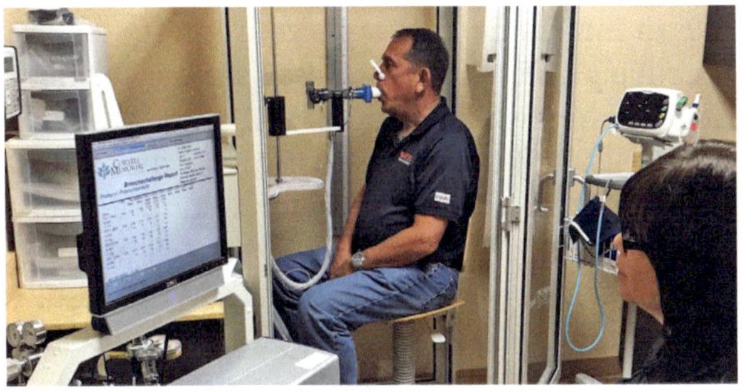

Figure 11.15. Advanced pulmonary function testing in a clinical setting.

Source: https://windsorpulmonaryfibrosis.org/wp-content/uploads/2021/03/Lung-function-test-banner.jpg.

11.6. Advances in Pulmonary Function Testing

The landscape of PFT has evolved considerably in recent years, with advances in technology enhancing diagnostic capabilities. For a long time, spirometry has been the primary method for assessing lung function; however, new imaging techniques are now altering the way we approach this evaluation. Notably, hyperpolarized 129Xe ventilation magnetic resonance imaging (MRI) offers the advantage of visualizing gas distribution within the lungs, allowing for the identification of ventilation defects that standard PFTs may overlook. Combining these methods can provide a clearer view of lung health, especially in cases of ILD, where early detection is crucial for effective management. Using advanced imaging techniques in conjunction with regular tests, healthcare providers can gain a deeper understanding of a patient's condition and select the most suitable care for them. Researchers are intensively studying how imaging biomarkers compare to standard pulmonary function tests, primarily to distinguish between different ILD subtypes. Studies have shown that while traditional spirometry cannot effectively differentiate between various forms of ILD, techniques like dynamic oxygen-enhanced MRI (OE-MRI) have demonstrated potential in this regard. Recent studies, for example, those comparing hyperpolarized 129Xe MRI and OE-MRI to standard PFT, have found that the results do not match up. In a group of ILD patients, imaging revealed that each disease type had its own distinct pattern of ventilation; however, this did not impact the overall lung function observed on spirometry. Due to this disconnect, it is evident that further research is necessary to determine the utility of imaging biomarkers in tracking ILD progression. Although there are difficulties in using advanced imaging in routine healthcare, its advantages are easy to see. With the advancement of pulmonary function testing, clinicians should start using both new imaging tools and traditional methods. As a result, healthcare providers can learn more about lung diseases and how the disease will affect the patient. Although 129Xe MRI and OE-MRI are not as replacements for PFTs today, they are currently used as alternatives to PFTs and provide important information about lung function that could influence future diagnostic methods. Using these advanced tools will help doctors manage patients with pulmonary diseases more effectively, which in turn leads to better health and quality of life for those affected.

11.6.1. Technological Innovations in PFTs

In recent years, advancements in technology have significantly transformed the landscape of PFTs, making them more efficient and accessible. The old PFTs, which were heavy and costly, have become easier to use and smaller in size. With smartphone-connected spirometers, patients can conduct tests at home, which reduces pressure on healthcare centers and provides healthcare providers with quick and reliable data. As a result of these changes, both patient compliance and remote monitoring have improved so that lung function can be checked regularly without many clinic visits. Due to these technological advancements, it is essential to utilize modern tools in daily medical practice to effectively manage chronic respiratory diseases and enhance patient care. In addition, the use of AI and machine learning in PFT interpretation has significantly improved the process of making diagnoses. They can study large sets of data more accurately than people, finding patterns that might be hard for humans to notice. Using algorithms, it is possible to distinguish between different respiratory illnesses based on slight changes in lung function data. As a result, doctors can offer patients more accurate and personalized care. Data analytics can also help identify public health trends and groups that may require healthcare, supporting the need to take action before problems arise. Adding AI to PFTs is a significant development that also alters the way respiratory health is managed, providing doctors with improved tools to treat patients and make more informed decisions. Additionally, online health communities have introduced a new dimension to the way patients learn about and engage in care for pulmonary conditions.

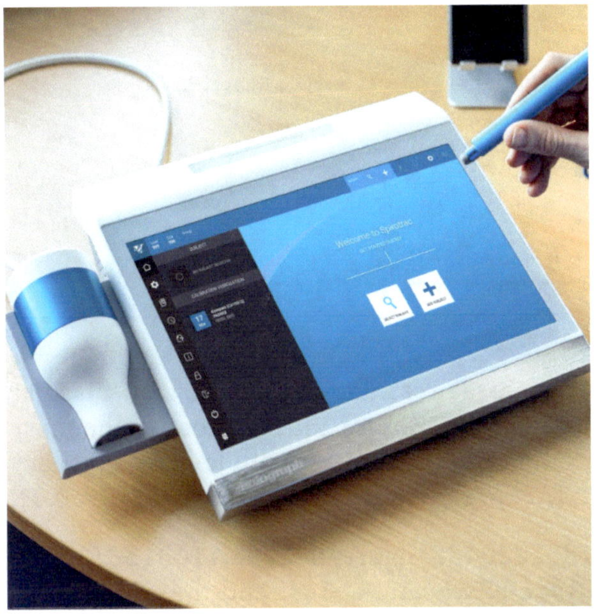

Figure 11.16. Touchscreen-based spirometry system for advanced pulmonary diagnostics.

Source: https://vitalograph.com/img/9194ad1a-e215-4aa0-b307-415a79b14311/img-3193-screen-scaled.webp?fm=webp&q=100&fit=crop&crop=1707%2C1707%2C238%2C0.

Patients now have more ways to talk about their health, get advice, and share what they go through. According to research, many community resources are utilized by patients in conjunction with medical advice, which means healthcare professionals should be aware of them, as evidenced by the investigation into the use of community resources by COPD patients. Talking with patients in these communities can reassure them, help them stick to their treatment, and encourage them to discuss how PFT results can be used in their care. Nevertheless, guide patients toward credible sources of information, enhancing their ability to navigate the wealth of information available and promoting informed health decisions, as illustrated by recent findings on patient participation in online health discussions (Boyce et al., 2020) (Figure 11.16).

11.6.2. Emerging Research and Methodologies

The landscape of PFTs is undergoing a significant transformation driven by emerging research and innovative methodologies. Experts in the field are focusing on enhancing the accuracy and utility of current PFT methods for diagnosis. For example, combining advanced imaging and AI with PFT results could significantly enhance how clinicians assess lung function. They make it possible to understand pulmonary conditions more thoroughly, which helps in early detection and gives patients the right therapies for their needs. Emphasizing care that puts patients first, with the help of new techniques, can greatly benefit pulmonary medicine and result in better outcomes and improved living standards. As new research emerges, clinical practice should also evolve to incorporate these techniques into regular assessments. Increasingly, emerging techniques are focusing on comprehensive and all-encompassing methods to assess the lungs. Still, the use of biomarkers in conjunction with PFTs is likely to provide new insights into lung diseases. Studies have proven that some biomarkers can help predict the outcome of diseases such as pulmonary hypertension, and this can be used along with traditional PFT measures. Studies have demonstrated that the TAPSE/sPAP ratio is a key prognostic factor in patients with systemic sclerosis and pulmonary hypertension, so using novel biomarkers in PFTs is promising. Due to this shift, pulmonary medicine is now transitioning towards personalized care, which utilizes both traditional methods and new scientific discoveries to optimize patient management. It is crucial to have standardized protocols and guidelines to facilitate the transition of new research into clinical practice. A recent group of specialists from diverse backgrounds proposed key strategies for managing complex lung diseases through innovative approaches and collaborative teamwork. The guidelines support doing literature reviews and reaching an agreement to guide how to diagnose and treat illnesses linked to PFT results. Such actions aim to connect advanced research with everyday medical practice, promoting a consistent approach to patient care across various settings. Ultimately, by prioritizing emerging research and establishing robust methodologies, the field of pulmonary function testing can elevate its role in delivering effective and responsive healthcare solutions to individuals with pulmonary conditions, thereby improving overall patient outcomes and quality of life (Figure 11.17).

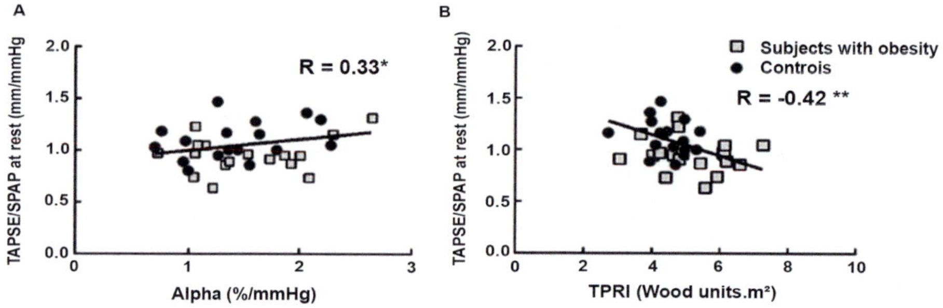

Figure 11.17. Correlation between the TAPSE/sPAP ratio at rest and the pulmonary vascular distensibility coefficient alpha-total during exercise (A); and exercise indexed total pulmonary vascular resistance (TPRi) at normalized maximal common QI (B). Subjects with lower pulmonary vascular distensibility and higher TPRi present lower TAPSE/sPAP ratios. *P < 0.05 and **P < 0.01.

Source: https://www.researchgate.net/publication/362820432/figure/fig3/AS:11431281187292191@1694168912982/Correlation-between-the-TAPSE-sPAP-ratio-at-rest-and-the-pulmonary-vascular.tif.

11.6.3. Future Directions in Pulmonary Diagnostics

New developments in pulmonary diagnostics are focusing on methods that do not require invasive procedures and enhance the accuracy of disease detection. Looking at the composition of exhaled breath could open up new opportunities here. Research has demonstrated that exhaled air contains volatile organic compounds (VOCs) that can indicate pathological conditions, particularly in chronic diseases such as COPD. Utilizing advanced methodologies like electronic noses and gas chromatography–mass spectrometry (GC-MS), studies have successfully identified specific VOCs associated with COPD. It appears that using breath analysis may help identify health issues early in individuals who are at risk. Ultimately, the integration of these non-invasive methods into routine clinical practice could revolutionize the detection and monitoring of pulmonary conditions, ensuring patients receive timely and appropriate care and potentially improving overall patient outcomes in pulmonary health (Bergamini et al., 2015). As personalized medicine becomes more important, it will impact the development of future pulmonary diagnostic methods. It is important to find biomarkers in respiratory diseases, especially in ILDs linked to autoimmune disorders, to guide personalized treatment. When clinical and biological predictors of disease progression are identified, healthcare professionals can monitor patients more closely and assess the effectiveness of their current treatments. Recently, experts have pointed out that having guidelines for screening and monitoring in newly diagnosed autoimmune-related ILDs is very important. When clinicians apply knowledge from pulmonology and rheumatology, they can both enhance their ability to diagnose cases and manage the most challenging patients. This integrative approach signifies a shift towards more holistic and customized care for patients suffering from pulmonary disorders (Good et al., 2024). Improvements in imaging and diagnostic tools will enhance the accuracy and efficiency of pulmonary diagnostics. Innovations in imaging modalities, such as HRCT and positron emission tomography (PET), allow for more detailed visualization of lung pathology. Because of these advancements, it becomes easier to identify conditions that are not always easy to detect, which helps doctors make more accurate predictions. AI and machine learning are now being used in data analysis, which makes it simpler to interpret various types of data, including those from radiology and spirometry. When these technologies are often and more widely in clinics, they are expected to make pulmonary diagnostics more precise and efficient. The combination of technology and clinical work in pulmonary diagnostics could significantly improve the way patients are cared for.

SUMMARY

Evaluating respiratory health and disease depends largely on PFTs. With these tools, it is possible to thoroughly examine lung function, which supports the diagnosis and management of COPD and asthma. Their role is not limited to diagnosis; PFTs can help choose the proper treatment and direct medical decisions. For instance, findings from PFTs can influence the approach to managing patients with advanced COPD, as high attenuation areas identified through quantitative CT analysis have been correlated with parameters of lung function, underscoring the importance of integrating imaging findings with respiratory assessments (Doellinger et al., 2019). Additionally, the use of PFTs in operations affects patient outcomes, particularly in surgical settings. Research has found that performing PFTs before surgery can help predict complications afterward, which is very important for handling patients well. FVC and FEV1 are used to identify patients who may experience respiratory issues after a major procedure, such as coronary artery bypass grafting. Studies emphasize the benefits of targeted preoperative interventions based on PFT results, as demonstrated in patients undergoing various cardiac surgeries (Lopez-Fagin et al., 1996). Therefore, incorporating PFTs into respiratory care enhances the effectiveness and safety of treatment for patients. The impact of PFTs in current clinical care is very significant. They are used to diagnose respiratory diseases and to help determine how patients will react to treatment and surgery. Due to new technologies and techniques, PFTs are now more accurate and reliable, underscoring their importance in the field of respiratory medicine. As new research investigates how lung function metrics affect health outcomes, PFTs are likely to evolve further, providing us with more information about lung diseases and potential treatments. Because they help evaluate lung function, PFTs are crucial for healthcare professionals who aim to provide optimal care for patients with breathing problems. Assessing PFTs is necessary for finding and treating different respiratory illnesses. They measure airflow, the amount of air the lungs can hold, and gas exchange to provide important information about lung health. When a baseline of lung function is set, doctors can detect signs of asthma, COPD, and pulmonary fibrosis. Having knowledge of FVC and FEV1, which are measured by PFTs, allows clinicians to read test results better and design the right treatment plan for each patient. With careful analysis, it is possible to tell apart obstructive from restrictive lung diseases, which highlights the role of PFTs in health care. Following the latest guidelines when performing and interpreting PFTs is necessary to maintain the highest level of respiratory care. New developments in treating lung diseases now emphasize the use of evidence-based methods, reflecting a deeper understanding of how the lungs function. A group made up of pulmonologists, respiratory therapists and other healthcare workers is important in making sure PFTs are correctly used. The focus on structured recommendations matches today's approach which puts patient safety and effectiveness first, over the traditional way. Additionally, new developments in technology and diagnosis necessitate regular updates to the guidelines, ensuring that healthcare professionals are informed about the latest best practices in pulmonary health. Understanding the broader context of pulmonary physiology helps you interpret PFT findings more effectively. PFT abnormalities may indicate underlying health issues that require further evaluation. For example, changes in PFT results can appear in heart failure, which highlights the link between the respiratory and cardiovascular systems. Guidelines such as those from the European Society of Cardiology and the European Respiratory Society further emphasize the importance of this relationship by providing updated strategies for managing pulmonary hypertension and related conditions, as noted in recent publications (Humbert et al., 2022).

CLOSER LOOK

PLETHYSMOGRAPHY

Plethysmography is a method doctors use to measure changes in the size of a body part, primarily to assess blood flow or lung capacity. It requires the use of devices called plethysmographs to detect these changes in volume, typically by measuring pressure or flow rate. It helps in the diagnosis of blood clots, lung function and venous insufficiency.

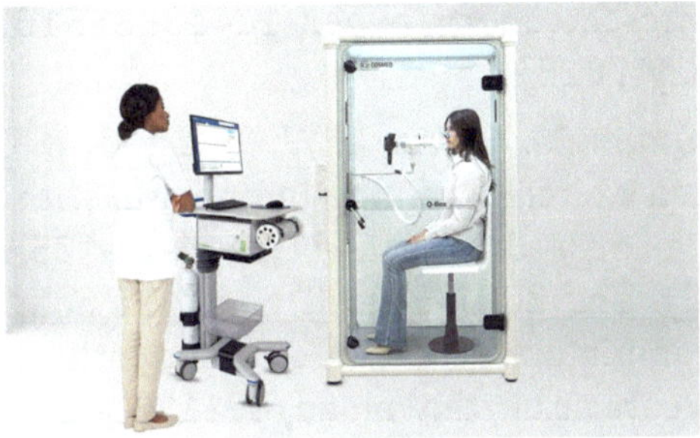

1. **Types of Plethysmography**

- **Body plethysmography:** Measures changes in lung volumes and airway resistance, helping o diagnose conditions such as COPD and other lung diseases.
- **Pulse Plethysmography:** Measures changes in volume associated with arterial blood flow, often used in pulse oximetry and other medical applications.
- **Venous Plethysmography:** Assesses blood flow in veins, which can be used to evaluate venous insufficiency.
- **Penile Pulse Volume Recording:** A specific type of plethysmography used to measure changes in penile volume during sexual arousal.

2. **Applications**

- **Lung Function Testing:** Body plethysmography is used to determine lung volumes, airway resistance, and other lung function parameters.
- **Diagnosis of Blood Clots:** Plethysmography can help detect blood clots in the legs and arms by measuring changes in volume.
- **Venous Insufficiency Assessment:** Venous plethysmography is used to evaluate venous function and identify conditions like varicose veins.
- **Monitoring Blood Flow:** Pulse plethysmography is used in pulse oximetry to measure oxygen saturation and monitor blood flow in various parts of the body.

3. **Procedure**

- **Body Plethysmography:** The patient sits in a sealed box or chamber while their breathing patterns are monitored.
- **Pulse Plethysmography:** A plethysmograph, often a pressure sensor or a light-emitting device, is placed on the body (e.g., finger) to measure changes in blood flow.

REFERENCES

1. Adegunsoye, A., Boctor, N., Chung, J. H., DiGeronimo, et al. (2019). *Diagnostic Test Interpretation and Referral Delay in Patients with Interstitial Lung Disease.* https://core.ac.uk/download/323068477.pdf (accessed on 31st May 2025).
2. Álvarez, T. J., Porto, F. Ó., Fernández, V. M., Gómez, C. L., Soto, A. C., Martínez, R. E., Sorriguieta, T. R., et al. (2024). Evaluating the diagnostic and prognostic utility of serial KL-6 measurements in connective tissue disease patients at risk for interstitial lung disease: Correlations with pulmonary function tests and high-resolution computed tomography. *BMC Pulmonary Medicine, 24.* https://www.semanticscholar.org/paper/1d4d3d855167f45458eaf5699e7281bd178da5be (accessed on 31st May 2025).
3. Amin, S., Abrazado, M., Quinn, M., Storer, T. W., Tseng, C., & Cooper, C. B. (2014). A controlled study of community-based exercise training in patients with moderate COPD. *BMC Pulmonary Medicine, 14*(1). https://doi.org/10.1186/1471-2466-14-125Adang, L. A., Aletaha, D., Armangue, T., Barchus, et al. (2022). The 2021 EULAR and ACR points to consider for diagnosis and management of autoinflammatory type I interferonopathies: CANDLE/PRAAS, SAVI and AGS. *Ann. Rheum Dis.* https://core.ac.uk/download/491172842.pdf (accessed on 31st May 2025).
4. Barkous, B., Briki, C., Boubakri, S., Abdesslem, M., Ben, A. N., Ben, H. W., Ben, S. H. (2024). Routine pulmonary lung function tests: Interpretative strategies and challenges. *Chronic Respiratory Disease, 21.* https://www.semanticscholar.org/paper/d647fa30f783df28c370735da63293b6c1359da8 (accessed on 31st May 2025).
5. Bergamini, A., Calzetta, L., Capuano, R., Cazzola, M., et al. (2015). *Analysis of Exhaled Breath Fingerprints and Volatile Organic Compounds in COPD.* https://core.ac.uk/download/572838474.pdf (accessed on 31st May 2025).
6. Bertolaccini, L., Camilleri, L., Casha, A. R., Dudek, M., et al. (2018). *Pathophysiological Mechanism of Post-Lobectomy Air Leaks.* https://core.ac.uk/download/322748695.pdf (accessed on 31st May 2025).
7. Bhakta, N. R., Bime, C., Kaminsky, D. A., McCormack, M. C., Thakur, N., Stanojevic, S., Baugh, A., et al. (2023). Race and ethnicity in pulmonary function test interpretation: An official American Thoracic Society statement. *American Journal of Respiratory and Critical Care Medicine, 207,* 978–995. https://doi.org/10.1164/rccm.202302-0310st (accessed on 31st May 2025).
8. Bianchi, S., Bruce, I. N., Chaudhuri, N., Eaden, J., et al. (2022). Imaging biomarkers of lung ventilation in interstitial lung disease from ^{129}Xe and oxygen enhanced ^{1}H MRI. *Journal of Magnetic Resonance Imaging.* https://core.ac.uk/download/541106286.pdf (accessed on 31st May 2025).
9. Bianchi, S., Bruce, I. N., Chaudhuri, N., Eaden, J., et al. (2023). Imaging biomarkers of lung ventilation in interstitial lung disease from ^{129}Xe and oxygen enhanced ^{1}H MRI. *Magnetic Resonance Imaging* https://core.ac.uk/download/541738102.pdf (accessed on 31st May 2025).
10. Bonner, S. N., Lagisetty, K., Reddy, R., Engeda, Y., Griggs, J., & Valley, T. (2023). Clinical implications of removing race-corrected pulmonary function tests for African American patients requiring surgery for lung cancer. *JAMA Surgery.* https://www.semanticscholar.org/paper/be2ed19fdde544964714a774d1cd875b60608c89 (accessed on 31st May 2025).

11. Borg, B., Osadnik, C., Adam, K., Chapman, D., Farrow, C., Glavas, V., Hancock, K., et al. (2022). Pulmonary function testing during SARS-CoV-2: An ANZSRS/TSANZ position statement. *Respirology (Carlton, Vic.)*, *27*, 688–719. https://www.semanticscholar.org/paper/0e7f8f5847b3df9dd54eb0fd3f3413b5480a4944 (accessed on 31st May 2025).

12. Boyce, L. K. (2020). *Examination of Online Health Information Seeking Effectiveness: Case Studies of Online Health Communities in COPD Patients.* https://core.ac.uk/download/392378708.pdf (accessed on 31st May 2025).

13. Carl, J., Cheplygina, V., De Bruijne, M., Paschaloudi, A., et al. (2018). *Automatic Emphysema Detection Using Weakly Labeled HRCT Lung Images.* https://core.ac.uk/download/161520273.pdf (accessed on 31st May 2025).

14. Chaithanya, K. S., Basti, A. R. S., & Prabhu, S. M. (2024). Pattern of pulmonary function tests in subjects recovered from COVID-19 infection. *National Board of Examinations Journal of Medical Sciences.* https://www.semanticscholar.org/paper/6e733d911f474b43cec837b845f3e698dfe745c0 (accessed on 31st May 2025).

15. Cheng, Y. T. (2014). Investigation of physiological responses during pulmonary and exercise stress tests and validity of the Wheel Perceived Exertion Scale among adolescents and adults with spina bifida. https://core.ac.uk/download/33560864.pdf (accessed on 31st May 2025).

16. Choi, J., Yang, Z., Lee, J. W., Lee, J. H., Kim, H. K., Yong, H., & Lee, S. Y. (2021). Usefulness of pulmonary rehabilitation in non–small cell lung cancer patients based on pulmonary function tests and muscle analysis using computed tomography images. *Cancer Research and Treatment: Official Journal of Korean Cancer Association*, *54*, 793–802. https://www.semanticscholar.org/paper/1c97a290eb2b7e6ed3d4471772b7ea702f5e1e01 (accessed on 31st May 2025).

17. Chung, J. H., & Goldin, J. G. (2018). Interpretation of HRCT scans in the diagnosis of IPF: Improving communication between pulmonologists and radiologists. *Lung*. https://core.ac.uk/download/323079221.pdf (accessed on 31st May 2025).

18. Dent, R., Greenhalgh, T., Griffin, M., & Parkes, et al. (2008). Effect on smoking quit rate of telling patients their lung age: The Step2quit randomized controlled trial. *BMJ*. https://core.ac.uk/download/1684974.pdf (accessed on 31st May 2025).

19. Digambiro, R. A., Parwanto, E., Tjahjadi, D., & Ditriana, D. (2025). Analysis of pulmonary function between e-cigarette users and non-smokers aged 20–30 years in Jakarta. *Jurnal Respirologi Indonesia*. https://www.semanticscholar.org/paper/55bca9551c77ae558e5edc10b3b38b2fcc3b8182 (accessed on 31st May 2025).

20. Docherty, A. B., Harrison, E. M., Green, C., Hardwick, H., Pius, R., Norman, L., Holden, K., et al. (2020). Features of 20,133 UK patients in hospital with COVID-19 using the ISARIC WHO Clinical Characterization Protocol: Prospective observational cohort study. *BMJ*. https://doi.org/10.1136/bmj.m1985 (accessed on 31st May 2025).

21. Doellinger, F., Feldhaus, F. W., Hubner, R. H., Kuhnigk, et al. (2019). Quantitative CT analysis in patients with pulmonary emphysema: Is lung function influenced by concomitant unspecific pulmonary fibrosis? *International Journal of Chronic Obstructive Pulmonary Disease.* https://core.ac.uk/download/228064807.pdf (accessed on 31st May 2025).

22. Fenech, M., Gouder, C., & Montefort, S. (2012). *Interstitial Lung Disease in Malta.* https://core.ac.uk/download/46602323.pdf (accessed on 31st May 2025).

23. Galić, I., Habijan, M., Leventić, H., & Romić, K. (2023). Machine learning empowering personalized medicine: A comprehensive review of medical image analysis methods. *Electronics, 12*, 4411. https://doi.org/10.3390/electronics12214411 (accessed on 31st May 2025).

24. Good, S., Sparks, J., & Volkmann, E. (2024). Screening, diagnosis, and monitoring of interstitial lung disease in autoimmune rheumatic diseases: A narrative review. Revista Colombiana de Reumatología. https://core.ac.uk/download/618291919.pdf (accessed on 31st May 2025).

25. Hasan, A. A., Hussoon, S. M., Muslim, T. M., & Mohammed, R. M. (2024). Correlation between smoking status and respiratory health among healthcare workers in hospitals of Mosul City/Iraq. *Indonesian Journal on Health Science and Medicine.* https://www.semanticscholar.org/paper/df3d0585ae14d99991e94121a7260f2d2aa8c3ec (accessed on 31st May 2025).

26. Heyer, J. H., Wisch, J. L., Nagra, K. K., Thakur, A., Hillstrom, H. J., Groisser, B. N., Zucker, C. P., et al. (2024). Novel surface topographic assessment of lung volume and pulmonary function tests in idiopathic scoliosis: A preliminary study. *Journal of Pediatric Orthopedics, 44*, 366–372. https://www.semanticscholar.org/paper/bf2f89a05882ff935499a6ff0aa45998bf53afd5 (accessed on 31st May 2025).

27. Humbert, M., Kovács, G., Hoeper, M. M., Badagliacca, R., Berger, R. M. F., Brida, M., Carlsen, J., et al. (2022). 2022 ESC/ERS guidelines for the diagnosis and treatment of pulmonary hypertension. *European Respiratory Journal, 61*, 2200879. https://doi.org/10.1183/13993003.00879-2022 (accessed on 31st May 2025).

28. Khurana, H. S., Kamath, S., Ghosh, K., Biswas, A., & Dasgupta, C. (2024). A study on the outcome of preoperative pulmonary function tests on a patient undergoing rheumatic mitral valve surgery. *Journal of Anesthesiology, Clinical Pharmacology, 40*, 470–477. https://www.semanticscholar.org/paper/e40971533ac302100a24895eb518701e79449f6c (accessed on 31st May 2025).

29. Lehmann, A., Gysan, M., Bernitzky, D., Bal, C., Prosch, H., Zehetmayer, S., Milos, R., et al. (2022). Comparison of pulmonary function test, diffusion capacity, blood gas analysis and CT scan in patients with and without persistent respiratory symptoms following COVID-19. *BMC Pulmonary Medicine, 22*. https://www.semanticscholar.org/paper/559d8f570bd15cbf56a996dc1b6e8f52d1ee93a8 (accessed on 31st May 2025).

30. Li, B., Liu, J., Cao, Y., Wang, Y., Wu, S., Hu, H., Xiao, X., et al. (2025). Multi-omics characterization of early chronic obstructive pulmonary disease. *Respiratory Research, 26*. https://www.semanticscholar.org/paper/5275fe423ff215e30d759315e7ac8a6976b80818 (accessed on 31st May 2025).

31. Liem, R. I., Lanzkron, S., Coates, T. D., DeCastro, L., Desai, A. A., Ataga, K. I., Cohen, R. T., et al. (2019). American Society of Hematology 2019 guidelines for sickle cell disease: Cardiopulmonary and kidney disease. *Blood Advances, 3*, 3867–3897. https://doi.org/10.1182/bloodadvances.2019000916 (accessed on 31st May 2025).

32. Lin, C. H., Cheng, S. L., Chen, C. Z., Chen, C. H., Lin, S. H., & Wang, H. C. (2023). Current progress of COPD early detection: Key points and novel strategies. *International Journal of COPD, 18*, 1511–1524. https://doi.org/10.2147/copd.s413969 (accessed on 31st May 2025).

33. Lopez-Fagin, L. S. (1996). Can target volume breathing exercises taught preoperatively decrease postoperative pulmonary complications for cardiac surgery patients? https://core.ac.uk/download/217400229.pdf (accessed on 31st May 2025).

34. Murphy, E. K., Doussan, A. F., Verga, S., Stommel, E. W., McIlduff, C., Halter, R. J., & Rutkove, S. (2024). Assessing pulmonary function in ALS using electrical impedance tomography. *2024 46th Annual International Conference of the IEEE Engineering in Medicine and Biology Society (EMBC)*. https://www.semanticscholar.org/paper/6ae95f5e79418d451f0fea16ae8ba79e047b3311 (accessed on 31st May 2025).

35. Nelson, R. E., & Richards, J. (2023). Breathing, obstruction, restriction, and gas exchange: A pulmonary function testing interpretation framework for novice learners. *ATS Scholar, 4*, 230–240. https://www.semanticscholar.org/paper/501c7e1cc7e99cc9bde717f733a6c924a5b22a3a (accessed on 31st May 2025).

36. Page, M. J., Moher, D., Bossuyt, P. M., Boutron, I., Hoffmann, T., Mulrow, C. D., Shamseer, L., et al. (2021). PRISMA 2020 explanation and elaboration: Updated guidance and exemplars for reporting systematic reviews. *BMJ*. https://doi.org/10.1136/bmj.n160 (accessed on 31st May 2025).

37. Petersson Sjögren, M. (2023). *Structure of the Distal Lung Studied with Inhaled Nanoparticles*. https://core.ac.uk/download/558638873.pdf (accessed on 31st May 2025).

38. Rex, D. K., Schoenfeld, P., Cohen, J., Pike, I. M., Adler, D. G., Fennerty, B., Lieb, J., et al. (2014). Quality indicators for colonoscopy. *The American Journal of Gastroenterology, 110*, 72–90. https://doi.org/10.1038/ajg.2014.385 (accessed on 31st May 2025).

39. Rossaint, R., Afshari, A., Bouillon, B., Černý, V., Cimpoeşu, D., Curry, N., Duranteau, J., et al. (2023). The European guideline on management of major bleeding and coagulopathy following trauma: Sixth edition. *Critical Care, 27*. https://doi.org/10.1186/s13054-023-04327-7 (accessed on 31st May 2025).

40. Santos, C. S., Retuerto, M., Sierra, L., Calleja, A. S., Bollo De, M. E., Ordas, M. J., De La Calle, L. J., et al. (2025). P135: KL-6 and IL-18 biomarkers in systemic sclerosis-associated interstitial lung disease: Enhancing prognostic insights into early detection, progression, lung volume changes, and mortality risk. *Rheumatology*. https://www.semanticscholar.org/paper/d58475b7c2264c5bcbc1ff67f7d9131fc28e3c02 (accessed on 31st May 2025).

41. Short, C., Semple, T., Abkir, M., Padley, S., Rosenthal, M., McNally, P., Tiddens, H., et al. (2024). Silence of the lungs: Comparing measures of slow and noncommunicating lung units from pulmonary function tests with computed tomography. *Journal of Applied Physiology, 137*, 883–891. https://www.semanticscholar.org/paper/06f67ace4c151507fc92cd73ff3b3fedb2e4f304 (accessed on 31st May 2025).

42. Spinella, A., Guerra, A. F., Mattioli, A. V., Ferri, C., Giuggioli, D., Lumetti, F., Coppi, F., et al. (2024). The predictive role of the TAPSE/sPAP ratio for cardiovascular events and mortality in systemic sclerosis with pulmonary hypertension. *Front. Cardiovasc. Med.* https://core.ac.uk/download/638790873.pdf (accessed on 31st May 2025).

43. Torregiani, C., Reale, M., Confalonieri, M., Dore, F., Crisafulli, C., Baratella, E., Salton, F., et al. (2024). Cardiopulmonary exercise testing complements both spirometry and nuclear imaging for assessing sarcoidosis stage and for monitoring disease activity. *Sarcoidosis, Vasculitis, and Diffuse Lung Diseases, 41*. https://www.semanticscholar.org/paper/8a4e88bd6b33538943ba12b800bf1533203aa4a5 (accessed on 31st May 2025).

44. Vahanian, A., Beyersdorf, F., Praz, F., Milojevic, M., Baldus, S., Bauersachs, J., Capodanno, D., et al. (2021). 2021 ESC/EACTS Guidelines for the management of valvular heart disease.

European Heart Journal, 43, 561–632. https://doi.org/10.1093/eurheartj/ehab395 (accessed on 31st May 2025).

45. Vicente, B. A., Sebastião, R., & Sencadas, V. (2024). Wearable devices for respiratory monitoring. *Advanced Functional Materials*. https://www.semanticscholar.org/paper/776918c8bb699efac7314413b4ae2fd759cccac7 (accessed on 31st May 2025).
46. Wen, G., Meng, J., Wang, H., Peng, P., Xu, Y., Wang, R., Yan, Z., et al. (2025). Prevalence of chronic obstructive pulmonary disease in high-risk populations at low, intermediate, high altitudes: A population-based cross-sectional study in Yunnan Province, China. *BMC Pulmonary Medicine, 25*. https://www.semanticscholar.org/paper/5a72d9cfbd45d8e059564fff8c61b8759b774e1a (accessed on 31st May 2025).
47. Yang, X., Wei, Y., Zhao, J., & Bai, Y. (2025). Correlation of lung function and sarcopenia in elderly patients with chronic obstructive pulmonary disease and analysis of factors influencing sarcopenia. *American Journal of Translational Research, 17*(1), 358–376. https://www.semanticscholar.org/paper/ffd257513e25294b6b556a6e21a648f4f9166aad (accessed on 31st May 2025).
48. Zamora, A. C., Jokerst, C., Yaddanapudi, K., Chaudhary, S., & Nagaraja, V. (2024). Imaging innovations in the screening, diagnosis, and monitoring of systemic autoimmune disease-related interstitial lung disease. MJ Radiology. https://core.ac.uk/download/620324047.pdf (accessed on 31st May 2025).
49. Zhou, J., Cai, Q., Zhao, Z., Dai, M., & Liang, Y. (2024). Decreases in lung volume and lung height among ankylosing spondylitis patients with pulmonary function impairment: A 3D CT investigation. *Journal of Orthopedic Surgery and Research, 19*. https://www.semanticscholar.org/paper/6392df2a9a0d76dbac4395da8f43e0ee7dd8e506 (accessed on 31st May 2025).
50. Zhou, L., Zhang, H., Yang, H., Li, Z., Han, C., Zhang, Y., & Hai, Y. (2023). Evaluation of pulmonary function after halo-pelvic traction for severe and rigid kyphoscoliosis utilizing CT with 3D reconstruction. *The Journal of Bone and Joint Surgery, 105*, 1793–1800. https://www.semanticscholar.org/paper/c458aeebf2c716cc300a71f97ad50972dbcfefa8 (accessed on 31st May 2025).

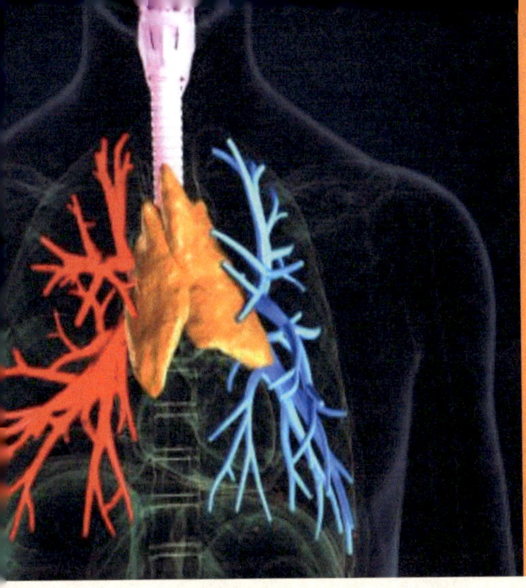

Chapter 12

NON-RESPIRATORY FUNCTIONS OF THE LUNG

Contents

Introduction

The lungs are primarily known for their role in breathing, but they also play a crucial part in several other vital functions essential for overall health and bodily balance. It is important to know these functions, because they show that lungs do more than just exchange gases. Lung tissue is involved in immune protection, control over inflammation, and making different bioactive substances. This is most evident in respiratory illnesses, where problems with other systems can exacerbate the primary condition. Recognizing these points enables more comprehensive medical care that considers the lungs from various perspectives. The lungs are involved in the endocrine system, a clear indication of their additional functions. The lungs make and release hormones and signaling molecules, and these play a role in cardiovascular health, fluid balance, and metabolism. For instance, angiotensin-converting enzyme (ACE), primarily known for its role in blood pressure regulation, is also produced in the lungs, indicating the organ's influence on systemic vascular health. Because of these details, the lungs are recognized as important in many bodily functions, which means treatment should address both their respiratory and non-respiratory roles. In addition, research in biomedicine is starting to show that lung-derived stem cells and organoids may be functional in regenerative medicine and for studying diseases. They give new insights into lung diseases and also lead to new ways of treating them. As researchers have been able to grow human airway organoids from lung tissue for a long time, they can study CF and check how drugs affect the disease. Due to these developments, it is clear that the lung is important for health and disease, and understanding its other roles is necessary for progress in medicine and better patient care. Studying all aspects of lung function, not just those related to breathing, remains crucial due to its current application in medical practice.

Definition of Lung Functions

Lung functions are not limited to just the usual ideas related to breathing. The lungs primarily function by allowing oxygen into the blood and removing carbon dioxide. However, new studies reveal that the lungs have vital functions beyond breathing, which contribute to maintaining overall systemic health. Among its functions are the regulation of acid-base balance, the modulation of the immune response, and the synthesis of specific bioactive molecules. The lungs play a crucial role in maintaining the body's metabolic balance by regulating pH levels through gas exchange. Such findings alter the conventional view of lung function, suggesting that it is important for homeostasis and immunity, not just for breathing. In addition to facilitating gas exchange and balance, the lungs play a crucial role in the body's immune system. Immune cells in the lymph nodes respond to pathogens, allergens, and other stimuli that trigger inflammation. The pulmonary microenvironment enables the body to detect harmful substances and organize immune responses that prevent infections from occurring. As alveolar macrophages are present in the lungs, this proves that the body has a strong defense against infections and illnesses. Such immune actions point out that the lungs are involved in more than just the transport of oxygen.

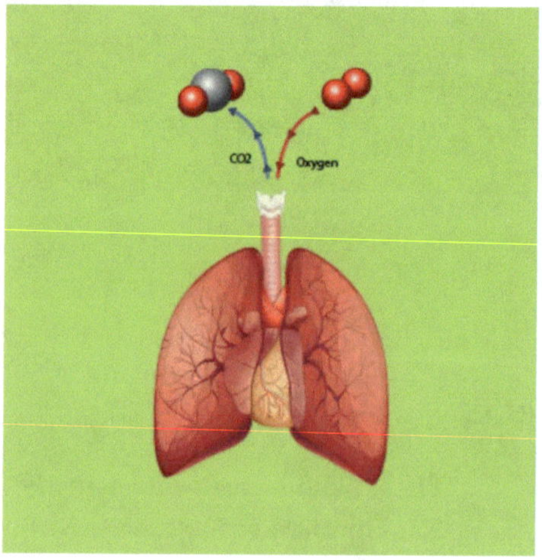

Figure 12.1. Lung functions.

Source: https://www.breathefree.com/-/media/project/breathefree/images/lung-health/how-lungs-look-and-function/function-of-the-lungs-1-2.png?updated=20241115050247.

So, they are involved in the immune system, and this involvement makes their other functions important for understanding lung health and diseases in general, biomedical terms. New research is uncovering the role that lungs play in metabolizing and activating hormones and regulatory molecules, which adds to our understanding of the lungs' functions. For instance, the conversion of angiotensin II (a potent vasoconstrictor) into angiotensin (1–7) is facilitated by the lungs, influencing blood pressure regulation and vascular tone. Since the lungs are involved in metabolism, they support heart health, which is especially evident in conditions such as COVID-19, where vascular problems have been observed. Studies demonstrate that COVID-19 can trigger distinct patterns of acute respiratory distress syndrome (ARDS), characterized by significant endothelial involvement, indicating a nuanced relationship between lung functions and systemic vascular health (Nilam et al., 2020). Thus, understanding the non-respiratory functions of the lung is crucial for advancing therapeutic strategies and improving patient care in both respiratory and systemic diseases (Figure 12.1).

Overview of Respiratory vs. Non-Respiratory Functions

The lungs are primarily known for their role in respiration, which involves exchanging oxygen and carbon dioxide in the blood. Still, the many other important jobs they do prove their significance to health. In addition to gas exchange, the lungs are involved in metabolic activities, including the regulation of hormones, such as angiotensin II, which helps control blood pressure. Also, the pulmonary circulation helps to filter out small blood clots and microbes, which protects the body from infections. The lungs play a crucial role in numerous immune functions, underscoring their significant contribution to maintaining the body's balance. Therefore, a comprehensive understanding of pulmonary function should encompass more than just breathing and include these key non-breathing roles, highlighting the complexity of the lungs. for the body's immune system. There are many innate immune cells in the respiratory epithelium, such as macrophages and dendritic cells, that react rapidly to inhaled pathogens. Due to this, the lungs help manage immune functions within the lungs and throughout the body, which helps prevent many respiratory infections. Mucus is also produced, which traps particles and pathogens and helps them be removed from the airways. Because the respiratory and immune systems depend on each other, lung health is crucial for both breathing and preventing diseases, such as pneumonia and COPD. This way, the lungs serve as a crucial link between the respiratory and non-respiratory systems in the human body. Additionally, the lungs have been found to play a role in regulating overall health by affecting blood pressure. Angiotensin I becomes angiotensin II, which is a potent vasoconstrictor in the pulmonary capillaries. It shows that the lungs help regulate the heart and stress their role in preserving the stability of the vascular system. Additionally, lung conditions, such as interstitial lung disease (ILD) or sarcoidosis, can have a cascading effect on other organ systems, often due to underlying systemic inflammation or impaired gas exchange. The non-respiratory functions of the lungs also extend to their interaction with conditions like primary Sjögren's syndrome, where lung involvement significantly impacts patient morbidity and mortality (Duarte et al., 2019). Therefore, understanding how lung physiology affects the rest of the body highlights the importance of non-respiratory functions, making it necessary to investigate their role in overall health.

Importance of Studying Non-Respiratory Functions

It is essential to understand how the lungs function besides breathing, especially when dealing with new respiratory diseases. The lungs primarily facilitate gas exchange, but they also play a role in controlling inflammation and maintaining the stability of the immune system. Recent studies have found that lung problems associated with COVID-19 affect more than just breathing, so a comprehensive approach to treatment and management is necessary. Those who have recovered from COVID-19 have shown several health problems, such as reduced mental abilities and less physical fitness, even after their acute respiratory symptoms have eased. This underscores the fundamental need to study and recognize non-respiratory functions, as neglecting these may lead to unaddressed health challenges and diminished quality of life for affected individuals (Johnsen et al., 2021). Furthermore, the way microRNAs affect chronic respiratory diseases underscores the importance of investigating their roles in other bodily systems. MicroRNAs help control important processes in the body, such as inflammation and cell differentiation, which are key to how the lungs function.

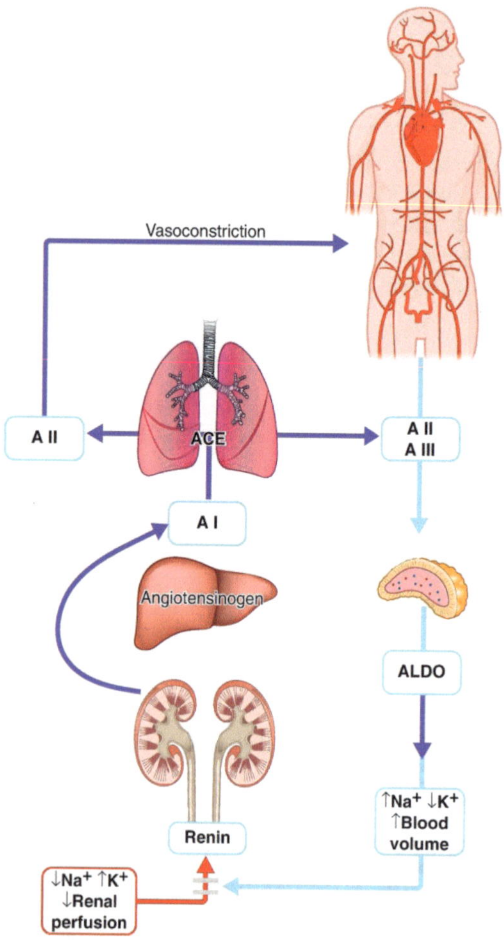

Figure 12.2. Non-respiratory functions.

Source: https://media.springernature.com/lw685/springer-static/image/chp%3A10.1007%2F978-3-030-00859-8_7/MediaObjects/185149_2_En_7_Fig2_HTML.jpg.

They can cause and influence diseases, which means they are important for respiratory issues as well as for conditions affecting other organ systems. For chronic conditions such as asthma, COPD, and idiopathic pulmonary fibrosis (IPF), alterations in microRNA expression can lead to dysregulated inflammation, ultimately impacting respiratory function and overall health. Studying these regulatory processes could lead to the development of new therapies and biomarkers to enhance the management of lung diseases. Thus, the study of non-respiratory functions is paramount to advancing comprehensive lung disease management (Lindsay et al., 2017). Additionally, examining non-respiratory lung functions aids in public health efforts and the prevention of various diseases. Since lung health affects the whole body, learning about non-respiratory functions can help find diseases earlier, sort patients by risk, and choose the right treatments. It is particularly important in chronic respiratory diseases, where prompt treatment may help prevent complications that affect more than just breathing. If healthcare providers understand the various functions of the lungs, they can develop more effective ways to prevent and treat diseases that also improve patients' overall well-being. As the burden of chronic respiratory diseases continues to grow globally, prioritizing research and advocacy surrounding the non-respiratory functions of the lung will be essential for improving patient outcomes and public health (Lindsay et al., 2017) (Figure 12.2).

12.1. Filtration of Particulate Matter

The lungs are primarily known for gas exchange, but they also play a role in filtering particles from the air. The filtration process helps keep the respiratory system and the whole body safe from inhaled pollutants outside. The lungs are composed of a tracheobronchial tree and mucous membranes that contain ciliated epithelial cells, which serve as a barrier. The cells hold inhaled particles, pathogens, and dust, so they do not reach the alveoli, where breathing takes place. Removing pollutants from the air, the lungs help both the respiratory and overall health of the body. In addition to using mechanical filtration, the lungs employ biochemical methods to deal with particles. Alveolar macrophages which live in the lungs, work to swallow and destroy small particles and germs that escape the first stages of filtration.

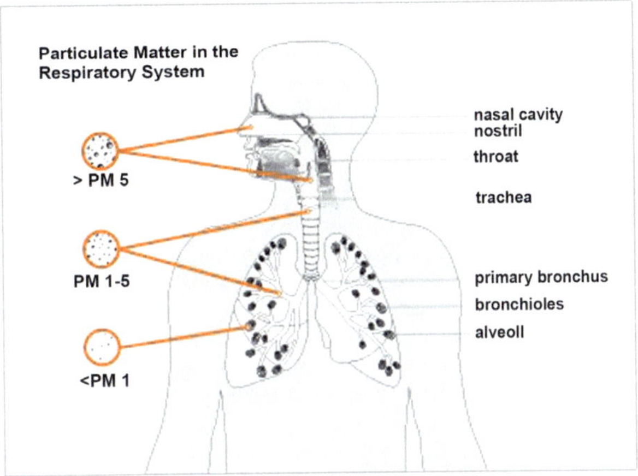

Figure 12.3. Particulate matter in the respiratory system.

Source: https://alen.com/pages/everything-you-need-to-know-about-airborne-particulate-matter.

This immune response is crucial, especially given the potential for particulate matter to induce inflammation and exacerbate respiratory conditions such as asthma and chronic obstructive pulmonary disease (COPD). The innate immune functions of the lungs are underscored by research such as the Global Burden of Diseases, Injuries, and Risk Factors Study, which highlights the impact of environmental risks on lung health and the systemic effects of particulate matter exposure (Gakidou et al., 2017). Additionally, removing particulate matter from the air is crucial for maintaining respiratory health and supporting other bodily functions. Proper filtering of harmful particles by the lungs decreases the body's overall inflammation and oxidative stress, which can prevent many diseases not related to the lungs. For instance, chronic exposure to fine particulate matter is associated with cardiovascular diseases (CVDs), underscoring the importance of lung filtration in maintaining overall health. Furthermore, the interaction of lung-derived substances, such as exosomes, with systemic circulation indicates a sophisticated communication network that may involve waste disposal and signaling functions beyond respiration (Gurunathan et al., 2019). Thus, the lungs' ability to filter particulate matter plays a crucial role in promoting not only respiratory but also systemic health (Figure 12.3).

12.1.1. Mechanisms of Filtration in the Lungs

The lungs are important for more than just breathing, primarily because they filter out harmful substances. The pulmonary system checks the air we breathe and collects any harmful particles or microorganisms it finds. Nasal turbinates, mucous, and cilia in the lungs all operate together to catch foreign particles. By filtering air in various ways, the process ensures that the lower respiratory tract is safe and the alveoli are protected from toxins and germs. Being able air matters a lot, as it helps both lung health and can impact diseases caused by environmental factors. The interaction between the lungs and the immune system is a significant aspect of pulmonary filtration. Pathogens removed by the lungs can trigger an immune system response, leading to inflammation. Although fighting infections requires this response from the immune system, excessive or uncontrolled activity can result in a cytokine storm, which is commonly observed in severe COVID-19 cases. This shows that the lungs act to keep out harmful elements and also add to inflammation in the body. Recent studies have shown that such immune reactions can be particularly detrimental, leading to acute lung injury (ALI) and respiratory failure. Understanding the complex interplay between filtration mechanisms and immune responses is vital for developing therapeutic interventions that mitigate lung injury while preserving the protective functions of the respiratory system, as demonstrated by the role of ACE2 in modulating these responses (Monteil et al., 2020). Additionally, understanding how the lungs filter air is crucial for comprehending various respiratory diseases and their corresponding treatments.

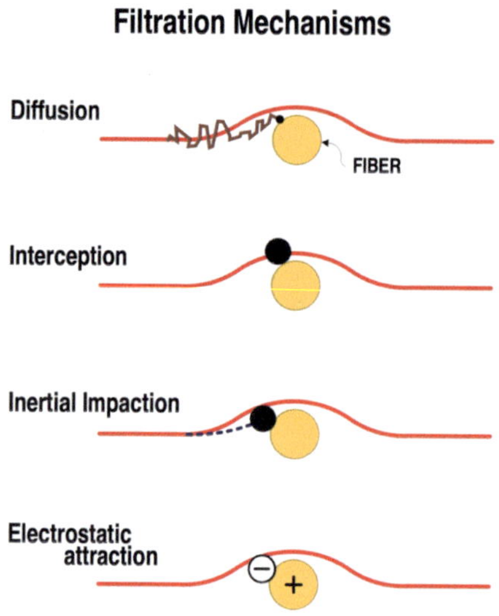

Figure 12.4. Filtration mechanisms.

Source: https://cdn.breathesafeair.com/wp-content/uploads/2020/07/Respirator-Filtration-Mechanisms-768x894.png?strip=all&lossy=1&ssl=1.

For instance, the expression of angiotensin-converting enzyme 2 (ACE2) in the lungs not only serves as a receptor for SARS-CoV and SARS-CoV-2 but also plays a protective role by enhancing local immune responses and mitigating inflammation (Monteil et al., 2020). Due to these numerous factors, it is crucial to investigate the impact of lung filtering on the risk of viral infections and associated health issues. Observations in clinical settings during the pandemic have highlighted the importance of these mechanisms, particularly in cases of cytokine storms observed in severely ill patients. Hence, an integrated understanding of pulmonary filtration and its non-respiratory functions is crucial for advancing therapeutic strategies that safeguard pulmonary health while addressing the challenges posed by viral pathogens (Figure 12.4).

12.1.2. Role of Mucus and Cilia in Trapping Particles

The mucosal lining of the respiratory tract plays a pivotal role in the non-respiratory functions of the lung, particularly in trapping airborne particles and pathogens. Mucus, which is made by goblet cells, is the main defense against harmful substances, allergies, and infections. It traps the inhaled particles, so they do not reach the sensitive parts of the lungs. The important components of mucus are glycoproteins, water, salts, and antimicrobial peptides, which make it more protective. By maintaining a hydrophilic environment, mucus not only captures and isolates foreign particles but also facilitates their expulsion from the airways through cilia-mediated transport, thereby playing a crucial role in lung health and defense against infections, especially under conditions such as those exacerbated by SARS-CoV-2 targeting respiratory mucosal cells, a concern underscored in recent studies (Simukoko et al., 2021) (Figure 12.5). Mucus and cilia, which are found along the respiratory lining, work together to remove debris that enters the lungs.

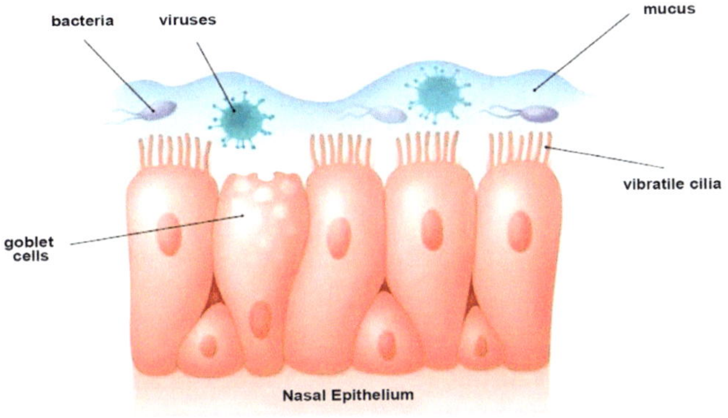

Figure 12.5. Nasal mucus: The nose is the first line of defense.

Source: https://ik.imagekit.io/rinosol2act/come_funziona_il_naso/nasal-mucus.jpg?updatedAt=1630005969699.

They move in a coordinated way, bringing the mucus up to the pharynx, which is called mucociliary clearance. The mechanism helps remove trapped particles and also supports the balance of the respiratory tract by controlling how pathogens and particulates are handled.

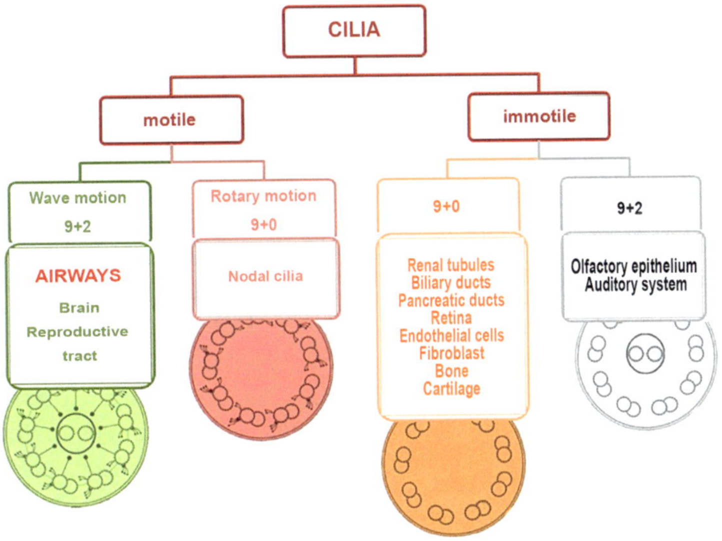

Figure 12.6. Cilia.

Source: https://www.frontiersin.org/files/Articles/516741/fphar-11-00609-HTML/image_m/fphar-11-00609-g001.jpg.

In conditions such as COPD and cystic fibrosis (CF), the efficiency of this system can be significantly disrupted. Due to inflammation, the mucus and cilia in these diseases do not function properly, which causes the airways to narrow and increases the likelihood of infections. The role of mucus and cilia is critical, as any dysfunction can compromise the lungs' ability to defend against environmental insults, emphasizing the importance of understanding these mechanisms (Bhongir et al., 2017). Additionally, the interaction between mucus and cilia is crucial for the overall immune response in the respiratory system. Mucus holds pathogens and also includes immunoglobulins and other immune factors that work against microorganisms. If the mucosal layer is weakened, as occurs in various lung diseases, the body's innate immune system must contend with new challenges. For example, when there is inflammation, the mucus might thicken, which stops ciliary movement and leaves the airways exposed to germs for longer. This link becomes particularly important when discussing severe breathing problems and infections, as poor mucociliary function increases a person's likelihood of developing ARDS and bronchitis. Understanding how mucus and ciliary action intersect with immune functions provides insight into potential therapeutic interventions targeting these non-respiratory functions of the lung (Simukoko et al., 2021) (Figure 12.6).

12.1.3. Impact of Air Quality on Lung Filtration Efficiency

The lung's ability to filter out particles to modulate inhaled air quality further underscores the lung's importance to other physiological tasks, aside from breathing. The lungs are essential for breathing and also play a crucial role in defending the body against harmful particles in the air. Having poor air quality, full of particles, toxic gases, and other pollutants, can seriously reduce the lungs' ability to clean the air we breathe. A decline in filtration makes it easier for harmful materials to reach the bloodstream, which can harm the body. Additionally, exposure to these pollutants can lead to ongoing inflammation and changes in the lungs, making it more difficult for the lungs to function and potentially leading to lung diseases that also impact non-breathing tasks. Understanding these factors is crucial for developing effective public health plans that improve air quality and protect people's lungs. Besides trapping particles, the lungs help control several key biochemical and physiological activities that are necessary for a healthy body. These activities are affected when air quality is poor. Pollutants are often the cause of disruptions in non-respiratory functions, which can influence the production and regulation of surfactants and other substances necessary for healthy lungs. It affects the way the lungs work as well as their ability to control inflammation and protect the body. A lack of clean air might disrupt the secretion of exosomes, which are important for intercellular communication and the movement of molecules that can control inflammation and injury in the lungs. As highlighted in current literature, understanding the implications of these changes is pressing for further research in pulmonary health (Zhang et al., 2020). Reducing the negative impact of air pollution on lung filtration efficiency requires measures that combine increased public awareness with targeted actions. Efforts to reduce emissions and improve air quality can significantly enhance lung health. Protocols designed for people recovering from surgery, such as those for airway care, can be helpful after exposure to poor air quality. For instance, recommendations for nutritional screening and prehabilitation for high-risk individuals may mitigate the effects of exposure on lung function, thereby preserving filtration efficiency (Batchelor et al., 2018). Through a combination of public health strategies and personal health initiatives, it is possible to protect the lung's vital non-respiratory functions, improving both individual and community health amidst ongoing air quality challenges (Figure 12.7).

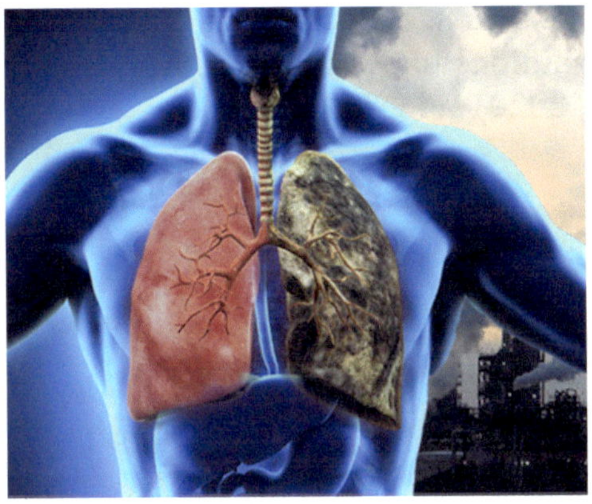

Figure 12.7. Comparative visualization of healthy and polluted lungs highlighting the impact of air quality on lung filtration efficiency.

Source: https://www.lifelinecelltech.com/wp-content/uploads/2021/03/lung-Smog-image-blog.jpg.

12.2. Immune Defense Mechanisms

The immune defense mechanisms of the lungs play a critical role beyond the respiratory functions traditionally associated with this organ. Development of the BALT begins at a young age in birds and it is a significant part of the immune system. BALT has organized B and T cells that help the immune system combat various pathogens. BALT is important because it supports the growth and specialization of lymphocytes, which are needed for a strong immune response. Because of this arrangement, the immune system can react quickly to germs in the lungs and prevent them from spreading to other areas of the body. These mechanisms explain the various ways the lungs support the immune system, which is essential for maintaining good health and combating diseases. Besides BALT, the lungs are defended by tissue macrophages and lymphocytes, which play a crucial role in identifying and combating infectious agents. When there is no inflammation, the number of macrophages on the respiratory surface is low, which reflects regular immune monitoring. Even so, adding live bacteria can prompt many active macrophages and heterophils to move into the lung and quickly deal with infection. Being able to mobilize immune cells highlights the key role of innate immunity and demonstrates that the lungs play an active role in maintaining the body's balance. So, making sure immune cells are present but not overly active is necessary for the lungs to function well, showing its importance in non-respiratory roles. The complexity of immune responses within the lung is further exemplified in bovine respiratory disease (BRD), where a diverse range of viral and bacterial pathogens interact with lymphoid tissues. It has been found that the transcriptional changes in the lungs and nearby lymph nodes, such as the bronchial and retropharyngeal lymph nodes, are distinct from each other. Based on the kind of pathogen, the immune system responds differently, and this affects the whole immune response network. Specific immune genes are found to coordinate the activity of other genes, which help the body fight against BRD pathogens. Understanding these intricate immune mechanisms paves the way for innovative therapeutic approaches and highlights the significance of the lungs' role in systemic immune regulation, further illustrating the non-respiratory functions of this vital organ (Dalamani et al., 2006; Behura et al., 2017).

12.2.1. Presence of Immune Cells in Lung Tissue

In addition to gas exchange, the lungs play a vital role in the body's immune response. Lung tissue has immune cells that are the first to stop viruses, bacteria and fungi from causing illness. For example, macrophages, dendritic cells, and lymphocytes are placed in the mucous membranes and air sacs, which allows them to identify and respond to threats in the air quickly. These immune cells in the lungs demonstrate that the lungs have functions beyond breathing, and they play a crucial role in both innate and adaptive immune responses. Understanding how these immune cells interact with pathogens is essential not only for grasping lung function but also for devising strategies to combat respiratory infections, particularly those caused by novel viruses like SARS-CoV-2, which has been shown to elicit significant immune responses in lung tissues (Hu et al., 2020). Studies of the lungs' immune profile show that several immune cells work together, especially when the body is affected by infections like COVID-19. In the most severe cases, immune cells, particularly macrophages and T lymphocytes, found in lung tissue are associated with harmful changes in the lungs, such as ARDS. Sometimes, these immune responses are not appropriately controlled, which results in more inflammation and damage to tissues. Studies indicate that the presence of high numbers of immune cells in the bronchoalveolar lavage fluid (BALF) of COVID-19 patients may signify an ongoing and, at times, overwhelming immune response. The implications of such findings extend beyond the immediate effects of viral infections, as they also raise questions about the long-term sequelae of lung-immune interactions, particularly regarding the development of chronic lung diseases following acute respiratory infections (Maggi et al., 2020). Moreover, having immune cells in the lungs highlights their key role in managing the local immune response, which can result in protection or in disease. In this way, the body recruits neutrophils, macrophages, and T cells to fight pathogens, which may result in both clearing the infection and causing some local inflammation. The inflammatory response is crucial for initiating repair, but if it persists for too long, it can cause significant damage to the lungs. Examining how immune cells behave in the lungs during disease is crucial for developing treatments that maintain the immune system's activity while also promoting healing. Such therapies would help mitigate the often devastating effects of viral infections on lung tissue, underscoring the need for comprehensive investigations into the multifunctional roles of immune cells in the pulmonary system and their contributions to overall respiratory health (Hu et al., 2020) (Figure 12.8).

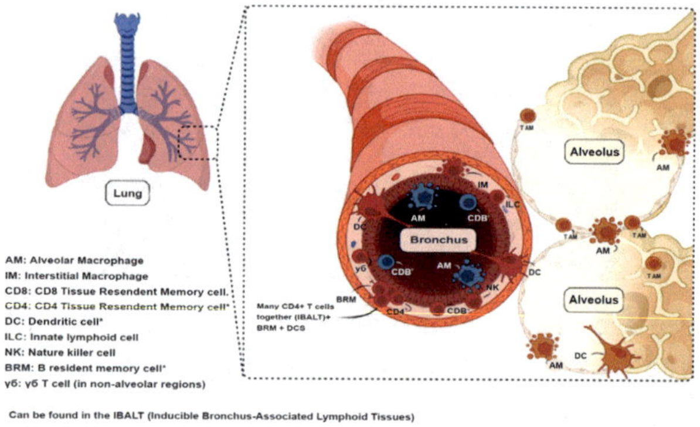

Figure 12.8. Location of immune tissue-resident cells in the lungs (alveoli and bronchus).

Source: https://www.researchgate.net/publication/364821458/figure/fig1/AS:11431281103640797@1669776975217/Location-of-immune-tissue-resident-cells-in-the-lungs-alveoli-and-bronchus-Created.png.

12.2.2. Role of the Lungs in the Body's Immune Response

Besides their primary job of exchanging gases, the lungs are important in the body's immune functions. They serve as a link between the outside world and the body's systems, containing many immune cells that are constantly searching for pathogens. The respiratory epithelium produces defensins and collectins, which help prevent the growth of invading microorganisms. Additionally, resident macrophages are present in the alveoli, where they can remove pathogens and debris, initiating the immune response. This interaction between the lungs and immune cells demonstrates that the lungs play a crucial role in defending the body against various infections and in controlling inflammation, thereby maintaining the body's normal functioning during potential invasions by pathogens. The lungs play a crucial role in regulating the body's overall immune response. For example, the lungs can direct immune cells to various parts of the body by producing chemokines and cytokines, which are essential for the movement and activation of immune cells. When pathogens or inflammation affect the lungs, lung cells release these signals to draw immune cells from the blood into the lung tissue. It stresses that both local and systemic immunity can be affected by the lungs. Changes in immune responses in the lungs can significantly impact the immune system's effectiveness during respiratory tract infections. Since the lungs face numerous pathogens, it is crucial for their immune system to function effectively to prevent excessive inflammation and tissue damage. Evidence suggests that lung-mediated immune responses can be highly complex, particularly during viral infections. Building models that demonstrate how viruses impact the immune system highlights the significance of an early immune response during infections. They help explain the specific jobs of different immune cells and the guidelines that affect their actions. It is now thought that the connection between the lungs and the immune system is significant for treating infections and for developing new drugs. By identifying differences in viral dynamics and immune responses in the upper versus the lower respiratory tract, researchers are better equipped to develop targeted therapeutic strategies for lung diseases and bolster the immune defenses therein, echoing the versatile non-respiratory functions of this vital organ (Suflita et al., 2012; Giegold et al., 2018).

12.2.3. Interaction Between Respiratory and Immune Systems

The lungs serve a critical dual role, functioning not only in respiration but also as a key player in the immune system. Since the respiratory tract is constantly exposed to airborne germs, allergens, and particles, it requires a robust defense mechanism. The first layer of protection is composed of lung epithelial cells, which also produce substances that prevent microbes and trap harmful particles. The mucosal area contains a lot of immune cells, such as macrophages and dendritic cells, that are in close contact with inhaled substances. As a result of these interactions, the immune system can effectively deal with infections at the local site and also regulate overall immunity to prevent pathogens from spreading. Thus, the lungs demonstrate how respiratory and immune functions are closely linked, illustrating their importance in defending the body against threats. The lungs, besides their protective role, play a crucial part in adapting the immune system. If pathogens enter the respiratory epithelium, dendritic cells migrate to nearby lymph nodes and instruct naïve T cells to respond. When considering respiratory infections such as tuberculosis, the lung's involvement is crucial because it depends on a strong immune response to be contained. Based on recent research, mucosal vaccines targeting Mycobacterium tuberculosis appear to elicit a stronger immune response than traditional vaccines, suggesting that the respiratory system can be effectively utilized. These developments underline the dynamic interplay between pulmonary function and immune modulation, reinforcing the lungs' central position in orchestrating overall body immunity (WR et al., 2019). Additionally, the interaction between the immune system and the respiratory system can play a role in the development of respiratory diseases. An example of this is equine herpesvirus type 1, which can complicate disease progression due to these interactions. It utilizes the mucosal epithelium and nearby immune cells, which cause damage and swelling that disrupts the lungs' function. Recent studies have demonstrated that in vitro models that mimic tissue interactions are highly useful for investigating the relationships involved in infection. They enable us to learn more about diseases and also aid in the design of new drugs and improved methods for their management. Consequently, the integration of respiratory and immune functions in health and disease underscores the importance of understanding their intricate interaction, particularly in the context of non-respiratory functions of the lung (Azab et al., 2019).

12.3. Metabolism of Bioactive Substances

Bioactive substances are metabolized by the lung, which is important for its non-breathing functions and overall health. Many beneficial effects on physiology are achieved by bioactive substances, such as organic acids and amino acids, primarily by regulating the immune system. For example, organic acids are known to kill bacteria, which benefits the gut by lowering the pH and increasing enzyme production. They are important for digestion as well as for supporting the immune system, illustrating the close connection between the lungs and stomach. Enhanced immune functions reduce susceptibility to infections, illustrating how the metabolism of bioactive substances can bolster defenses against respiratory pathogens by acting on both mucosal and systemic immunity, aligning with the growing understanding of the lung's roles beyond respiration (Bosi et al., 2009). In addition, how bioactive compounds such as essential oils and immunonutritional components are processed by the body can significantly impact lung health during both disease and recovery. Some bioactive substances have antimicrobial properties, which increase their value in preventing and treating respiratory infections. For example, immunonutrition is being investigated as a means to enhance the body's immune response to viruses like SARS-CoV-2. Immunonutrition helps regulate the immune system and facilitates faster recovery from respiratory diseases in patients. Therefore, incorporating bioactive substances into our meals may be crucial for maintaining lung health, underscoring their potential role in treating lung diseases. The ability of these compounds to enhance both local and systemic immunity underscores their importance in the non-respiratory functions of the lung (Acevedo-Espinola et al., 2022). Besides boosting immunity, the breakdown of bioactive substances affects bodily processes that support respiratory health. The way amino acids and proteins in bovine colostrum and spray-dried plasma interact suggests they may help improve lung function. Such proteins and amino acids may influence inflammation and tissue repair, which is crucial for mitigating lung injury and infection. With more research on these mechanisms, having a diet rich in bioactive substances can support the health of the gut, lungs, and the immune system. By elucidating these pathways, scientists can gain a deeper understanding of how dietary interventions can serve as both preventive and therapeutic measures in respiratory health, highlighting the crucial intersection between nutrition, metabolism, and lung function (Bosi et al., 2009).

12.3.1. Conversion of Angiotensin I to Angiotensin II

The conversion of angiotensin I to angiotensin II represents a critical process within the renin-angiotensin system (RAS), which has significant implications beyond pulmonary function and directly correlates with non-respiratory roles of the lung. Angiotensin I, an inactive precursor, is transformed into angiotensin II primarily by the action of angiotensin-converting enzyme (ACE), mainly located in the endothelial cells of the lungs. It is necessary to convert angiotensin I to angiotensin II, since angiotensin II strongly affects blood pressure, fluid balance, and the balance of electrolytes in the body. Because angiotensin II can constrict blood vessels, it can affect the body's overall circulation, which can influence pulmonary capillary function, illustrating the relationship between lung health and heart health. Additionally, angiotensin II helps increase aldosterone, leading to sodium retention and the reabsorption of more water by the kidneys. The conversion of angiotensin I to angiotensin II by the lung is part of the body's efforts to maintain balance how these interactions balance can be significant, especially when the heart or body is under stress. Notably, the classical renin-angiotensin pathway has negative adverse effects, including the induction of inflammation and fibrosis, which are significant issues in chronic lung diseases. Understanding how these pathways function may lead to new treatments that mitigate these harmful effects and enhance overall health. Recent research further highlights the significance of the alternative axis of the RAS, where ACE2 and its associated peptide, angiotensin-(1-7), play protective roles against the harmful effects of angiotensin II. As new health crises arise such as the COVID-19 pandemic, the relationship between these factors is more significant, as it leads to increased inflammation and blood clots. Due to the fact that circulating angiotensin II can cause harm – particularly during a state when ACE2 is reduced, it is crucial to investigate this process and its effects on the lung beyond its role in respiration. Therefore, it becomes evident that the RASs' influence extends well beyond traditional notions of respiratory physiology, implicating a broader spectrum of bodily systems and their interactions (Galarza et al., 2020; Ivanchenko et al., 2023) (Figure 12.9).

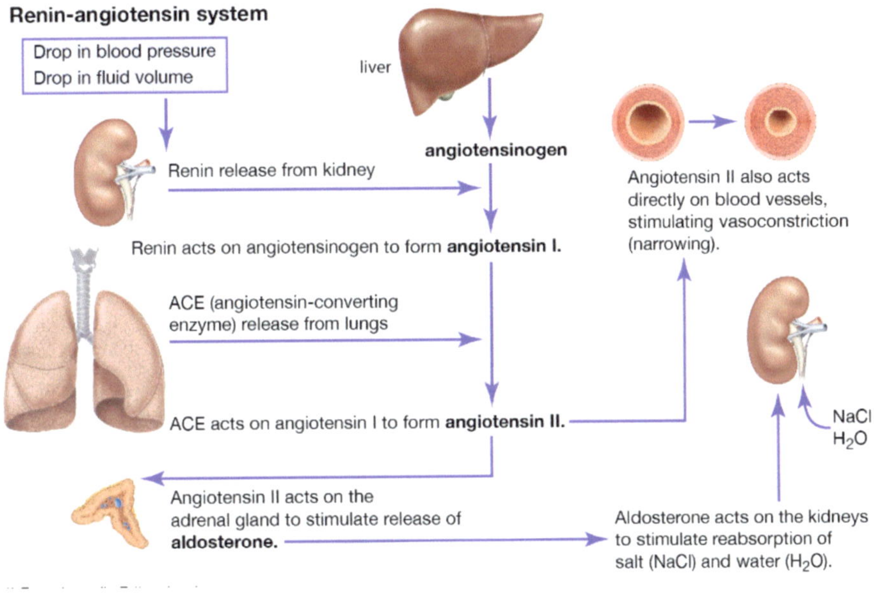

Figure 12.9. Renin angiotensin system (RAS).

Source: https://cdn.britannica.com/21/185321-050-9EA74796/Renin-angiotensin-system.jpg.

12.3.2. Role of the Lungs in Drug Metabolism

The lungs, traditionally recognized for their respiratory functions, also play a crucial role in drug metabolism, influencing the pharmacokinetics of various medications. The lungs can alter drugs by enzymatic processes using specialized cells, which may change how the drugs are absorbed and how well they work. The pulmonary tissue contains cytochrome P450 and other enzymes that help change xenobiotics. The lungs can either convert prodrugs into active compounds or facilitate the removal of active compounds, highlighting their crucial role in drug metabolism. It is important to understand these processes, especially when drugs are given by inhalation, because they can change the expected drug effects. Moreover, the presence of dipeptidyl peptidase 4 (DPP4) within lung tissues highlights another dimension of pulmonary drug metabolism. DPP4 is crucial for metabolizing certain drugs and has been identified as playing a significant role in lung disease. It helps control energy use in the body, affects inflammation, and is involved in immunity, which changes how lungs deal with drugs when someone is sick. With COVID-19, the increased presence of inflammatory mediators can make DPP4 affect how drugs are handled by the body, which could result in different treatment outcomes for patients. Due to this complex relationship, it is essential to continue researching how lung metabolism affects drug efficacy. It is also crucial to understand the relationship between inflammation, drug metabolism, and lung function, particularly in cases of severe respiratory diseases. Inflammation in the lungs, which is common in many lung diseases, can influence the activity of metabolic enzymes in the area. During acute lung infections, cytokines can increase, which may lower the activity of metabolic pathways, as was seen during the COVID-19 pandemic. Such changes may affect how inhaled drugs or systemic drugs metabolized in the lungs are cleared, so treatment plans may be adjusted to ensure the best results and minimize harm. Overall, recognizing the lungs' role in drug metabolism enriches our comprehension of non-respiratory functions and their implications for clinical practice (Figure 12.10).

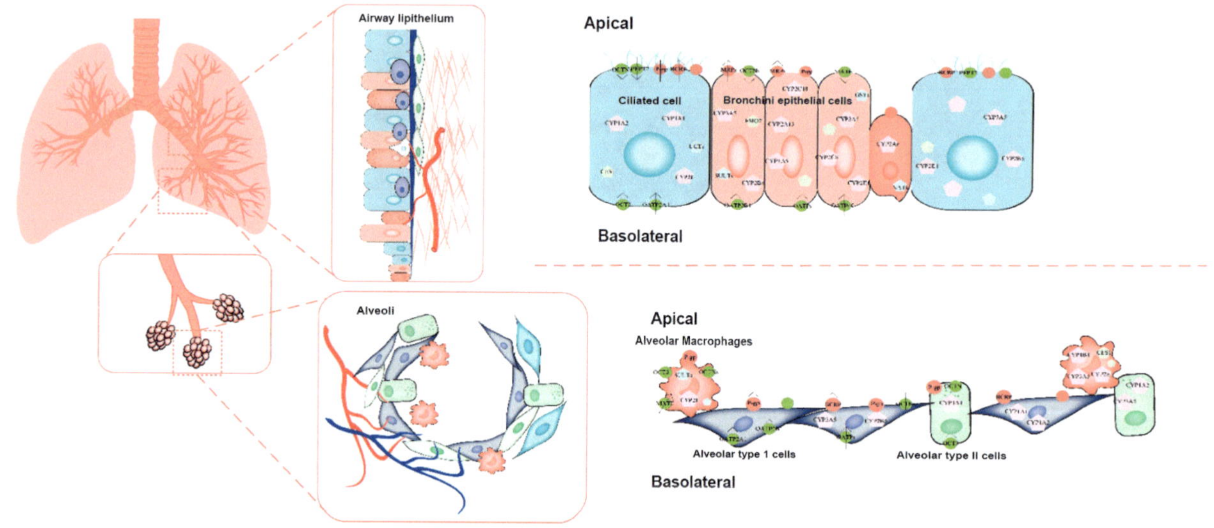

Figure 12.10. Pulmonary drug transporters and metabolic enzymes. (Green circles indicate uptake transporters and red circles indicate efflux transporters; pentagons indicate metabolic enzymes).

Source: https://www.mdpi.com/ijms/ijms-25-04671/article_deploy/html/images/ijms-25-04671-g002.png.

12.3.3. Influence of Lung Metabolism on Systemic Circulation

The interaction between the lungs and blood circulation highlights the lungs' other important roles. The lungs primarily exchange gases, but they also participate in metabolic activities that can have a significant impact on the cardiovascular system. Enzymes in the lungs can influence the amounts of bioactive substances, such as nitric oxide, which helps control the diameter of blood vessels.

The lungs help regulate blood pressure and perfusion throughout the body by influencing the availability of these compounds in the circulation, which is crucial for maintaining homeostasis, in addition to respiration. Therefore, understanding how lung metabolism and systemic circulation work together is necessary for incorporating pulmonary health into cardiovascular evaluations. Examining trace gas levels during respiration helps reveal the metabolic activities in the lungs and their impact on the entire body. Determining exhaled nitric oxide has recently become important in clinical practice, as it reveals acute changes in inflammation and blood vessel reactions in the lungs. Furthermore, ongoing research into other volatile organic compounds (VOCs) in exhaled breath may enhance our comprehension of the influence of lung metabolism on systemic parameters. Changes in the levels of these metabolites can indicate how the body is functioning and how it responds to stresses, such as exercise. The incorporation of quantifiable breath analysis expands our understanding of how lung-derived metabolic products can impact systemic circulation, indicating a need for more standardized protocols in clinical practice (Amann et al., 2010). Besides, compartment models can connect the way we analyze breath with the actual metabolism in the lungs and systemic circulation. For example, changes in breath acetone are mainly caused by how the airways take up the gas, rather than by changes in the overall body concentration. This means that the gas content in exhaled breath, especially when someone is in different physiological states, can show metabolic activity that is not easily seen with standard monitoring. Based on these findings, the lungs are crucial for systemic circulation due to their metabolic functions. The elucidation of these pathways has crucial implications for developing interventional strategies aimed at improving systemic health outcomes based on pulmonary function (N/A, 2025).

12.4. Regulation of Blood Pressure

The regulation of blood pressure involves a complex interplay between various systems within the body, including significant contributions from the respiratory system, notably the lungs. As non-respiratory functions of the lung, the production of ACE plays a crucial role in the renin-angiotensin-aldosterone system (RAAS), which is essential for regulating blood pressure. The conversion of angiotensin I to angiotensin II, which leads to an increase in blood pressure, is mainly done by the lungs. This action by the enzyme is needed to maintain blood pressure and also to respond when blood pressure is high or low. Pulmonary function plays a role in cardiovascular health by controlling blood gases, which in turn affect blood vessel tone and volume, illustrating the connection between the respiratory and cardiovascular systems in regulating blood pressure. When someone has SARS-CoV-2 infection, which affects the lungs, it can cause changes in their blood pressure and heart function. In the context of COVID-19, severe acute respiratory syndrome coronavirus 2 (SARS-CoV-2) disrupts normal physiological processes, leading to inflammation and vascular complications beyond the lungs. The inflammation associated with the disease can exacerbate breathing problems and may also cause blood pressure instability due to issues with endothelial cells and increased blood vessel resistance. Understanding these interactions is crucial for developing effective therapies that mitigate complications arising from both respiratory and cardiovascular compromise in patients affected by these diseases (Tay et al., 2020). Also, the link between lung function and blood pressure is important in the treatment of different types of CVDs. Since the lungs do much more than just help with breathing, healthcare providers are paying more attention to how respiratory therapies can aid in blood pressure control. For example, interventions like continuous positive airway pressure (CPAP) in patients with obstructive sleep apnea not only improve respiratory function but also lower blood pressure, highlighting the therapeutic potential of targeting respiratory mechanisms to benefit cardiovascular health. Additionally, the use of mechanical ventilation in critically ill patients demonstrates how improved lung function can help maintain blood pressure. As research progresses, further elucidation of these pathways offers promising avenues for integrating respiratory health into CVD management (Zheng et al., 2020) (Figure 12.11).

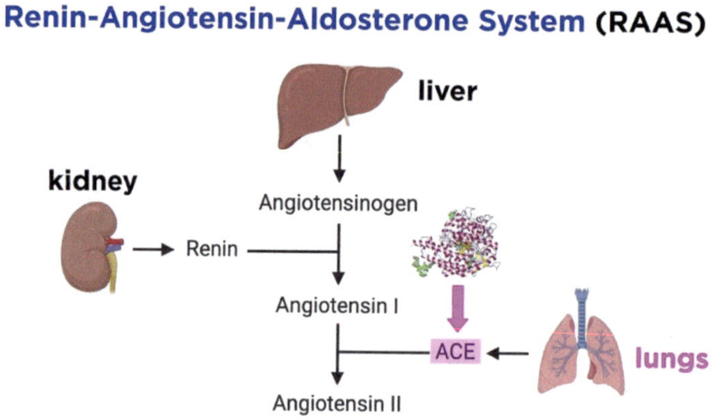

Figure 12.11. Renin-angiotensin-aldosterone system (RAAS).

Source: https://i.ytimg.com/vi/4NYVBtt0ioI/maxresdefault.jpg.

12.4.1. The Role of the Lungs in the Renin-Angiotensin System

The lungs are important in the RAS, which is a series of hormones that control blood pressure and fluid levels in the body. Although they are mainly known for their role in breathing, lungs also help RAS by expressing ACE2, which helps control the effects of angiotensin II, which causes blood vessels to narrow. ACE2 acts by converting angiotensin II into angiotensin (1-7), which promotes vasodilation and exhibits beneficial effects on cardiovascular health. The presence of ACE2 in the lung alveolar epithelial cells signifies a dual function of the lungs, not only in gas exchange but also as a central player in cardiovascular regulation, thus highlighting their importance beyond mere respiration (Pillay et al., 2021). Recent studies have also shown that problems in the RAS, particularly those involving ACE2, may contribute to several health issues. Elevated levels of angiotensin II are associated with increased pulmonary vascular resistance (PVR) and hypertension, which may exacerbate conditions like ARDS. The lungs play a key role in the RAS, which is important in cases of COVID-19, where the virus reduces the amount of ACE2. This disruption not only affects blood pressure regulation but also exacerbates pulmonary inflammation and injury, illustrating the critical interplay between the lungs and the RAS during respiratory infections and their systemic implications (Pillay et al., 2021). ACE2 in the lung plays a crucial role in various physiological functions, making it essential to investigate its role in both health and disease. In addition to shielding the lungs and heart from damage, ACE2 plays a role in maintaining stable water levels in the body and regulating inflammation. It has been found that mice lacking the ACE2 enzyme are more susceptible to hypertensive nephropathy and lung diseases, which suggests the enzyme's protective role in non-respiratory functions of the lungs. The lungs are recognized in the RAS framework for their importance in maintaining bodily balance, and this approach also highlights ways to treat diseases by targeting this system, demonstrating that the lungs have multiple roles.

12.4.2. Effects of Pulmonary Circulation on Systemic Blood Pressure

The pulmonary circulation plays a crucial role in regulating systemic blood pressure, acting as a distinct segment of the cardiovascular system that finely tunes hemodynamic responses. Blood in the lungs participates in gas exchange and undergoes changes in structure and function, which impact systemic vascular resistance. The pulmonary circulation typically has lower pressures, averaging around 10–15 mmHg, which helps maintain low vascular resistance and facilitates optimal gas exchange. When blood moves from the lungs back into the systemic circulation, the point where these systems meet is vital for cardiovascular health; any issues here can cause secondary problems in arterial pressure and flow. Additionally, the relationship between pulmonary vascular pressures and systemic blood pressure highlights the lungs' role in functions beyond breathing. If pulmonary artery pressure increases, as occurs in pulmonary hypertension, it can cause the right ventricle to generate more pressure, which may affect the pressure in the systemic arteries. There is a connection whereby changes in systemic blood pressure affect pulmonary blood flow—higher systemic resistance can cause the pulmonary artery pressure to increase. Understanding this relationship is crucial for treating both lung diseases and other illnesses that can arise when hemodynamics are disrupted, highlighting the interconnectedness of these systems. Biochemical activities in the pulmonary circulation also help control systemic blood pressure by releasing substances that affect blood vessels. The lungs produce endothelin and nitric oxide, which are hormones and mediators that control the tightness of blood vessels and resistance in the circulatory system. They are necessary for keeping homeostasis because they control vasodilation and vasoconstriction in various parts of the body. Modifying these substances can cause changes in blood pressure, which is clear in conditions such as sepsis, where the inflammatory response can alter PVR and impact the entire system. Thus, a comprehensive understanding of the pulmonary circulation's effects on systemic blood pressure provides critical insights into the non-respiratory functions of the lungs, encapsulating their integral role in overall cardiovascular stability (Danaei et al., 2018; Rhodes et al., 2017) (Figure 12.12).

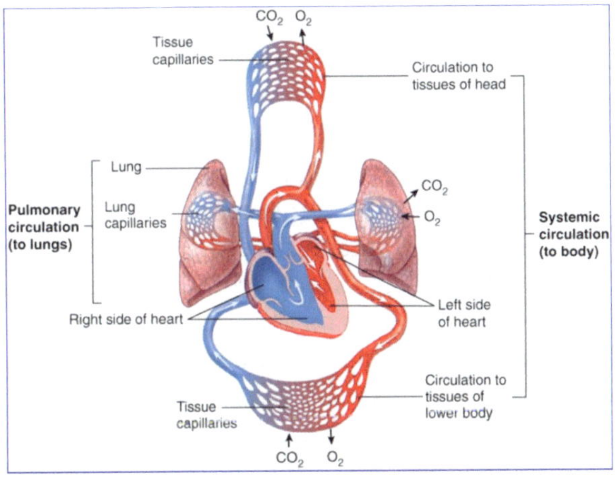

Figure 12.12. Systemic and pulmonary circulation.

Source: https://www.researchgate.net/profile/Azza-Jabbar/publication/311274630/figure/fig37/AS:1003049124392967@1616155955090/Figure-61-Systemic-and-pulmonary-circulation-Marieb-ENand-Hoehn-KAnatomy-and.png.

12.4.3. Clinical Implications of Lung-Related Blood Pressure Regulation

The way the lungs regulate blood pressure has major clinical significance for studying different heart problems. The lungs play a crucial role in producing and regulating angiotensin II, a hormone that helps control blood pressure. It is important for maintaining stable blood pressure and may also suggest a relationship between lung problems and hypertension. Also, since lung function is linked to vascular health, respiratory health plays a key role in preventing CVD. Problems with lung-related blood pressure can worsen heart complications, which is why treating both the lungs and heart together is important in clinical care. Therefore, focusing on these interactions can lead to new treatment methods that benefit people with chronic respiratory diseases and related cardiovascular issues. Increasing research is indicating that alterations in the lung microbiota may contribute to blood pressure regulation and increase the risk of cardiovascular issues. Lung microbiome research shows that the lungs have important roles in the immune system, apart from breathing. Dysbiosis may cause chronic inflammation, which has been connected to the development of hypertension and other CVDs. Therefore, understanding how the lung microbiota affects blood pressure is crucial. Treatments that focus on the microbiota, such as modulation and fecal microbial transplantation, appear effective in dealing with dysbiosis and its effects on blood pressure. As studies continue to explore this intricate connection, the potential for integrating microbiota-focused therapies into traditional treatment regimens offers a novel avenue for managing hypertension and potentially other related health issues (Hou et al., 2022). The effects of blood pressure regulation in the lungs are especially noticeable when someone is infected with COVID-19. It appears that SARS-CoV-2 infection may cause the immune system to become unbalanced which can harm breathing and affect how the heart functions. The interaction between this virus and the immune system highlights the intimate connection between lung health and systemic health, particularly in relation to blood pressure regulation during viral infections (Tay et al., 2020). A good understanding of these dynamics is necessary to develop effective therapies for addressing issues related to breathing and heart problems caused by these infections. As the lungs are involved in regulation, doctors are now treating respiratory and vascular issues in patients with acute respiratory illnesses together. Viewing things from this broad perspective is essential for delivering better patient care and advancing knowledge of the lungs' additional functions.

12.5. Acid-Base Balance

The lungs' primary function has often been associated with gas exchange; however, its role in maintaining acid-base balance is equally crucial within the context of non-respiratory functions. Acid-base balance refers to the mechanisms the body employs to regulate its pH levels, maintaining homeostasis despite fluctuations resulting from metabolic activities and environmental factors. Of significant importance is the involvement of the bicarbonate buffer system – a physiological process which assists in controlling the concentration of carbon dioxide (CO_2) in the blood. Through respiration, the lungs facilitate the exchange of a key byproduct of cellular metabolism, which is primarily carbon dioxide (CO_2). By effectively eliminating CO_2, the lungs help prevent acidosis, a condition characterized by excessive acidity in bodily fluids, thereby supporting various enzymatic functions and metabolic pathways essential for life. Further elaborating on the acid-base regulation, the lungs respond to acid-base disturbances by adjusting the rate and depth of breathing. In conditions where the blood becomes too acidic, such as metabolic acidosis, the respiratory system increases ventilation to expel carbon dioxide, leading to a decrease in hydrogen ion concentration and a corresponding rise in blood pH. Conversely, during states of alkalosis, where there is insufficient acidity, the lungs may reduce respiratory rates to retain CO_2, ultimately aiding in correcting the elevated pH levels. The ability of the lungs to rapidly adjust to metabolic changes through respiratory compensation exemplifies the significance of this organ in contributing to acid-base homeostasis. This adaptive response plays a pivotal role in sustaining bodily functions, emphasizing the complex interplay between respiratory and metabolic processes. In addition to its respiratory functions, the lungs contribute to acid-base balance through involvement in metabolic processes.

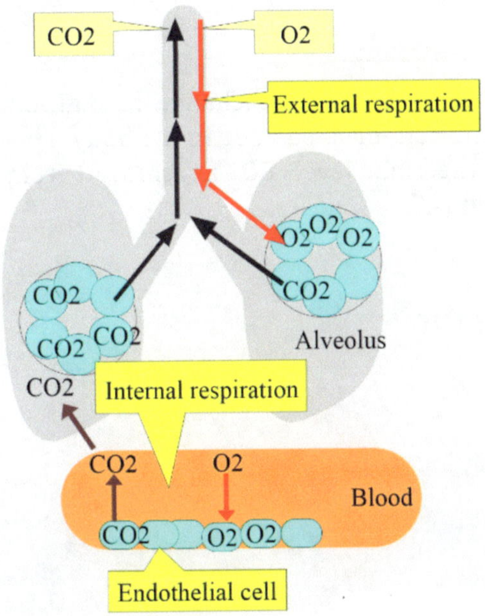

Figure 12.13. Acid-base role of lung respiration.

Source: https://labpedia.net/wp-content/uploads/2020/01/Acid-base-lung-role-respiration-2.jpg.

The metabolic activities within lung tissues, including the synthesis and degradation of various compounds, can influence local and systemic pH levels. For instance, specific lung cells can produce bicarbonate ions, which contribute to the blood's buffering capacity. Moreover, factors such as inflammation and infection can alter the lungs metabolic landscape, potentially impacting acid-base status. During respiratory diseases such as COVID-19, the lungs role in acid-base balance can be severely affected. Abnormalities in CO_2 elimination due to impaired gas exchange can precipitate respiratory acidosis, highlighting the vital importance of lung function not merely in respiration but also in maintaining overall acid-base equilibrium and homeostasis within the body (Cuadrado et al., 2020; Liona et al., 2020) (Figure 12.13).

12.5.1. Mechanisms of CO_2 Exchange and Its Effect on pH

The lungs play a crucial non-respiratory role in maintaining acid-base balance within the body, primarily through the exchange of carbon dioxide (CO_2). This gas exchange occurs in the alveoli, where carbon dioxide diffuses from the blood into the alveolar space, while oxygen is simultaneously absorbed. The removal of CO_2 is critical because it contributes to the bicarbonate buffering system, which helps regulate blood pH. As CO_2 levels rise in the blood, it reacts with water to form carbonic acid (H_2CO_3), which dissociates into bicarbonate and hydrogen ions, lowering pH and leading to acidosis if not correctly managed. Therefore, efficient CO_2 removal is essential not only for respiratory health but also for cardiovascular and neurological stability, as alterations in blood pH can significantly impact overall metabolic function. The mechanisms underlying CO_2 exchange are intricately linked to neural and chemical signaling, which carefully regulate ventilation patterns in response to metabolic demands. Chemoreceptors in the medulla oblongata and peripheral arteries detect variations in CO_2 and pH, prompting adjustments in respiratory rate and depth. When CO_2 levels increase, this triggers an increase in tidal volume and respiratory rate, facilitating enhanced elimination of CO_2. Conversely, during hyperventilation, excessive CO_2 removal can lead to respiratory alkalosis, characterized by elevated blood pH. Therefore, the body's ability to modulate ventilation based on real-time feedback from these chemoreceptors is essential for maintaining homeostasis, reflecting the lungs' significant role not only in gas exchange but also in pH regulation through these feedback mechanisms. Furthermore, the clinical implications of CO_2 exchange and pH regulation extend beyond normative physiology into various pathological conditions. For instance, in states of acute respiratory failure, as seen in conditions like COPD, the inability to expel CO_2 efficiently can lead to hypercapnia and subsequently respiratory acidosis, necessitating interventions such as high-flow nasal cannula (HFNC) therapy to enhance ventilation and CO_2 clearance (Oczkowski et al., 2021). The management of arterial blood gases (ABGs), including CO_2 and pH levels, becomes a focal point in treating patients with respiratory distress, emphasizing the interconnectedness of respiratory functions with systemic health outcomes. Thus, understanding the mechanisms of CO_2 exchange and their physiological implications is essential for addressing the non-respiratory functions of the lung in clinical practice, reinforcing the significance of these processes in maintaining metabolic balance and overall health (Claassen et al., 2021).

12.5.2. Role of the Lungs in Maintaining Homeostasis

The lungs have several other roles besides their primary job of gas exchange in maintaining homeostasis. It is imperative that they help to maintain the acid-base balance in the body. Through respiration, the amount of CO_2 in the blood is kept at the right level. CO_2 is removed from the blood in exhalation, which helps prevent respiratory acidosis.

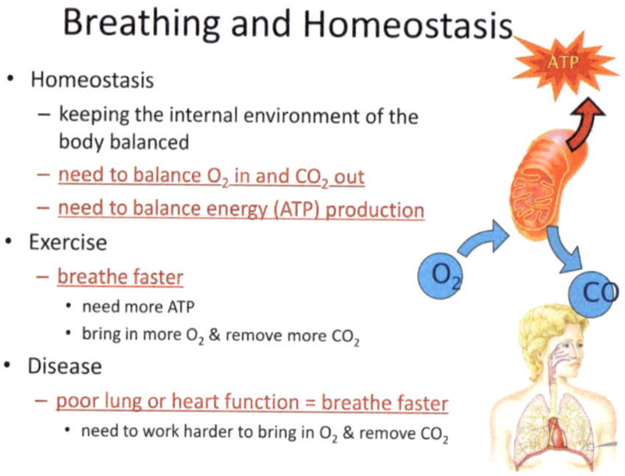

Figure 12.14. Breathing and homeostasis.

Source: https://slideplayer.com/slide/12891111/78/images/2/Breathing+and+Homeostasis.jpg.

If breathing is not working correctly, CO_2 builds up and makes the body more acidic, which can harm how cells function. Therefore, the lungs are crucial for preventing significant changes in blood pH, underscoring their key role in maintaining balance during metabolism and exercise. Besides breathing, the lungs play a crucial role in the body's immune response, which helps maintain homeostasis. Type I and type II cells in the alveolar epithelium defend the body against inhaled bacteria and debris. Gas exchange in the lungs is helped by pulmonary surfactant, which also has properties that support the local immune system. This surfactant, acting at the air-liquid interface in the alveoli, engages with inhaled pathogens and promotes their clearance, thereby protecting the body's internal environment (Hegermann et al., 2020). The lungs help prevent infections by regulating the immune response, which helps maintain bodily balance and promotes overall health. Apart from facilitating gas exchange and immunity, the lungs also regulate fluid balance in the body, a crucial function for maintaining overall bodily balance. The alveolar-capillary barrier helps maintain fluid balance by preventing pulmonary edema and regulating the movement of fluids through the lung epithelium. The presence of surfactant and the glycocalyx of the alveolar epithelium is critical in maintaining alveolar structure and function, preventing excessive fluid accumulation (Hegermann et al., 2020). This system is crucial for enabling the alveoli to function properly in gas exchange and for reducing the risk of lung problems associated with excessive fluid accumulation. Thus, the lungs' role extends into fluid management, underscoring the complexity of their contributions to maintaining a stable internal environment amidst various physiological challenges (Figure 12.14).

12.5.3. Consequences of Lung Dysfunction on Acid-Base Balance

The lungs are important for maintaining acid-base balance, primarily by regulating the amount of CO_2 in the blood. Problems with how the lungs function or with gas exchange can disrupt the balance, leading to respiratory acidosis or alkalosis. When someone has COPD or pulmonary fibrosis, their lungs do not function as well, and they are less able to remove CO_2. Having too much CO_2 in the blood causes a decrease in pH, leading to acidosis. Due to this imbalance, the respiratory system is put under stress, and other body parts that rely on a stable pH for proper function are also affected. The outcomes are important, which means it is necessary to understand how problems in the lungs can affect other parts of the body. Additionally, the way acid-base disturbances occur in lung dysfunction can lead to the kidneys and other systems making adjustments to compensate. When respiratory acidosis occurs, the kidneys typically increase the amount of bicarbonate they reabsorb to mitigate the acidosis. If lung dysfunction is not resolved, the kidneys may be unable to cope, which can lead to persistent imbalances that exacerbate the original respiratory problem. Due to this complexity, it is evident that the various organ systems rely on one another for maintaining homeostasis. Additionally, when acid-base balance is disrupted, it can significantly impact metabolism and exacerbate both lung diseases and non-lung-related illnesses. Understanding the relationships between these conditions can inform more effective treatments for lung dysfunction. Increased oxidative stress caused by ongoing lung dysfunction provides a deeper understanding of the long-term health effects. Reactive oxygen and nitrogen species (RONS) are often produced as byproducts of chronic lung diseases, contributing to systemic inflammation and tissue damage. A high level of RONS compared to antioxidants is of great concern because it is related to aging and many health problems such as those affecting the heart and the brain. Because lung health and systemic oxidative stress are interconnected, it is clear that addressing both local and systemic issues following lung dysfunction is necessary. Consequently, measures aimed at enhancing lung function should include strategies to restore acid-base balance, while also considering the management of oxidative stress (Liguori et al., 2018; Zheng et al., 2020).

12.6. Vocalization and Sound Production

Sound and voice are produced by the lungs, which are essential for speaking and communicating. Speech is possible because respiratory functions and precise body movements work together. The lungs help move air out when people speak, which is required for phonation. The function depends closely on the neural mechanisms involved in making speech. It has been found that certain brain growths, such as those in cerebello-cerebral circuitry, support learning to predict body movements and actions, which help with speaking and control of voice. Such neurological adaptations underscore the evolutionary significance of vocalization, positioning it as a crucial mechanism for social interaction and cognitive development in humans (John, 2008). Also, the connection between gestures and talking demonstrates how well the respiratory and motor systems cooperate to produce sounds. Often, people use gestures that are in rhythm with their speech, making the interaction more engaging. This can be explained by examining vocal-entangled gestures, which integrate movements, breathing, and speaking. As explained, these gestures demonstrate how body movements and speech are closely linked, making speech more expressive.

Infants start by babbling with their voices, which helps them later use gestures as a form of communication. The foundational role of these vocal-entangled processes in facilitating sound production is mirrored in non-human animals, revealing an evolutionarily deep-rooted aspect of vocal communication (Fuchs et al., 2022). Investigating vocalization as a non-breathing lung function also involves examining its mental effects. The ability to use complex vocalizations is linked to improved cognitive abilities, including attention and executive function. Because of these skills, people can handle complex social situations and create detailed ways of communicating. Combining motor movements, breathing, and thinking skills gives voice a key role in human interactions. Improving how we articulate words through practice and thought helps the connections between speech and other mental functions become clearer. This interplay suggests that the evolution of vocalization not only facilitated basic communication needs but also played a pivotal role in the advancement of human cognition and social organization, thus emphasizing the comprehensive importance of the lungs beyond respiratory purposes (John, 2008).

12.6.1. Anatomy of the Larynx and Its Function in Sound Production

The larynx (or voice box) is very important, essential for making sounds, which is one of the non-respiratory roles of the lungs. The larynx is found at the point where the pharynx and trachea join and it is made up of several cartilages that help it be both strong and flexible. The thyroid, cricoid, and arytenoid cartilages are the main ones, and they help keep the vocal cords in the correct position and at the proper tension. As air leaves the lungs, it goes through the larynx which makes the vocal folds vibrate. The vibration produces sound, and changes in pitch and volume occur when muscles in the vocal cords are contracted. Thus, the larynx includes many important structures that support breathing and are involved in speaking and expressing feelings. The way the larynx works in conjunction with other body parts enables it to produce a wide range of sounds. In the larynx, the vocal folds can be stretched or relaxed by muscles, which help create many different vocal sounds. Also, the larynx and respiratory system work closely together; when we swallow, the larynx closes to prevent food or liquid from entering the lungs and disturbing sound production. The way respiration and phonation rely on the larynx highlights its importance in many ways. As identified in the literature, various vocal qualities can be produced by manipulating the air pressure and flow from the lungs, emphasizing the larynx's significance not only in respiration but also in artistic and expressive forms of communication (Homberger et al., 2017). Additionally, the larynx is designed to support the various ways people use their voices. The different ways we sing, shout, or whisper show how the larynx adjusts the way we produce sound according to what we need to do. Studies have found that the way a person speaks can cause different emotions in listeners. As explored in studies analyzing the connection between voice modulation and audience engagement, the anatomical features of the larynx play a pivotal role in shaping how sound is perceived (Gasc et al., 2018). This understanding of the larynx's role in communication further underscores its importance as a non-respiratory function within the broader context of lung physiology (Figure 12.15).

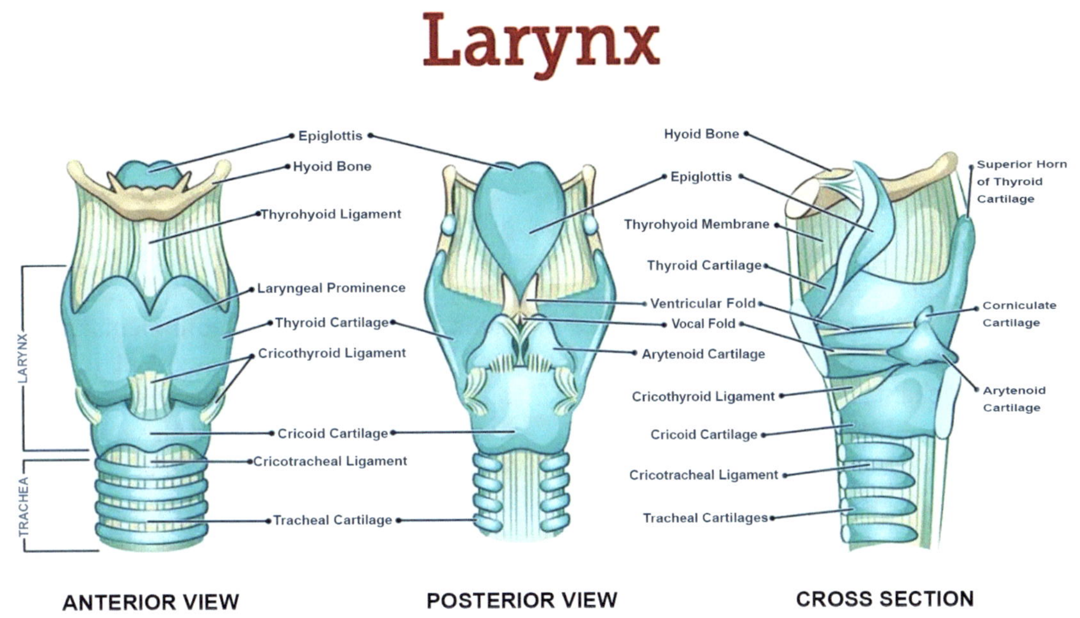

Figure 12.15. Larynx anatomy.

Source: https://speechfit.io/_next/image?url=https%3A%2F%2Fimages.prismic.io%2Fspeechfit%2Fa76af431-7a6d-4588-8978-a060c6b23845_1675511253036%2B%25281%2529.jpeg%3Fauto%3Dcompress%2Cformat&w=3840&q=75.

12.6.2. Role of Airflow in Speech and Vocalization

The way air moves through the lungs when we speak highlights their role in producing speech, which is not limited to breathing. Sound is created in vocalization by air that comes out of the mouth. The larynx is very important because it holds the vocal folds, which vibrate as air passes through, turning air into sound. This is achieved through the coordinated action of muscles that regulate air pressure and flow in the lungs. You can see the accuracy of this system in the way we speak, from soft whispering to loud shouting, which all involve different ways the vocal folds move and breathe. For this reason, controlling airflow is important for music, speech, and good communication. This multifaceted engagement underlines the significance of the lungs in activities beyond mere respiration, suggesting a broader functional scope within vocalization (Gonz et al., 2024). Moreover, the complexity of speech production is further demonstrated by the involvement of the central nervous system (CNS) in regulating airflow and laryngeal function. The laryngeal motor cortex (LMC) orchestrates the interplay between breathing and vocalization, ensuring that airflow is appropriately modulated for speech. It demonstrates the importance of airflow in speaking and expressing ideas. This neural pathway which includes the mesencephalic periaqueductal grey matter, allows the body to keep a balance between breathing and speaking. Because of this, the risk of sudden stops in speech due to a lack of air is reduced, allowing communication to flow smoothly. This intricate orchestration reveals the lungs' non-respiratory role, highlighting how sophisticated neural interactions influence our capacity to vocalize effectively (Gonz et al., 2024). Speech-generated airflow is important not only for talking, but also for understanding how respiratory diseases can be transmitted, which is especially relevant during recent health crises. Scientific studies on the spread of droplets when we speak show that using a mask can influence the chances of spreading airborne pathogens. For example, differences in mouth shape and the volume of speech can lead to the production of more airborne droplets, which means even silent communication could be risky. If researchers understand airflow in these situations, they can develop more effective ways to prevent respiratory infections. Additionally, this information highlights the importance of airflow for both speech and public health, underscoring the significant roles the lungs play beyond their primary function of breathing.

12.6.3. Impact of Lung Health on Voice Quality

Lung health plays a crucial role in determining voice quality, as the respiratory system provides the fundamental support necessary for phonation. Voice production depends on the lungs working well to provide the breath that causes the vocal cords to vibrate. COPD or asthma can limit the ability to breathe properly which can impact the quality and strength of someone's voice. Reduced lung capacity or blocked airways can make it harder to support breathing, which weakens or strains the voice. Such individuals, including educators, singers, and public speakers, may experience significant impacts on their job performance, communication, and self-confidence. In addition to the way we produce sound, the quality of our voice can be shaped by the environment, especially by the quality of the air. Living in areas with high pollution for a long time, which is common in industrial regions, can cause breathing problems that reduce singing ability. Evidence shows that exposure to air pollution leads to an increase in cases of respiratory diseases, which can weaken the lungs and reduce the clarity and strength of a person's voice. Having healthy lungs is necessary for singing well, which is why everyone should support efforts to keep the air clean. Furthermore, ongoing legislative actions and health initiatives aimed at improving air quality are necessary not just for respiratory health but for preserving the quality of voice, with a substantial ripple effect on overall social interaction and cultural expression (Chamola et al., 2020). Recognizing what the lungs do beyond breathing reveals the strong connection between lung health and vocal quality. When lung health is poor, people may experience hoarseness, get tired when using their voice, and find their vocal range is smaller. Such vocal problems can significantly impact a person's job and personal life, making it more challenging for voice professionals to perform their duties effectively and causing increased frustration during regular conversations. It is clear that robust public health efforts are necessary to safeguard the lungs and maintain clean air, given the economic implications of declining voice quality. Efforts by organizations and governments to reduce air pollution and improve respiratory health are not just beneficial for physical well-being. However, they are vital for enhancing one of humanity's essential forms of expression (Crystal et al., 2019). Since lung health significantly impacts voice quality, it is crucial to prioritize environmental conservation and public health.

SUMMARY

Having looked at the non-respiratory functions of the lung, it is evident that they serve many important roles outside of gas exchange. The lungs help regulate acid-base balance, influence metabolism, and support the body's immune system. It opposes the main idea that the body's primary function is breathing. A recent area of research has shown that the lungs play a crucial role in regulating blood pressure and fluid balance by producing angiotensin II from angiotensin I. These functions are important to understand because chronic conditions and external pressures can make these roles more challenging, which may result in poor health outcomes and increase the risk of diseases. In addition, studies have shown that smoking harms lung function, which highlights important issues for public health. Tobacco use has adverse effects on the lungs that go beyond breathing problems and can worsen other health problems, too. Research on Sri Lankan smokers found that regular smoking leads to poor lung function, as shown by decreases in FVC and peak expiratory flow rates, and this is connected to more respiratory problems and a lower quality of life. Improving lung health by addressing harmful habits should remain important in healthcare programs, especially in areas where smoking is common and research is limited. Studies on ECMO outcomes reveal how lung function changes after treatment. Studies have found that ECMO can assist patients with acute respiratory failure; however, the recovery of lung function over time is similar to that seen with conventional mechanical ventilation. This highlights the importance of ongoing research into how various treatments affect the lungs' different functions over time. Being aware of these functions, in addition to breathing, is vital for everyone involved in lung healthcare. As we learn more about these factors, it will help us find better ways to prevent and treat diseases and demonstrate the importance of the lungs to the entire body. Besides gas exchange, the lungs have important functions in the body. A key role in regulating fluid balance in the body is played by the RAS. The lungs make angiotensin II, which helps manage blood pressure and fluid balance in the body. It stimulates blood vessels to narrow, which increases systemic vascular resistance. In addition, the lungs play a role in breaking down substances such as hormones and vasoactive peptides, which affect both the heart and the body's circulation. By helping to produce angiotensin II from angiotensin I, the lungs demonstrate their crucial role in maintaining the cardiovascular system and fluid balance. The lungs are also important for immune defense functions. The respiratory epithelium and its associated immune cells, such as alveolar macrophages, play a crucial role in protecting the body by removing pathogens and particles from the air. The presence of the lungs in the body enhances the production of immunoglobulins and immune mediators, which aid the body in fighting infections. They are also able to control systemic inflammation, which is associated with numerous chronic diseases, such as COPD. Studies indicate that infections such as Helicobacter pylori can adversely impact lung function, underscoring the intricate relationship between lung health and systemic inflammatory responses (Ra et al., 2017). This indicates that the lungs play a crucial role in maintaining breathing and regulating the body's immune response. The lungs are important for metabolizing drugs and natural substances, which affect both drug actions and body functions. The body needs to use this function for both activating drugs and removing toxins. The lungs contain certain enzymes that can activate or deactivate the actions of pharmacologically important substances. The enzymes in the lungs can affect how well certain medications work, particularly for individuals with asthma or COPD. Furthermore, emerging research suggests that the interaction between coffee consumption and renal function may be influenced by pulmonary health, indicating that the lungs may modulate the systemic effects of dietary components (Mazidi et al., 2021).

CLOSER LOOK

HYPERCAPNIA

Hypercapnia, also known as hypercarbia, is a condition where there is an abnormally high level of CO_2 in the blood. This buildup occurs when the body is unable to remove CO2 from the bloodstream effectively. Hypercapnia can range in severity, from mild to acute, and can lead to a variety of symptoms, including lethargy, headache, and even confusion or disorientation, depending on the CO_2 level (Figure 12.16).

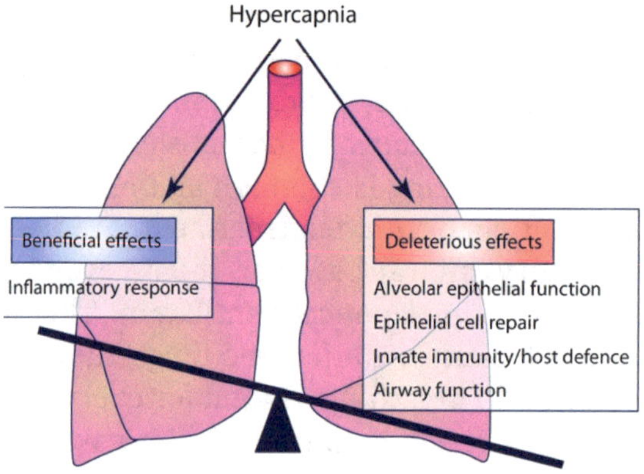

Figure 12.16. Dual effects of hypercapnia on pulmonary function.

Source: https://physoc.onlinelibrary.wiley.com/cms/asset/8f0b2aa2-6c19-4d83-a972-dbe9a7052fd5/tjp12194-gra-0001-m.jpg.

1. **Signs and Symptoms:** Hypercapnia can develop due to an existing health condition, and its symptoms may be linked to either the condition or the hypercapnia itself. Specific symptoms attributable to early hypercapnia are dyspnea (breathlessness), headache, confusion, and lethargy. Clinical signs include flushed skin, full pulse (bounding pulse), rapid breathing, premature heartbeats, muscle twitches, and hand flaps (asterixis). There is a greater chance of dangerous heart rhythm problems. Another cause of hypercapnia is when the breathing gas contains carbon dioxide or when the rate of gas exchange cannot keep up with the carbon dioxide produced by the body, which may happen when ventilation is limited by the density of the gas at high ambient pressures.
2. **Causes:** Carbon dioxide is a byproduct of metabolism, but if it is produced more quickly than the body can remove it, it will accumulate. When you exercise intensely, your body produces significantly more carbon dioxide than when you are at rest. Blood carries carbon dioxide, and it is removed from the body when we breathe out. Hypoventilation, lung disease, or a decrease in consciousness are the usual causes of hypercapnia. It sometimes comes from breathing in areas with very high carbon dioxide, such as those affected by volcanic or geothermal activity, or from breathing in your own exhaled air. Respiratory acidosis can also happen together with hypercapnia in this condition.

Acute hypercapnic respiratory failure may occur in acute illness caused by COPD, chest wall deformity, some forms of neuromuscular disease (such as myasthenia gravis), and obesity hypoventilation syndrome. AHRF may occur in any case of respiratory failure, especially if the muscles used for breathing become worn out, such as in severe pneumonia and acute severe asthma. It can also happen when there is a severe loss of consciousness, such as from an opioid overdose.

3. **Mechanism:** A reflex is triggered by hypercapnia, which makes breathing faster and helps the body obtain more oxygen, such as when waking up and turning the head during sleep. A lack of this reflex can be dangerous, such as in cases where it contributes to sudden infant death syndrome.

   Hypercapnia can induce increased cardiac output, an elevation in arterial blood pressure (higher levels of carbon dioxide stimulate aortic and carotid chemoreceptors with afferents -CN IX and X- to medulla oblongata with following chrono- and inotropic effects), and a propensity toward cardiac arrhythmias. Hypercapnia may increase pulmonary capillary resistance.

4. **Treatment:** The treatment for acute hypercapnic respiratory failure depends on the underlying cause, but may include medications and mechanical respiratory support. In those without contraindications, NIV is often used in preference to invasive mechanical ventilation. In the past, the drug doxapram (a respiratory stimulant), was used for hypercapnia in acute exacerbation of COPD. However, there is little evidence to support its use compared to NIV, and it does not feature in recent professional guidelines.

   Very severe respiratory failure, which may also be accompanied by hypercapnia, is often treated with ECMO, a technique that adds oxygen to and removes carbon dioxide directly from the blood.

   A relatively novel modality is extracorporeal carbon dioxide removal ($ECCO_2R$). This techniquc removes CO_2 from the bloodstream and may reduce the time mechanical ventilation is required for those with AHRF; it requires smaller volumes of blood flow compared to ECMO.

REFERENCES

1. Acevedo-Espinola, R., & Torres-Obregon, S. (2022). Immunonutrition as a potential strategy to prevent and cope with coronavirus disease (COVID-19). *Food Research, 6*(3), 429–434. https://doi.org/10.26656/fr.2017.6(3).346Amann, A., Amann, A., Lumb, A. B., Schrikker, A. C., Mörk, A. K., Mörk, A. K., Amann, A., et al. (2010). *A Mathematical Model for Breath Gas Analysis of Volatile Organic Compounds with Special Emphasis on Acetone.* http://arxiv.org/abs/1003.4475 (accessed on 31st May 2025).
2. Azab, W., Kamel, M., Osterrieder, K., Pavulraj, et al. (2019). *EHV-1 Pathogenesis: Current in Vitro Models and Future Perspectives.* https://core.ac.uk/download/227044277.pdf (accessed on 31st May 2025).
3. Barclay, W. R., Stylianou, E., McShane, H., Paul, M. J., Reljic, R., Resende Co, T., Rodriguez, A., et al. (2019). *Mucosal Delivery of Tuberculosis Vaccines: A Review of Current Approaches and Challenges.* https://core.ac.uk/download/286270868.pdf (accessed on 31st May 2025).
4. Batchelor, T., Rasburn, N., Abdelnour-Berchtold, E., Brunelli, A., Cerfolio, R. J., Gonzalez, M., Ljungqvist, O., et al. (2018). Guidelines for enhanced recovery after lung surgery: Recommendations of the Enhanced Recovery After Surgery (ERAS®) Society and the European Society of Thoracic Surgeons (ESTS). *European Journal of Cardio-Thoracic Surgery, 55*, 91–115. https://doi.org/10.1093/ejcts/ezy301 (accessed on 31st May 2025).
5. Behura, S. K., Gershwin, L. J., Grupioni, N. V., Kim, et al. (2017). Tissue tropism in host transcriptional response to members of the bovine respiratory disease complex. Scientific Reports. https://core.ac.uk/download/323067894.pdf (accessed on 31st May 2025).
6. Bhongir, R. K. V. (2017). *On Dysregulated Inflammation and Airway Host Defense.* https://core.ac.uk/download/83761398.pdf (accessed on 31st May 2025).
7. Bosi, P., Janczyk, P., Koopmans, S. J., Lalles, et al. (2009). Impact of bioactive substances on the gastrointestinal tract and performance of weaned piglets: A review. *Animal.* https://core.ac.uk/download/pdf/29247139.pdf (accessed on 31st May 2025).
8. Brito-Zerón, P., Gracia-Tello, B., Robles, Á., Alguacil, A., Bonet, M., De-Escalante, B., Noblejas-Mosso, A., et al. (2021). Characterization and outcomes of SARS-CoV-2 infection in patients with sarcoidosis. *Viruses, 13.* https://www.semanticscholar.org/paper/8fb2677abf3adda60d272e6edfaaa7bcbaf72b01 (accessed on 31st May 2025).
9. Brown, R. L., & Clarke, T. B. (2016). *The Regulation of Host Defenses to Infection by the Microbiota.* https://core.ac.uk/download/77016328.pdf (accessed on 31st May 2025).
10. Chamola, V., Hassija, V., Gupta, V., & Guizani, M. (2020). A comprehensive review of the COVID-19 pandemic and the role of IoT, drones, AI, blockchain, and 5G in managing its impact. *IEEE Access, 8*, 90225–90265. https://doi.org/10.1109/access.2020.2992341 (accessed on 31st May 2025).
11. Claassen, J. A. H. R., Thijssen, D. H. J., Panerai, R. B., & Faraci, F. M. (2021). Regulation of cerebral blood flow in humans: Physiology and clinical implications of autoregulation. *Physiological Reviews, 101*, 1487–1559. https://doi.org/10.1152/physrev.00022.2020 (accessed on 31st May 2025).
12. Cuadrado, A., Pajares, M., Benito, C., Jiménez-Villegas, J., Escoll, M., Fernández-Ginés, R., García-Yagüe, Á. J., et al. (2020). Can activation of NRF2 be a strategy against COVID-19?

Trends in Pharmacological Sciences, 41, 598–610. https://doi.org/10.1016/j.tips.2020.07.003 (accessed on 31st May 2025).

13. Dalamani, G., Kaspers, B., & Reese, S. (2006). *The Avian Lung-Associated Immune System*. https://core.ac.uk/download/12174987.pdf (accessed on 31st May 2025).
14. Danaei, M., Dehghankhold, M., Ataei, S., Hasanzadeh, D. F., Javanmard, R., Dokhani, A., Khorasani, S., et al. (2018). Impact of particle size and polydispersity index on the clinical applications of lipidic nanocarrier systems. *Pharmaceutics, 10*, 57. https://doi.org/10.3390/pharmaceutics10020057 (accessed on 31st May 2025).
15. Deb, S., & Arrighi, S. (2021). Potential effects of COVID-19 on cytochrome P450-mediated drug metabolism and disposition in infected patients. *European Journal of Drug Metabolism and Pharmacokinetics, 46*, 185–203. https://doi.org/10.1007/s13318-020-00668-8 (accessed on 31st May 2025).
16. Dickson, K. J., Hess, E., Powers, J. V., Wallace-Robinson, et al. (2025). Publications of the Space Physiology and Countermeasures Program, Cardiopulmonary Discipline: 1980–1990. https://core.ac.uk/download/pdf/42809290.pdf (accessed on 31st May 2025).
17. Duarte, A., Cordeiro, A., & Santos, M. (2019). AB0503 the lung in Sjögren's syndrome patients – an overview of clinical characteristics and disease outcome. *Annals of the Rheumatic Diseases, 78*, 1714–1715. https://www.semanticscholar.org/paper/d3711bb84aec43dc30947c7865f6881f2ee3422a (accessed on 31st May 2025).
18. Fondevila, G. J. F., Martorell Castellano, C. (Coordinador), Miotto, G., Polo López, et al. (2018). *Advertising and Evaluation of Voice Through Digital Media*. https://core.ac.uk/download/250239174.pdf (accessed on 31st May 2025).
19. Fuchs, S., & Pouw, W. (2022). *Origins of Vocal-Entangled Gesture*. https://core.ac.uk/download/541698163.pdf (accessed on 31st May 2025).
20. Gakidou, E., Afshin, A., Abajobir, A. A., Abate, K. H., Abbafati, C., Abbas, K., Abd-Allah, F., et al. (2017). Global, regional, and national comparative risk assessment of 84 behavioral, environmental and occupational, and metabolic risks or clusters of risks, 1990–2016: A systematic analysis for the Global Burden of Disease Study 2016. *The Lancet, 390*, 1345–1422. https://doi.org/10.1016/s0140-6736(17)32366-8 (accessed on 31st May 2025).
21. Galarza, N. C., & Monge Condori, M. D. L. A. (2020). *Model of Trigger Mechanisms of SARS CoV-2 Infections*. https://core.ac.uk/download/539911324.pdf (accessed on 31st May 2025).
22. Giegold, M. (2018). *Modeling of the Immune Response During Virus Infection of the Human Respiratory* tract. https://core.ac.uk/download/pdf/289960831.pdf (accessed on 31st May 2025).
23. González-García, M., Carrillo-Franco, L., Morales-Luque, C., Dawid-Milner, M. S., & López-González, M. V. (2024). Central autonomic mechanisms involved in the control of laryngeal activity and vocalization. *Biology, 13*, 118. https://doi.org/10.3390/biology13020118 (accessed on 31st May 2025).
24. Gurunathan, S., Kang, M. H., Jeyaraj, M., Qasim, M., & Kim, J. H. (2019). Review of the isolation, characterization, biological function, and multifarious therapeutic approaches of exosomes. *Cells, 8*, 307–307. https://doi.org/10.3390/cells8040307 (accessed on 31st May 2025).

25. Hegermann, J., Kuebler, W. M., Lopez-Rodriguez, E., Matuszak, et al. (2020). *On Top of the Alveolar Epithelium: Surfactant and the Glycocalyx.* https://core.ac.uk/download/323256852.pdf (accessed on 31st May 2025).

26. Herath, P., Wimalasekera, S., Amarasekara, T., Fernando, M. S., & Turale, S. (2025). Comparison of respiratory symptoms and pulmonary functions of adult male cigarette smokers and non-smokers in Sri Lanka: A comparative analytical study. *PLOS ONE, 20.* https://www.semanticscholar.org/paper/12b705006225b5733873342b540d01814d4a0608 (accessed on 31st May 2025).

27. Homberger, D. G. (2017). The avian lingual and laryngeal apparatus within the context of the head and jaw apparatus, with comparisons to the mammalian condition: Functional morphology and biomechanics of evaporative cooling, feeding, drinking, and vocalization. The Biology of the Avian Respiratory System. https://core.ac.uk/download/373117495.pdf (accessed on 31st May 2025).

28. Hou, K., Wu, Z. X., Chen, X. Y., Wang, J. Q., Zhang, D., Xiao, C., Zhu, D., et al. (2022). Microbiota in health and diseases. *Signal Transduction and Targeted Therapy, 7.* https://doi.org/10.1038/s41392-022-00974-4 (accessed on 31st May 2025).

29. Hu, B., Guo, H., Zhou, P., & Shi, Z.-L. (2020). Characteristics of SARS-CoV-2 and COVID-19. *Nature Reviews Microbiology, 19,* 141–154. https://doi.org/10.1038/s41579-020-00459-7 (accessed on 31st May 2025).

30. Ivanchenko, S., Kovalyova, O., & Zhuravlyova, A. (2023). *Renin-Angiotensin System: A Review of Historical Perspectives.* https://core.ac.uk/download/574566620.pdf (accessed on 31st May 2025).

31. Johnsen, S., Sattler, S. M., Miskowiak, K. W., Kunalan, K., Victor, A., Pedersen, L., Andreassen, H. F., et al. (2021). Descriptive analysis of long COVID sequela identified in a multidisciplinary clinic serving hospitalized and non-hospitalized patients. *ERJ Open Research, 7,* 00205–2021. https://doi.org/10.1183/23120541.00205-2021 (accessed on 31st May 2025).

32. Liguori, I., Russo, G., Curcio, F., Bulli, G., Aran, L., Della-Morte, D., Gargiulo, G., et al. (2018). Oxidative stress, aging, and diseases. *Clinical Interventions in Aging, 13,* 757–772. https://doi.org/10.2147/cia.s158513 (accessed on 31st May 2025).

33. Maggi, E., Canonica, G. W., & Moretta, L. (2020). COVID-19: Unanswered questions on immune response and pathogenesis. *Journal of Allergy and Clinical Immunology, 146,* 18–22. https://doi.org/10.1016/j.jaci.2020.05.001 (accessed on 31st May 2025).

34. Mangalmurti, N. S., Reilly, J., Cines, D., Meyer, N., Hunter, C., & Vaughan, A. (2020). COVID-19–associated acute respiratory distress syndrome clarified: A vascular endotype? *American Journal of Respiratory and Critical Care Medicine, 202,* 750–753. https://www.semanticscholar.org/paper/a2c12e5d364296d00b061f087a801b1b036cdae3 (accessed on 31st May 2025).

35. Mazidi, M., Dehghan, A., Mikhailidis, D., Jozwiak, J., Covic, A., Sattar, N., Banach, M., et al. (2021). The association between coffee and caffeine consumption and renal function: Insight from individual-level data, Mendelian randomization, and meta-analysis. *Archives of Medical Science: AMS, 18,* 900–911. https://www.semanticscholar.org/paper/8e477e6b4f2a5c204b6fa3e010c91058720dc448 (accessed on 31st May 2025).

36. Monteil, V., Kwon, H., Prado, P., Hagelkrüys, A., Wimmer, R., Ståhl, M., Leopoldi, A., et al. (2020). Inhibition of SARS-CoV-2 infections in engineered human tissues using clinical-grade soluble

human ACE2. *Cell, 181*, 905–913.e7. https://doi.org/10.1016/j.cell.2020.04.004 (accessed on 31st May 2025).

37. Murga, A., Bale, R., Li, C. G., Ito, K., & Tsubokura, M. (2023). Large eddy simulation of droplet transport and deposition in the human respiratory tract to evaluate inhalation risk. *PLoS Computational Biology*, *19*, e1010972. https://doi.org/10.1371/journal.pcbi.1010972 (accessed on 31st May 2025).

38. Murray, C. J. L., Ikuta, K. S., Sharara, F., Swetschinski, L. R., Robles, A. G., Gray, A. P., Han, C., et al. (2022). Global burden of bacterial antimicrobial resistance in 2019: A systematic analysis. *The Lancet*, *399*, 629–655. https://doi.org/10.1016/s0140-6736(21)02724-0 (accessed on 31st May 2025).

39. N/A. (2025). *Aerospace Medicine and Biology: A Continuing Bibliography with Indexes, Supplement 130, July 1974*. https://core.ac.uk/download/pdf/42893215.pdf (accessed on 31st May 2025).

40. North, C. M., Rice, M. B., Ferkol, T. W., Gozal, D., Hui, C., Jung, S. H., Kuribayashi, K., et al. (2019). Air pollution in the Asia-Pacific Region. *Respirology*, *24*, 484–491. https://doi.org/10.1111/resp.13531 (accessed on 31st May 2025).

41. Oczkowski, S., Ergan, B., Bos, L. D. J., Chatwin, M., Ferrer, M., Gregoretti, C., Heunks, L., et al. (2021). ERS clinical practice guidelines: High-flow nasal cannula in acute respiratory failure. *European Respiratory Journal*, *59*, 2101574. https://doi.org/10.1183/13993003.01574-2021 (accessed on 31st May 2025).

42. Pillay, T. S., Wiese, O., & Zemlin, A. E. (2021). *Molecules in Pathogenesis: Angiotensin Converting Enzyme 2 (ACE2)*. https://core.ac.uk/download/528259406.pdf (accessed on 31st May 2025).

43. Poon, L. C., Yang, H., Dumont, S., Lee, J. C. S., Copel, J. A., Danneels, L., Wright, A., et al. (2020). *ISUOG* Interim guidance on coronavirus disease 2019 (COVID-19) during pregnancy and puerperium: Information for healthcare professionals – an update. *Ultrasound in Obstetrics and Gynecology*, *55*, 848–862. https://doi.org/10.1002/uog.22061 (accessed on 31st May 2025).

44. Ra, S., Sze, M., Lee, E. C., Tam, S., Oh, Y., Fishbane, N., Criner, G., et al. (2017). Azithromycin and risk of COPD exacerbations in patients with and without *Helicobacter pylori*. *Respiratory Research, 18*. https://www.semanticscholar.org/paper/145751aba285fe92efeaf0640c3ad7975eb2612f (accessed on 31st May 2025).

45. Rhodes, A., Evans, L., Alhazzani, W., Levy, M. M., Antonelli, M., Ferrer, R., Kumar, A., et al. (2017). Surviving Sepsis Campaign: International Guidelines for Management of Sepsis and Septic Shock: 2016. *Critical Care Medicine*, *45*, 486–552. https://doi.org/10.1097/ccm.0000000000002255 (accessed on 31st May 2025).

46. Sachs, N., Papaspyropoulos, A., Zomer-Van, O. D. D., Heo, I., Böttinger, L., Klay, D., Weeber, F., et al. (2019). Long-term expanding human airway organoids for disease modeling. *The EMBO Journal, 38*. https://doi.org/10.15252/embj.2018100300 (accessed on 31st May 2025).

47. Simukoko, H. (2021). *Refocusing Functional Anatomy and Immunology of the Respiratory Mucosa in the Advent of COVID-19*. https://core.ac.uk/download/387220020.pdf (accessed on 31st May 2025).

48. Skoyles, J. R. (2008). Respiratory, postural and spatio-kinetic motor stabilization, internal models, top-down timed motor coordination and expanded cerebello-cerebral circuitry: A

review. Nature Preceedings. https://core.ac.uk/download/pdf/1569872.pdf (accessed on 31st May 2025).

49. Sparano, C., Maggi, M., & Petrone, L. (2022). Response to Letter to the Editor from Lui et al.: 'Euthyroid sick syndrome as an early surrogate marker of poor outcome in mild SARS-CoV-2 disease': Prognostic significance of non-thyroidal illness syndrome in the whole spectrum of COVID-19 severity. *Journal of Endocrinological Investigation, 45*, 903, 904. https://www.semanticscholar.org/paper/adb06c377cd948e3f8be3f5c8b11082e5c619ca4 (accessed on 31st May 2025).

50. Stolzenburg, L. R., & Harris, A. (2017). The role of microRNAs in chronic respiratory disease: Recent insights. *Biological Chemistry, 399*, 219–234. https://doi.org/10.1515/hsz-2017-0249 (accessed on 31st May 2025).

51. Suflita, N. (2012). *Multimodality in the Science Classroom: A Focus on Multimedia Representations and How Students Learn.* https://core.ac.uk/download/233569821.pdf (accessed on 31st May 2025).

52. Tay, M. Z., Poh, C. M., Rénia, L., MacAry, P. A., & Ng, L. F. P. (2020). The trinity of COVID-19: Immunity, inflammation and intervention. *Nature Reviews Immunology, 20*, 363–374. https://doi.org/10.1038/s41577-020-0311-8 (accessed on 31st May 2025).

53. Wang, B., & Ye, X. (2024). Long-term lung function recovery after ECMO versus non-ECMO management in acute respiratory failure: A systematic review and meta-analysis. *BMC Pulmonary Medicine, 24.* https://www.semanticscholar.org/paper/3385eb0aaff86dd00c759ce0b117c5b63392212f (accessed on 31st May 2025).

54. Ye, Q., Wang, B., & Mao, J. (2020). The pathogenesis and treatment of the 'cytokine storm' in COVID-19. *Journal of Infection, 80*, 607–613. https://doi.org/10.1016/j.jinf.2020.03.037 (accessed on 31st May 2025).

55. Zhang, T., Xiang, T., Zhang, S., Wang, D., Wang, L., Wang, Q., & Fan, H. (2021). The roles of dipeptidyl peptidase 4 (DPP4) and DPP4 inhibitors in different lung diseases: New evidence. *Frontiers in Pharmacology, 12.* https://doi.org/10.3389/fphar.2021.731453 (accessed on 31st May 2025).

56. Zhang, Y., Bi, J. Y., Huang, J., Tang, Y., Du, S., & Li, P. (2020). Exosome: A review of its classification, isolation techniques, storage, diagnostic and targeted therapy applications. *International Journal of Nanomedicine, 15*, 6917–6934. https://doi.org/10.2147/ijn.s264498 (accessed on 31st May 2025).

57. Zheng, D., Liwinski, T., & Elinav, E. (2020). Interaction between microbiota and immunity in health and disease. *Cell Research, 30*, 492–506. https://doi.org/10.1038/s41422-020-0332-7 (accessed on 31st May 2025).

58. Zheng, M., Boni, L., & Fingerhut, A. (2020). Minimally invasive surgery and the novel coronavirus outbreak: Lessons learned in China and Italy. *Annals of Surgery, 272*, e5, e6. https://doi.org/10.1097/sla.0000000000003924 (accessed on 31st May 2025).

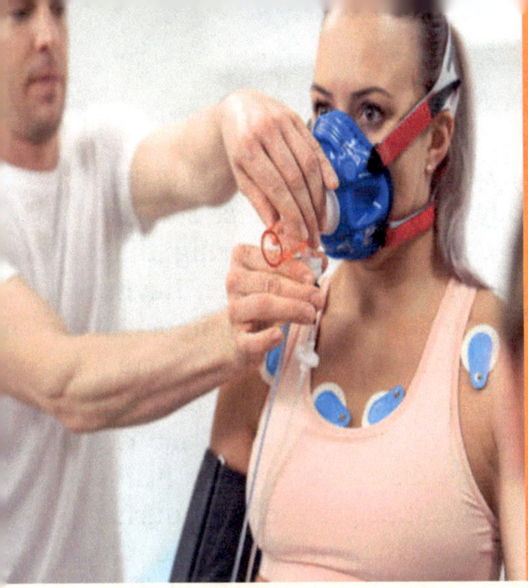

Chapter 13

RESPIRATORY ADJUSTMENTS IN EXERCISE

Contents

Introduction

Respiratory changes during exercise are crucial in understanding how the body responds to increased physical effort. As the intensity of exercise increases, the muscles require more oxygen, which means the body needs to breathe faster and more efficiently. A combination of nerve and hormone signals controls how the heart and lungs work during exercise. The autonomic nervous system (ANS) plays a pivotal role in this adjustment, wherein sympathetic activation occurs alongside parasympathetic withdrawal, ensuring that adequate blood flow and oxygen delivery to working muscles are maintained. In this way, respiration is an active process that utilizes different body systems to improve how long and well we can exercise, highlighting the connections between various parts of our physiology. Besides exercise, respiratory adaptations can also explain and prevent various health problems. Noticing how breathing changes during exercise can guide training and rehabilitation, mainly for those with heart or lung conditions. According to research, using proper breathing techniques can help athletes and fitness enthusiasts take in more oxygen and recover more quickly, making them beneficial for anyone looking to improve their health. It is also important to study these changes, since proper actions are needed to protect crew members from health problems in space, as microgravity can be similar to the stress of intense exercise. By studying how our bodies react and how this response is utilized in various environments, we recognize the importance of understanding changes in breathing during exercise. The primary reason for studying these changes is to enhance performance in sports and to gain a deeper understanding of how the heart and lungs respond to stress. Exploring this area can help find out how respiratory function works which in turn helps develop better strategies for health care. For example, research has found that the exercise pressure reflex is crucial for maintaining a stable heart rate during physical activity, ensuring that vital organs are well perfused. Also, research from spaceflights points out that being flexible is important in different gravity conditions, which leads scientists to explore ways to keep astronauts healthy both during and after missions. Exploring these dimensions highlights the critical nature of respiratory adjustments within exercise contexts and encourages a holistic approach to optimizing health and performance in various settings (Crisafulli et al., 2014).

Definition of Respiratory Adjustments

Respiratory adjustments encompass the various changes that occur in the respiratory system when the body requires more energy, such as during exercise. Such changes in breathing are made by adjusting both the rate and depth and the nervous system and muscles regulate these changes. When exercise becomes more intense, the body requires more oxygen and must remove more carbon dioxide, which necessitates the lungs working harder and more efficiently. Due to this, muscles are supplied with enough oxygen when needed, which helps them perform at their best. Additionally, respiratory adjustments help maintain the body's acid-base balance stability during intense exercise, underscoring their importance for overall bodily balance. Having a clear idea of these adjustments is important because it highlights how the respiratory system can handle and meet the needs of physical activity. Besides breathing in more air, the lungs also adjust the distribution of air inside them, which helps facilitate gas exchange during exercise. While physical activity continues, the body uses several parts of the lungs to help take in more oxygen and eliminate more carbon dioxide. This recruitment demonstrates that the body can manage blood flow and breathing, so that the parts of the lungs with the most blood are also well ventilated. Moreover, research indicates that the release of cell-derived microvesicles (MVs) during exercise may also influence respiratory adjustments. These MVs, shed by various cells in response to physical stress, can carry bioactive agents that modulate physiological responses, thus contributing to the adaptations in respiratory function observed during and after exercise (Mourot et al., 2018). Understanding these processes helps explain how cells signal the entire body during intense exercise. Besides oxygen, the changes in breathing during exercise are important for understanding how the heart reacts. When you start exercising more, your heart and lungs work harder to give your muscles the oxygen they need. Nerve signals, hormones, and changes in blood vessel resistance from the cardiovascular system help it adapt to the changes happening in the respiratory system. Studies suggest that mathematical modeling can further elucidate the dynamics of cardiovascular adjustments during exercise, providing insights into the interplay between heart rate, blood pressure, and ventilation during varied intensity levels (Mitchell et al., 2025). Due to these detailed models, we can observe how the body responds to exercise by adjusting its breathing patterns.

Importance of Respiratory Function During Exercise

The respiratory system helps the body meet its increased energy needs during exercise. When a person exercises harder, the body needs to take in more oxygen and get rid of more carbon dioxide. As a result of this exchange, the body can maintain balance and utilize oxygen to produce energy efficiently. The brain controls breathing rate and depth to ensure there is enough air for exercise, adjusting accordingly to the intensity of the person's work. The brain gives orders, and chemoreceptors detecting changes in blood gases provide feedback, which helps regulate these processes. These interactions not only enhance respiratory function but also support cardiovascular stability during exertion, underscoring the respiratory system's integral role in overall exercise performance and endurance (Crisafulli et al., 2014). Additionally, if breathing is impaired, it can lead to significant issues, particularly for individuals with pre-existing health conditions. Chronic heart failure can cause people to tire easily and find it hard to exercise, and this may be due to problems in the body and the lungs. Problems with breathing can make it harder for the heart to function properly, leading to reduced exercise tolerance and increased fatigue. Understanding these phenomena relies a lot on the effects of muscle receptors sending signals back to the brain. Too much signaling from group III/IV muscle afferents can cause the body to respond poorly to exercise, which leads to both central and peripheral fatigue. As such, the interplay between respiratory and cardiovascular functions is vital for optimizing exercise tolerance and performance in those with compromised health status (Angius et al., 2020). Besides improving your performance, focusing on respiratory function during exercise is crucial for your overall health in the long run. Regular exercise can help improve lung function, enhance oxygen utilization, and increase the efficiency of lung function. On a larger scale, exercise enhances the coordination between the lungs and heart, which in turn lowers the risk of chronic diseases. Importantly, interventions aimed at improving respiratory mechanics may serve as therapeutic strategies to counteract adverse conditions such as chronic obstructive pulmonary disease (COPD) and heart failure. By focusing on enhancing respiratory function, individuals not only improve their capacity for physical activity but also fortify their cardiovascular health, illustrating the vital importance of respiratory adjustments during exercise (Crisafulli et al., 2014) (Figure 13.1).

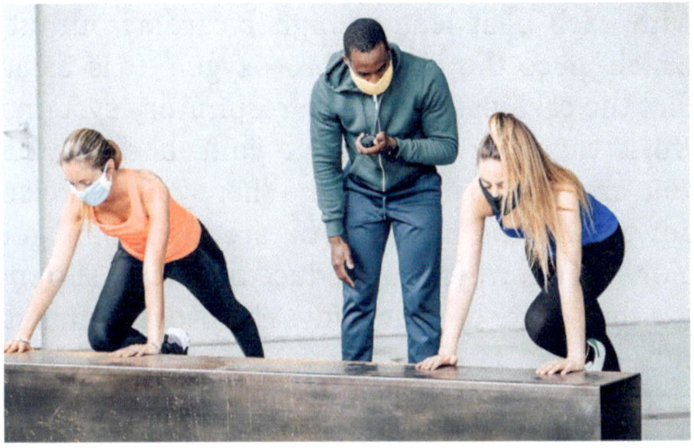

Figure 13.1. Masked physical training during the COVID-19 pandemic.

Source: https://media-cldnry.s-nbcnews.com/image/upload/t_fit-1500w,f_auto,q_auto:best/newscms/2021_12/3457424/210316-trainer-masks-bd-2x1.jpg.

13.1. Physiological Responses to Exercise

When people exercise, their bodies respond in several ways to give more oxygen to the muscles. In this adaptation, the respiratory system is crucial because it facilitates increased airflow in and out of the body. While exercising, the body breathes much more quickly and deeply, a phenomenon known as hyperpnea. As a result of this adjustment, more oxygen is delivered to the blood and more carbon dioxide is removed from it. In addition, these changes in breathing are maintained by both nerve and hormone signals to ensure tissues receive enough oxygen, even when there is insufficient oxygen in the air. The ability to modulate ventilation in response to the body's needs is not only crucial for performance but also underscores the respiratory system's adaptability in various environmental conditions and during exercise (Webb et al., 2022). When we exercise, both the heart and blood vessels change in response to our breathing, demonstrating the body's teamwork. The rise in heart rate and the amount of blood pumped with each beat lead to higher cardiac output, which gives the body more oxygen. It is clear that the cardiovascular and respiratory systems work together to support your body when you are physically active. When you exercise powerfully, the muscles you are using may get more blood, which can reduce the blood supply to other parts of your body. The process makes sure oxygen is delivered to the most valuable places, which increases metabolism and helps the body function. Interestingly, studies suggest that individuals with adaptations such as high hemoglobin-oxygen affinity can experience differing cardiorespiratory responses during hypoxic conditions, raising critical questions about the efficiency of oxygen transport in various physiological states and its implications for exercise (Zhao et al., 2020). Besides the quick changes in your body during exercise, the long-term ones are also significant for improving your performance. Training often improves the amount of oxygen your lungs can take in and how efficiently they use it. Regular aerobic activities build up the strength of the respiratory muscles, which improves the mechanics of breathing. Additionally, as you train, your resting heart rate decreases, and your stroke volume increases, which helps you stay active for a longer period during exercise. Due to these adaptations, both athletes and recreational exercisers can maintain their endurance for an extended period without becoming too tired. Furthermore, understanding how these physiological responses evolve with exercise has potential implications for rehabilitation protocols and exercise recommendations, particularly for populations with specific health challenges or recovery needs (Webb et al., 2022).

13.1.1. Increased Respiratory Rate During Physical Activity

When we exercise, our bodies undergo numerous changes to provide the extra oxygen required. An increase in respiratory rate is important because it allows the body to get more oxygen to its working muscles. As exercise intensity increases, the brain's breathing centers prompt us to breathe both faster and deeper. This change makes sure that the lungs can remove carbon dioxide, which builds up during intense exercise. Improved breathing during exercise supports energy production and helps maintain the body's acid-base balance, highlighting the integrated role of the respiratory system in sustaining physical performance. Along with the rapid breathing that occurs immediately, the increase in respiratory rate during exercise is influenced by various metabolic processes. When muscles need more oxygen and produce more carbon dioxide, the body increases the rate of breathing. While metabolic changes are significant, competing can also increase heart and breathing rates, sometimes more than expected. When a person is stressed, their heart rate increases, and they need more oxygen. This prompts them to breathe faster, as they require more oxygen. This phenomenon illustrates the connection between stress and respiratory efficiency, as emotional and psychological factors intertwine with physiological adjustments during physical activity, creating a multifaceted response to exertion (Allen et al., 2009). Respiratory rate affects exercise differently for each person and activity. Since endurance athletes are efficient at utilizing oxygen, they typically breathe more effectively during exercise. Untrained individuals may experience greater increases in their breathing rate during exercise, suggesting that their bodies are not adapting well to exercise. The cause of these differences is varied, including differences in lung capacity, muscle oxygen use, and general cardiovascular fitness. Thus, understanding the nuances of respiratory adjustments, including the increase in respiratory rate, offers valuable insights into both sports performance and the physiological mechanisms underlying exercise responses (de Jonge et al., 2009) (Figure 13.2).

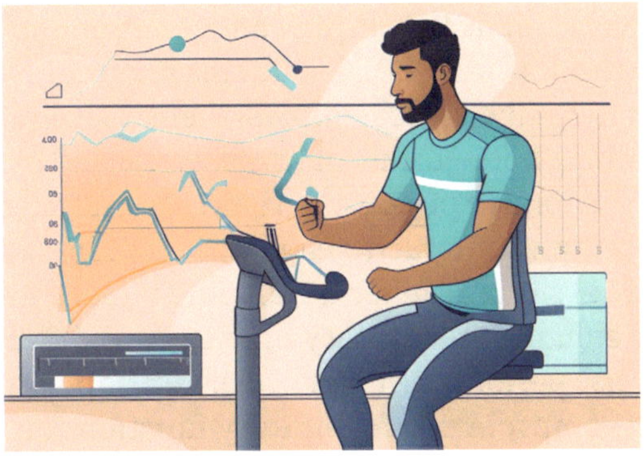

Figure 13.2. Increased respiration during physical activity.

Source: https://koala.sh/api/image/v2-csq46-wrenk.jpg?width=1216&height=832&dream.

13.1.2. Changes in Tidal Volume and Minute Ventilation

As individuals engage in exercise, the physiological demands placed on the respiratory system result in notable changes in tidal volume (TV) and minute ventilation (VE). The amount of air inhaled or exhaled in a single breath is called TV, and the total amount of air taken in during one minute is called minute ventilation. The muscles need extra oxygen during physical activity to work correctly. Therefore, the lungs inhaled. It is necessary for effective gas exchange because it directly controls the amount of oxygen for muscles and the amount of carbon dioxide removed. In some situations, tight clothing may prevent the lungs from working as well as they could, which can affect both tidal volume and minute ventilation. For example, a study found that when sports bras were tighter, the underband pressure resulted in less tidal volume at the peak of exercise. In this research, participants exhibited a higher breathing frequency when underband tightness increased, leading to a significant enhancement in minute ventilation despite a reduced tidal volume (Kipp et al., 2024).

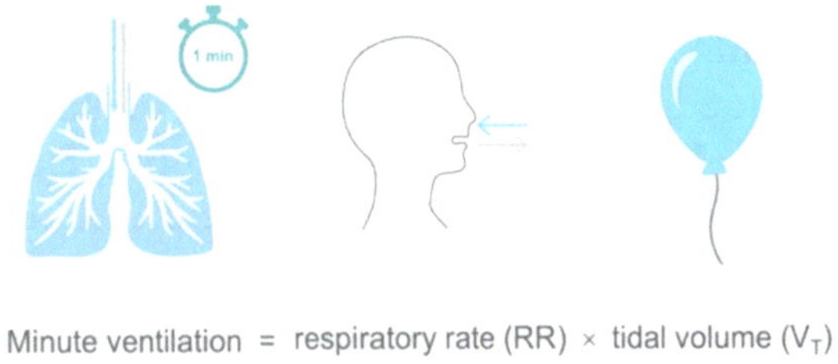

Figure 13.3. Ventilation minute.

Source: https://d25iein5sonfaj.cloudfront.net/v1/public-drupal-medmastery-assets-production/migrated-images/noninvasive-ventilation-minute-calculation-illustrated.png?cfg=eyJ3aWR0aCI6NjAwLCJoZWlnaHQiOjQwMCwib3V0cHV0Ijoid2VicCJ9.

It demonstrates that the body can adapt to challenging conditions, although it also raises questions about how effectively oxygen is utilized during strenuous activities. Moreover, a person's overall health and fitness can affect their breathing, which can make it harder to understand tidal volume and minute ventilation. A study assessing deployed veterans reported reduced breathing frequencies alongside increased dyspnea ratings during maximal exercise testing relative to non-deployed controls, indicating altered ventilatory mechanics under physical stress (Alexander et al., 2023). Therefore, existing health problems can make it difficult for the lungs to adjust tidal volume and minute ventilation, which affects both exercise ability and general respiratory health. Recognizing these variances is crucial for developing effective exercise programs and interventions tailored to individual needs, ultimately promoting better respiratory adjustments during physical activity (Figure 13.3).

13.1.3. Role of Chemoreceptors in Regulating Breathing

Chemoreceptors play a crucial role in regulating breathing, particularly during exercise when metabolic demands shift significantly. These specialized sensory receptors are sensitive to changes in the chemical composition of the blood, specifically the levels of carbon dioxide (CO_2), oxygen (O_2), and pH. Central chemoreceptors (located in the medulla oblongata) predominantly respond to elevated CO_2 levels, thereby stimulating increased ventilation to expel excess carbon dioxide. In contrast, peripheral chemoreceptors situated in the carotid and aortic bodies respond to decreases in O_2 and increases in CO_2 and acidity. This dual feedback mechanism ensures that adequate oxygen delivery and metabolic waste removal are maintained during physical exertion, thus highlighting the critical function of chemoreceptors in sustaining homeostasis under varying physiological conditions. As exercise intensity increases, the demand for oxygen rises, leading to a concomitant elevation in both ventilation rate and depth, known as hyperpnea. This phenomenon is carefully orchestrated by chemoreceptors, which detect the accumulating CO_2 resulting from increased metabolic activity. Research indicates that during mild or moderate exercise, alveolar ventilation adjusts in direct proportion to metabolic rate, effectively regulating arterial CO_2 levels near resting thresholds (Mitchell et al., 2024). Due to the relationship between central and peripheral chemoreceptors, breathing can change rapidly, ensuring that muscles receive sufficient oxygen. In addition, these receptors can adjust their sensitivity depending on different stimuli, which helps them fit well into the respiratory control system needed for maintaining performance during prolonged exercise. Besides reacting to immediate breathing needs, chemoreceptors are involved in long-term changes in breathing control that happen with exercise training. These receptors activate specific neural pathways within the central command system, preparing the respiratory muscles for the demands of exercise. Furthermore, emerging evidence suggests that the cerebellum may play a significant role in fine-tuning this respiratory response through learning mechanisms, highlighting the interplay between sensory input and motor output (Mitchell et al., 2024). Chemoreceptors can adjust easily, which allows them to regulate breathing both quickly during exercise and over a more extended period. Therefore, understanding the complex interactions within chemoreceptor pathways is crucial for developing interventions that enhance respiratory efficiency and overall exercise performance, particularly in populations with compromised respiratory function (Figure 13.4).

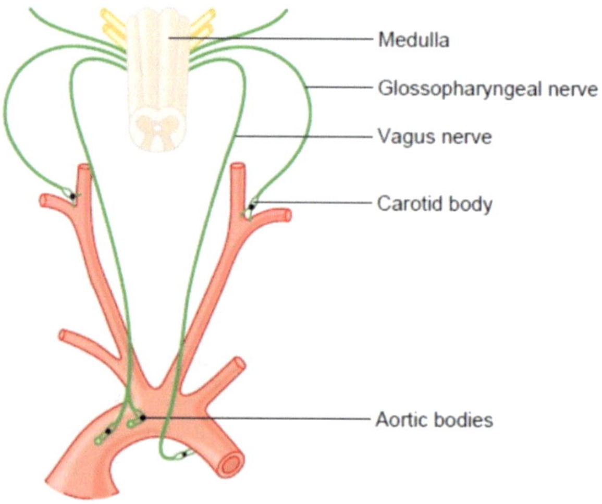

Figure 13.4. Respiratory control by peripheral chemoreceptors in the carotid and aortic bodies.

Source: https://img.brainkart.com/imagebk20/2eHUDzN.jpg.

13.2. Impact of Exercise Intensity on Respiration

When you exercise harder, the respiratory system has to work harder, which changes both your breathing rate and depth. At the beginning of moderate exercise, people take in and release more air with each breath. As a result of this adjustment, oxygen can enter the blood more easily, and carbon dioxide can leave it at a faster rate. When exercise intensity increases to vigorous levels, the body requires more oxygen, and consequently, the respiratory rate increases. The relationship between tidal volume and respiratory rate demonstrates that the respiratory system responds to various physical situations, which is crucial for athletes to understand. Also, the ANS plays a more important role as the intensity of exercise increases. When we engage in intense activities, the sympathetic nervous system activates, which increases our heart rate and enhances ventilation to ensure we receive sufficient oxygen. Certain reflexes, such as the exercise pressor reflex, ensure that blood flow and oxygen reach important tissues and help remove carbon dioxide. Such neural changes are necessary, primarily in dynamic activities, as the heart and lungs must work together to maintain performance. By knowing how these systems work together, we can use training to help the body make better respiratory and heart changes during strenuous exercise, which results in higher athletic performance and endurance. Furthermore, the management of exercise intensity is integral to training regimens aimed at optimizing athletic performance while minimizing risks of maladaptation, such as unexplained underperformance syndrome (UUPS). Sports scientists and coaches advise athletes to use well-structured training that combines progressively more challenging exercises with enough time for rest to improve their performance. Depending on how hard an athlete exercises, the stress on the respiratory system can either help or harm, especially if they do not allow their body to rest properly. It is important for athletes and coaches to closely monitor training, as well as sleep, nutrition, and mental state, to help with respiratory responses. This interdisciplinary approach to sports science, emphasizing the complex interactions between exercise intensity and respiratory adjustments, underscores the necessity for tailored training strategies that optimize health and performance outcomes in competitive environments (Crisafulli et al., 2014; Collins et al., 2015).

13.2.1. Differences between Aerobic and Anaerobic Exercise

The distinction between aerobic and anaerobic exercise lies primarily in the energy systems utilized during physical activity. Aerobic exercises are those that are performed at a moderate pace and require oxygen to support the body's energy production, such as running, swimming, or cycling. While performing these exercises, the body utilizes both carbohydrates and fats through aerobic pathways, which helps the heart and lungs function more efficiently. It encourages changes in the heart and lungs, which help oxygen move through the body more efficiently. Higher oxygen uptake and utilization result in improved endurance and overall fitness. Unlike aerobic exercise, anaerobic exercise involves quick, high-energy movements such as sprinting or lifting weights and the body uses stored energy in the muscles instead of oxygen right away. So, knowing these differences helps you decide on the proper training and what health benefits you can expect. These different energy systems also affect the body's response to the intensity and duration of exercise. To meet the body's increased need for oxygen, aerobic exercise gradually makes your heart and lungs work harder. On the other hand, anaerobic exercise brings about sudden and sharp changes in breathing patterns, as the body begins to produce lactic acid during anaerobic metabolism. Due to this metabolic change, the body requires more oxygen to recover after exercise, which in turn causes the lungs to work harder and breathe faster. Additionally, these distinctions are significant for therapy, particularly when working with individuals in clinical settings. For instance, Bonini et al. (2017) highlight that physical activity functions as an effective tool for preventing cardiovascular risk, a consideration particularly relevant for patients with varying aerobic capacities. Additionally, understanding the differences between aerobic and anaerobic exercise can inform training plans tailored to your specific goals. To improve aerobic capacity, some people prefer steady-state workouts that help them use oxygen effectively and build cardiovascular strength. Those who want to improve their strength and power may concentrate on anaerobic exercises, which require quick, intense bursts of energy. According to research, factors such as temperature can impact the amount of work a person can perform in both aerobic and anaerobic exercise. According to Newton et al. (2025), variations in body temperature can impact exercise output, suggesting a complex relationship between environmental conditions and exercise performance. Thus, recognizing how these forms of exercise engage different metabolic pathways reinforces the importance of tailored exercise programming in promoting overall health and performance (Figure 13.5).

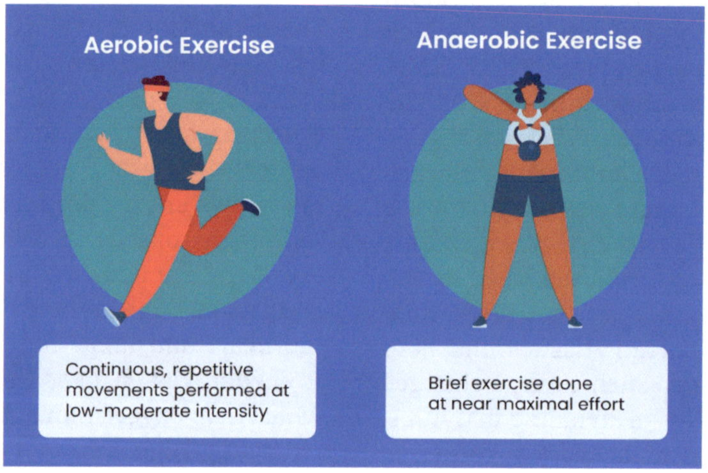

Figure 13.5. Aerobic and anaerobic exercise.

Source: https://images.ctfassets.net/yixw23k2v6vo/2akPh7ZPkfEDuOy8ROc16x/ebed7e9e6e1f760e4f6b3cfa8324de83/large-GettyImages-1369420657-aerobic-vs-anaerobic.jpg.

13.2.2. Thresholds of Exercise Intensity and Respiratory Response

Understanding the thresholds of exercise intensity is critical for comprehending how the respiratory system adapts during physical activity. A higher level of exercise requires the body to use more oxygen, resulting in a faster and deeper breathing rate. This happens mainly at the anaerobic threshold, which is a key point where the body switches from using oxygen to using energy without oxygen, because there is not enough oxygen available. As lactic acid builds up in the muscles at this point, the body attempts to remove the excess carbon dioxide produced by anaerobic metabolism, which strengthens breathing. As a result, experts say that being aware of this threshold helps them design better workouts and enhance performance by being more careful about how hard they exercise and how their breathing changes. It is clear from studying the respiratory system during exercise that several physiological processes are involved. Initially, breathing adjusts to match the activity's energy needs, as indicated by a steady increase in ventilation as oxygen consumption increases. Still, after reaching a particular exercise intensity, the relationship is no longer linear, suggesting metabolic acidosis is starting, which leads to more breathing adjustments. Due to this shift, athletes, individuals undergoing rehabilitation, and those with respiratory issues are all affected.

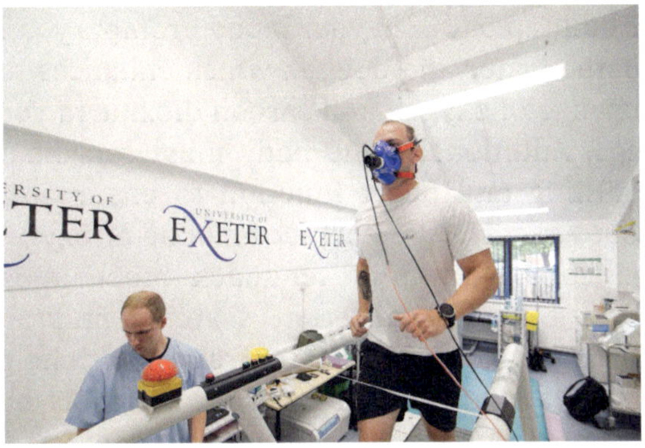

Figure 13.6. VO_2 max testing during treadmill exercise at the University of Exeter.

Source: https://images.squarespace-cdn.com/content/v1/5f2b2d504703b3643016bffd/1600986808691-H4M5Y2VA1L899VNP8SD1/VO2MAX4729.jpg.

Learning about how exercise intensity affects breathing can guide the creation of safe exercise guidelines for all groups, which helps people become fitter while avoiding problems related to breathing or injury during intense activities. Also, how hard a person exercises and the resulting changes in breathing differ significantly from one person to another due to age, level of fitness, and health issues. For this reason, using exercise testing to check these limits is helpful in both medical and sports settings. Assessments may show how much aerobic capacity a person has and the point at which ventilation becomes too much for the body. When creating personal workout plans, such assessments are necessary to ensure optimal results and prevent overexertion of the body. Therefore, knowledge of these thresholds not only aids in understanding the respiratory adjustments that occur during exercise but also has substantial implications for improving training methodologies and promoting better health outcomes across diverse populations (Eldridge et al., 2016; Matthew et al., 2021) (Figure 13.6).

13.2.3. Adaptations in Respiratory Function with Training

Respiratory function undergoes significant adaptations with consistent training, ultimately enhancing an individual's overall exercise capacity. A key adaptation is increased pulmonary ventilation, which is the amount of air breathed in and out by the lungs. The muscles that aid breathing, such as the diaphragm and intercostal muscles, become stronger and function more effectively as athletes continue to exercise. This change in breathing lets you take in more air, which increases the amount of oxygen you get and the amount of carbon dioxide you get rid of. Through such training, athletes can perform better in endurance sports and utilize energy more efficiently, demonstrating that the body can adapt well to training focused on respiratory improvement. Training also alters how blood flows through the lungs, making it easier for the lungs to take in oxygen during exercise. Frequent exercise causes more capillaries to develop in the lungs, thereby increasing the area where gas exchange occurs. It helps the most when the body needs of oxygen, such as during strenuous exercise. Additionally, a better match between air in the alveoli and blood in the pulmonary capillaries occurs, which is crucial for gas exchange. These adjustments not only support improved athletic performance but also serve a protective role in individuals with conditions that compromise cardiovascular stability, as evidenced by some studies highlighting the role of physical training in mitigating exercise intolerance and fatigue (Angius et al., 2020). Respiratory mechanics are enhanced in numerous ways, and this highlights the importance of systematic training. Neural control of breathing during training is also significant for seeing the bigger effects exercise has on the body. Training strengthens the central command, which makes it easier for the body to regulate breathing during physical activity. exercising. Over time, a close connection forms between the part of the brain that controls breathing and the intensity of the body's exercise. The way feedback from muscles changes also develops, which explains why people with chronic heart failure may find it harder to exercise after the pathways are interrupted. Therefore, the integration of respiratory adaptations through training can significantly benefit cardiovascular health, suggesting that even those with pre-existing conditions may enjoy improvements with regular exercise (Dickson et al., 2025). Such findings underscore the profound impact of exercise training on respiratory adjustments, further affirming its importance in health and performance contexts (Figure 13.7).

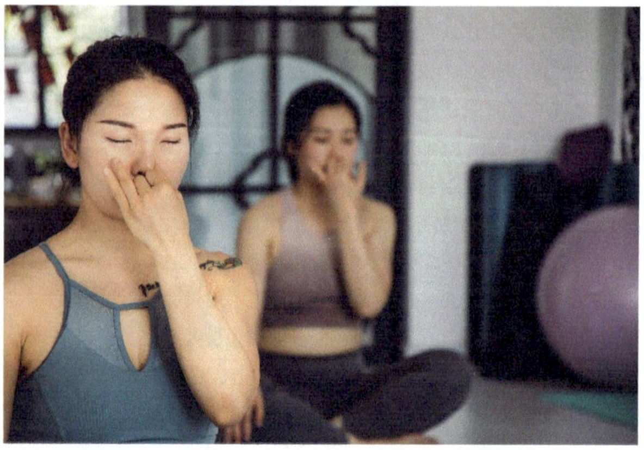

Figure 13.7. Breathing exercise.

Source: https://www.health.com/thmb/h12xcDa-0Sh6ryHyM8NsjLA0sx8=/6720x0/filters:no_upscale():max_bytes(150000):strip_icc()/Health-GettyImages-1314942804-9d5921c70058438ea6397a1b12f61455.jpg.

13.3. Factors Influencing Respiratory Adjustments

When we exercise, our bodies undergo several respiratory changes to ensure the muscles receive sufficient oxygen. Central to these adjustments are chemoreceptors that monitor blood gases, particularly carbon dioxide (CO_2) and oxygen (O_2) levels. As you exercise harder, the buildup of CO_2 in your blood prompts you to breathe faster and deeper, which enhances the exchange of oxygen and carbon dioxide in your lungs. Additionally, the body must coordinate breathing and heart function to ensure that tissues receive the correct amount of oxygen. The combination of feedback mechanisms points out how different systems must be carefully balanced during exercise which helps increase endurance and performance. As our understanding of these processes deepens, it becomes clear that specific factors, such as fitness level and health status, can further complicate respiratory responses to exercise (Angius et al., 2020). Muscle afferent feedback is critical in guiding changes in breathing. Group III and IV afferent fibers, which arise from skeletal muscle, convey information about muscle metabolic status and joint position to the central nervous system (CNS). It becomes essential during exercise because it affects both breathing and blood circulation. A strong reaction from these nerves may cause breathing difficulties, particularly in individuals with chronic heart failure, who often experience fatigue early on. This dysfunctional feedback can cause a downward spiral, limiting exercise capacity and exacerbating feelings of exertion and breathlessness (Angius et al., 2020). Because afferent signaling is crucial for respiratory regulation, targeting exercise training can help alleviate some of the limitations to respiratory changes. Additionally, the environment and altitude can significantly impact the breathing changes that occur during exercise. At higher altitudes, because there is less oxygen, the body must make bigger changes in how it breathes. People may start breathing faster to compensate for the lack of oxygen, which causes them to rely more on anaerobic metabolism. Additionally, the conditions of temperature, humidity, and air quality can impact how effectively the body absorbs and releases oxygen. Due to these external challenges, the body requires a robust respiratory response system, which means that factors affecting breathing extend beyond internal processes and also include environmental factors. Recognizing these various influences is crucial for developing effective training and enhancing performance in diverse situations.

13.3.1. Age and Its Effects on Respiratory Efficiency

As people age, their breathing ability typically decreases due to changes in their bodies. The primary reason for this less efficient breathing is that the lung tissue becomes less elastic, resulting in smaller lung volumes and a reduced ability to exchange gases. Consequently, older adults may experience a decrease in forced expiratory volume (FEV) and vital capacity (VC), which can adversely affect their ability to perform strenuous physical activities. Age also results in the chest wall becoming stiffer and the rib cage less flexible, making it harder to breathe effectively. These changes in the body can lead to difficulties in breathing properly when exerting oneself, which can make it harder for older individuals to obtain sufficient oxygen and eliminate carbon dioxide. Therefore, it is essential to understand how aging affects breathing, as this knowledge informs more effective exercise plans for seniors. Age can also bring changes to the brain's control of breathing, which affects how well the body handles exercise. The CNS helps control breathing, and the aging process may reduce the strength of these controls. More specifically, chemoreceptors may become less sensitive to changes in carbon dioxide and oxygen, resulting in inadequate lung response to increased effort. Thus, this problem can make exercising more challenging for older people, as poor respiratory function may limit their ability to maintain activity for an extended period. Also, as people age, they may be more likely to get obstructive and restrictive lung diseases, which can make their brain problems worse. Knowing how aging affects both the physical and nervous system components of breathing is essential for creating suitable exercise plans for older individuals. Due to these changes, we should seek ways to help maintain respiratory function as people age.

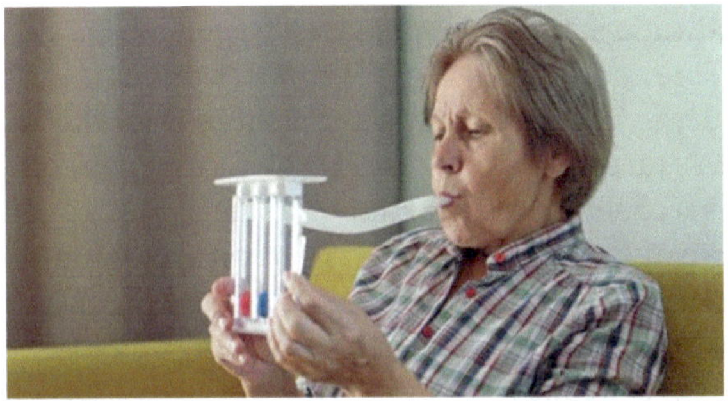

Figure 13.8. An elderly woman engaged in a health exercise, blowing into a spirometer a device designed to measure lung capacity and strengthen respiratory muscles.

Source: https://elements-resized.envatousercontent.com/elements-video-cover-images/d61cd0aa-a65a-4e2c-bc92-634090fe039e/video_preview/video_preview_0000.jpg?w=500&cf_fit=cover&q=85&format=auto&s=7e74b4e2ab16d553adcea79757ccde5e5e50ec293220f27b63b59694f148e648.

Numerous studies have demonstrated that respiratory muscle training and aerobic exercises can enhance breathing in individuals of all ages. These programs can make respiratory muscles stronger and more enduring, which benefits lung function and gas exchange in older people. Also, these interventions can enhance the heart's responses to exercise, which helps deliver more oxygen to the body. Additionally, considering the impact of nutrition and supplementation—such as the effects observed with citrulline malate and beetroot juice, which can influence blood flow and metabolic efficiency—could be essential for enhancing exercise performance in older adults (Eric et al., 2019). Consequently, addressing the multifaceted nature of age-related respiratory changes through targeted strategies holds promise for improving exercise tolerance and quality of life among older individuals (Figure 13.8).

13.3.2. Altitude and Its Impact on Oxygen Availability

Altitude significantly impacts oxygen availability, profoundly affecting respiratory adjustments during exercise. As altitude increases, the air pressure decreases, resulting in a corresponding decrease in the partial pressure of oxygen. Because oxygen is not as readily available, the body struggles to deliver enough oxygen to meet its needs during physical activity. At high altitudes, the air contains less oxygen, which reduces the lungs' ability to function effectively and lowers exercise capacity. Athletes must adjust their bodies by breathing more deeply and changing their blood chemistry to help oxygen reach and be used by the muscles. To improve performance at high altitudes, it is essential to understand these adaptations, which highlight the link between altitude, oxygen, and exercise physiology. In addition to the immediate problems caused by reduced oxygen, prolonged exposure to high altitudes can lead to significant bodily changes over time. The body goes through acclimatization, which results in producing more RBCs to help with oxygen transportation. It is important because it helps athletes maintain their performance in places with low oxygen levels. Additionally, research indicates that mastering the art of training at different altitudes can help athletes perform at their peak in major events by optimizing their training and recovery. This notion aligns with findings related to UUPS, which underscore the importance of a multifaceted approach to training, encompassing not only physical parameters but also factors such as nutrition, sleep, and psychological well-being (Collins et al., 2015). Furthermore, the problems caused by high altitude are significant for both astronauts and athletes. NASAs explorations emphasize the significance of managing oxygen availability in environments such as lower atmospheric pressure during extravehicular activities (EVA). By carefully selecting suitable atmospheric conditions—such as the recommended 8.0 psia with 32% oxygen for EVA missions—the potential risks of hypoxia and related physiological disturbances are mitigated (Arias et al., 2025). This highlights that altitude affects oxygen levels in both terrestrial activities and space missions. Exploring these dynamics will not only enhance our understanding of performance limitations induced by altitude but also advance the strategies employed to overcome these challenges, thereby ensuring optimal outcomes in diverse high-stakes environments (Figure 13.9).

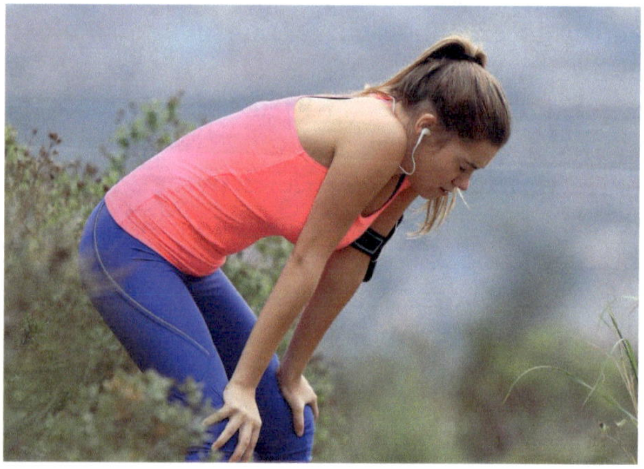

Figure 13.9. Runner experiencing breathlessness during outdoor exercise.

Source: https://runningplanetjournal.com/wp-content/uploads/2021/11/frustrated-runner-wordpress-1280x640.jpg.

13.3.3. Environmental Factors Such as Temperature and Humidity

Changes in temperature and humidity in the environment are significant for how breathing adjusts during exercise. When it is very hot, the body's metabolism speeds up, and with increased humidity, its ability to regulate its temperature is significantly affected. The need for oxygen increases during exercise in hot weather, causing people to breathe faster and more deeply to maintain their oxygen levels. As the body attempts to dissipate heat, the breathing rate adjusts to meet both the body's energy needs and cooling requirements. These changes are necessary, especially when exercising for an extended period, to prevent overheating or dehydration.

When it is very humid, the body has a harder time cooling down by sweating. As a result, the heart and lungs are subjected to greater pressure. When the air is humid, people often report that they have to work harder and feel more tired while exercising. Studies have found that people experiencing heat stress may breathe harder and faster to prevent hypoxemia, which can result from intense exercise. This response is further complicated by the body's efforts to maintain homeostasis, necessitating a complex series of adjustments that underscore the importance of environmental awareness during physical activities (Mitchell et al., 2025).

Research on acclimatization provides additional insight into how temperature and humidity impact exercise performance. The body uses short-term adaptations to handle heat stress, which helps improve how it breathes. Studies have emphasized the significance of thermoregulation and hydration as pivotal components of acclimation (Fox et al., 2025). These changes in the body help people survive and also do better in competitions. Also, adapting to heat can lead to better sweat response and stronger heart function, which are important for athletes training in various climates. All this evidence suggests that environmental factors should be incorporated into training and strategies for achieving peak performance during exercise.

13.4. Respiratory Conditions and Exercise

It is challenging for individuals with respiratory conditions to exercise due to the impact of these conditions on physical activity. Problems with airflow and oxygen exchange in COPD and asthma can make it difficult for someone to exercise correctly. When dyspnea is a common factor, patients find it more stressful to engage in exercise, which makes their breathing problems worse. Even with these difficulties, engaging in regular physical activity is crucial for maintaining good heart health and overall fitness. Programs created for people with respiratory conditions can boost their lung strength, help them exercise longer, and use oxygen more efficiently, which improves their daily living. As people exercise, they may notice their breathing improves, which can help them overcome previous breathing difficulties, proving that regular exercise is essential for respiratory health. During exercise, the body requires more oxygen, which means people with respiratory conditions must adjust their breathing a lot. Moving from rest to physical activity, people's bodies make many adjustments, such as using more oxygen and producing more carbon dioxide, which can make it harder for those with respiratory issues. Healthy individuals typically maintain arterial blood gas (ABG) homeostasis throughout submaximal exercise by efficiently matching cardiovascular and respiratory responses to metabolic demands. However, people with lung or breathing problems may not be able to make these changes, which can result in breathing difficulties or failure during intense activities. Sensory feedback from contracting muscles plays a crucial role in regulating these adjustments; for instance, group III and IV sensory fibers help inform respiratory neurons of the metabolic state of exercising muscles, which is particularly important in patients with compromised respiratory systems who require precise management of oxygen delivery to avoid hypoxia and other complications (Gomes et al., 2022). Improved respiratory assistance technology makes it easier for individuals with chronic lung conditions to engage in exercise. Using portable oxygen breathing devices can help patients breathe in more oxygen while moving, thereby preventing them from becoming short of breath. The addition of modern monitoring tools such as machine learning and biosensors has greatly improved portable oxygen therapy by making it possible to adjust the oxygen supply based on each person's needs. These intelligent systems continuously monitor physiological parameters such as blood oxygen saturation and heart rate, ensuring that oxygen supplementation is optimally tailored to support varying levels of exertion (Zhang, 2024). For this reason, these technologies boost patients' exercise abilities and help them stick to their exercise plans which leads to better health outcomes.

13.4.1. Common Respiratory Conditions Affecting Exercise Performance

It is essential for physically active individuals to understand how common respiratory conditions impact their exercise performance. Asthma, COPD and exercise-induced bronchoconstriction seriously reduce a person's ability to do their best. As asthma can harm both short-term and long-term breathing, it may cause wheezing, shortness of breath, and chest tightness during exercise, which reduces the body's ability to use oxygen. In the same way, COPD, which often results from long-term exposure to irritants like tobacco smoke, causes ongoing inflammation and makes it hard to breathe, reducing how much exercise a person can do. Therefore, people should adjust their exercise routines to manage symptoms and incorporate proper warm-ups and cool-downs to prevent exacerbating their symptoms during intense workouts. In addition to structural changes in the airways, alterations in the nervous system significantly impact how people with respiratory illnesses breathe during exercise. For instance, during dynamic exercise, the autonomic nervous system (ANS) plays a critical role in regulating both cardiovascular and respiratory responses to meet the heightened metabolic demands of the muscles involved. The usual changes in the autonomic nervous system, significantly altered in individuals with chronic respiratory diseases, including parasympathetic withdrawal and sympathetic activation. If there is dysregulation, the body's ability to exchange gases and deliver oxygen to tissues can be impaired, which may affect how well and for how long a person can perform. As shown by research, these adjustments are necessary for maintaining blood pressure in the arteries at the right level and ensuring vital organs are supplied with blood when the body is under stress. Therefore, understanding these mechanisms is crucial for developing targeted exercise interventions for individuals affected by respiratory conditions (Crisafulli et al., 2014). The relationship between respiratory problems and physical activity highlights the importance of managing them effectively. Exercise plans made for asthma and COPD can boost lung function, improve fitness and reduce the adverse effects of these conditions. Using breathing techniques, interval training, and slowly increasing exercise can help reduce the triggers for symptoms so that individuals can exercise more easily. Additionally, monitoring pollen counts and air quality can help manage symptoms more effectively. New research is showing that rehabilitation programs help individuals with respiratory problems stick to their exercise plans. By fostering safer and more enjoyable exercise environments, healthcare providers can significantly enhance the quality of life for these individuals (N/A, 2025).

13.4.2. Strategies for Managing Asthma During Physical Activity

Effective management of asthma during physical activity requires a multifaceted approach that incorporates pre-exercise strategies and ongoing monitoring. It is important to use short-acting beta-agonists or bronchodilators before doing any physical activity to help relieve bronchoconstriction. As a result, people with asthma can exercise without worrying about their symptoms worsening. Also, knowing what causes your symptoms, such as pollen, cold air, or intense exercise, helps you adapt your environment and activities, which makes exercising more enjoyable and manageable. When you know what causes your asthma and use the right medicines, you can manage your asthma better when exercising. Maintaining regular contact with your healthcare team is an essential way to manage asthma while exercising. Following up regularly helps adjust the asthma plan to fit the current symptoms and the person's level of activity. Telling patients about the early symptoms of an asthma attack allows them to take action before the situation gets worse. A good warm-up routine can help the lungs get ready for exercise, slowly increase the heart rate, and boost airflow, which might help prevent exercise-induced bronchospasm. Regular check-ups and the use of preventive measures enable people with asthma to participate in activities safely and comfortably. Besides, the environment where exercise takes place is essential for managing asthma. It is essential for individuals to choose exercise locations that are not excessively polluted or experience significant temperature fluctuations. If pollen levels are high outside, exercising indoors can help prevent breathing problems. Another way to help is by practicing diaphragmatic breathing, which can support the lungs during physical activity. It helps you take in oxygen more efficiently, which may improve your endurance. Ultimately, a comprehensive strategy that encompasses medication adherence, environmental awareness, and physical preparedness equips individuals with asthma to manage their condition effectively while participating in regular exercise, aligning with the overarching goal of promoting health and fitness within this population (Dołęga et al., 2024; Hołownia et al., 2024) (Figure 13.10).

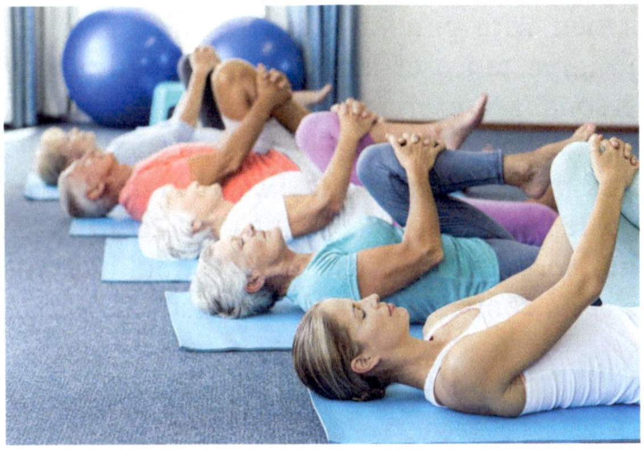

Figure 13.10. Exercise for managing asthma.

Source: https://www.crystalrunhealthcare.com/sites/default/files/Yoga-ideal-exercise-for-asthma.jpg.

13.4.3. Importance of Pulmonary Rehabilitation for Patients

The significance of pulmonary rehabilitation (PR) for patients with chronic respiratory conditions is widely recognized within the medical community. PR involves different methods to help people with diseases such as COPD feel better physically and mentally. Central to this program is the promotion of exercise, which has been shown to improve exercise capacity (EC), a critical outcome for COPD patients. Research indicates that the 6-minute walking test (6MWT) is not only easy to implement but also correlates strongly with patient prognosis and quality of life. Thus, PR programs that emphasize structured exercise training can significantly influence health outcomes, underscoring the need for healthcare professionals to advocate for such interventions as a key component in managing chronic respiratory diseases (Benzo et al., 2019). Moreover, a systematic approach to cardiopulmonary exercise testing (CPET) has become integral in evaluating the efficacy of PR. CPET enables exercise programs to be tailored to each patient, enhancing their adherence to the rehabilitation plan. The latest guidelines suggest using standardized testing to account for the differences in exercise response among patients with lung diseases, which helps studies and clinics compare their results. Due to standardization, CPET and other evaluation methods can be used reliably in various settings, providing valuable information to aid in rehabilitation improvement. By integrating patient feedback into CPET protocols, clinicians can further personalize rehabilitation plans, making them not only more effective but also more aligned with patient needs (Aguilaniu et al., 2019). Applying PR to respiratory care highlights the importance of facilitating the body's respiratory changes during exercise. If patients have a personalized exercise program, they typically find it easier to manage their condition, which may lead to improved lung health and increased endurance. PR also supports physical activity, which gives patients the confidence to manage their health independently. The primary goal is to help people live better by enabling them to manage their own affairs and utilize fewer healthcare services. Therefore, the emphasis on PR should be a focal point in the management of chronic respiratory disease, contributing to better patient outcomes and a higher standard of care (Figure 13.10).

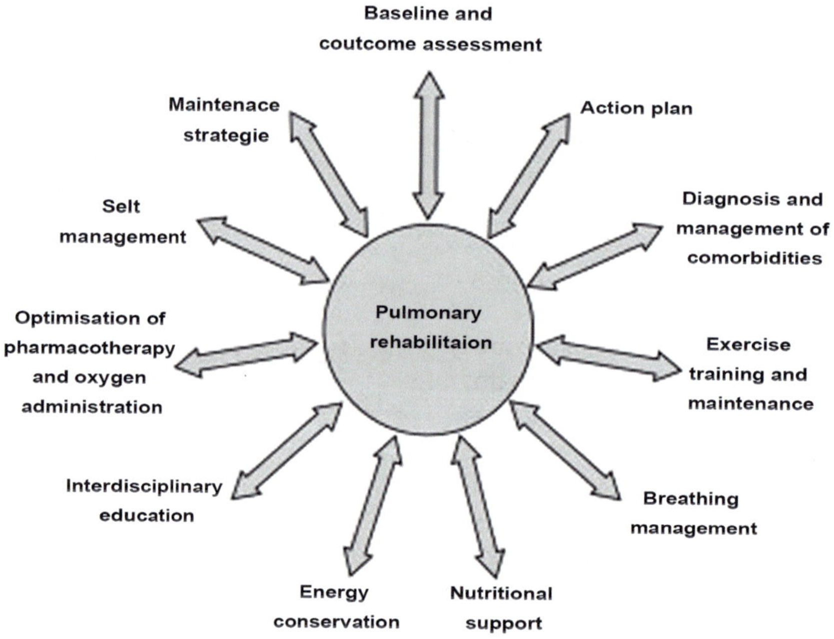

Figure 13.11. Key components of pulmonary rehabilitation.

Source: https://www.researchgate.net/profile/Fernanda-Ribeiro-23/publication/259988145/figure/fig2/AS:267562931978294@1440803382618/Key-components-of-pulmonary-rehabilitation.png.

13.5. Benefits of Exercise on Respiratory Health

Regular exercise is essential for improving respiratory health, as it affects the lungs and the whole breathing system. Being physically active encourages better breathing, which helps with gas exchange. The muscles used for breathing are also engaged during exercise, resulting in a higher volume of air inhaled and a faster breathing rate. It leads to stronger diaphragm and intercostal muscles and also helps to make lung tissues more flexible. Additionally, regular training can lead to changes in the respiratory system that enable the body to utilize oxygen more efficiently in both aerobic and anaerobic conditions.

As a result, people usually feel less breathless and can participate in physical activities for longer periods. Besides, exercise leads to positive changes in lung structure. Engaging in more physical activity helps reduce inflammation and clear mucus from the lungs, which is particularly important for individuals with long-term conditions such as asthma and COPD. When airways are open and lung function improves, there are fewer episodes of symptoms, which helps people with these illnesses continue with physical activities and have a better quality of life. Exercising regularly helps the heart and lungs, which improves breathing efficiency.

These improvements support each other, as observed in many studies. Exercising helps your body and also improves your mental well-being, which is good for your lungs. Exercising often can decrease anxiety, stress, and depression, which can significantly affect how the respiratory system works. Muscle tension caused by stress, including in the breathing muscles, may result in breathlessness or reduced airflow. Exercise lowers stress and improves mental health, which in turn helps people breathe more easily and relax, ultimately enhancing their respiratory health. In addition, exercising may motivate individuals to make better health choices, such as eating healthier and quitting smoking, which all help support lung health. Exercise benefits us in many ways, including helping to regulate our emotions and behaviors, which are vital for efficient breathing.

13.5.1. Improvement in Lung Capacity and Function

Improved lung function and capacity play a key role in understanding the changes that happen in the body during exercise. When people exercise, their need for oxygen increases, which causes changes in their respiratory system. Improved gas exchange and stronger ventilation are among the adaptations that help the animal perform better. Working out encourages the growth of type I muscle fibers, which helps the lungs function more efficiently and improves oxygen delivery. Thus, people usually breathe less often, but their oxygen intake remains the same or increases, demonstrating that regular exercise plays a significant role in improving lung function over time. Also, changing your diet can support the progress you make from exercising. A recent study found that beetroot juice, which contains dietary nitrate, can lower systolic blood pressure in patients with COPD and also boost their vascular function and exercise ability. This research highlights the role of nutritional strategies in enhancing respiratory health. By integrating dietary interventions alongside exercise regimens, individuals may not only comprehensive improvement in physical well-being (Andrew, 2024). Respiratory conditions, including post-COVID-19 pneumonia, greatly benefit from the lasting effects of effective rehabilitation programs. Studies done recently have pointed out that survivors have notable problems with lung function, as shown by lower FEV and VC during their recovery. Still, these patients made significant improvements in lung capacity and strength after three to six months of rehabilitation. It proves that specially designed exercise plans are necessary to improve lung function and general health. Integrating strength and aerobic training into rehabilitation not only enhances lung capacity but also improves quality of life, highlighting the necessity for ongoing assessment and intervention in post-recovery care (Ngamsutham et al., 2024) (Figure 13.12).

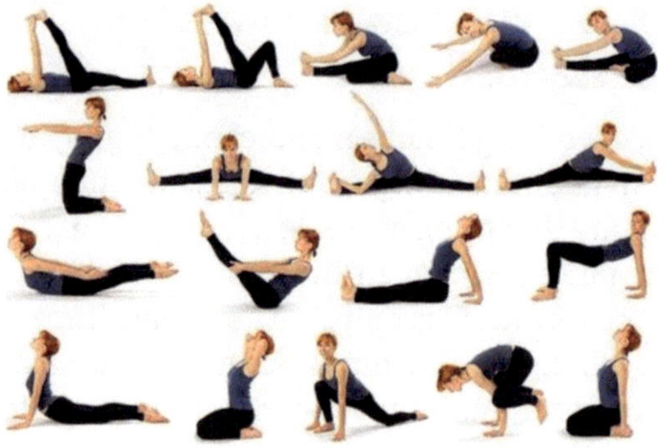

Figure 13.12. Cardio exercise improves the capacity of the lungs.

Source: http://www.trainer.ae/articles/wp-content/uploads/2016/04/cardio-exercise.jpg.

13.5.2. Enhanced Efficiency of Gas Exchange

The better gas exchange during exercise is essential for the respiratory system to give more oxygen to the active muscles. When the body moves more, it needs to take in more oxygen and expel more carbon dioxide. To adapt, the respiratory system takes in more air and breathes more often, which improves the exchange of gases in the alveoli. It is influenced by the intensity, duration, and level of fitness. Better gas exchange allows the body to use oxygen more effectively and delays tiredness, which boosts athletic performance. The incorporation of specific strategies, such as controlled hyperventilation or engaging in activities like sauna bathing, has been shown to improve cardiorespiratory fitness further, indicating a link between environmental stimuli and the physiological capacity for gas exchange enhancement (Kunutsor et al., 2024). It has been demonstrated in performance optimization that combining different treatments can enhance the process of gas exchange. For instance, a study examining athletes during high-intensity cycling interventions reported that a comprehensive approach, known as the enhanced recovery package (ERP), led to significant increases in performance metrics, including power output and heart rate, compared to a placebo. This increase was linked to improvements in respiratory parameters, such as breathing frequency and respiratory exchange ratio, illustrating a direct connection between systemic adjustments in gas exchange and athletic performance (Beltrami et al., 2024). For this reason, customized treatments that focus on specific physiological pathways can help improve exercise performance by enhancing gas exchange, highlighting the important role of respiratory changes in sports training and recovery. Besides making you feel stronger right away, improved gas exchange is also essential for lasting exercise improvements. Often, practicing in conditions that encourage gas exchange, such as high altitude or aerobic activities, can result in lasting benefits for your heart and lungs. Findings suggest that frequent engagement in such practices can elevate levels of cardiorespiratory fitness, resulting in sustained improvements in both maximal oxygen uptake and endurance performance (Kunutsor et al., 2024). Once the body is better at exchanging gases, athletes can train harder and are less likely to experience fatigue or injury. These long-term adaptations emphasize the importance of understanding gas exchange dynamics in the context of exercise, thereby informing best practices for athletic training and conditioning programs (Figure 13.13).

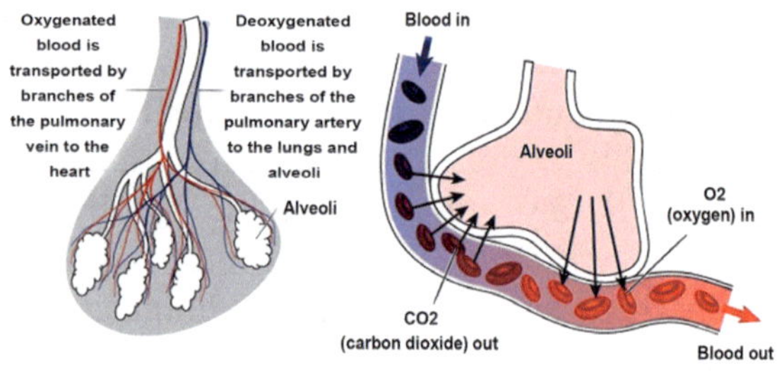

Figure 13.13. Gas exchange in the lungs.

Source: https://cdn.ps.emap.com/wp-content/uploads/sites/3/2018/01/Fig-2-Gas-exchange-in-the-lungs_660.jpg.

13.5.3. Long-Term Effects of Regular Exercise on Respiratory Diseases

Regular exercise has a substantial impact on respiratory health mainly because it reduces inflammation. Airway inflammation often makes chronic breathing diseases like asthma and COPD worse. Regular aerobic exercise helps reduce these inflammatory responses, which in turn improves lung function. Studies have found that the key mechanisms are boosting the body's inflammatory response and controlling the immune system, which together support better breathing health. Individuals with chronic respiratory conditions may experience fewer symptoms and an improved quality of life when they engage in regular aerobic exercise. The importance of these findings cannot be overstated, as they not only highlight the therapeutic benefits of exercise but also underscore the role of lifestyle modifications in managing respiratory diseases (Li et al., 2024). Moreover, the long-term effects of regular exercise extend beyond inflammation to encompass the benefits of pulmonary rehabilitation (PR). Being physically active regularly has been found to boost lung capacity and strengthen the muscles used for breathing, which are both key to respiratory health. People with asthma can gain more control over their symptoms by exercising regularly, which often results in fewer episodes and reduced medication use. Studies suggest that using exercise programs specifically designed for individuals with respiratory diseases can be highly beneficial. Exercise increases lung function and also improves heart health, both of which are essential for overall well-being. By understanding these correlations, medical professionals can identify exercise as a crucial component of effective treatment strategies for patients with respiratory impairments or diseases (Bonini et al., 2017). In addition, regular physical activity is linked to improved mental and social well-being, which can also benefit the lungs. The mental pressure on people with chronic respiratory diseases can make their symptoms worse and reduce their health. Doing regular physical activities can help manage stress and anxiety, which results in better mental health. When psychological well-being improves, it can help people stay more active, which over time leads to better breathing. Programs that help people maintain regular exercise over a long period address both the body and mind, making disease management more comprehensive. Therefore, recognizing the multifaceted benefits of exercise in improving respiratory outcomes proves essential for the effective treatment and management of chronic respiratory diseases, highlighting the need for an integrated approach in healthcare (Li et al., 2024) (Figure 13.14).

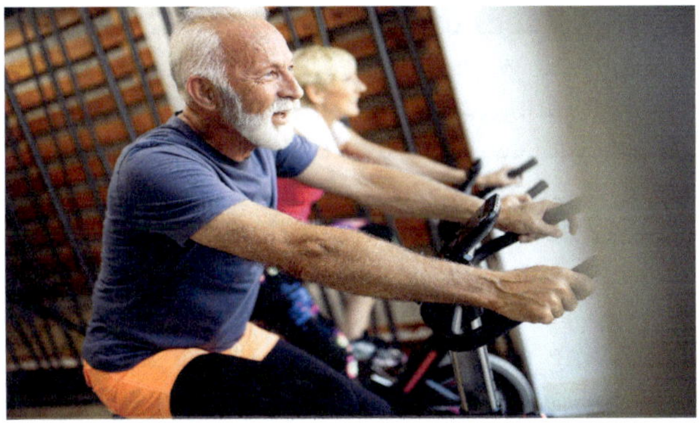

Figure 13.14. Older adults engaging in indoor cycling exercise to support cardiovascular and respiratory health.

Source: https://cdn.sanity.io/images/0vv8moc6/ajmc/512b482f73d3ec78bc3e80b853857e38590274e4-5162x3441.jpg?fit=crop&auto=format.

SUMMARY

Looking at the different ways the respiratory system changes with exercise, it is clear that these changes help the body function well and stay active. Particularly, high-intensity interval training (HIIT) has been shown to elicit significant improvements in cardiorespiratory adjustments, thus enhancing exercise performance. Studies show that people who engage in HIIT have higher minute ventilation and heart rates before and during intense exercise, allowing them to exercise longer. These findings underscore the significance of training intensity in fostering efficient pulmonary responses, indicating that targeted exercise regimens can promote significant improvements in respiratory capacity over time (Ito et al., 2024). The changes they make go further than just basic health, helping athletes perform better and stay healthier. Additionally, the way sports bras fit and function can significantly impact how well people breathe during physical activity. It has been shown that when underband tightness is increased for women, their breathing patterns become faster and their tidal volume decreases. It demonstrates how the design of equipment can affect female athletes' performance. The alteration in how oxygen consumption and work of breathing are manifested during exercise necessitates an awareness of how external factors, such as garment selection, can impact exercise dynamics (Kipp et al., 2024). Therefore, both athletes and designers should consider how biomechanics and comfort work together to achieve optimal performance. To develop effective training and perform well, it is essential to understand how breathing changes during exercise. Both the improvements from tough workouts and the risks of wearing unsuitable clothing for sports demonstrate that choosing the right approach to training and what to wear is crucial. As we can see significant changes in the body from rigorous training and the restrictions of clothing, it is evident that more research is needed. Such studies can illuminate the myriad ways athletes can maximize their performance through informed choices about both their training regimens and the equipment they use, ensuring that both respiratory efficiency and athletic success are achieved (Ito et al., 2024; Kipp et al., 2024). Understanding how breathing changes during exercise is essential to appreciate the body's responses to physical activity. When we exercise, our body needs more oxygen, so the breathing rate and depth increase. Thanks to this process, muscles get more oxygen and release more carbon dioxide, which is necessary for them to keep producing energy. Various changes occur in the nervous system and muscles to meet the increasing energy demands. As the intensity of exercise goes up, the activity of the respiratory muscles becomes stronger to supply the body with the oxygen it needs. In this context, the link between thermal regulation and respiratory changes is also considered very important. Research has found that systems meant to maintain body temperature, such as liquid-cooled clothes, can make a big difference in exercise performance. When subjects exercised at different intensities, having automated temperature control based on their sweat rates made them feel significantly more comfortable. Additionally, the use of head- and neck-cooling in these garments underscores the connection between regulating temperature and breathing. Appropriately managing body temperature not only enhances overall comfort but also optimizes respiratory function by reducing the additional strain on the respiratory system during strenuous activities (Blackaby et al., 2025). Besides, the effects of respiratory changes are also seen in the economy through their impact on human capital and health indicators. Pollution causes health problems and adds to respiratory stress, meaning that it is essential that national accounting includes these factors. Studying the damage caused by air pollutants helps us design actions to address the situation using suitable policies. Utilizing innovative tax systems for emissions may help address these issues and promote improved public health.

CLOSER LOOK

CARDIOPULMONARY EXERCISE TESTING (CPET)

CPET is a specialized stress test that evaluates how well your heart, lungs, and muscles work together during exercise. It measures your body's response to physical exertion, providing insights into your overall functional capacity and identifying potential issues (Figure 13.15).

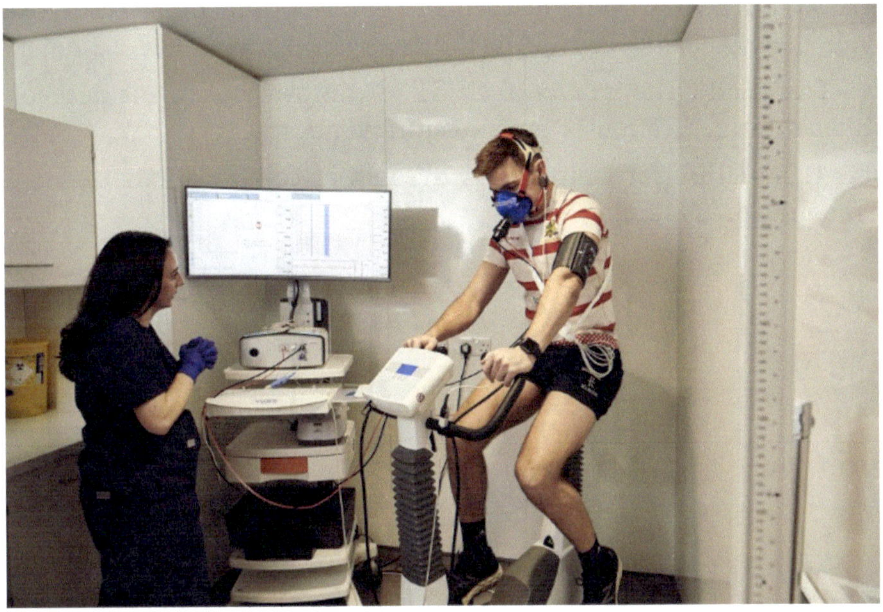

Figure 13.15. Cardiopulmonary exercise testing (CPET) using a stationary bike and metabolic mask.

Source: https://onewelbeck.com/media/onkiyhyx/_dsc8137-copy.jpg.

1. **Key Aspects of CPET**

- **Non-Invasive:** CPET is generally a non-invasive test that involves breathing into a mouthpiece while exercising, typically on a cycle ergometer or treadmill.
- **Comprehensive Assessment:** It assesses various aspects of your body's response to exercise, including ventilation, gas exchange, and cardiovascular and musculoskeletal function.
- **Diagnostic and Prognostic Tool:** CPET helps diagnose conditions like pulmonary and CVDs, assess exercise intolerance, and predict prognosis.
- **Individualized Therapy:** The information gathered from CPET can be used to create personalized exercise programs and rehabilitation plans.

2. **How is CPET Conducted?**

- **Graded Exercise:** CPET typically involves a progressive increase in exercise intensity until you reach your maximum capacity.

- **Monitoring:** During the test, several factors are monitored, including heart rate, blood pressure, oxygen saturation, and gas exchange.
- **Data Analysis:** The collected data is then analyzed to evaluate your body's response to exercise and identify any limitations or abnormal responses.

3. **Benefits of CPET:**

- **Determines Exercise Capacity:** CPET helps determine your functional capacity, which is the maximum amount of exercise your body can perform without fatigue.
- **Identifies Underlying Problems:** It can help pinpoint the cause of exercise intolerance, whether it's related to the heart, lungs, or other systems.
- **Guides Treatment:** The results of CPET can inform treatment decisions, such as adjustments to medication or surgical interventions.
- **Predicts Risk:** CPET can help assess the risk of complications during surgery or other medical procedures.

REFERENCES

1. Aguilaniu, B., Armstrong, H. F., Kampouras, A., Beaver, W. L., Bell, C., Borg, G., Boyce, M., et al. (2019). *ERS Statement on Standardization of Cardiopulmonary Exercise Testing in Chronic Lung Diseases.* https://core.ac.uk/download/286027730.pdf (accessed on 31st May 2025).
2. Alexander, T., Watson, M. A., Klein-Adams, J. C., Ndirangu, D. S., Serrador, J. M., Falvo, M. J., & Lindheimer, J. B. (2023). Deployed Veterans exhibit distinct respiratory patterns and greater dyspnea during maximal cardiopulmonary exercise: A case-control study. *PLoS ONE, 18*(5), e0286015. https://doi.org/10.1371/journal.pone.0286015Allen, M. T., Barnett, T., Blix, A., Brener, J., Brosschot, J. F., Carroll, D., Carroll, D., et al. (2009). *Metabolically Exaggerated Cardiac Reactions to Acute Psychological Stress Revisited.* https://core.ac.uk/download/pdf/8769379.pdf (accessed on 31st May 2025).
3. Angius, L., & Crisafulli, A. (2020). Exercise intolerance and fatigue in chronic heart failure: Is there a role for group III/IV afferent feedback? https://core.ac.uk/download/288430577.pdf (accessed on 31st May 2025).
4. Arias, D., Conkin, J., Fogarty, J., Huff, J. L., et al. (2025). *Effects of the 8 Psia / 32% O_2 Atmosphere on the Human in the Spaceflight Environment.* https://core.ac.uk/download/pdf/323104456.pdf (accessed on 31st May 2025).
5. Beltrami, F., Hanselmann, L., & Spengler, C. (2024). Effects of combined interventions to optimize performance during high-intensity exercise in trained individuals. *European Journal of Sport Science, 24*, 45–55. https://www.semanticscholar.org/paper/cf0162387bb555d8cbf47e8da075b23c1213d687 (accessed on 31st May 2025).
6. Benzo, R., Lam, N., NETT Research Group, Novotny, P., et al. (2019). *Low Income as a Determinant of Exercise Capacity in COPD.* https://core.ac.uk/download/323078876.pdf (accessed on 31st May 2025).
7. Blackaby, J. R., Chambers, A. B., & Miles, J. B. (2025). A study of thc thermoregulatory characteristics of a liquid-cooled garment with automatic temperature control based on sweat rate: Experimental investigation and biothermal man-model development. https://core.ac.uk/download/pdf/85232194.pdf (accessed on 31st May 2025).
8. Bonini, M., Filardi, T., Lenzi, A., Marinelli, L., et al. (2017). *Metabolic and Cardiovascular Response to Exercise in Patients with Type 1 Diabetes.* https://core.ac.uk/download/98335818.pdf (accessed on 31st May 2025).
9. Collins, D., Lewis, N. A., Pedlar, C. R., et al. (2015). Can clinicians and scientists explain and prevent unexplained underperformance syndrome in elite athletes: An interdisciplinary perspective and 2016 update. *BMJ Open Sport Exerc. Med.* https://core.ac.uk/download/42137754.pdf (accessed on 31st May 2025).
10. Crisafulli, A., Marongiu, E., Nobrega, A. C. L., O'Leary, D. S., et al. (2014). Neural regulation of cardiovascular response to exercise: Role of central command and peripheral afferents. *BioMed Research International.* https://core.ac.uk/download/pdf/54599119.pdf (accessed on 31st May 2025).
11. De Jonge, L., DeLany, J. P., Heilbronn, L. K., Martin, C. K., et al. (2009). Metabolic and behavioral compensations in response to caloric restriction: Implications for the maintenance of weight loss. *PLoS ONE.* https://core.ac.uk/download/12777241.pdf (accessed on 31st May 2025).

12. Dickson, K. J., Hess, E., Powers, J. V., Wallace-Robinson, M., et al. (2025). Publications of the Space Physiology and Countermeasures Program, Cardiopulmonary Discipline: 1980–1990. https://core.ac.uk/download/pdf/42809290.pdf (accessed on 31st May 2025).
13. Dołęga, J., Hudzińska, P., Krzykawski, K., Maciejczyk, M., et al. (2024). The role of pulmonary rehabilitation and physical activity in the prevention, treatment and management of respiratory diseases – A comprehensive review. Quality in Sport. https://core.ac.uk/download/636385575.pdf (accessed on 31st May 2025).
14. Eldridge, S., Chan, C., Campbell, M. J., Bond, C., Hopewell, S., Thabane, L., & Lancaster, G. (2016). CONSORT 2010 statement: Extension to randomized pilot and feasibility trials. *BMJ*. https://doi.org/10.1136/bmj.i5239 (accessed on 31st May 2025).
15. Fox, S. C., Greenleaf, J. E., Sciaraffa, D., Stockmann, M., et al. (2025). *Human Acclimation and Acclimatization to Heat: A Compendium of Research, 1968–1978.* https://core.ac.uk/download/pdf/42863127.pdf (accessed on 31st May 2025).
16. Gomes, F. S., & Lopes, T. R. (2022). What is behind the curtain? Revealing muscle metaboreceptor sensitization. *The Journal of Physiology, 600*. https://www.semanticscholar.org/paper/c63eba3cda8f5b85bd3b3d30a8eb0536a124e016 (accessed on 31st May 2025).
17. Hołownia, W., Krzesłowska, W. J., Pytel, P., Szewczyk, K., et al. (2024). *Physical Activity as a Trigger for Anaphylaxis: Understanding Food-Dependent Exercise-Induced Anaphylaxis.* https://core.ac.uk/download/613193166.pdf (accessed on 31st May 2025).
18. Huhtala, A., & Samakovlis, E. (2025). *Green Accounting, Air Pollution and Health.* https://core.ac.uk/download/pdf/6418030.pdf (accessed on 31st May 2025).
19. Ito, G., Feeley, M., Sawai, T., Nakata, H., Otsuki, S., Nakahara, H., & Miyamoto, T. (2024). High-intensity interval training improves respiratory and cardiovascular adjustments before and after initiation of exercise. *Frontiers in Physiology, 15*. https://www.semanticscholar.org/paper/c46aa5bae84dae57c269131a337ba625a088708e (accessed on 31st May 2025).
20. Kipp, S., Leahy, M. G., & Sheel, A. W. (2024). Sports bra restriction on respiratory mechanics during exercise. *Medicine & Science in Sports & Exercise, 56*, 1168–1176. https://www.semanticscholar.org/paper/f72a7a4c75e13cced68af5fb2006d5ab8f58ea0d (accessed on 31st May 2025).
21. Kunutsor, S., Isiozor, N., Kurl, S., & Laukkanen, J. (2024). Enhancing cardiorespiratory fitness through sauna bathing. *Journal of Cardiopulmonary Rehabilitation and Prevention, 44*, 295–300. https://www.semanticscholar.org/paper/1720f044eb67e9bd938627a24a3206e1015a32d8 (accessed on 31st May 2025).
22. Li, Z. (2024). *Anti-Inflammatory Effects of Regular Aerobic Exercise on Common Chronic Diseases and Their Mechanisms.* https://core.ac.uk/download/616936851.pdf (accessed on 31st May 2025).
23. Mitchell, G. S., & Welch, J. F. (2024). *Inaugural Review Prize 2023: The Exercise Hyperpnea Dilemma: A 21st-Century Perspective.* https://core.ac.uk/download/603470267.pdf (accessed on 31st May 2025).
24. Mitchell, J. W., Nadel, E. R., & Stolwijk, J. A. J. (2025). *Development of Mathematical Models of Environmental Physiology.* https://core.ac.uk/download/pdf/85233818.pdf (accessed on 31st May 2025).

25. Mourot, L., Rakobowchuk, M., & Wilhelm, E. N. (2018). *Exercise-Derived Microvesicles: A Review of the Literature.* https://core.ac.uk/download/288430488.pdf (accessed on 31st May 2025).

26. N/A. (2025). *Aerospace Medicine and Biology: A Continuing Bibliography with Indexes, Supplement 125.* https://core.ac.uk/download/pdf/42897953.pdf (accessed on 31st May 2025).

27. N/A. (2025). *Cardiopulmonary Discipline Science Plan.* https://core.ac.uk/download/pdf/42808701.pdf (accessed on 31st May 2025).

28. Newton, J. L., Robinson, S., & Sadowski, B. (2025). Part III – The effects of thermal stresses on the aerobic and anaerobic work capacities of men: Final scientific report. https://core.ac.uk/download/pdf/85247976.pdf (accessed on 31st May 2025).

29. Ngamsutham, T., Chaiwong, W., Dacha, S., Sitilertpisan, P., Pothirat, C., Duangjit, P., Deesomchok, A., et al. (2024). Pulmonary function, functional capacity, respiratory, and locomotor muscle strength after severe to critically ill COVID-19: A long-term study. *Tuberculosis and Respiratory Diseases, 87*, 532–542. https://www.semanticscholar.org/paper/b2de5af1d5fe779b45d5f4f928073ba73d966c7f (accessed on 31st May 2025).

30. Page, M. J., Moher, D., Bossuyt, P. M., Boutron, I., Hoffmann, T., Mulrow, C. D., Shamseer, L., et al. (2021). PRISMA 2020 explanation and elaboration: Updated guidance and exemplars for reporting systematic reviews. *BMJ*. https://doi.org/10.1136/bmj.n160 (accessed on 31st May 2025).

31. Trexler, E. T., Keith, D. S., Schwartz, T. A., Ryan, E. D., Stoner, L., Persky, A. M., & Smith-Ryan, A. E. (2019). Effects of citrulline malate and beetroot juice supplementation on blood flow, energy metabolism, and performance during maximum effort leg extension exercise. *The Journal of Strength and Conditioning Research, 33*, 2321–2329. https://doi.org/10.1519/jsc.0000000000003286 (accessed on 31st May 2025).

32. Webb, A. J. (2024). "Every beet you take": Lowering systolic blood pressure and improving vascular function/exercise capacity via the dietary nitrate–nitrite–NO pathway in patients with COPD. *European Respiratory Journal, 63*. https://www.semanticscholar.org/paper/62c7bfd33fe67b513277e0b9c8ed859b8d9b6229 (accessed on 31st May 2025).

33. Webb, K., Dominelli, P. B., Baker, S. E., Klassen, S. A., Joyner, M. J., Senefeld, J. W., & Wiggins, C. C. (2022). Influence of high hemoglobin-oxygen affinity on humans during hypoxia. *Frontiers in Physiology, 12*. https://doi.org/10.3389/fphys.2021.763933 (accessed on 31st May 2025).

34. Zhang, H. (2024). Portable oxygen breathing apparatus integrated with biosensors: Enabling intelligent monitoring and optimal oxygen provision for biomechanical homeostasis. *Molecular & Cellular Biomechanics*. https://www.semanticscholar.org/paper/3abd7a436940c73649cd2757709524bf060cf02b (accessed on 31st May 2025).

35. Zhao, L., Xie, Y. X., & Wang, C. (2020). Recommendations for respiratory rehabilitation in adults with coronavirus disease 2019. *Chinese Medical Journal, 133*, 1595–1602. https://doi.org/10.1097/cm9.0000000000000848 (accessed on 31st May 2025).

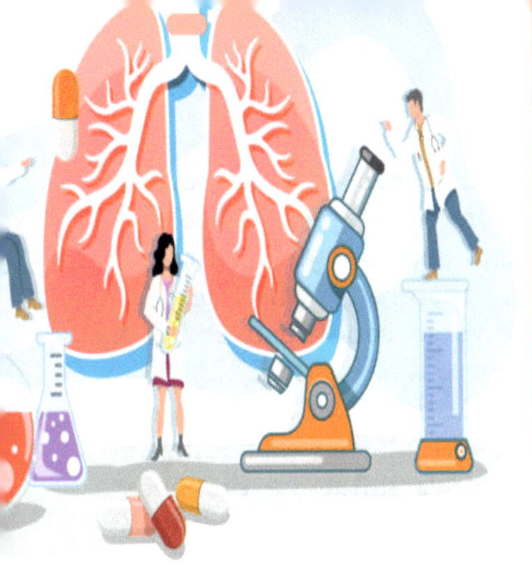

Chapter 14

DEVELOPMENTAL AND COMPARATIVE RESPIRATORY PHYSIOLOGY

Contents

Introduction

Respiratory physiology examines the intricate mechanisms by which organisms exchange gases, adapting to varying environments and energy demands. To see how species have adapted their respiratory systems, it is necessary to study developmental and comparative respiratory physiology. Respiration in mammals living on land and in aquatic organisms is very different, and this is affected by the temperature and amount of oxygen available. Due to the fact that climate change is causing habitats to change, studying these adaptations helps predict how species will respond to new environments. Connecting physiology and ecology allows us to see how species adapt fully and the effects these adaptations have on the environment. Additionally, examining the development of respiratory physiology reveals how both growth and environmental factors can alter an organism's respiratory capabilities. For example, the growth of a respiratory system often matches the environment where a species lives. For example, mammals have lungs that change in structure, and fish have gills, which help them exchange gas efficiently in different life stages or environments. Studies have found that the amount of oxygen organisms experience during their growth can affect their health and reproduction later in life. Studies on these developmental patterns indicate a strong connection between bodily changes and the environment, highlighting the importance of respiratory development in the face of rapid environmental changes. Comparative research on different species also helps explain the pressures that affect the development of respiratory systems. Examining many organisms enables scientists to identify common patterns in respiratory adaptation that are linked to their environments. The results of experiments on *Drosophila melanogaster* in different oxygen levels show that organisms raised in hypoxia may behave differently from those raised in normoxia or hyperoxia. The findings indicate that the amount of oxygen available during development can shape an organism's abilities, which suggests that adaptations usually happen as a result of pressures experienced throughout life. The nuances of these adaptations are crucial to understanding the challenges posed by hypoxia and thermal stress, directing future research that explores the implications of these findings for environmental change (Bahr et al., 2015; Angilletta et al., 2017).

Definition of Respiratory Physiology

Comparative physiology encompasses respiratory physiology, which examines how different organisms adapt their breathing to meet the metabolic needs of their bodies. It explores the mechanisms of gas exchange, air movement into and out of the lungs, and the processes that regulate them in different animals. Besides discussing the anatomy of the lungs and airways, respiratory physiology encompasses the biochemical and physical processes related to breathing and oxygen utilization. By examining both developmental and comparative aspects, researchers gain insights into how different species have evolved distinct respiratory strategies suitable for their environments and lifestyles, which aids in understanding respiratory disorders and adaptations in diverse conditions, including pregnancy and severe illness, as highlighted in recent studies (O'Neil et al., 2021). Respiratory physiology should be studied by examining how environmental factors influence the body's responses. A comparison of respiratory systems explains how differences in organs such as lungs, gills, or specialized air sacs change how efficiently gas exchange takes place—selective pressures, such as oxygen levels in water versus on land, influence these adaptations. As noted in the context of respiratory research's evolution, integrating functional genomics into the study of respiratory physiology allows scientists to explore the role of gene expression in these adaptations, ultimately fostering a deeper understanding of physiological processes at both the cellular and organismal levels (Dow, 2007).

This means that respiratory physiology links the genes of animals to their adaptations in the environment, providing a comprehensive understanding of how respiration changes among animals. In addition, the importance of developmental respiratory physiology is significant, particularly when examining how respiratory systems develop in various species. This branch examines how the respiratory system develops, from the embryo stage to adulthood, to meet the needs of different life stages and environments.

For example, in mammals, significant physiological shifts occur during gestation, as highlighted in studies surrounding the impacts of COVID-19 on pregnant women (O'Neil et al., 2021). Grasping these transitions is essential, as they influence medical care and environmental management, which in turn affect public health and policy. In summary, the definition of respiratory physiology encompasses a wide array of processes and adaptations that underscore the complexity and dynamic nature of respiration across the animal kingdom, thereby reinforcing its importance in both practical applications and theoretical discussions (Figure 14.1).

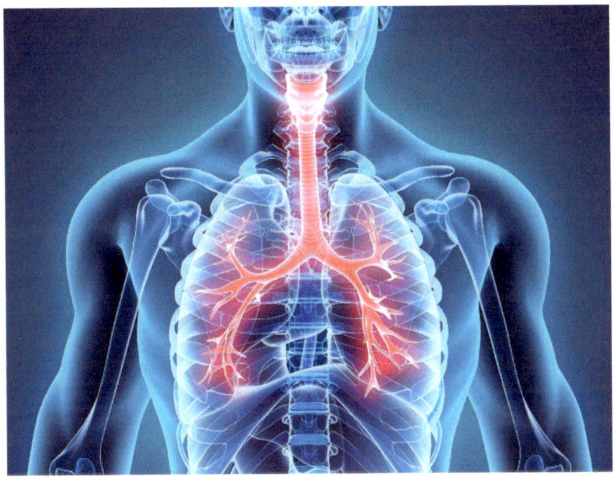

Figure 14.1. Anatomical illustration of the human respiratory system.

Source: https://ohmyfacts.com/wp-content/uploads/2024/06/45-facts-about-the-respiratory-system-1717844905.jpg.

Importance of Studying Developmental and Comparative Aspects

The value of studying developmental and comparative aspects in respiratory physiology lies in its ability to reveal how species have adapted for improved gas exchange. Scientists can see how various environmental factors affect the structure and function of the respiratory system. For example, the development of lungs in land animals is a significant change that enables them to obtain oxygen more easily, which is crucial for survival in areas with limited oxygen. With this knowledge, researchers can predict how organisms will react to new environmental changes, particularly in the context of climate change. The knowledge gained from examining different respiratory systems can inform conservation efforts and help explain how animals respond to environmental changes. Seeing how these systems are linked gives a fuller sense of biology, highlighting how development, environment, and evolutionary biology are related. Additionally, studying how respiratory physiology changes as organisms grow helps us identify key moments that shape their ability to perform and cope. For instance, the metabolic shifts observed during the development of grape berries are indicative of broader metabolic processes relevant in other organisms, including shifts in carbohydrate metabolism that may impact energy availability for respiration (Dai et al., 2013). Such changes in development can alter the way organisms respond to factors like temperature and oxygen levels. Researchers can determine the factors within the body responsible for survival and adaptation by comparing these processes across different species. Comparative studies of respiratory systems help us learn more about them and show the key factors that allow successful development in various habitats. Additionally, examining developments and comparisons in the field of respiratory physiology supports progress in biomedical research and its applications. Insights gained from model organisms, such as *Drosophila melanogaster*, have broad implications for understanding human health, particularly regarding how oxygen availability during developmental stages can influence later life performance (Angilletta et al., 2017). The way a person develops as a child can powerfully affect their breathing health and function in adulthood. When researchers understand the primary developmental windows and their effects, they may develop strategies to improve human respiratory diseases, potentially finding ways to prevent or treat them. In general, blending developmental and comparative studies helps us better understand evolution and also aids in addressing health issues faced by a variety of species, including humans.

14.1. Developmental Aspects of Respiratory Physiology

Respiratory physiology changes a lot as an organism grows from being an embryo to becoming an adult and these changes are significant to understand. A key example is in mammals, where the lung develops a lot from the pseudo-glandular stage to the alveolar stage, which involves both structural and functional changes. It includes changes in the structure and also in the way the body's systems work for better gas exchange. As the surfactant develops, it helps reduce tension on the alveoli, thereby improving lung function. These changes are extremely detailed, therefore it is clear that environmental factors such as gestational age and exposure to pollutants can affect respiratory health from before birth to after birth. Understanding these aspects of respiratory development can elucidate the mechanisms behind various respiratory disorders prevalent in early life stages (Bahr et al., 2015).

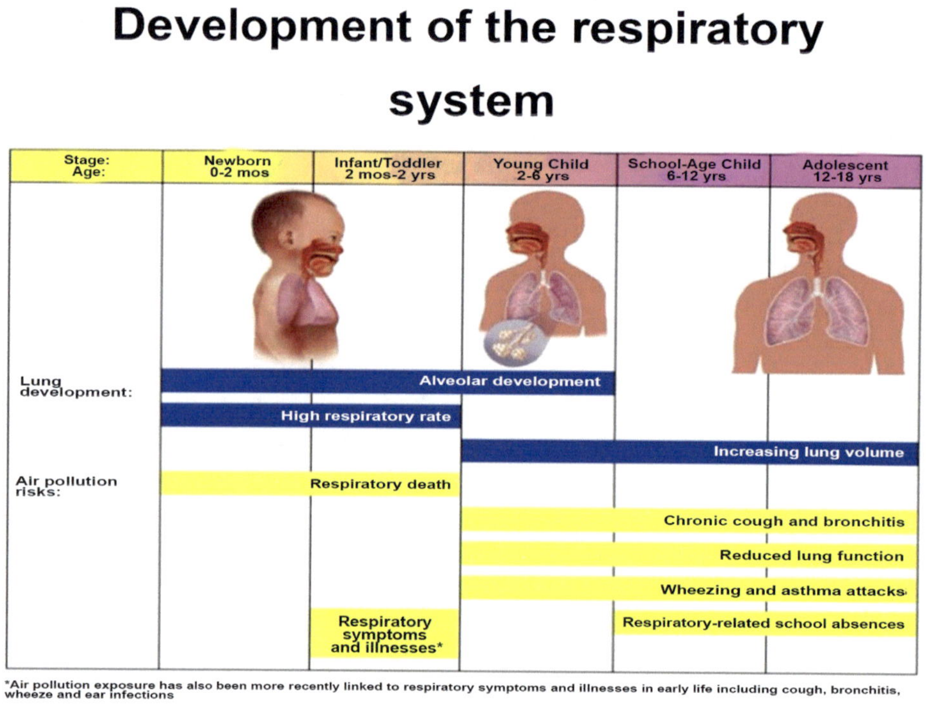

Figure 14.2. Development of respiratory system.

Source: https://image4.slideserve.com/9215480/development-of-the-respiratory-system-l.jpg.

Fish and other aquatic organisms, on the other hand, have special adaptations in their developmental physiology that fit their environment. Unlike land animals, fish use gills for their lungs, which allow them to breathe underwater. The shift from an embryo to a juvenile fish often involves the development of gill arches and lamellae, which help the fish obtain more oxygen from the water. Additionally, the immune system in fish related to respiration is flexible, and stress can have a significant impact on it. Research has shown that stress can alter the immune system of fish, potentially impacting their respiratory function. For instance, differential blood cell counts in fish exposed to pollutants reveal physiological alterations, highlighting the interconnectedness of respiratory development and systemic health within this group of vertebrates (Farley et al., 1994). Understanding the similarities and differences in respiratory development among species reveals how evolution and physiology interact. While mammals have a highly complex system for living on land, amphibians and reptiles exhibit transitional features that reflect their distinct lifestyles. Birds have specialized their respiratory system to meet the increased oxygen needs of their bodies, mainly during flight. Due to the presence of air sacs, air can move through the lungs smoothly, which is helpful for taking in oxygen and getting rid of carbon dioxide. By comparing different species, such studies reveal how respiratory systems have evolved and how evolutionary factors have influenced their development. Investigating these diverse respiratory adaptations deepens our understanding of how environmental contexts drive physiological development across the animal kingdom, offering crucial insights into potential vulnerabilities and adaptations in response to changing ecosystems (Bahr et al., 2015) (Figure 14.2).

14.1.1. Respiratory System Development in Embryos

Early in pregnancy, the respiratory system begins to develop and continues to evolve through several key phases. The respiratory diverticulum (the first sign of respiratory development) appears from the foregut endoderm in the fourth week of embryo development. As a result of this structure, trachea, bronchi, and lung buds are formed. The respiratory system undergoes significant changes as the embryo develops, including branching morphogenesis, which is essential for forming the lung's complex structure. By the end of the embryonic period, the airways are formed, which lay the foundation for their later development. Discovering these early steps is important since it highlights the importance of early embryonic growth for healthy respiration after birth. When the embryo develops into a fetus, the respiratory system undergoes significant changes in both structure and function. By the 16th week, the lungs separate into distinct lobes, and the alveoli begin to develop, a process that occurs when type I and type II pneumocytes are formed. They are needed to produce surfactant, which helps decrease surface tension in the lungs and allows for proper breathing after birth. Surfactant production begins around the 24th week of pregnancy, a key step in preparing the fetus for life outside the womb.

Additionally, proper lung growth and maturation depend on the optimal amount of amniotic fluid and intrauterine pressure, both of which are closely related to fetal growth. It demonstrates that respiratory development is influenced by other vital systems in the body, enabling the embryo to develop properly. In addition, understanding how the respiratory system develops can be gained by examining it through the lens of evolutionary biology, which reveals that many physiological adaptations are pleiotropic. Many genes in the respiratory system influence several traits, which are important for the evolution of complex respiratory systems. With the development of multicellular organisms, animals required new methods for breathing in various environments. It is clear from studying the embryonic development of respiration in various species that homologous structures, such as lungs, gills, and other respiratory surfaces, have evolved under different pressures. Such insights affirm that respiratory system development is a reflection of both phylogenetic and ontogenetic factors, thereby enriching our overall understanding of developmental and comparative respiratory physiology (Bahr et al., 2015; Torday et al., 2015) (Figure 14.3).

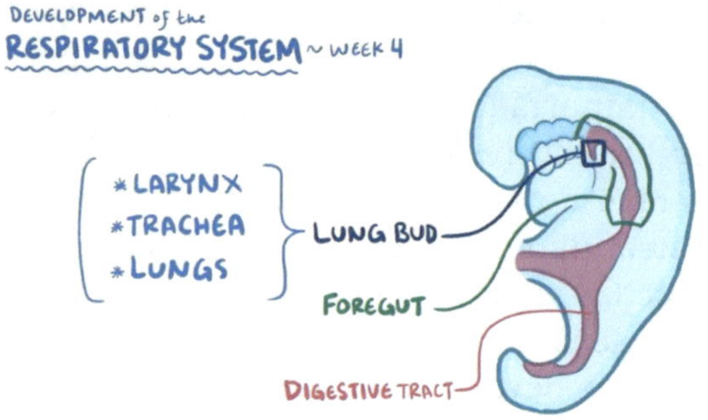

Figure 14.3. Development of the respiratory system.

Source: https://www.osmosis.org/_next/image?url=https%3A%2F%2Fd16qt3wv6xm098.cloudfront.net%2F-xfMgz8USTSOJsLU2MjoQF_SRYukc2TA%2F_.jpg&w=3840&q=75.

14.1.2. Changes in Respiratory Function During Growth

The changes in the respiratory system during growth are a major aspect of developmental physiology, illustrating how living organisms adapt their bodies to meet new needs. While a baby is still an infant, the lungs undergo significant development, enabling them to function correctly after birth. When a baby is born, it must start breathing and develop lung circulation, which are significant changes. Respiratory development during this stage varies significantly; mammals mature much faster and more noticeably than some aquatic species. As growth occurs, the lungs expand in size and their surface area increases, leading to biochemical changes that enhance gas exchange, a crucial process for meeting the increased metabolic needs of growth. While respiratory efficiency generally rises as a person matures, environmental conditions remain very important. Changes in temperature and oxygen levels can affect how well the lungs function, which in turn often alters the course of development. For instance, research has shown that high temperatures can exacerbate oxygen shortages, so the body requires more oxygen than it can obtain. It means that those who develop under hypoxia tend to have more difficulties during physical activities or when dealing with stress. Here, breathing conditions during development can influence how well an animal performs in adulthood, demonstrating that respiratory physiology is closely tied to its surroundings.

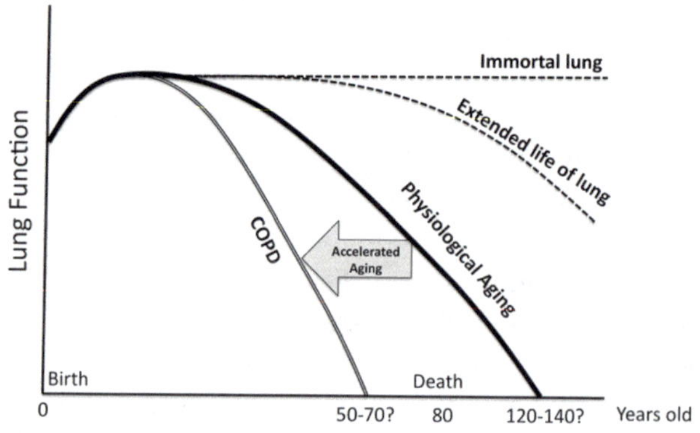

Figure 14.4. Changes of lung function with aging and its possible modification.

Source: https://www.researchgate.net/profile/Nicolas-Mercado/publication/261443085/figure/fig1/AS:608409925713922@1522067638639/Changes-of-lung-function-with-aging-and-its-possible-modification-Lung-function-is.png.

The implications of these adaptations are particularly evident in species that encounter varying oxygen levels and thermal stressors throughout their life cycles, underscoring the adaptability of respiratory systems in relation to environmental pressures (Angilletta et al., 2017). The relationship between growth, development, and respiratory function reveals significant insights into evolutionary physiology. Different species exhibit varying capacities for adjusting their respiratory systems to meet the challenges posed by their environments, including variations in oxygen availability and temperature. Research has shown that organisms raised in hyperoxic conditions may perform better under stress compared to those from normoxic or hypoxic backgrounds, indicating that the developmental environment plays a crucial role in determining respiratory efficiency. Consequently, understanding the nuances of these changes in respiratory function during growth not only provides insight into individual physiological adaptations but also sheds light on broader evolutionary trends among species. Such investigations can inform conservation strategies, particularly as environmental change continues to threaten the delicate balance of oxygen supply and demand essential for many species' survival (Bahr et al., 2015) (Figure 14.4).

14.1.3. Impact of Environmental Factors on Development

Environmental conditions are essential for the growth of respiratory physiology, affecting its structure and function. Lung growth and function are strongly affected by air quality, temperature and humidity. Exposure to various pollutants, including particles and VOCs, can disrupt the normal growth of the lungs in young children.

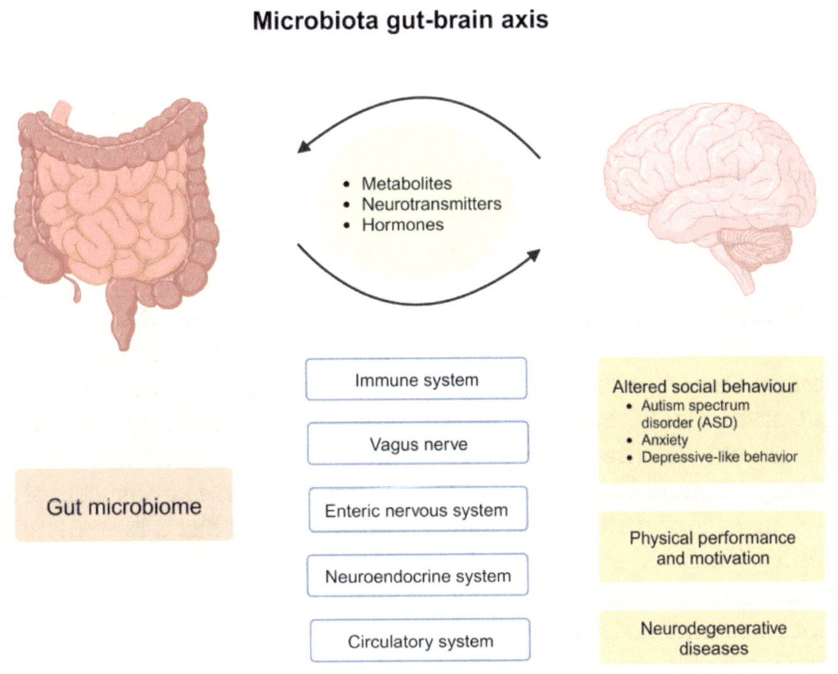

Figure 14.5. Microbiota-gut-brain axis.

Source: https://media.springernature.com/full/springer-static/image/art%3A10.1038%2Fs41392-024-01743-1/MediaObjects/41392_2024_1743_Fig1_HTML.png.

As well as causing immediate breathing problems, it can result in chronic lung diseases like COPD and asthma later on. In addition, environmental factors interact with an individual's genetic background, causing respiratory health to change over the course of a person's life. Knowing about these environmental factors is crucial for designing effective strategies and interventions to combat respiratory diseases and promote the development of healthy lungs. In respiratory health, microbial environments are critical because they help maintain the normal functioning of the respiratory system. It is now clear through research that the microbiota in the gut and respiratory tract work in tandem with the host's immune system to protect against infections and maintain bodily balance. When these microbial groups are upset due to antibiotics, a lack of good nutrition, or stressful conditions, it can cause dysbiosis, which may result in inflammation and harm to the development of the respiratory system. Such a balance is necessary, as when the microbiota is out of balance, it can result in asthma and allergic diseases, demonstrating that the environment can have a significant impact on the immune system. Additionally, understanding how these microbial interactions evolve during development can help identify early interventions to improve respiratory health and prevent diseases in children and other vulnerable populations. The effect of stress on the environment is significant when considering how it influences respiratory development. Both mental and physical stressors can cause significant changes in the body's control systems, which can impact respiration. In some cases, ongoing stress can make asthma symptoms worse and reduce how well the respiratory system works. The connection is formed by the way the nervous and immune systems interact, mainly through the microbiota-gut-brain axis. Elevated stress levels have been shown to alter microbial composition, affecting immune responses that play a crucial role in lung development and disease susceptibility (John et al., 2019). As scientific inquiry continues to explore these connections, it becomes increasingly evident that addressing environmental stressors is vital for promoting optimal respiratory development and reducing the burden of respiratory diseases throughout life (Figure 14.5).

14.2. Comparative Respiratory Physiology

The study of comparative respiratory physiology offers critical insights into the evolutionary adaptations of various vertebrates, revealing how different species have evolved unique respiratory mechanisms to suit their environments and metabolic demands. The patterns in which the bronchial tree branches have become a primary interest in this area, especially when looked at through fractal geometry. The approach demonstrates that the structure of the respiratory system is closely tied to the environment in which each species lives. For example, the fractal patterns found in horses (which are mammals) are related to their high metabolism and help them exchange gases efficiently. At the same time, iguanas and bullfrogs, which are ectothermic, have simpler breathing mechanisms, as they do not need to expend as much energy and are adapted in different ways to their habitats. This contrast underscores the significance of comparative respiratory physiology in understanding how form directly relates to function in the evolution of vertebrate life (Montgomery, 2024). The nasopharynx plays a crucial role in the overall functioning of the respiratory system. The development of the lung in both mammals and humans, as well as in other tetrapods, has been crucial for respiration and other bodily functions. Examining the nasopharynx reveals how we breathe, as well as how we speak and think, which are key aspects of being human. The nasopharynx has a long history, dating back to the earliest jawless fish. Its development involved many changes that made it useful for breathing and hearing in higher vertebrates. Recognizing the nasopharynx's evolutionary importance broadens the scope of comparative respiratory physiology, emphasizing the interconnectedness of invasive systems and highlighting the need for an interdisciplinary approach to understanding respiratory adaptations (Pagano et al., 2022). All in all, understanding comparative respiratory physiology helps reveal the details of evolutionary changes in vertebrates. Using fractal dimension calculations and similar approaches helps explain in more detail how respiratory systems adapt to their environment. They extend beyond just differences in body structure to encompass essential body functions necessary for survival and reproduction in a changing world. Researchers also learn that the nasopharynx and similar structures play a role in many key functions, not just breathing. The evolving nature of respiratory adaptations epitomizes the plasticity and resilience of life on Earth, underscoring the importance of ongoing studies in developmental and comparative respiratory physiology (Montgomery, 2024; Pagano et al., 2022).

14.2.1. Respiratory Adaptations in Aquatic vs. Terrestrial Animals

The respiratory adaptations of aquatic and terrestrial animals reflect the diverse environments in which they thrive. Fish and other water creatures use gills to draw oxygen from water which contains only about 30% as much oxygen as air. Gills work well because of countercurrent exchange, which brings oxygen-rich water in the opposite direction to the blood flow, helping the fish absorb more oxygen. Unlike aquatic animals, terrestrial animals must use air to breathe, so they need different body structures and methods. Lungs in mammals and many reptiles are designed to facilitate gas exchange, allowing them to inhale air rich in oxygen and exhale air with carbon dioxide. The fact that fish developed lungs instead of gills to live on land demonstrates how evolution adjusts when habitats change. A variety of features in the lungs of terrestrial vertebrates help them breathe more efficiently. Due to the numerous alveoli in mammalian lungs, more gas exchange can occur, allowing the body to absorb more oxygen and eliminate more carbon dioxide. Additionally, surfactant in the lungs reduces surface tension within alveoli, preventing them from collapsing and maintaining proper lung function. Alternatively, aquatic animals have special features such as a gill surface with many blood vessels, which helps them absorb oxygen from the water quickly. Amphibians, for example, can breathe through their gills or lungs, demonstrating how animals can transition from water to land. Such differences in respiratory systems highlight their importance in the metabolism of living organisms. Crocodilians are an interesting example since they can breathe like animals in the water and on land. As they live primarily in water, a crocodilian's lungs and four-chambered heart allow it to get more oxygen and release more carbon dioxide than other animals. According to research, crocodilians possess a neural control shunting mechanism that enables efficient oxygen utilization while diving, effectively bypassing the pulmonary circuit during prolonged underwater periods (Bennett-Stamper et al., 2004). This adaptation points out how the body can control the balance between its lungs and general blood circulation based on its surroundings. Ultimately, the comparative respiratory physiology of various animal groups illustrates how evolutionary pressures shape respiratory systems, optimizing survival in both aquatic and terrestrial realms (Campbell et al., 2008) (Table 14.1).

Table 14.1. Aquatic vs. Terrestrial Respiration

Aquatic respiration	Terrestrial respiration
Occurs in organisms living in water	Occurs in land organisms
Involve oxygen which is dissolved in water	Does not involved dissolved oxygen
Main respiratory organ is gills	Main respiratory organ is generally lungs
Gills are tough and spiny	Lungs are moist, slippery and soft
Breathing rate is comparatively higher	Breathing rate is comparatively lower

Source: https://betrained.in/All-In-One/10-Science/Life-Processes-B-Respiration-Solution.

14.2.2. Evolutionary Trends in Respiratory Systems

The way respiratory systems have evolved over time indicates the numerous ways organisms have adapted to their surroundings. When vertebrates moved from water to land, their breathing systems had to undergo significant changes. Early amphibians evolved to change their swim bladders into lungs, which enabled them to breathe air while still utilizing their moist skin for additional respiration. This ability to change demonstrates an important method of evolution. For instance, plants must be good at holding onto that which enables plants to cope with terrestrial habitats, where oxygen is readily available in the air. However, plants must also be adept at retaining moisture and exchanging gases. Due to these morphological changes, terrestrial vertebrates began to develop more efficient respiratory systems, which resulted in reptiles, birds, and mammals having lungs that support their metabolism in various settings. Another interesting example can be found in insects – which have evolved a system of tracheae that allows gas exchange directly within the cells. This design enables insects to distribute oxygen to every part of their body without the use of blood, which is particularly beneficial since their metabolism increases significantly when they are active. The success of this trait is apparent because they can live in both arid deserts and wet rainforests. Additionally, the impact of environmental conditions on the respiratory systems of insects is crucial, considering that climate change is altering their habitats. For instance, increased temperatures have been shown to influence insect metabolism and behavior, causing shifts in their respiratory efficiency and overall fitness as they cope with altered ecological dynamics (Daniel et al., 2010). Climate change has an influence on respiratory systems that extends beyond changes in body parts, impacting the way animals breathe. Organisms need to regulate their metabolism when temperatures and their environment change to survive. For example, insects need to use their resources carefully, mostly during diapause when there is little food available, by utilizing what they have stored. When temperatures rise, the metabolic processes are affected, which means the animal's reserves are used up faster than they should be. Similarly, plants are not immune to these changes, as trends indicate detrimental effects on growth and gas exchange efficiency under extreme conditions (Craita et al., 2013). Understanding these trends in evolution provides valuable insights for protecting and managing species as they adapt to rapid changes in the world. Studying these various respiratory adaptations helps us see how living things change over time due to their environment.

14.2.3. Case Studies of Specific Species

The study of respiratory physiology across various species reveals fascinating adaptations that inform our understanding of evolution and environmental interaction. Marine mammals such as whales and dolphins are good examples of how animals can adapt their bodies to fit life in the water. Dolphins (such as the bottlenose) can store oxygen, have high myoglobin levels, and use their lungs selectively, which helps them stay underwater for long periods without experiencing hypoxia.

The adaptations are necessary for dolphins to survive, as they enable them to hunt effectively at great depths and cope with the pressure changes that affect their bodies. In this way, this particular example helps explain how different species adapt their respiratory systems to their environments. The way birds breathe, for example, in the common ostrich, is an interesting contrast to that of marine mammals. Birds utilize air sacs to maintain airflow through their lungs, facilitating more efficient gas exchange. This change enables birds to maintain a high metabolism, which is necessary for flying, as it requires them to use a significant amount of oxygen during extended periods of flight. Additionally, studies suggest that avian lungs are designed in a manner that facilitates the birds' ability to take in oxygen, even at high altitudes where oxygen levels are lower in the air. The example of the common ostrich demonstrates that changes in bird anatomy, particularly in the respiratory system, have enabled birds to evolve and thrive in various habitats. Another compelling focus within the field of developmental and comparative respiratory physiology is the case study of amphibians, particularly the African clawed frog (*Xenopus laevis*). Amphibians are unique in their respiratory adaptations, as they inhabit both aquatic and terrestrial environments. As tadpoles, *Xenopus laevis* breathe with gills, but as adults they mostly use their skin and lungs to breathe. It demonstrates that organisms can adapt their breathing patterns to suit the environment they inhabit. Moreover, being able to live in different habitats depends on their versatility, which allows them to utilize both water and land resources. By examining the case of *Xenopus laevis*, researchers gain valuable insights into the evolutionary adaptations and physiological mechanisms that enable survival across diverse ecosystems, contributing to a deeper understanding of respiratory function among vertebrates (Figure 14.6).

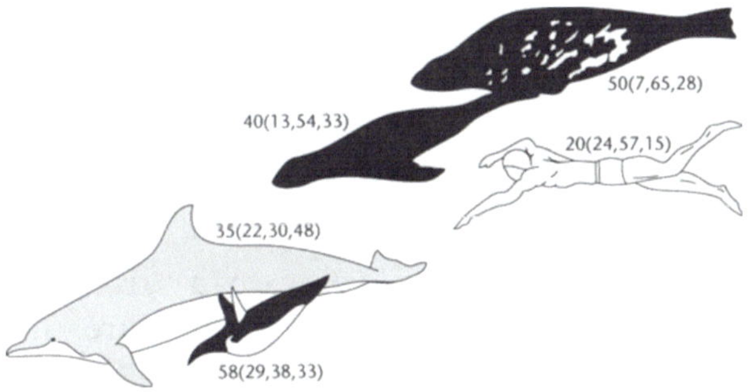

Figure 14.6. The oxygen stores of dolphins, sea lions, fur seals, true seals, humans, and penguins are provided in mL O_2 per kg body mass. The numbers in parentheses are the relative contribution of O2 stored in the lung, blood, and muscle.

Source: https://www.researchgate.net/profile/Daniel-Costa-12/publication/228053579/figure/fig2/AS:282652071481396@1444400913784/The-oxygen-stores-of-dolphins-sea-lions-and-fur-seals-true-seals-humans-and-penguins.png.

14.3. Mechanisms of Gas Exchange

The mechanisms by which gases are exchanged play a crucial role in understanding respiratory physiology in many organisms. In particular, the changes caused by evolution have given rise to the unique respiratory features found in different taxa. Gills in aquatic organisms allow them to take in oxygen using a large surface area, which reduces the energy needed for breathing. Unlike aquatic animals, terrestrial animals have lungs that help them take in oxygen from the air. This difference highlights that gas exchange relies on a thin layer that facilitates the rapid movement of gases and provides sufficient surface area to meet the body's needs. The detailed structure of these respiratory systems is guided by both the physical characteristics of gases and the conditions in which organisms have evolved which highlights the role of both development and comparison in this field. The movement of oxygen into and out of the body is significant for organisms responding to different environmental pressures. High temperatures may make it more difficult for the body to utilize oxygen, especially when there is insufficient oxygen. Research indicates that animals exposed to hypoxia may exhibit heightened sensitivity to thermal stress due to an increased oxygen demand that exceeds supply, creating a critical intersection between gas exchange mechanisms and environmental adaptability. This relationship is evident in the study of *Drosophila melanogaster*, where variations in oxygen concentration during developmental stages were found to significantly impact flight performance under thermal stress (Angilletta et al., 2017). It appears that fitness can be influenced by both immediate breathing and the conditions experienced throughout a person's entire life, which connects the study of developmental physiology to breathing efficiency. Additionally, analyzing how different species exchange gases can reveal insights into their ecological and evolutionary adaptations. Different animals use different methods to get oxygen, and this can determine their chances of survival and reproduction in various habitats. Some land animals use lungs, but others have developed alternative methods of breathing, such as cutaneous respiration, in challenging environments. Adaptations are formed because of selective pressures like how much oxygen is available, changes in temperature, and the amount of activity. In brief, efficient ways of exchanging gases help both individuals and entire species survive environmental changes. A comprehensive understanding of these processes can inform conservation strategies and management practices aimed at mitigating the effects of climate change and habitat loss (Bahr et al., 2015).

14.3.1. Diffusion and Partial Pressure Gradients

Respiratory physiology depends on the principles of diffusion and partial pressure gradients. Diffusion means that molecules move from a region with more of them to a region with fewer, which is very important for gas exchange in both water and land. How efficiently oxygen is picked up and carbon dioxide is removed in respiration depends mainly on the difference in partial pressure between the gases in the air and those in the blood. If the oxygen pressure in the air is greater than the oxygen pressure in the blood, oxygen will move into the bloodstream by itself. This is most noticeable in organisms that live at different altitudes or in various water environments, where the pressures of gases can change significantly and impact their mechanisms for transporting gases and adapting metabolically. Different organisms in developmental and comparative physiology exhibit special adaptations that facilitate diffusion. For example, people who live at high altitudes have features that help them absorb oxygen even when there is less of it available. They usually involve having more lung surface and stronger hemoglobin for oxygen, which allows efficient gas exchange at low oxygen levels. They demonstrate that diffusion is crucial in the respiratory system and that the environment can significantly impact the body's functioning. The ability to maintain aerobic metabolism under hypoxic conditions is an adaptive trait that results from both genetic evolution and environmental pressures, thereby highlighting the complex interplay between diffusion processes and respiratory adaptations across various species (Jay et al., 2019).

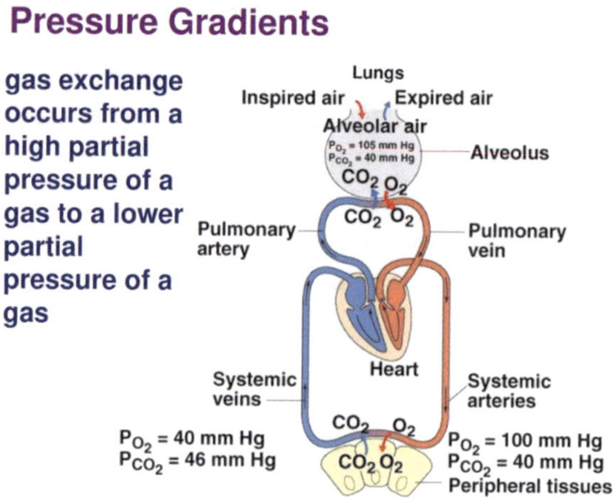

Figure 14.7. Pressure gradients.

Source: https://slideplayer.com/slide/12955466/79/images/16/Pressure+Gradients+gas+exchange+occurs+from+a+high+partial+pressure+of+a+gas+to+a+lower+partial+pressure+of+a+gas.jpg.

Additionally, understanding how diffusion and partial pressure gradients function is crucial for advancements in medicine and ecology. For example, new approaches to managing pulmonary hypertension can rely on these basic concepts, particularly when addressing issues that impede regular gas exchange. Recent guidelines emphasize the significance of optimizing oxygen delivery in patients with compromised respiratory function (Humbert et al., 2022). In addition, research on hypoxia in many organisms indicates that changes in oxygen transport can enhance metabolic efficiency. Because of this, looking into these physiological processes helps us understand comparative respiratory physiology and also supports medical and conservation efforts for species under hypoxic stress. The ongoing exploration of diffusion and partial pressure gradients underscores their crucial role in shaping respiratory strategies in response to environmental challenges (Figure 14.7).

14.3.2. Role of Hemoglobin and Other Respiratory Pigments

Hemoglobin, which is present in vertebrates, plays a crucial role in carrying oxygen and releasing carbon dioxide, thereby influencing respiratory physiology. It grabs oxygen molecules in the lungs and then transports them to tissues throughout the body. Because hemoglobin binds cooperatively, it can easily pick up and release oxygen; each oxygen molecule that sticks to hemoglobin makes it want to grab more.

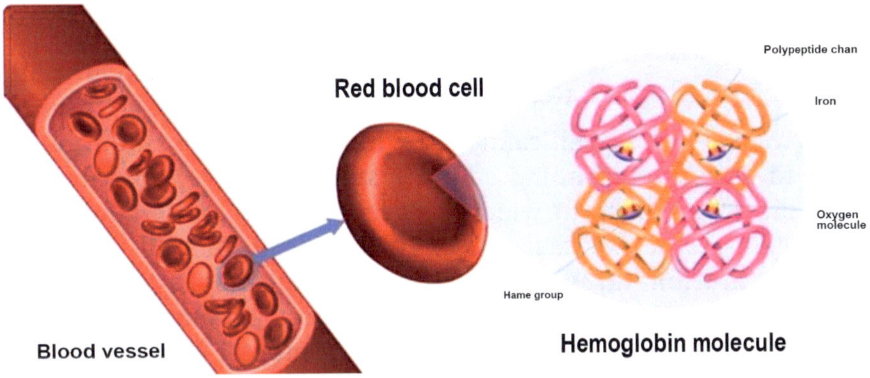

Figure 14.8. Respiratory pigments.

Source: https://www.zoologytalks.com/wp-content/uploads/2023/06/IMG_2904-768x330.jpeg.

This property ensures that oxygen is delivered effectively and that aerobic metabolism, necessary for energy production, occurs in tissues. Moreover, variations in hemoglobin structure among species highlight evolutionary adaptations to diverse environmental conditions, demonstrating how respiratory physiology has evolved to meet the varying metabolic demands of different organisms. This highlights the significance of hemoglobin in comparative respiratory physiology (Anderson et al., 2018). As well as hemoglobin, myoglobin and hemocyanin help different organisms exchange gases. Myoglobin, primarily found in muscle, stores oxygen for when it is needed, enabling marine mammals to dive for extended periods. Hemocyanin, which has copper rather than iron, is the primary oxygen carrier in many invertebrates, including mollusks and crustaceans. The presence of various types of respiratory pigments demonstrates how living things have adapted to the challenges of oxygen shortage or fluctuations in oxygen levels. Understanding these variations not only provides insights into specific adaptations but also emphasizes the importance of respiratory pigments in maintaining homeostasis across diverse biological systems (Karen et al., 2017). Respiratory pigments are important for more than gas exchange; they also play a role in metabolism and how well the organism performs. The fact that hemoglobin can interact with carbon dioxide and organic phosphates is involved in the Bohr effect, which increases oxygen availability in active tissues when carbon dioxide levels rise. Due to this mechanism, tissues always get enough oxygen even when conditions change. Due to respiratory pigments, organisms can respond to environmental stresses, including oxygen shortages and temperature fluctuations. By examining the roles of hemoglobin and other respiratory pigments within the broader context of developmental and comparative respiratory physiology, one can appreciate their critical contributions to the evolutionary success and adaptability of various species in response to their ecological niches (Anderson et al., 2018) (Figure 14.8).

14.3.3. Comparative Analysis of Gas Exchange in Different Organisms

The method of gas exchange varies significantly from one organism to another, depending on their evolution and the environment in which they live. The primary types of gas exchange mechanisms include diffusion through cell membranes, specialized structures such as gills and lungs, and tracheal systems. For example, fish breathe through gills, which are specially designed to absorb dissolved oxygen from the water, as the water contains less oxygen than air. Alternatively, mammals that live on land, such as humans, have lungs that help them take in oxygen and eliminate carbon dioxide through surfactant and alveolar ventilation. This comparison highlights the various ways in which organisms exchange gases, resulting in adaptations that make respiration more efficient in different environments, and demonstrating the principles of respiratory physiology across many species. By comparing gas exchange, we can observe the challenges organisms face in living in extreme environments. For example, some types of mice living in high altitudes have special adaptations that enable them to thrive in areas with lower oxygen levels. Studies indicate that these adaptations include an enhanced alveolar surface area and improved oxygen extraction mechanisms, allowing them to thrive where other species, such as rats, exhibit maladaptive physiological traits, including excessive erythrocytosis and right ventricular hypertrophy (Lemoine et al., 2016). This demonstrates that the ability to change in response to the environment and adapt through evolution is crucial for various organisms, as their gas exchange strategies significantly influence their success in different habitats. Moreover, the Krogh principle demonstrates how certain organisms can serve as models for studying gas exchange in living organisms. The principle posits that certain organisms are particularly suited for addressing specific biological questions due to their distinctive traits and physiological mechanisms (Ankeny et al., 2018). It is most noticeable in comparative respiratory physiology, where selecting animals with different and noticeable gas exchange systems allows researchers to identify general rules about how organisms adapt to various environments. Researchers can use these comparisons to better understand how respiratory mechanisms work, which helps both developmental physiology and evolutionary biology.

14.4. Pathophysiology of Respiratory Disorders

Respiratory disorders develop due to a combination of anatomical, physiological, and biochemical factors, which lead to problems with gas exchange and lung function. Pulmonary hypertension and COPD demonstrate that underlying diseases can interfere with the usual way the lungs work. The high pressure in the lungs' blood vessels in pulmonary hypertension causes the right ventricle to work harder, which can result in heart failure—classifying pulmonary hypertension, including those caused by left heart disease or respiratory disease such as hypoxia, aids in understanding the multifactorial nature of this disorder (Abbott et al., 2020). When these groups are recognized, doctors can design treatments that address both the symptoms and the causes, which can help patients improve. Research into how respiratory physiology changes over time offers an important understanding of the different ways respiratory disorders can appear at different ages.

For instance, neonates have underdeveloped lungs, making them particularly susceptible to acute respiratory distress syndrome (ARDS). Asthma in children may be caused by inherited traits or by things in the environment that make the airways overly sensitive and cause inflammation. Adults experience changes in their lungs and the way they exchange gases, which can be serious health concerns.

It is essential to recognize that these changes underscore the importance of considering respiratory disorders throughout a person's entire life, as adapting to various body changes during development is crucial for maintaining respiratory health. Comparative respiratory physiology helps us understand how different animals react differently to problems with breathing. Studying how animals adapt to high altitudes, such as their enhanced oxygen uptake, can provide insights into human respiratory problems. For example, insights gained from studying pulmonary hypertension in dogs reveal similarities in disease mechanisms and progression that can be extended to human cases (Abbott et al., 2020). Additionally, understanding the relationship between neurons and metabolism in relation to breathing performance, as demonstrated by studies on energy metabolism in stressful situations, helps us comprehend how environmental factors impact respiratory health. Such a comparison is necessary to develop new approaches for diagnosing and treating respiratory diseases in diverse populations.

14.4.1. Common Respiratory Diseases and Their Impact

Many people around the world suffer from respiratory diseases, which cause both health problems and deaths. Asthma, COPD, and pneumonia are common respiratory diseases that cause a big strain on healthcare services. Asthma, which involves the airways becoming inflamed and narrowed, affects millions worldwide and often leads to emergency room visits and hospitalizations. COPD, which is mainly caused by smoking and environmental pollution, causes the lungs to function less well over time, making symptoms worse and shortening life expectancy. Understanding how these diseases develop and spread helps design more effective interventions and public health policies to mitigate their impact. More attention has been given to the relationship between respiratory diseases and environmental problems in recent years. The severity and frequency of respiratory problems often depend on air quality, allergens, and changes in climate. For instance, elevated levels of pollen from plants such as *Kentucky bluegrass* and white birch can exacerbate allergic responses in susceptible individuals, contributing to asthma attacks and respiratory distress (Gevaert et al., 2019). Climate change is expected to cause an increase in pollen production and alter the air quality, potentially leading to more respiratory health issues. For this reason, studying how respiratory physiology responds to external factors is important to find ways to support and strengthen respiratory health in a world that is constantly changing. Also, respiratory diseases have a major significant effect on the economy, which highlights the need for a full range of healthcare services. Hospital stays, medicine, and outpatient care for COPD and asthma are very expensive, and families and communities also face extra costs due to lost work and the burden of caregiving. Existing studies indicate that the economic burden of respiratory diseases underscores the need for increased public health funding and targeted educational initiatives to improve disease management and prevention (Aristarán et al., 2016). Addressing these common respiratory conditions requires a multidisciplinary approach that integrates clinical expertise, community engagement, and policy advocacy to create healthier environments and improve the overall quality of life for affected individuals (Figure 14.9).

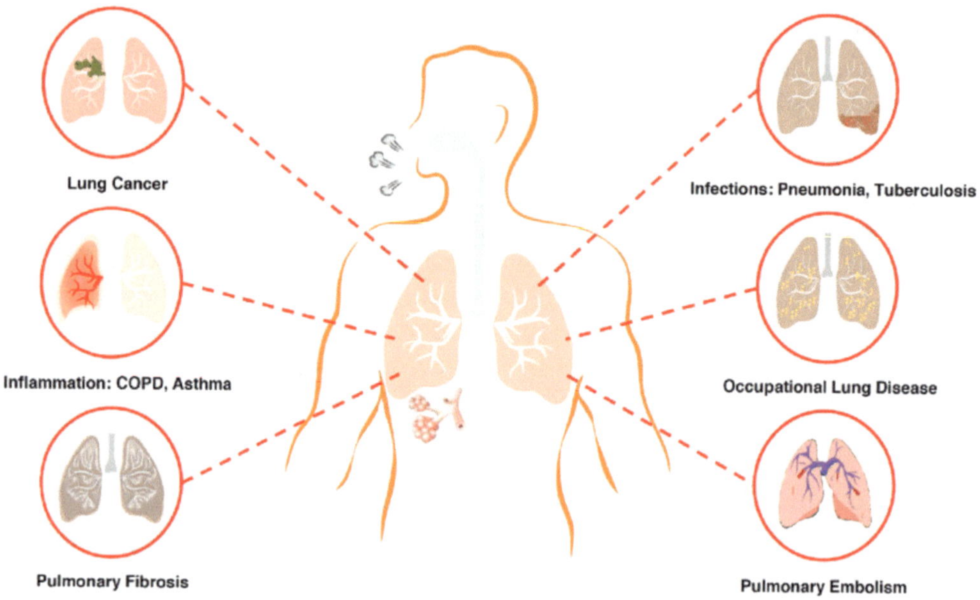

Figure 14.9. Common respiratory diseases: respiratory diseases are among the leading cause of deaths worldwide. Chronic respiratory conditions including COPD and asthma affect most people. All respiratory diseases have symptoms varying from mild to severe and can also be life-threatening.

Source: https://www.researchgate.net/profile/Jesus-Shrestha/publication/338429576/figure/fig1/AS:847043081797634@1578962216226/Common-respiratory-diseases-respiratory-diseases-are-among-the-leading-cause-of-deaths.png.

14.4.2. Developmental Disorders Affecting Respiration

Respiratory function is greatly affected by developmental disorders, mainly in babies born early and teenagers. The impact of such disorders can manifest in various forms, including obstructive sleep apnea (OSA), asthma, and other conditions that affect respiratory function. At this stage, internalizing disorders can develop, particularly due to the additional demands placed on the respiratory system. Because lung health and developmental issues are closely linked, it is essential to utilize different specialties in both research and care. By understanding how genetic, cognitive, and environmental factors contribute to these disorders, researchers can better identify at-risk populations and tailor interventions to improve respiratory outcomes (Vidal, 2025). It has been found that early support is important for premature newborns to deal with breathing problems linked to developmental disorders. A study on physiotherapy for newborns found that those who received respiratory therapy showed better oxygen saturation and heart rate. It involved helping babies lie in positions similar to being in the uterus, which supports better breathing. The results indicated that premature infants who participated in these programs not only showed enhanced respiratory stability but also regular neurological assessments, underscoring the necessity of immediate preventative measures (Chatzopoulou et al., 2024). Due to these results, it is crucial for healthcare professionals to prioritize respiratory health when developing strategies for vulnerable newborns. Besides affecting infants, developmental disorders can also influence respiration in later life, so ongoing monitoring and interventions are needed. Because these disorders change, the treatment must also change to suit the individual's development. Proper management of respiratory illnesses associated with these disorders can improve quality of life and prevent serious health problems in the future. Future studies should focus on long-term research that examines the interplay between development and respiratory health, adapting approaches to utilize a variety of samples and situations. Such investigations are crucial for developing effective public health policies and intervention programs that aim to improve respiratory outcomes across diverse populations facing developmental challenges (Vidal, 2025) (Figure 14.10).

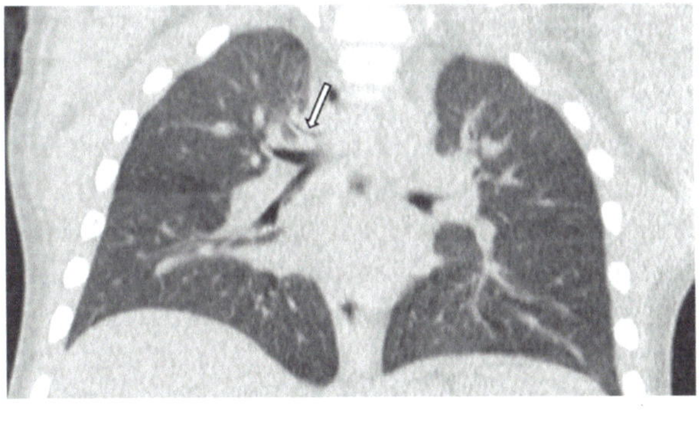

Figure 14.10. Tracheal bronchus, indicated by the arrow, in a child with Down syndrome.

Source: https://www.mdpi.com/children/children-11-00246/article_deploy/html/images/children-11-00246-g003.png.

14.4.3. Comparative Analysis of Respiratory Disorders Across Species

Studying respiratory disorders involves examining different species, which helps us understand how they are adapted and what makes them vulnerable. An example is that mammals have a well-developed diaphragm and a detailed lung system that helps them exchange gases efficiently. Alternatively, birds have special respiratory traits, such as air sacs and one-way airflow, which help them take in oxygen during both inhalation and exhalation. It demonstrates that the various types of respiratory systems are closely tied to the needs of each species in its environment and for energy production. Comparative analyses draw attention to these differences and also reveal how respiratory disorders manifest differently across various taxa, as well as how they respond to pathogens or environmental changes, which contributes to our understanding of respiratory physiology. Comparisons between species have helped identify the factors that influence respiratory diseases. Studying congenital heart disease has been greatly aided by the findings from genetic research conducted on various animals. As noted in recent studies, innovations in molecular testing techniques have expanded our understanding of the genetic contributions to respiratory pathologies, such as asthma and COPD, in humans (Pierpont et al., 2018). Using such animal models, scientists can study the causes of respiratory diseases and investigate the role of genes in these conditions. This demonstrates the importance of comparative studies in identifying the various factors contributing to respiratory health and disease in different species, as well as in understanding the interplay between genetics and environmental effects. Respiratory disorders are interesting because they involve the relationship between microbes and the respiratory system, which crosses species lines. It has been demonstrated that the gut-brain connection, influenced by the gut microbiota, plays a crucial role in respiratory balance, as alterations in the microbiota can exacerbate respiratory conditions. This aspect of respiratory physiology reflects a holistic view where the microbiome's influence is evident across different species, potentially informing therapeutic strategies (John et al., 2019). Further investigations into this axis show that they play a key role in asthma and lung infections, which suggests that changing the microbiota could be a new way to treat respiratory diseases. Therefore, comparing different respiratory conditions improves our knowledge and encourages new studies and treatments in respiratory health.

14.5. Technological Advances in Respiratory Physiology

New technologies in respiratory physiology have significantly transformed the way medicine and research are conducted, enabling a deeper understanding of the respiratory system's functions at various stages of life. A significant advancement is the use of high-throughput genetic screening methods, such as CRISPR/Cas9 and single-cell RNA sequencing, which enable researchers to study respiratory diseases at a highly detailed level. These technologies enable the modeling of congenital diseases in organisms such as zebrafish, thereby facilitating comparative studies that reveal critical insights into human respiratory disorders (Figure 14.11).When scientists study the genetic and physical similarities between zebrafish and humans, they can discover common pathways that regulate the development and function of the respiratory system. As a result, using these tools together enhances basic science and helps translate discoveries into therapies for respiratory illnesses. Another substantial advancement is the utilization of extracorporeal membrane oxygenation (ECMO), particularly in neonatal care for conditions such as congenital diaphragmatic hernia. This method dramatically improves the support of newborns with severe respiratory failure by giving them the oxygen and blood pressure they need. Reports show that the survival chances and outcomes of babies receiving ECMO have improved significantly due to new advancements in the method and in how it is managed before and after the procedure. On the other hand, there are still difficulties, for example, deciding which patients are suitable and handling possible complications such as bleeding and blockages.

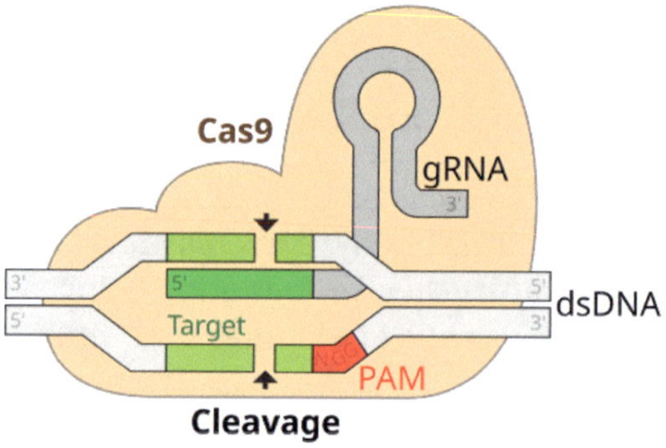

Figure 14.11. CRISPR-Cas9.

Source: https://upload.wikimedia.org/wikipedia/commons/thumb/5/57/GRNA-Cas9.svg/1024px-GRNA-Cas9.svg.png.

Continuous research focusing on optimizing ECMO protocols alongside ongoing technological innovations is vital for further improving outcomes in this vulnerable population (Miranda et al., 2020). Biotechnology continues to drive the study of respiratory physiology by enabling the monitoring and treatment of patients in real-time. New technologies, such as wearable sensors and advanced imaging, enable clinicians to monitor respiratory function in real-time and without invasive procedures, allowing them to select the most effective treatment options. Using data analytics and machine learning, these systems can predict when respiratory events are likely to occur, enabling early intervention and reducing the risk of complications. Moreover, these technologies make it possible to follow how respiratory function changes over time in different life stages, which improves our knowledge of comparative respiratory physiology. As technology advances, it holds the potential to revolutionize both our understanding of respiratory systems and the treatment and management of respiratory diseases in developmental medicine, thereby bridging the gap between basic research and clinical application (Kumar et al., 2023) (Figure 14.12).

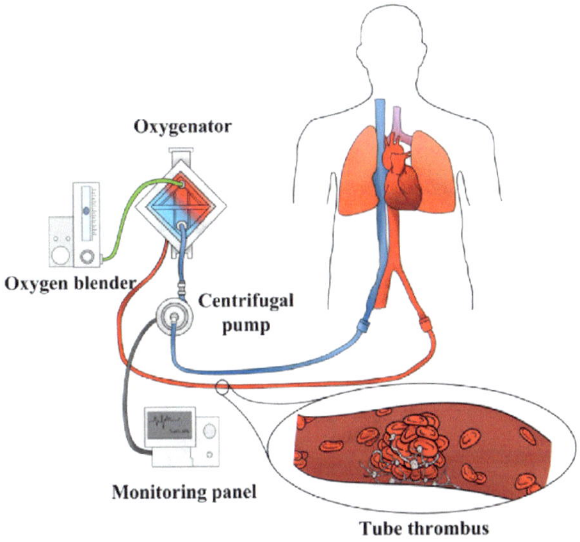

Figure 14.12. Extracorporeal membrane oxygenation (ECMO) is composed of five parts: a centrifugal pump, an oxygenator, tube, an oxygen blender and a monitoring panel.

Source: https://www.researchgate.net/profile/Wei-Tong-16/publication/372196708/figure/fig1/AS:11431281175616740@1689836926458/Extracorporeal-Membrane-Oxygenation-ECMO-is-composed-of-five-parts-a-centrifugal-pump.png.

14.5.1. Innovations in Respiratory Monitoring and Assessment

Innovations in respiratory monitoring and assessment have played a pivotal role in advancing our understanding of respiratory physiology across various species. The use of modern technology, such as wearable devices and mobile health apps, supports continuous tracking of tidal volume, respiratory rate, and oxygen saturation. Due to these developments, researchers and clinicians can now collect and analyze data on respiratory health in real-time. In addition, nanotechnology has made it possible to create biosensors that can detect specific biomarkers in exhaled air, which provides a non-invasive way to evaluate lung function. As noted in recent studies, these advancements not only enhance diagnostic capabilities but also contribute to individualized treatment plans, particularly in chronic respiratory diseases where conventional assessment methods may fall short (Joseph et al., 2023). Therefore, respiratory monitoring is continuing to develop, leading to further improvements in healthcare and research.

The Polyvagal Theory enables us to understand how various physiological states impact the functioning of the lungs. This theory emphasizes how autonomic nervous system (ANS) responses influence feelings of safety, which, in turn, may impact respiratory patterns. It proposes that the body's internal states can be measured objectively, thereby enabling more targeted therapeutic interventions (Stephen, 2022). By applying these new strategies, researchers can examine how stress and emotions affect breathing, which proves why assessing respiration is important for overall health. Additionally, incorporating psychosocial aspects into respiratory monitoring can help clinicians effectively manage the various aspects of respiratory diseases.

So, more people are realizing that progress in respiratory assessment should consider the connections among physiology, psychology, and environmental elements. Emerging technologies, including machine learning and artificial intelligence (AI), have the potential to revolutionize respiratory monitoring beyond traditional methods. These techniques enable the study of extensive information from respiratory tests, identify patterns, and make accurate predictions. For example, using predictive algorithms can help identify the early signs of worsening in patients with COPD or asthma, allowing for prompt treatment and improved care. Additionally, using automated methods to interpret data reduces errors and makes clinical decisions more reliable. As digital health becomes increasingly prevalent in healthcare, utilizing new respiratory assessment tools can help manage patients more effectively and inform public health strategies. In essence, the continual evolution of respiratory monitoring tools is not only advancing the field of developmental and comparative respiratory physiology but also improving patient outcomes through more informed and proactive care (Figure 14.13).

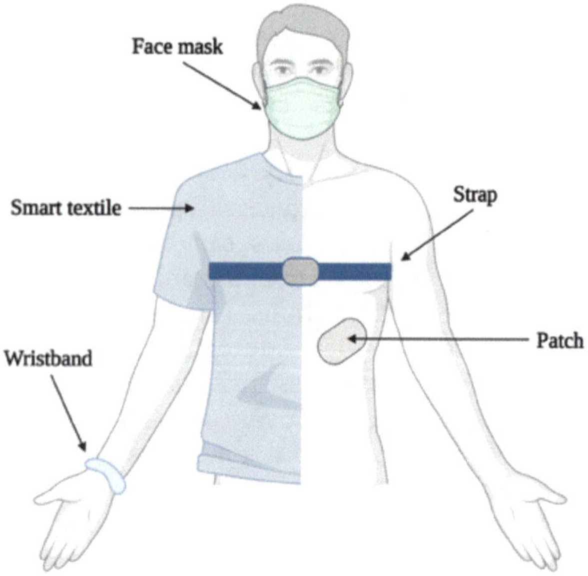

Figure 14.13. Schematic representation of wearable devices that allow the monitoring of respiratory data.

Source: https://www.researchgate.net/publication/381323945/figure/fig3/AS:11431281288447279@1730731751563/Schematic-representation-of-wearable-devices-that-allow-the-monitoring-of-respiratory.png.

14.5.2. Role of Biotechnology in Understanding Respiratory Systems

Biotechnology is becoming increasingly important in the study of respiratory systems, particularly in the areas of developmental and comparative physiology. Through advanced genetics, scientists can study how breathing works in various species. By utilizing biotechnologies such as CRISPR and genetic sequencing, scientists can identify pathways crucial to the efficiency of respiration. Also, biotechnology allows scientists to change respiratory genes to learn how they help organisms adapt to different places which gives us knowledge about evolution. They enhance our understanding of respiratory physiology and contribute to the development of new treatments for diseases that affect humans and animals. Additionally, some organisms possess impressive adaptations in their respiratory systems that can be studied using biotechnology. For example, *Pichia anomala* is interesting because it can handle many metabolic tasks and is resilient against environmental pressures. Researchers can utilize the cellular and physiological traits of P. anomala to understand how its respiratory system functions in various situations, which may aid in discovering new applications for it in both environmental and industrial contexts. The biotechnological insights gained from such studies can significantly contribute to the design of biomimetic systems that replicate efficient respiratory mechanisms, offering practical applications in biotechnology, particularly in bioremediation and agricultural biological control strategies (Walker et al., 2010). Integrating respiratory physiology and biotechnology demonstrates the interdisciplinary approach now common in biology. Additionally, space biology utilizes biotechnology to investigate how respiratory systems operate in extreme environments. Studies on how people and animals breathe in space and at varying air pressures are crucial for planning long-duration missions. Biotechnology enables the monitoring of physiological changes and gene expression in response to these unique environments, contributing to our understanding of cardiovascular and respiratory adaptations (Garshnek et al., 2025).

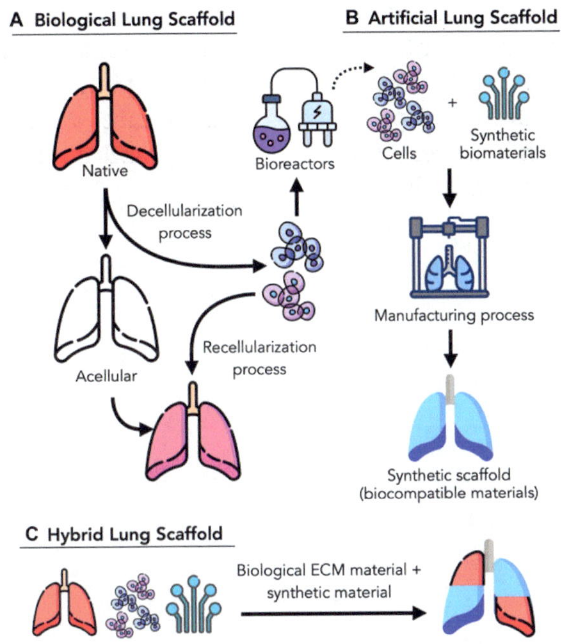

Figure 14.14. Lung tissue scaffolds can be bioengineered in different ways. (A) Biological lung scaffolds can be obtained from humans and animals; (B) Artificial scaffolds can be manufactured based on a variety of methods (e.g., 3D bioprinting, electrospinning), utilizing synthetic biomaterials, cells, and bioinks; and (C) By combining biological components such as cells and ECMs, hybrid scaffolds can be manufactured in combination with biocompatible materials.

Source: https://www.frontiersin.org/files/Articles/1011800/fbioe-10-1011800-HTML/image_m/fbioe-10-1011800-g001.jpg.

Having this understanding is crucial for ensuring the effective operation of life support systems and maintaining the health and well-being of astronauts. The integration of biotechnological methodologies with physiological studies not only enhances our comprehension of respiratory systems but also aids in optimizing health strategies for humans exposed to extraterrestrial conditions, thereby expanding the practical applications of respiratory physiology research (Figure 14.14).

14.5.3. Future Directions in Respiratory Research

As more research is conducted in respiratory science, incorporating microbiome studies will play a crucial role in understanding respiratory physiology. It appears that the gut microbiota plays a crucial role in both digestive health and the health of the respiratory system, influencing it through the microbiota-gut-brain connection. Due to this interaction, immune responses in the lungs and respiratory function may be affected, potentially leading to new treatments for respiratory diseases. Future research will likely focus on elucidating the mechanisms through which microbial metabolites, such as short-chain fatty acids, affect respiratory physiology, as well as their implications for conditions like asthma and COPD (John et al., 2019). Researchers can utilize this approach to develop more effective methods for preventing and treating respiratory diseases, ultimately benefiting patients. Genetic and epigenetic factors play a crucial role in the development and functioning of the lungs, and they are expected to be further studied in the future. Due to advancements in gene editing and sequencing, researchers can now investigate genetic variations associated with respiratory diseases. Learning about the genetic causes of congenital adrenal hyperplasia and their effects on respiratory function might help doctors choose better personalized therapies. Also, factors related to epigenetics, which are affected by pollution and lifestyle, are being recognized for their impact on lung health and disease risk. This multifactorial approach will enable scientists to delineate the underlying biological pathways and mechanisms that contribute to respiratory health, potentially guiding the development of targeted therapies

(Speiser et al., 2018). The field is changing and focusing on genetics and epigenetics will be necessary to understand respiratory physiology fully. Going forward, respiratory research likely concentrate more on creating new treatments, with the help of advanced technologies, focusing on developing new treatments. Due to precision medicine, treatments can now be tailored to fit each patient's specific situation, which is particularly beneficial for many respiratory conditions. Work on inhaled treatments, gene therapies, and interventions guided by biomarkers will result in better ways to treat CF and asthma. The increasing use of telemedicine and remote monitoring technologies opens up new ways to manage respiratory health, ensure patients follow their treatment plans, and gather real-time information for researchers. By leveraging technology, future respiratory research is poised to transform clinical practice, resulting in improved outcomes and quality of life for patients with respiratory ailments (John et al., 2019). Ultimately, by employing innovative research and prioritizing patient care, we can transform respiratory physiology and address related health issues.

SUMMARY

After studying developmental and comparative respiratory physiology, it is evident that the field helps us understand how respiratory systems have evolved in many different species. The way the body is built, how it functions, and the environment it inhabits demonstrate the wide range of respiratory adaptations. For example, the different ways aquatic and terrestrial organisms breathe highlight how habitats influence their evolution. They provide insights into the workings of the body and stress the role these systems play in an organism's health and chances of survival. Thus, respiratory physiology is important for biology, medicine, and environmental science. In addition, utilizing the latest research, including microbiota studies, provides a different perspective on how the respiratory system functions in both health and disease. The way microbiota helps keep the body stable and regulates the immune system may play a significant role in respiratory health. Problems with the microbiome or dysbiosis may be linked to chronic respiratory diseases, proving that the microbiome affects respiratory health. The field stresses the importance of seeing respiratory functions as a whole, which includes anatomical, physiological, and microbial aspects. Earlier research has shown that these systems interact in many ways, and imbalances can cause serious, profound changes in the body, which is why more studies are needed. In short, the diverse ways respiratory systems function in various species demonstrate how evolution and the environment play a crucial role in establishing physiological standards. The relationship between how the respiratory system is built and how it works explains both its complexity and its important role in nature and evolution. Moving forward, further research on this subject, particularly regarding the role of microbiota as described in the literature, will be necessary to enhance respiratory health. When these areas are connected, researchers can gain a deeper understanding of the reasons behind normal and abnormal breathing, which may lead to the development of new treatments and informed public health plans. To achieve this, bringing together research results from various scientific fields will be crucial for gaining a deeper understanding of respiratory physiology and its impact on health. When examining how respiration develops and differs among species, we find that respiratory systems are remarkably complex. It has been observed that the structure of respiratory systems often reveals how they have evolved in response to environmental changes over time. For example, the way lungs work and are built differs between terrestrial and aquatic organisms, allowing them to exchange gases efficiently in their respective habitats. It is clear from comparative studies that respiratory changes have been important for both survival and the variety of species. The connection between respiratory physiology and ecological niches is a key aspect of understanding evolutionary biology, demonstrating how external conditions can influence internal systems over multiple generations. More research on microbiota reveals how respiratory health is linked to the rest of the body. It has been observed that microbiota play a crucial role in maintaining the healthy function of organs that facilitate breathing. An imbalance in the microbiota has been tied to worse respiratory diseases and increased inflammation in the body, which may be due to changes in the immune system and metabolic processes. Understanding the impact of microbiomes on respiratory function enables us to recognize how alterations in microbes can contribute to disease development and progression. The results point to a link between microbial health and lung function which should lead to more research on ways to treat microbiota. Finally, the research has highlighted the role of the gut-brain axis in respiratory physiology, demonstrating that there is significant two-way communication between the gut and the respiratory system. It points out that microbial metabolites can alter respiratory health by affecting the immune system or nerves, which may in turn influence airflow and gas exchange.

CLOSER LOOK

NASOPHARYNX

The nasopharynx is the uppermost portion of the pharynx, a passageway connecting the nasal cavity to the oropharynx. It is located behind the nasal cavity and is lined with respiratory epithelium. Key structures within the nasopharynx include the soft palate, uvula, adenoids (pharyngeal tonsils), and openings of the Eustachian tubes (Figure 14.15).

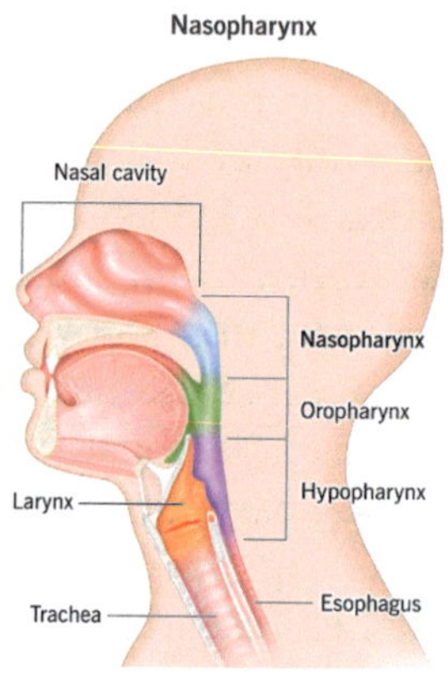

Figure 14.15. Anatomical regions of the upper respiratory tract, including the nasopharynx.

Source: https://my.clevelandclinic.org/-/scassets/images/org/health/articles/22376-nasopharynx.

- **Anatomy and Location**
  - Superior Boundary: Skull base., Inferior Boundary: Soft palate.
  - Posterior Wall: Contains the pharyngeal tonsils (adenoids).
  - Lateral Walls: Include the Rosenmüller's fossa., Connects: Nasal cavity to oropharynx.
  - Contains: Openings of the Eustachian tubes, which connect to the middle ear
- **Function**
  - **Respiratory:** Lined with respiratory epithelium, facilitating air passage from the nose to the respiratory tract.
  - **Pharyngeal Tonsils:** Help protect the body against infection.
  - **Swallowing:** The soft palate raises to close off the nasopharynx during swallowing, preventing food from entering the nasal cavity.
- **Clinical Significance**
  - **Nasopharyngeal Cancer:** A relatively rare head and neck cancer that originates in the nasopharynx.
- **Adenoid Hypertrophy:** Enlargement of the adenoids, particularly in children, which can cause airway obstruction.

REFERENCES

1. Angilletta, M. J. Jr., Le Vinh Thuy, J., Shiehzadegan, S., Szabla, D., et al. (2017). More oxygen during development enhanced flight performance but not thermal tolerance of *Drosophila melanogaster. PLoS ONE.* https://core.ac.uk/download/161347574.pdf (accessed on 31st May 2025).
2. Ankeny, R., Dietrich, M. R., Green, S., Leonelli, S., et al. (2018). *'Extreme' Organisms and the Problem of Generalization: Interpreting the Krogh Principle.* https://core.ac.uk/download/pdf/295731996.pdf (accessed on 31st May 2025).
3. Aristarán, M., Guevara, M. R., Hartmann, D., Hidalgo, C., et al. (2016). The research space: Using the career paths of scholars to predict the evolution of the research output of individuals, institutions, and nations. Scientometric. http://arxiv.org/abs/1602.08409 (accessed on 31st May 2025).
4. Bahr, C., Romanini, C. E. B., Berckmans, D., Decuypere, E., Bergoug, H., McGonnell, I. M., Molenaar, R., et al. (2015). *Higher Levels of CO_2 During Late Incubation Alter the Hatch Time of Chicken Embryos.* https://core.ac.uk/download/36778323.pdf (accessed on 31st May 2025).
5. Bennett-Stamper, C., Carrier, D., Grigg, G., Johnston, S., et al. (2004). *Evidence for Endothermic Ancestors of Crocodiles at the Stem of Archosaur Evolution.* https://core.ac.uk/download/12728201.pdf (accessed on 31st May 2025).
6. Bita, C. E., & Gerats, T. (2013). Plant tolerance to high temperature in a changing environment: Scientific fundamentals and production of heat stress-tolerant crops. *Frontiers in Plant Science, 4.* https://doi.org/10.3389/fpls.2013.00273 (accessed on 31st May 2025).
7. Campbell, A., Hemmingsen, E., Kay, R., Knox, D., Louw, G., McNab, B., Schmidt-Nielsen, K., et al. (2008). *General Ecology: Animal Physiology*. https://core.ac.uk/download/195676680.pdf (accessed on 31st May 2025).
8. Chatzopoulou, A., Xinias, S., Papadopoulou, O., Trevlakis, E., Chalkia, A., Xinias, G., Xinias, I., et al. (2024). The impact of physiotherapy on the developmental progress of preterm infants hospitalized in the intensive care unit. FYSIKOTHERAPIA. https://www.semanticscholar.org/paper/e5cb2f65787eac427d386f6305dac6ea41fdccb6 (accessed on 31st May 2025).
9. Cryan, J. F., O'Riordan, K. J., Cowan, C. S. M., Sandhu, K. V., Bastiaanssen, T. F. S., Boehme, M., Codagnone, M. G., et al. (2019). The microbiota-gut-brain axis. *Physiological Reviews, 99*, 1877–2013. https://doi.org/10.1152/physrev.00018.2018 (accessed on 31st May 2025).
10. Dai, Z., Delrot, S., Feil, R., Gomes, E., et al. (2013). Metabolic profiling reveals coordinated switches in primary carbohydrate metabolism in grape berry (*Vitis vinifera* L.), a non-climacteric fleshy fruit. *Journal of Experimental Botany*. https://core.ac.uk/download/210621820.pdf (accessed on 31st May 2025).
11. Dow, J. (2007). Integrative physiology, functional genomics and the phenotype gap: A guide for comparative physiologists. *Journal of Experimental Biology, 210*, 1632–1640. https://www.semanticscholar.org/paper/c52a9bbb2048d04f3b51e278c9f9d04bd32c7fc8 (accessed on 31st May 2025).
12. Farley, S., Lemaire-Gony, S., & Pulsford, A. L. (1994). *Effects of Stress on the Immune System of Fish.* https://core.ac.uk/download/11020744.pdf (accessed on 31st May 2025).

13. Garshnek, V., Hooke, L. R., Radtke, M., Rowe, D., et al. (2025). *USSR Space Life Sciences Digest, Issue 3*. https://core.ac.uk/download/pdf/42842161.pdf (accessed on 31st May 2025).

14. Gevaert, K., Impens, F., Laval, K., Nauwynck, H., et al. (2019). *Pollens Destroy Respiratory Epithelial Cell Anchors and Drive Alphaherpesvirus Infection*. https://core.ac.uk/download/222452376.pdf (accessed on 31st May 2025).

15. Hahn, D. A., & Denlinger, D. L. (2010). Energetics of insect diapause. *Annual Review of Entomology, 56*, 103–121. https://doi.org/10.1146/annurev-ento-112408-085436 (accessed on 31st May 2025).

16. Hou, K., Wu, Z. X., Chen, X. Y., Wang, J. Q., Zhang, D., Xiao, C., Zhu, D., et al. (2022). Microbiota in health and diseases. *Signal Transduction and Targeted Therapy, 7*. https://doi.org/10.1038/s41392-022-00974-4 (accessed on 31st May 2025).

17. Humbert, M., Kovács, G., Hoeper, M. M., Badagliacca, R., Berger, R. M. F., Brida, M., Carlsen, J., et al. (2022). 2022 ESC/ERS guidelines for the diagnosis and treatment of pulmonary hypertension. *European Respiratory Journal, 61*, 2200879. https://doi.org/10.1183/13993003.00879-2022 (accessed on 31st May 2025).

18. Joseph, T. M., Mahapatra, D. K., Esmaeili, A., Piszczyk, Ł., Hasanin, M. S., Kattali, M., Haponiuk, J. T., et al. (2023). Nanoparticles: Taking a unique position in medicine. *Nanomaterials, 13*, 574. https://doi.org/10.3390/nano13030574 (accessed on 31st May 2025).

19. Kumar, M., Kim, C. H., & Singla, N. (2023). Editorial: Zebrafish as a model for human congenital disorders. *Frontiers in Cell and Developmental Biology, 11*. https://www.semanticscholar.org/paper/c2c848312240f71cc8fbb1b9cb06bfc5e28e59b0 (accessed on 31st May 2025).

20. Lemoine, A. (2016). The influence of environmental hypoxia in the physiological responses of laboratory rats and mice during postnatal life and adulthood. https://core.ac.uk/download/442621756.pdf (accessed on 31st May 2025).

21. Matthews, K. A., Croft, J. B., Yong, L., Lu, H., Kanny, D., Wheaton, A. G., Cunningham, T. J., et al. (2017). Health-related behaviors by urban-rural county classification — United States, 2013. *MMWR Surveillance Summaries, 66*, 1–8. https://doi.org/10.15585/mmwr.ss6605a1 (accessed on 31st May 2025).

22. Miranda, M., Abecasis, F., Almeida, S., Tôrres, É., Boto, L., Camilo, C., Neves, J., et al. (2020). ECMO in neonates with congenital diaphragmatic hernia: The experience of a Portuguese ECMO referral center. *Acta Medica Portuguesa, 33*(12), 819–827. https://www.semanticscholar.org/paper/76739e6b4a93d54aeaeab7d475db406a730da8dd (accessed on 31st May 2025).

23. Montgomery, R. M. (2024). Fractal geometry in vertebrate respiratory systems: A comparative analysis of branching patterns across species. *Political Science International*. https://www.semanticscholar.org/paper/b43b453d4ac4481b0721dc0e5d6c3165fa2e47b3 (accessed on 31st May 2025).

24. O'Neil, E., Lin, H., Shamshirsaz, A. A., Naoum, E. E., Rycus, P., Alexander, P., Ortoleva, J., et al. (2021). Pregnant and peripartum women with COVID-19 have high survival with extracorporeal membrane oxygenation: An Extracorporeal Life Support Organization registry analysis. *American Journal of Respiratory and Critical Care Medicine, 205*, 248–250. https://www.semanticscholar.org/paper/d93168333ddb16ac4efd6223b47a5965e9e9ced1 (accessed on 31st May 2025).

25. Pagano, A., & Márquez, S. (2022). The nasopharynx as a window to half a billion years of evolutionary change to the upper respiratory tract. *The Anatomical Record, 305*, 1829–1841. https://www.semanticscholar.org/paper/48342109f9077d591bdb2c6991fd0e2de273dab1 (accessed on 31st May 2025).

26. Pierpont, M. E., Brueckner, M., Chung, W. K., Garg, V., Lacro, R. V., McGuire, A. L., Mital, S., et al. (2018). Genetic basis for congenital heart disease revisited: A scientific statement from the American Heart Association. *Circulation, 138*. https://doi.org/10.1161/cir.0000000000000606 (accessed on 31st May 2025).

27. Porges, S. W. (2022). Polyvagal theory: A science of safety. *Frontiers in Integrative Neuroscience, 16*. https://doi.org/10.3389/fnint.2022.871227 (accessed on 31st May 2025).

28. Reinero, C., Visser, L. C., Kellihan, H. B., Masseau, I., Rozanski, E., Clercx, C., Williams, K., Abbott, J., Borgarelli, M., & Scansen, B. A. (2020). ACVIM consensus statement guidelines for the diagnosis, classification, treatment, and monitoring of pulmonary hypertension in dogs. *Journal of Veterinary Internal Medicine, 34*(2), 549–573. https://doi.org/10.1111/jvim.15725Anderson, H. L., Brodsky, I. E., & Mangalmurti, N. S. (2018). The evolving erythrocyte: Red blood cells as modulators of innate immunity. *The Journal of Immunology, 201*, 1343–1351. https://doi.org/10.4049/jimmunol.1800565 (accessed on 31st May 2025).

29. Speiser, P., Arlt, W., Auchus, R. J., Baskin, L. S., Conway, G. S., Merke, D. P., Meyer-Bahlburg, H. F. L., et al. (2018). Congenital adrenal hyperplasia due to steroid 21-hydroxylase deficiency: An Endocrine Society clinical practice guideline. *The Journal of Clinical Endocrinology & Metabolism, 103*, 4043–4088. https://doi.org/10.1210/jc.2018-01865 (accessed on 31st May 2025).

30. Storz, J. F., & Scott, G. R. (2019). Life ascending: Mechanism and process in physiological adaptation to high-altitude hypoxia. *Annual Review of Ecology, Evolution, and Systematics, 50*, 503–526. https://doi.org/10.1146/annurev-ecolsys-110218-025014 (accessed on 31st May 2025).

31. Sünwoldt, J. (2018). *Neuronal Culture Microenvironments Determine Preferences in Bioenergetic Pathway Use*. https://core.ac.uk/download/199423644.pdf (accessed on 31st May 2025).

32. Torday, J. S. (2015). *Pleiotropy as the Mechanism for Evolving Novelty: Same Signal, Different Result*. https://core.ac.uk/download/323075977.pdf (accessed on 31st May 2025).

33. Vidal-Ribas, P. (2025). Editorial: A granular approach to internalizing disorders in adolescents: Examining developmental pathways and environmental influences to identify high-risk youth. *JCPP Advances, 5*. https://www.semanticscholar.org/paper/c5da7e83a4d03204aacd06ebca2072072734433c (accessed on 31st May 2025).

34. Walker, G. M. (2010). *Pichia Anomala: Cell Physiology and Biotechnology Relative to Other Yeasts*. https://core.ac.uk/download/228176756.pdf (accessed on 31st May 2025).

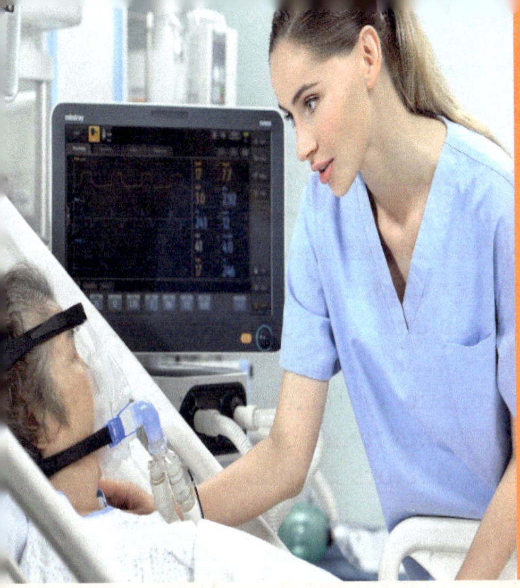

Chapter 15

PATHOPHYSIOLOGY OF COMMON RESPIRATORY DISORDERS

Contents

Introduction

It is essential to learn about respiratory disorders to manage and treat them effectively. Respiratory disorders encompass a spectrum of conditions, ranging from obstructive diseases, such as chronic obstructive pulmonary disease (COPD) and asthma, to restrictive disorders like pulmonary fibrosis and acute respiratory distress syndrome (ARDS). Different factors cause all these disorders, but they often have similar symptoms, for example, dyspnea, wheezing and chronic cough. Inflammation and changes to the airways are caused by COPD, which is primarily due to smoking or exposure to environmental pollutants. These changes lead to reduced airflow. Alternatively, asthma leads to airways that become overly sensitive, causing them to narrow and produce excessive mucus. Correctly understanding these differences enables doctors to select the most effective approach for diagnosing and treating patients with various respiratory illnesses, thereby enhancing their quality of life and improving their chances of recovery. When examining specific respiratory disorders, it is essential to acknowledge the complexities associated with conditions such as bronchiolitis obliterans (BO). This less frequent condition makes it difficult to diagnose because its symptoms are similar to those of COPD. The literature indicates that BO is caused by fibrosis in the small airways, which occurs when the bronchiolar epithelium is damaged and excessive granulation tissue growth occurs. The symptoms and signs on imaging tests can be similar to those in COPD, which can make the diagnosis harder. In addition, BO can be caused by toxic exposures and autoimmune diseases, which shows why healthcare providers should be aware of it. Understanding these connections ensures timely intervention and improves the management of respiratory disorders that may initially appear to be straightforward cases of COPD or other common conditions (King et al., 1989). Effective management of respiratory disorders often incorporates advanced treatments such as non-invasive ventilation (NIV), which has become a cornerstone in the care of patients experiencing respiratory failure. NIV is a significant change from intubation, since it offers support without the usual dangers of intubation, such as tracheal injury or infections. It works best in acute cases, such as COPD exacerbations and ARDS, as prompt respiratory support can significantly impact the patient's recovery. NIV allows patients to avoid surgery and still receive help with breathing, which has proven to be very helpful in both short-term and long-term situations. As non-invasive approaches continue to evolve and expand in their applications, they serve as a vital resource for healthcare professionals aiming to optimize care and enhance quality of life in individuals affected by a range of respiratory disorders (Kumar et al., 2022).

Definition and Significance of Respiratory Disorders

Many respiratory disorders can significantly impact breathing, leading to a reduced oxygen supply and difficulty expelling carbon dioxide. Due to being complex and long-lasting, COPD, asthma, ARDS, and pulmonary fibrosis cause difficulties for both patients and the healthcare system. Respiratory disorders are defined as more than just problems with breathing; they also consider the various causes, which can be environmental, genetic, or related to lifestyle. Understanding the underlying causes of these disorders enables doctors to diagnose them early and manage them effectively, ultimately improving patients' lives and reducing healthcare costs. Respiratory conditions are also a significant concern worldwide since they increase the risk of illness and death, so it is important to carry out extensive public health actions and keep researching their causes. Recognizing and addressing respiratory disorders is crucial because they are closely linked to gas exchange and maintaining a stable metabolism. Problems with respiration can result in hypoxemia and hypercapnia, which can harm different parts of the body. For instance, chronic diseases like COPD and asthma can precipitate respiratory failure, which is categorized into Type I (hypoxemic) and Type II (hypercapnic) respiratory failure. Since these disorders can have a serious impact on the body, it is crucial to provide close monitoring and support, particularly in emergency settings. Additionally, current pulmonology practice suggests that using corticosteroids helps reduce inflammation and improve the airways' response. Corticosteroids have diverse applications, addressing reactive airway diseases and chronic inflammation, but also necessitating careful consideration of their adverse effects on a patient's health (Baloch et al., 2017). Treating respiratory disorders now focuses more on providing individualized care that targets the unique causes in each patient. With the help of precision medicine and technological progress, it has become possible to make better diagnoses and develop targeted drugs. Asthma management, for instance, has benefited from identifying various types of the disease which has resulted in new biologic agents that can be used to treat each patient more effectively. Also, it is now crucial in critical care to understand when to use ventilatory support, invasive or non-invasive, to help patients survive. As research progresses, the integration of emerging therapeutic modalities will be crucial in addressing the complexities of respiratory disorders, ultimately leading to improved patient outcomes and a deeper understanding of their pathophysiology (Grobler et al., 2012) (Figure 15.1).

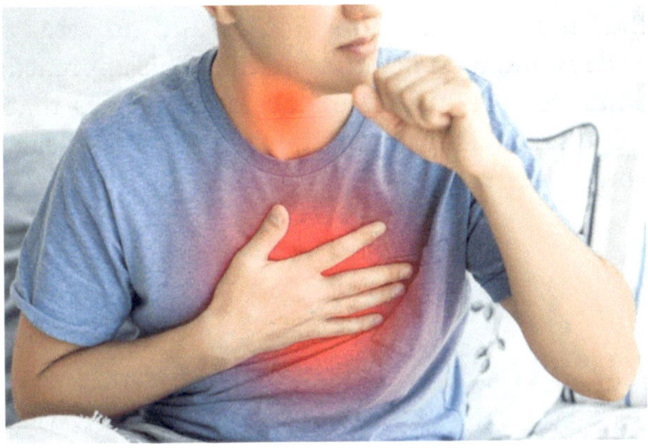

Figure 15.1. Representation of respiratory distress in an individual, highlighting key symptoms such as chest discomfort and persistent coughing.

Source: https://www.shutterstock.com/image-photo/sore-throat-cough-man-lung-600nw-2089273759.jpg.

Overview of Common Respiratory Disorders

There are many types of respiratory disorders, and each one can have a significant effect on breathing. COPD is recognized as a primary reason for sickness and death around the world. COPD causes chronic bronchitis and emphysema, which result in a chronic cough, phlegm, and difficulty breathing. Because the disease worsens over time, it becomes increasingly challenging to maintain quality of life; therefore, we should focus on its underlying causes, which are airflow blockage and inflammation in the airways. On the other hand, asthma is a condition where airways become blocked and then open again, typically due to environmental factors such as allergens or irritants. Many patients experience episodes of wheezing and difficulty breathing, underscoring the need for prompt diagnosis and efforts to control airway inflammation and constriction. ARDS and pulmonary fibrosis reveal another aspect of respiratory disorders, with ARDS typically triggered by acute lung injury (ALI) from various causes, including pneumonia, trauma, or sepsis. The primary feature of ARDS is that it causes severe breathing difficulties and low oxygen levels rapidly, due to increased permeability of the alveolar-capillary membrane, which leads to pulmonary edema. Those who are affected usually need immediate medical care, which can include putting them on a ventilator to help them breathe properly. Pulmonary fibrosis refers to a group of lung diseases in which the tissue in the lungs becomes scarred, over time reducing the exchange of oxygen and carbon dioxide. The leading causes are often chronic inflammation and scarring, which damage the typical structure of the lungs, so it is important to catch this condition early and provide treatment. There are two kinds of respiratory failure: Type I, which is hypoxemic and involves low oxygen levels, and Type II, which is hypercapnic and involves too much carbon dioxide in the body. These failures can arise from various underlying conditions, including COPD exacerbations, severe pneumonia, and central nervous system (CNS) depression. The need for urgent care, such as oxygen or ventilation, is often necessary because these conditions can quickly lead to more serious problems. It is essential for healthcare providers to understand the pathophysiology of these disorders because it shapes the way ventilatory support is chosen. Consequently, mastery of ventilatory concepts, as outlined in clinical literature, such as those found in Drasovean et al. (2023), is essential in improving patient outcomes in the context of these common respiratory disorders. Furthermore, ongoing research, as presented in Cross et al. (2011), highlights the importance of comprehensive surveillance and intervention frameworks in enhancing respiratory health, particularly among high-risk populations.

Importance of Understanding Pathophysiology

Pathophysiology is important in treating respiratory illnesses because it helps identify the primary causes of the disease. This helps healthcare providers understand the changes in the body that happen in COPD and Asthma, which share similar but not identical inflammatory processes. If clinicians understand these pathways, they can give patients the best treatment options. For instance, corticosteroids are frequently used in managing these conditions due to their ability to modulate the inflammatory response. The efficacy of this treatment hinges on an in-depth understanding of how glucocorticoids interact with immune cells, as noted in recent literature (Baloch et al., 2017). Recognizing these difficulties, clinicians can more accurately predict how the disease will progress and take targeted steps to manage symptoms. Pathophysiology also plays a crucial role in the development of new treatments. Special interventions, often including ventilators, are usually needed for respiratory problems such as ARDS and Pulmonary Fibrosis. Knowledge of the pathophysiological changes in lung function informs which types of ventilatory modes are most suitable, such as pressure-controlled versus volume-controlled ventilation (Falkenström et al., 2010). allows researchers to search for innovative ways to treat them, for example, with biologics that can control Taking this approach helps shift care from treating symptoms alone to focusing on the whole patient, so each person gets the best and most personalized treatment. Additionally, possessing a strong knowledge of pathophysiology is crucial for informing patients and their families about respiratory diseases. Teaching patients is vital for following treatment plans, particularly in chronic diseases such as COPD and Asthma, where modifying their lifestyle is crucial for managing the disease. When patients know the reasons behind their health problems, they are more involved in their treatment, which helps them recover better. If patients understand how their diseases work, they are more likely to recognize when symptoms worsen and when they should consult their doctor. In addition, clinicians can build a team-like relationship with their patients, helping them make decisions that include what they prefer and how they understand their health condition. This approach enhances the quality of care and ensures that treatment plans align with each patient's goals and objectives.

15.1. Chronic Obstructive Pulmonary Disease (COPD)

COPD is a significant health issue worldwide, causing ongoing breathing problems and limited airflow because of problems in the airways and alveoli. Chronic inflammation is the leading cause of COPD which is primarily triggered by inhaling harmful particles or gases, mainly from cigarette smoke. Due to the ongoing inflammation, the airways narrow and their elasticity decreases, which adds to the obstructive ventilatory defect. As these changes continue, the body may become more susceptible to infections and pollutants, which can exacerbate the disease. The ongoing impact of these processes reduces lung function and causes many health problems, which call for proper management strategies to help patients with COPD. Effective management and rehabilitation strategies are crucial in addressing the complexities associated with COPD, which often coexists with multiple comorbidities such as cardiovascular disease (CVD) and diabetes. Pulmonary rehabilitation (PR) has emerged as a cornerstone of COPD management, emphasizing a multifaceted approach that combines exercise training, education, and self-management strategies. The latest guidance recommends employing personalized PR strategies to enhance patient care. COPD patients have shown improvement in physical activity and overall well-being with water-based rehabilitation and Tai Chi. After an exacerbation or lung volume reduction surgery, rehabilitation becomes very important. The tailored intervention not only enables patients to achieve greater lung capacity and endurance but also fosters a more active lifestyle after rehabilitation, underscoring the essential role that physical activity plays in managing COPD effectively (Candemir et al., 2017). Furthermore, it is critical to recognize that the clinical presentation of COPD can share similarities with other respiratory disorders, such as bronchiolitis obliterans (BO), complicating diagnostic efforts. BO is less frequent and causes fibrosis in the small airways, which can result in both obstructive and, occasionally, restrictive breathing problems. Due to this overlap, COPD may be misdiagnosed when both inflammation and fibrosis are found. Being aware of these details helps healthcare providers give the proper care to patients who suffer from toxic fumes or autoimmune diseases. A proper diagnosis is necessary, as incorrectly labeling respiratory problems can result in incorrect treatment, which can significantly impact the patient's life. Therefore, a comprehensive approach that integrates diagnostic precision with effective rehabilitation strategies is fundamental to managing patients with COPD and ensuring optimal care outcomes (King et al., 1989).

15.1.1. Definition and Classification of COPD

COPD is a condition that gets worse over time, causing airflow limitation because of chronic bronchitis and emphysema. When people are exposed to harmful particles or gases for a long time, usually from smoking cigarettes, this can cause both diseases. Because of the inflammation in COPD, the airways and the pulmonary parenchyma are structurally altered, and this leads to obstruction and reduced gas exchange. Because COPD is composed of different components, its definition highlights the complexity of the illness and underscores the need to investigate how the disease develops and impacts multiple bodily functions. Due to this complexity, accurate classification is crucial for selecting the appropriate treatment and management plan for patients with this condition. The classification of COPD primarily revolves around the Global Initiative for Chronic Obstructive Lung Disease (GOLD) framework, which incorporates assessments of airflow limitation, symptoms, and a history of exacerbations. The severity of airflow limitation is categorized using post-bronchodilator spirometry results, with stages ranging from mild (GOLD 1) to very severe (GOLD 4). Additionally, the assessment of symptoms is supported by tools such as the Modified Medical Research Council (mMRC) dyspnea scale and the COPD Assessment Test (CAT). Healthcare providers can create personalized treatment plans when they utilize these elements in combination. With this knowledge, doctors can identify diseases more easily, track how the disease progresses, and use treatments that fit the patient's individual needs, ultimately benefiting the patient. Additionally, it is crucial to assess and classify COPD in greater detail than just through clinical evaluation. Managing COPD effectively requires understanding the various risk factors, including exposure to pollutants, genetic predisposition, and other underlying health conditions. When healthcare professionals identify these risk factors, they can recommend prevention strategies and ways to mitigate risks for individuals at risk of developing COPD, which is crucial for addressing the public health impact of the disease. As scientists learn more about how diseases interact, they may develop more effective ways to classify them and discover new treatments. Thus, recognizing the definition and classifications of COPD serves as a foundational aspect in the broader context of respiratory disorders, echoing the need for continued education and awareness surrounding this prevalent chronic illness (Figure 15.2).

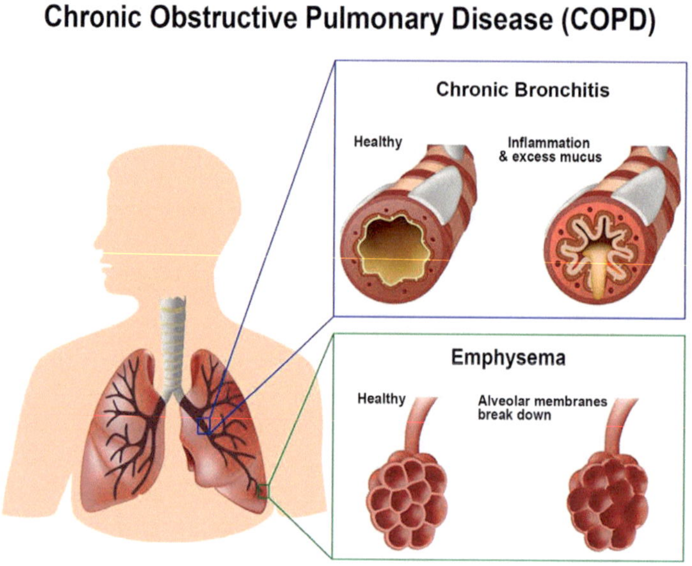

Figure 15.2. Chronic obstructive pulmonary disease (COPD).

Source: https://images.theconversation.com/files/51298/original/5vq77fd6-1402980783.jpg?ixlib=rb-4.1.0&q=45&auto=format&w=754&fit=clip.

15.1.2. Pathophysiological Mechanisms Involved

Common respiratory diseases, such as COPD and asthma, are caused by the interaction of inflammation, oxidative stress, and changes in the airways. COPD is caused by inhaling pollutants and cigarette smoke, which result in a constant inflammatory process that damages the lungs and changes the airways. The nuclear factor erythroid 2-related factor (Nrf2) pathway plays a pivotal role in protecting against oxidative stress. Usually, this transcriptional activator increases cell defenses; however, when there is excessive oxidative stress, it disrupts the balance, allowing cells to be damaged, which facilitates the progression of diseases. Changes in the Keap1-Nrf2 signaling pathway have been identified in various respiratory diseases, suggesting that restoring Nrf2 activity could serve as a therapeutic target for managing symptoms of COPD and asthma (Lee et al., 2021). In addition to COPD and asthma, acute respiratory distress syndrome (ARDS) and pulmonary fibrosis also demonstrate distinct pathophysiological mechanisms anchored in inflammatory responses and fibrotic processes. The primary feature of ARDS is widespread damage to the alveoli, leading to increased vascular permeability and hindering gas exchange. Neutrophils and pro-inflammatory cytokines are released in large numbers during the acute inflammatory response, exacerbating lung injury. Pulmonary fibrosis occurs when the body heals from repeated lung damage by depositing excessive collagen, which reduces the lungs' ability to function properly. A proper balance between the two types of factors is necessary because a disruption can lead to ongoing changes in the tissue. Studying how these pathways interact gives us ideas for treatments that may reduce fibrosis and help patients with these severe conditions—in addition, knowing how respiratory failure, especially Types I and II, works is vital for choosing the right management strategies, such as using NIV. In type I respiratory failure, there is low oxygen in the blood but normal carbon dioxide levels, which often happens in pneumonia or ARDS, due to difficulty with gas exchange. In Type II respiratory failure, the ventilation and perfusion are not balanced, which results in hypercapnia and is commonly linked to flare-ups of COPD. NIV usage results in lower rates of endotracheal intubation and its associated problems. Evidence suggests that early intervention with NIV in immobilized patients, especially during severe COPD exacerbations or acute cardiogenic pulmonary edema, leads to improved outcomes and a decrease in hospital stays (Navarra et al., 2020). Hence, an in-depth understanding of these mechanisms is crucial for optimizing therapeutic strategies and improving patient care in respiratory disorders (Figure 15.3).

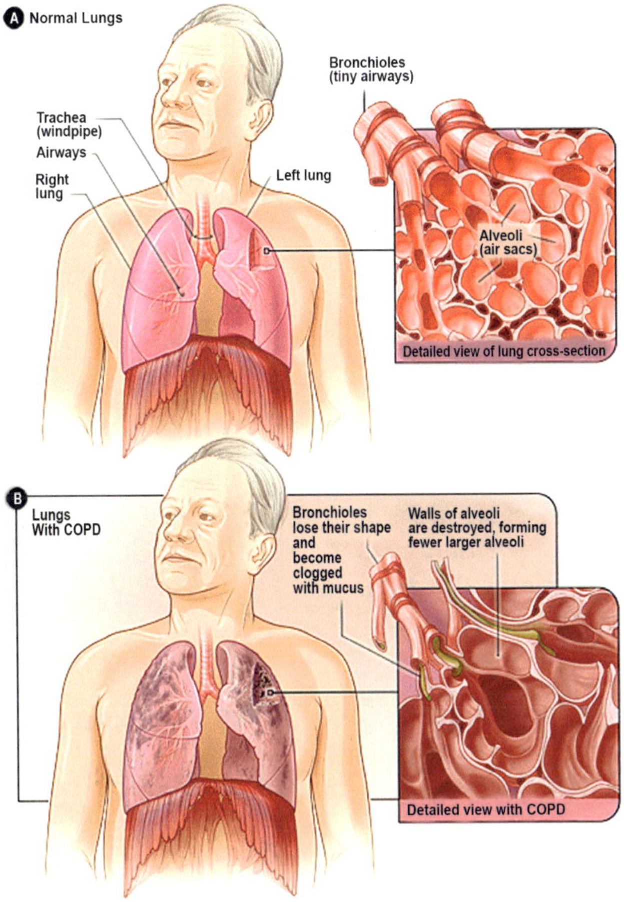

Figure 15.3. Normal lungs shown in upper diagram. Lungs damaged by COPD in lower diagram with an inset showing a cross-section of bronchioles blocked by mucus and damaged alveoli.

Source: https://upload.wikimedia.org/wikipedia/commons/9/93/Copd_2010.jpg.

15.1.3. Clinical Manifestations and Diagnosis

Common respiratory disorders are often recognized through their clinical signs, which are important for making a diagnosis and planning treatment. Common symptoms of COPD include a persistent cough, wheezing, and difficulty breathing, which tend to worsen over time. Asthma usually causes episodes of difficulty breathing, tightness in the chest, and increased mucus production, which is triggered by environmental factors. Alternatively, ARDS is often linked to severe respiratory failure that shows up fast with symptoms such as dyspnea, cyanosis, and hypoxemia. Recognizing these clinical features is vital for healthcare providers, as they guide the differential diagnosis, which distinguishes these conditions from others that might exhibit similar symptoms but require different therapeutic approaches, potentially affecting treatment outcomes (Yuri and Leonid, 2020). A respiratory disorder is typically diagnosed by carefully reviewing the patient's medical history, conducting a physical examination, and utilizing various diagnostic tests. Usually, clinicians assess the patient's symptoms, medical background and any factors in the environment that could worsen breathing problems. Pulmonary function tests (PFTs), including spirometry, are instrumental in quantifying airflow limitation, particularly in COPD and asthma, enabling an objective assessment of disease severity. Tests such as chest X-rays and CT scans are used to gain a deeper understanding of pathological changes, particularly in cases of pulmonary fibrosis or ARDS. Blood gas tests also check the amounts of oxygen and carbon dioxide, which help identify respiratory failure. These diagnostic avenues, when combined with clinical evaluations, form a holistic approach to understanding the underlying pathophysiological processes of respiratory disorders (Baloch et al., 2017). It is crucial to diagnose respiratory problems promptly and accurately for effective care. If a diagnosis is incorrect, the patient may not receive the correct treatment at the right time, which could exacerbate their condition. An example is when bronchodilators are relied on without corticosteroids to treat asthma, which can actually make the disease worse. When ARDS is diagnosed quickly, ventilatory support can be initiated, and the underlying cause, such as infection or trauma, can be treated. Understanding the symptoms of COPD enables healthcare providers to teach patients how to manage their symptoms and prevent them from worsening. Ultimately, an acute awareness of the clinical features and diagnostic methods is essential for optimizing outcomes in patients with common respiratory disorders (Yuri and Leonid, 2020) (Figure 15.4).

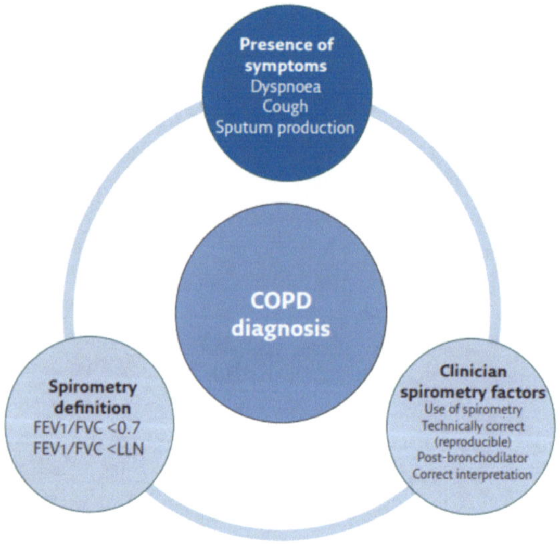

Figure 15.4. Components of a COPD diagnosis.

Source: https://www.researchgate.net/publication/332482825/figure/fig2/AS:748868861976576@1555555658515/Components-of-a-COPD-diagnosis.png.

15.2. Asthma

The primary feature of asthma is inflammation in the airways, which causes intermittent airflow obstruction and leads to breathing difficulties.

Eosinophils, mast cells, T-lymphocytes, and epithelial cells are some of the cellular parts that are linked in this pathology. Such interactions cause the airways to become overly sensitive and alter their structure, leading to bronchoconstriction, mucus overproduction, and swelling of the airways. The changes in the airways lead to the main symptoms of asthma, such as wheezing, shortness of breath, chest tightness, and coughing, which are often worse at night or in the early morning. The way asthma develops is important, critical because it helps identify what causes the disease and leads to finding treatments that reduce inflammation and lower the risk of future exacerbations, which improves both the quality of life and health outcomes for patients. Due to recent advancements in understanding asthma, doctors can now utilize a range of new treatments that necessitate individualized care.

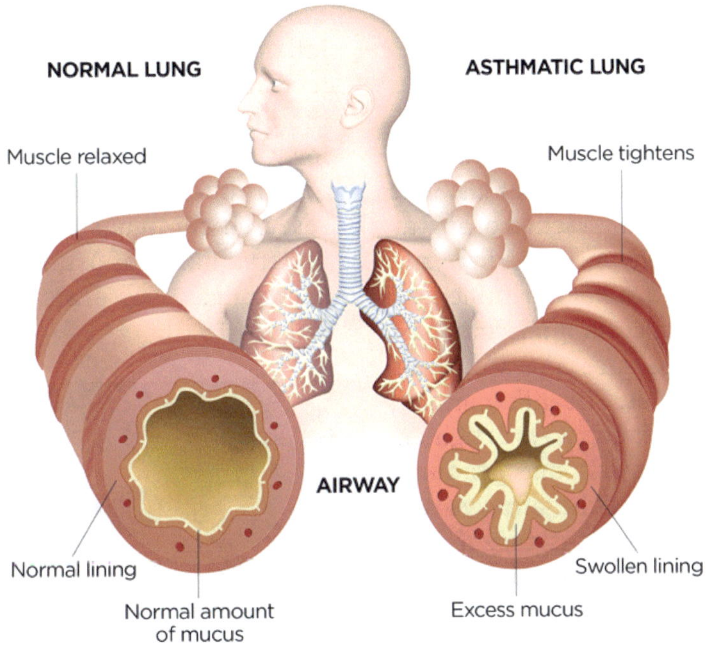

Figure 15.5. Normal vs. asthma lung.

Source: https://irp.cdn-website.com/2e75da1a/dms3rep/multi/normal-vs-asthma-lung.png.

Biologics that target specific pathways in allergic asthma have been studied, and those that block interleukin-5 and other cytokines have proven to be highly effective. They work by tackling the inflammation that causes the disease, not only by reducing the symptoms. In addition, managing asthma effectively involves controlling the environment and educating patients, as avoiding allergens and irritants supports the use of medications. Recent research highlights the potential for interventions like bronchial thermoplasty, which offers a novel approach by precisely targeting airway smooth muscle to reduce hyperreactivity, marking a paradigm shift in the therapeutic landscape for asthma treatment (Toma, 2005). An asthma exacerbation can cause severe breathing problems and requires understanding how it happens and what can be done to help. Asthma has a strong effect on the lungs, and research shows that people with uncontrolled asthma may gradually lose lung function. In addition, asthma often leads to increased use of medical services and expenses, particularly when individuals require emergency care or are hospitalized. Severe asthma attacks can lead to respiratory failure, which shows how asthma and other respiratory problems are connected. Timely and effective management strategies are crucial for mitigating the risk of respiratory failure and enhancing overall patient outcomes, underscoring the importance of comprehensive asthma care within the broader scope of respiratory pathophysiology (Figure 15.5).

15.2.1. Definition and Types of Asthma

Asthma is a condition in which the airways become inflamed, causing people to experience repeated episodes of wheezing, difficulty breathing, chest tightness, and coughing. The symptoms are caused by the interaction of airway inflammation, bronchial hyperreactivity, and airflow obstruction. The primary pathological process is the activation of eosinophils and mast cells which then releases substances such as histamines and leukotrienes. The inflammation causes the muscles around the airways to tighten, makes the airway linings swell, and produces more mucus, which narrows the airways and makes it difficult to breathe. It is essential to understand the definition and the underlying processes of asthma to effectively manage it and help patients lead better lives. Depending on their causes, triggers, and how they are treated, asthma can be put into several distinct types. The most common forms include allergic (extrinsic) asthma, which is often triggered by environmental allergens such as pollen, dust mites, or pet dander, and non-allergic (intrinsic) asthma, which respiratory infections, stress, or exposure to cold air may induce. Many people with asthma experience exercise-induced bronchoconstriction, which occurs during physical activity. Asthma symptoms may be triggered in some workers by certain substances found in their workplaces, which can result in occupational asthma. All in all, understanding these types of asthma helps doctors choose management strategies that target each patient's specific causes and triggers. Due to the fact that asthma is a complex condition, it is essential to employ effective methods for diagnosing and treating it in the clinic. Recognizing that inflammation makes the airways more reactive and prone to narrowing is an important part of managing asthma. Usually, ICSs are used to address inflammation, and bronchodilators are given to help relax the airway muscles and ease symptoms. Additionally, new treatments for asthma have prompted scientists to investigate the molecular mechanisms underlying airway inflammation and remodeling. It appears that focusing on specific inflammatory pathways in therapy could lead to more effective treatments for various types of asthma, benefiting patients and reducing the need for healthcare. As research continues to evolve, a more nuanced understanding of asthma will further enhance personalized care practices in respiratory health (Figure 15.6).

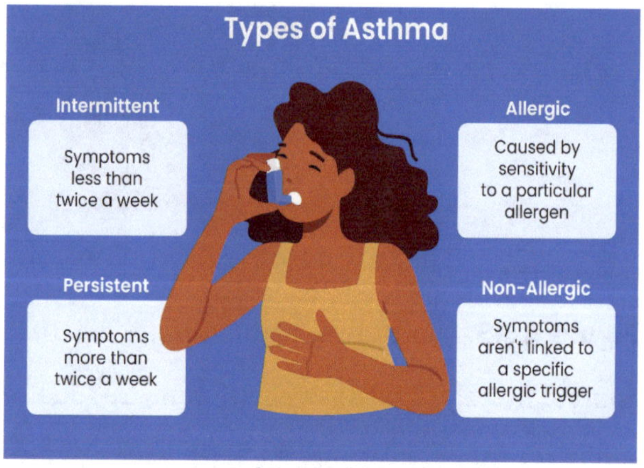

Figure 15.6. Types of asthma.

Source: https://images.ctfassets.net/yixw23k2v6vo/1dHP21MpLyIqnNxG2NTO2N/6880d4d362a80ed4c1be5a7fa262bd89/Gettyimages-1453953402-asthma-types.jpg.

15.2.2. Pathophysiological Changes During an Asthma Attack

During an asthma attack, the main changes happen because of inflammation and constriction of the airways, which come from an overactive immune system reacting to different triggers. If the airway epithelium is exposed to allergens, irritants, or viruses, it gets activated and releases histamine, leukotrienes, and cytokines. They cause inflammatory cells, especially eosinophils and mast cells, to gather, which results in swelling of the airway walls. The process causes the bronchi to narrow, which makes it harder for air to move and is a main reason for the symptoms of asthma, such as wheezing and shortness of breath.

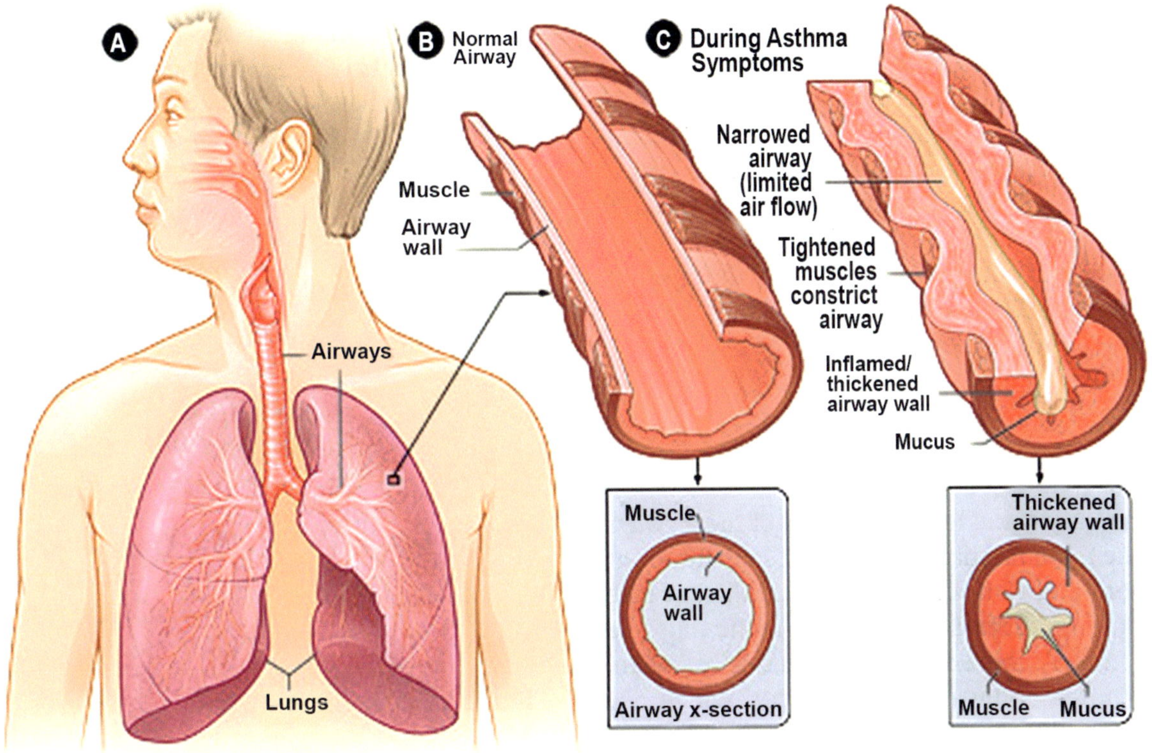

Figure 15.7. (A) shows the location of the lungs and airways in the body; (B) shows a cross-section of a normal airway; and (C) shows a cross-section of an airway during asthma symptoms.

Source: https://upload.wikimedia.org/wikipedia/commons/4/4a/Asthma_attack-illustration_NIH.jpg.

The inflammation can cause the airways to change over time, leading to long-term changes in lung function and increasing the difficulty of managing asthma. The airways become increasingly blocked during an asthma attack as the bronchial muscles contract, resulting in difficulty breathing. When there is inflammation, the bronchial tissues become more sensitive to any additional stimuli, which makes bronchoconstriction worse. Additionally, producing excessive mucus is common, which narrows the airways and makes breathing more difficult. The combination of inflamed bronchial tissue and tightened muscles causes a cycle that makes the asthma attack continue. These events can cause immediate breathing problems and also make the airways more sensitive, which may lead to long-term lung issues. If triggers are present all the time and treatment is lacking, it can cause serious health problems and risk respiratory failure in the worst cases. All of these changes eventually lead to a severe breathing problem characterized by difficulty exhaling. If airflow remains obstructed, hypoxemia may develop due to poor oxygen exchange, which can cause the body to respond with actions that put more strain on the heart and lungs. Also, a brutal asthma attack can result in anxiety and a faster heart rate, as the body tries to manage its reduced oxygen supply. Even though there are drugs to help with asthma symptoms, keeping up with these treatments is crucial to prevent further health problems from asthma. Further exploration of treatment efficacy, particularly in the context of emerging respiratory challenges, highlights the need for meticulous clinical management in conditions like coronavirus disease 2019 (COVID-19), where overlap of pathophysiological mechanisms can pose significant therapeutic challenges (Calzetta et al., 2020; Yuri & Leonid, 2020) (Figure 15.7).

15.2.3. Triggers and Risk Factors Associated with Asthma

Inflammation and hyperreactivity of the airways are the main features of asthma. Many different triggers and risk factors play a significant role in making asthma worse and managing the condition. Asthma often develops due to pollen, dust mites, mold, and pet dander, which are common environmental allergens. In addition, factors such as tobacco smoke, strong odors, and air pollution can exacerbate symptoms, highlighting the importance of understanding how environmental influences affect disease progression. Programs that reduce contact with these triggers play a key role in improving asthma results and reducing the serious health problems linked to the disease, mainly for more vulnerable people. Because these environmental factors can lead to asthma symptoms, it is important to take action to improve living conditions, which might help reduce the number of asthma attacks and improve life for those affected. Along with environmental causes, personal health details give valuable information about asthma. Having a family history of the disease greatly increases the chances of developing it, which is why genetic predisposition is considered an important risk factor. Having allergic rhinitis and eczema with asthma may indicate that all three share a similar immune system, which can make symptoms worse. Also, being overweight and leading a sedentary life are among the factors that raise the number of asthma cases and make the condition worse. Obesity has been found to make airway inflammation and responsiveness worse, which can make it harder to treat patients.

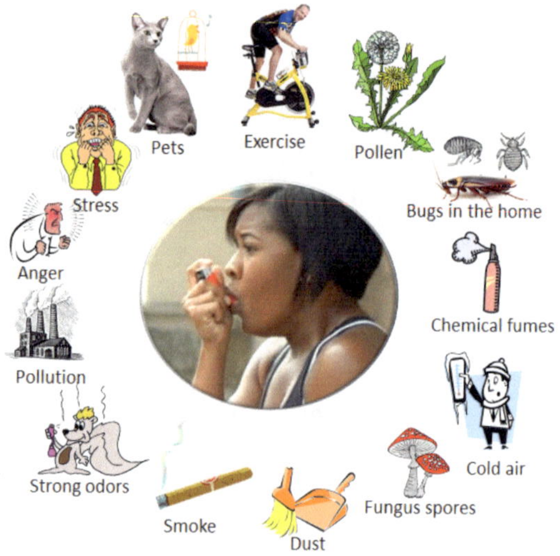

Figure 15.8. Asthma triggers.

Source: https://upload.wikimedia.org/wikipedia/commons/9/97/Asthma_triggers_2.PNG.

Understanding these related health conditions is crucial for guiding doctors in managing asthma, as it indicates that a multifaceted approach is necessary, considering both genetic and lifestyle factors. Due to the COVID-19 pandemic, there are now additional challenges related to asthma risk factors. Researchers have found that patients with previous respiratory problems are more likely to suffer severe consequences if they get SARS-CoV-2, although the details are still not fully understood. When asthma patients contract viral infections, it can lead to more severe symptoms, so their condition needs to be monitored more closely during outbreaks of respiratory viruses. Also, changes brought about by the pandemic (such as being inside more and feeling more stress) could lead to increased exposure to things that irritate the lungs, making asthma harder to control. As highlighted in recent medical literature, including insights from the European Respiratory Society, understanding how such global health crises impact chronic respiratory disorders is vital for developing targeted health policies and interventions tailored to this vulnerable population (Emiralioğlu et al., 2022; Awatade et al., 2023) (Figure 15.8).

15.3. Acute Respiratory Distress Syndrome (ARDS)

ARDS is a critical condition characterized by widespread pulmonary inflammation and increased permeability of the alveolar-capillary membrane, which leads to severe hypoxemia and respiratory failure. ARDS occurs when inflammation, stress on the lungs, and cellular damage interact. When pneumonia, sepsis, or trauma occur, they kickstart the immune system, which then releases pro-inflammatory cytokines. The result is not only fluid in the lungs but also a decrease in gas exchange, which leads to serious oxygen problems for the patient. It is essential to understand the causes of ARDS so that treatments can be designed to reduce inflammation and help patients recover. Since the syndrome has multiple causes, it needs to be managed by addressing the onset of inflammation and its subsequent effects. Recent studies have highlighted that oxidative stress plays a significant role in the development of ARDS. Elevated levels of reactive oxygen species (ROS) can exacerbate lung injury, leading to further complications. Notably, antioxidant therapies, particularly N-acetylcysteine (NAC), have shown promise in ameliorating oxidative stress-related damage in ARDS patients. Research indicates that intravenous NAC administration improves oxygenation and lowers mortality rates among those affected by acute lung injury (ALI) and ARDS when compared to control groups. Due to the impact of genetic variations in glutathione-S-transferase on oxidative stress, doctors should consider personalized treatments.

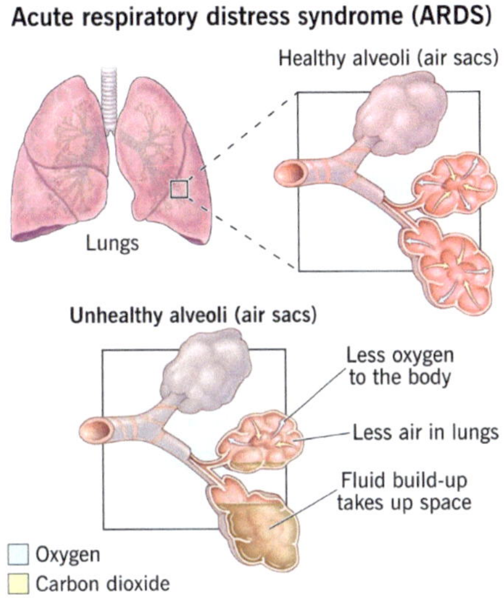

Figure 15.9. Acute respiratory stress syndrome (ARDS).

Source: https://my.clevelandclinic.org/-/scassets/images/org/health/articles/acute-respiratory-stress-syndrome.

As ongoing investigations continue to elucidate the mechanisms of oxidative stress in ARDS, a more nuanced understanding can inform clinical practice and enhance therapeutic interventions (Ghahremani et al., 2009). Because COVID-19 is a relatively new cause of ARDS, researchers and doctors are now studying how it differs from influenza in this regard. Investigations have found that, although COVID-19-related ARDS is characterized by higher compliance and minute ventilation, there are no significant changes in the P/F ratio when compared to ARDS resulting from influenza. Notably, the management of mechanically ventilated patients with COVID-19 has raised questions about the effectiveness of low driving pressures (ΔP) in improving outcomes. It appears that these strategies may, in fact, cause the lungs to lose their ability to function effectively with ventilators over time. So, healthcare providers should adjust their intensive care treatment for patients with COVID-19-related ARDS. An understanding of these differences is crucial for formulating clinical strategies that can optimize patient care in this evolving landscape (Bals et al., 2022) (Figure 15.9).

15.3.1. Definition and Causes of ARDS

ARDS causes the lungs to become severely inflamed very quickly, which leads to significant difficulties in breathing. ARDS is clinically defined by acute onset, pulmonary infiltrates visible on imaging, and decreased oxygenation, typically assessed through the ratio of arterial oxygen to the fraction of inspired oxygen (PaO_2/FiO_2).

The syndrome can occur as a result of many direct and indirect lung problems, such as pneumonia, sepsis, trauma, and swallowing gastric contents. Because of risk factors such as being elderly and having other health problems, it is important to diagnose and treat acute respiratory failure as soon as possible. There are several factors involved in ARDS, including the activation of inflammation, which causes the alveolar-capillary membrane to become more permeable. Because the blood vessels are highly permeable, protein-rich fluid moves into the alveoli, causing pulmonary edema and reducing the lungs' flexibility. At the same time, neutrophils and macrophages enter the area and release substances that sustain the inflammation. If there is a higher number of pro-inflammatory mediators than anti-inflammatory ones, it may cause the lungs to become damaged and fibrotic, which often leads to bad outcomes. To develop the right therapies and supportive care, it is essential to understand how these pathogenic mechanisms interact. The causes of ARDS are either direct lung injuries or indirect injuries, and each situation has its own clinical features. Pneumonia, toxic inhalation and pulmonary contusions are examples of conditions that can cause direct lung injuries because they directly affect the lung parenchyma. In some cases, indirect damage to the lungs is caused by conditions like sepsis or pancreatitis, which eventually interfere with lung function.

The various reasons for ARDS highlight the importance of early detection and appropriate care tailored to the underlying cause. Research continues to identify potential therapeutic interventions, such as corticosteroids, which may modulate the inflammatory response and improve outcomes in ARDS patients (Baloch et al., 2017). Furthermore, ongoing studies are exploring the implications of ARDS in the context of COVID-19, underlining the urgency in understanding its pathophysiology to enhance clinical practices (Yuri & Leonid, 2020) (Table 15.1).

Table 15.1. Common Causes of ARDS

Infections	Inhalation of toxic fumes	Others
Tuberculosis Malaria Leptospirosis Scrub typhus Enteric fever Dengue haemorrhagic fever	Chlorine Methyl isocyanate Nitrogen dioxide Paraffin flames Methylene chloride	Severe pneumonia Aspiration Drowning Fat embolism Acute pancreatitis
Poisoning and Toxins Organophosphours compounds Paraquat	**Obstetric causes** **Heat stroke**	

Source: https://www.researchgate.net/profile/Ashesh-Dhungana/publication/318853135/figure/tbl1/AS:614184219852806@1523444337191/Common-causes-of-ARDS-in-the-tropics.png.

15.3.2. Pathophysiological Processes in ARDS

Several processes in the body become active in ARDS, such as those caused by pneumonia, trauma, and sepsis. Disruption of the alveolar-capillary barrier is a leading cause of ARDS, which results in increased fluid in the lungs. Due to this disruption, proteins and fluid move into the alveoli, which hinders the exchange of gases and leads to atelectasis. Due to hypoxemia, patients with ARDS often require mechanical ventilation, which shows how important it is to know the causes of ARDS. When these inflammatory mediators are released due to injury, they exacerbate the condition, which can lead to lung fibrosis if not addressed early, highlighting the importance of early diagnosis and treatment in this disease. The lungs in ARDS are filled with neutrophils and macrophages, which release cytokines and chemokines. These mediators contribute to further damage to the alveolar epithelium and also facilitate the formation of hyaline membranes, which impede gas exchange. The inflammatory cytokine storm in ARDS patients may cause problems in several organs which makes it harder to treat. The relationship between the immune response and ventilatory mechanics highlights the need for tailored therapeutic approaches, such as the application of low tidal volume strategies in mechanical ventilation to reduce ventilator-induced lung injury (VILI). It is still a significant concern in modern critical care medicine for clinicians to reduce the number of deaths caused by ARDS. ARDS can also result in lung fibrosis, which explains why it is often considered a continuum from ALI to chronic lung illnesses. This series of events highlights the importance of understanding the cellular and molecular processes involved. For example, BO can resemble ARDS and COPD in its symptoms and changes in the body which may lead to confusion in making the correct diagnosis. Being aware of these complexities helps doctors distinguish ARDS from other diseases and also highlights the important steps in monitoring and treating the disease as it progresses. As such, research continues to emphasize elucidating these pathways to enhance both prevention and treatment strategies for ARDS, particularly in the context of emerging respiratory challenges due to viral infections like COVID-19, as noted in studies addressing Cor pulmonale and its related complications (King et al., 1989; Yuri and Leonid, 2020) (Figure 15.10).

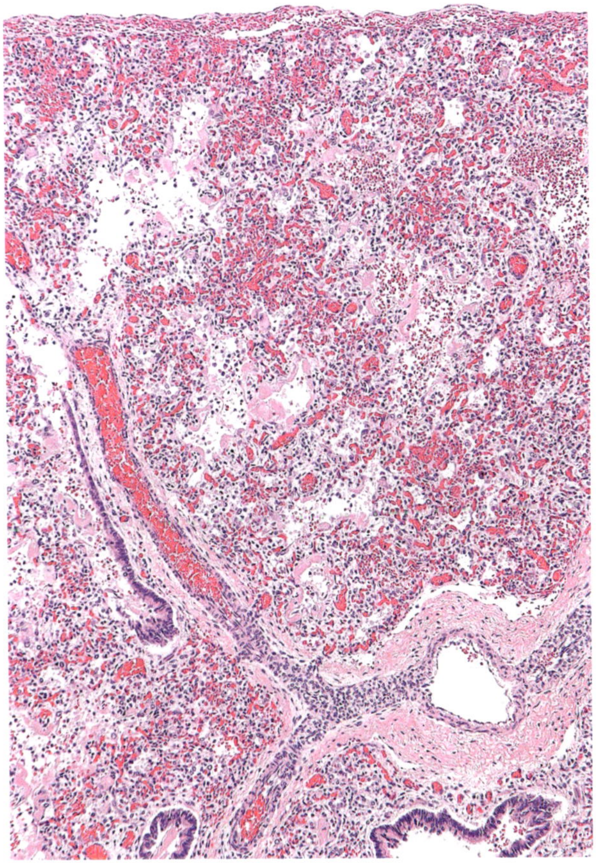

Figure 15.10. Micrograph of diffuse alveolar damage, the histologic correlate of ARDS.

Source: https://upload.wikimedia.org/wikipedia/commons/thumb/4/44/Hyaline_membranes_-_intermed_mag.jpg/800px-Hyaline_membranes_-_intermed_mag.jpg.

15.3.3. Clinical Features and Diagnostic Criteria

COPD, asthma, and ARDS have many common symptoms, which means it is important to assess patients to make an accurate diagnosis carefully. In COPD, a chronic cough and the production of sputum are common, and these symptoms usually get worse as breathing difficulties increase, especially when someone is active. Alternatively, asthma patients may experience reversible airway blockage, causing wheezing, chest tightness, and shortness of breath, which can change in intensity and frequency. Clinical criteria for diagnosing these conditions often include lung function tests, such as spirometry, which measure forced expiratory volume in one second (FEV1) and forced vital capacity (FVC). According to the GOLD guidelines, managing COPD requires monitoring symptoms and lung function to assess the severity of the disease. Respiratory disorders are typically diagnosed using a combination of clinical exams, imaging, and laboratory results. For ARDS, the Berlin Definition sets out specific criteria, which are an acute onset, bilateral opacities seen on chest X-rays, and the presence of pulmonary edema that is not entirely due to heart failure or too much fluid. In patients with pulmonary fibrosis, high-resolution computed tomography (HRCT) plays a pivotal role in identifying the characteristic interstitial patterns that aid in diagnosis. A person's chances of getting these lung conditions are increased by growing older, having smoked before and being exposed to pollutants. As these methods encompass many aspects, practitioners can distinguish between various respiratory disorders and design tailored treatment plans for each patient. Joining clinical signs with diagnostic criteria is very important for the proper management of respiratory illnesses. The use of corticosteroids, while beneficial in reducing inflammation in conditions such as asthma and COPD, must be carefully monitored due to their potential long-term adverse effects on health, including metabolic disturbances and increased susceptibility to infections (Baloch et al., 2017). As more is learned about the causes of these disorders, doctors should employ an assessment approach that aligns with both the symptoms and the test results. It enables doctors to utilize standard treatment plans while still tailoring them to meet the unique needs of each patient, thereby improving clinical outcomes. As emphasized in recent studies, attention to such clinical nuances is vital in addressing the complexities of conditions like respiratory failure, thereby enhancing the overall efficacy of ventilatory support interventions (Yuri and Leonid, 2020) (Figure 15.11).

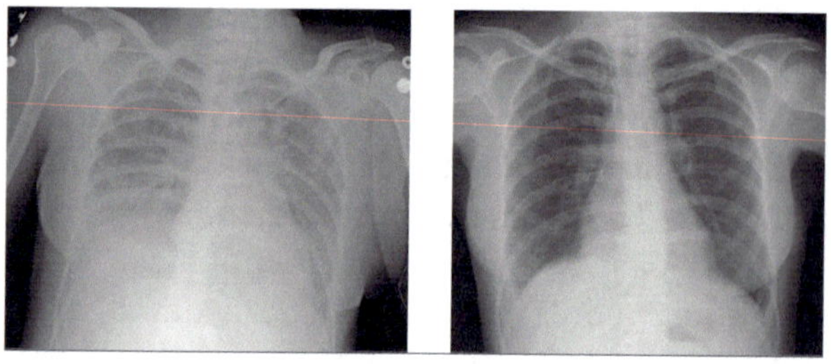

Figure 15.11. A chest X-ray of transfusion-related acute lung injury (left) which led to ARDS. Right is the same patient with resolved injury 72 hours after ventilator support.

Source: https://upload.wikimedia.org/wikipedia/commons/7/73/Transfusion-related_acute_lung_injury_chest_X-ray.gif.

15.4. Pulmonary Fibrosis

Pulmonary fibrosis is understood by examining its leading causes, which include the progressive scarring of lung tissue that eventually deforms the alveoli. Due to this change, gas exchange is disrupted, resulting in blood that lacks sufficient oxygen and can cause symptoms such as dyspnea and chronic cough. The factors that can lead to pulmonary fibrosis are environmental exposures, autoimmune diseases, and certain drugs. The cellular response to lung injury triggers an aberrant healing process that involves the proliferation of fibroblasts and excessive deposition of extracellular matrix (ECM) proteins. Over time, this fibrotic remodeling significantly compromises lung compliance, which in turn contributes to restrictive lung disease—a condition often confused with other respiratory disorders such as COPD (King et al., 1989). Pulmonary fibrosis brings more problems than just breathing difficulties, as it also worsens a patient's quality of life and causes much morbidity. Many patients notice that they become less able to exercise as their lungs are not flexible enough to expand appropriately. Additionally, if breathing becomes more difficult, patients may require supplemental oxygen to manage low oxygen levels and enhance their daily activities. Even with new drugs designed to control fibrosis, there is still a great need for better treatments. The management of pulmonary fibrosis can be complex, requiring a multidisciplinary approach that encompasses pulmonologists, radiologists, and primary care providers, along with the use of tools such as lung function tests and high-resolution computed tomography (HRCT) to monitor disease progression (Kumar et al., 2022). In advanced cases of pulmonary fibrosis, the risk of respiratory failure increases, necessitating interventions such as non-invasive ventilation (NIV) to alleviate symptoms and enhance respiratory support. NIV is now considered a main approach for treating respiratory distress, since it is not as invasive as intubation. NIV can assist in improving ventilation and oxygenation in patients experiencing respiratory failure because of fibrotic lung diseases. The use of non-invasive techniques not only minimizes the risk of complications but also enhances patient comfort, thereby improving treatment adherence (Kumar et al., 2022). As the field of pulmonary medicine evolves, ongoing research is crucial for deepening our understanding of pulmonary fibrosis and refining therapeutic approaches, ultimately aiming for improved patient outcomes in this challenging respiratory disorder (Figure 15.12).

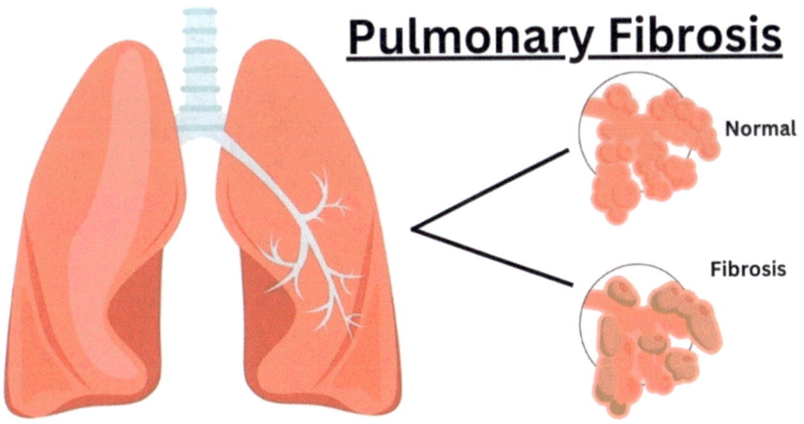

Figure 15.12. Pulmonary fibrosis.

Source: https://drsyedarshadhusainpulmonologist.com/wp-content/uploads/2024/05/7-Things-About-Pulmonary-Fibrosis.jpg.

15.4.1. Definition and Types of Pulmonary Fibrosis

Pulmonary fibrosis is caused by the scarring of lung tissue, resulting in less effective lung function and symptoms such as shortness of breath and a persistent cough. This disease can be classified into various forms, including idiopathic pulmonary fibrosis (IPF), which arises without a known cause, and secondary pulmonary fibrosis, which stems from identifiable factors such as environmental exposure, autoimmune diseases, or drug toxicity. There is an imbalance in pulmonary fibrosis between epithelial cell injury, inflammation, and fibrosis, leading to unusual repair and the accumulation of extra ECM components. Understanding the various forms of pulmonary fibrosis is crucial for treating patients and enhancing their outcomes in lung disorders with fibrosis. One of the primary forms of pulmonary fibrosis, IPF, is difficult because the cause is not well understood. It usually impacts older people and causes worsening breathing problems, which result in a reduced quality of life and higher death rates. Usually, IPF is diagnosed by combining HRCT scans and lung biopsies to spot reticular patterns and honeycombing. On the other hand, secondary pulmonary fibrosis is often linked to connective tissue diseases, chronic hypersensitivity pneumonitis, and exposures at work. Because pulmonary fibrosis is so complex and varies, its management depends on the type and can include antifibrotic drugs or lung transplantation for advanced disease. Although different types of pulmonary fibrosis share common traits, understanding the underlying causes of inflammation and tissue structural changes is crucial for developing effective treatments. Fibroblasts are regularly active and produce more fibrous tissues, which is a key feature of the disease. It has been found that persistent inflammation contributes to the development of pulmonary fibrosis, and unbalanced immune reactions prolong the disease's duration. Insights into mechanisms such as apoptosis and efferocytosis reveal how failure to resolve inflammation can lead to chronic changes in lung tissue, emphasizing the interplay between inflammation and fibrosis in pulmonary disorders (Caudrillier et al., 2016; Husebø et al., 2021). This understanding not only enhances knowledge of pulmonary fibrosis but also promotes the exploration of novel treatment modalities that may mitigate progression and alleviate symptoms (Figure 15.13).

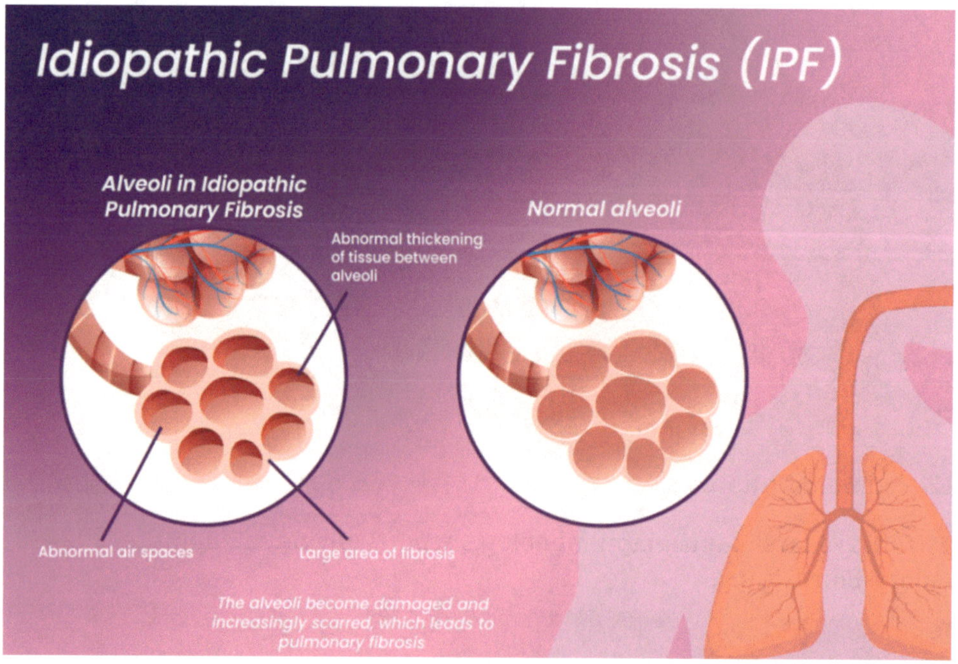

Figure 15.13. Idiopathic pulmonary fibrosis (IPF).

Source: https://www.cambridgenetwork.co.uk/sites/default/files/styles/article_main/public/Idiopathic%20Pulmonary%20Fibrosis.png?itok=v5VdxaH_.

15.4.2. Pathophysiological Mechanisms Leading to Fibrosis

Fibrosis happens when there is too much ECM in the lungs, which results in scarring and stiffness. COPD and asthma, which are common respiratory disorders, cause chronic inflammation that leads to a series of actions that make tissue damage and fibrosis worse. The inflammation occurs because there are more pro-inflammatory mediators than anti-inflammatory ones, which leads to fibroblasts and myofibroblasts becoming active. Such cells are important for making collagen and other proteins in the ECM, which help repair tissue, but can also result in too much fibrotic tissue if not controlled. Recognizing this imbalance is crucial for understanding the causes of fibrotic lung diseases and for developing treatments that help restore balance in the body's inflammatory responses. Researchers have given considerable attention to the role that oxidative stress plays in initiating and progressing fibrosis. ROS produced during inflammation can damage cells and at the same time stimulate ongoing inflammation, which is a leading cause of fibrosis. The Nrf2 signaling pathway is critical here since it helps protect cells from oxidative stress. Under typical conditions, the Kelch-like ECH-associated protein 1 (KEAP1) regulates Nrf2 activity, but severe oxidative stress can disrupt this pathway, leading to unchecked inflammation and subsequent fibrotic changes in lung tissue. Studies have demonstrated that alterations in the Keap1-Nrf2 signaling may contribute directly to respiratory diseases, including ARDS and pulmonary fibrosis, reinforcing the critical impact of oxidative stress in these processes (Lee et al., 2021). The recent spread of COVID-19 has made it clear that understanding fibrosis in viral respiratory infections is significant. An infection with SARS-CoV-2 can cause severe inflammation, which is sometimes called a cytokine storm, and this can result in ARDS. Inflammation mediated by cytokines such as interleukin-6 (IL-6) and IL-1 not only exacerbates ALI but also has been implicated in the fibrotic remodeling of lung tissue. Lung tissue from patients with fibrosis shows many destroyed pneumocytes and the presence of a hyaluronan membrane, which are the prominent signs of fibrosis. The interplay between persistent inflammation and the fibrotic remodeling observed in COVID-19 underscores the need for therapeutic strategies that target inflammatory pathways to prevent or mitigate the development of fibrosis in patients with severe respiratory viral infections (Azimi et al., 2020).

15.4.3. Symptoms and Diagnostic Approaches

The identification of symptoms in respiratory disorders is crucial for effective diagnosis and management. Common symptoms across various respiratory disorders such as COPD, asthma, ARDS, and pulmonary fibrosis include dyspnea, cough, and wheezing. These symptoms can vary significantly in their presentation and severity, often complicating the diagnostic process. For instance, in COPD, patients typically experience a progressive decline in respiratory function characterized by chronic cough and sputum production. Conversely, asthma manifests primarily as intermittent wheezing and shortness of breath, which specific triggers can exacerbate. Understanding these symptoms is essential, as early recognition can lead to timely interventions and reductions in morbidity associated with these conditions (Bogun et al., 2017). The clinical context in which these symptoms occur also plays a vital role in informing the diagnostic approach adopted by healthcare practitioners. Diagnostic approaches for respiratory disorders necessitate a comprehensive evaluation, including a thorough patient history, physical examinations, and various diagnostic tests (Figure 15.14). Many doctors rely on spirometry to aid in the diagnosis of COPD and asthma by assessing lung function. The outcomes determine the seriousness of the disease and help decide on treatment. Radiographic imaging, particularly chest X-rays and computed tomography (CT) scans, is also essential in diagnosing pulmonary fibrosis and ARDS, where structural lung changes can be visualized. Furthermore, arterial blood gas (ABG) analysis is crucial for identifying the degree of respiratory failure, whether Type I or Type II, by assessing oxygenation and carbon dioxide levels (Emiralioğlu et al., 2022).

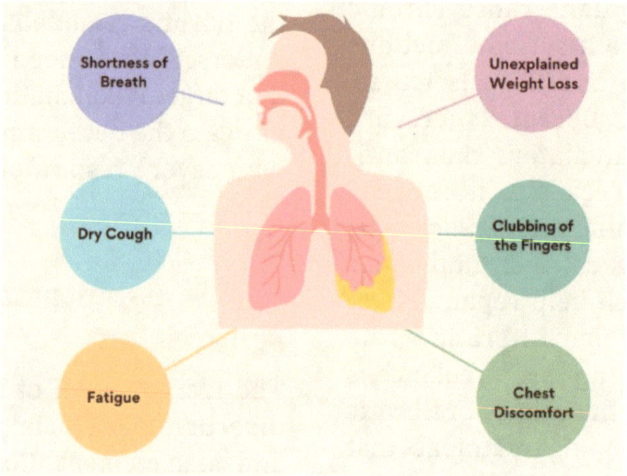

Figure 15.14. Symptoms of idiopathic pulmonary fibrosis (IPF).

Source: https://continentalhospitals.com/uploads/mceu_70013423511734338323837.jpg.

By pulling together information from patients and test results, healthcare providers can make an accurate diagnosis and develop a treatment plan tailored to each patient. Additionally, the use of diagnostic guidelines has made it easier to identify and treat respiratory disorders.

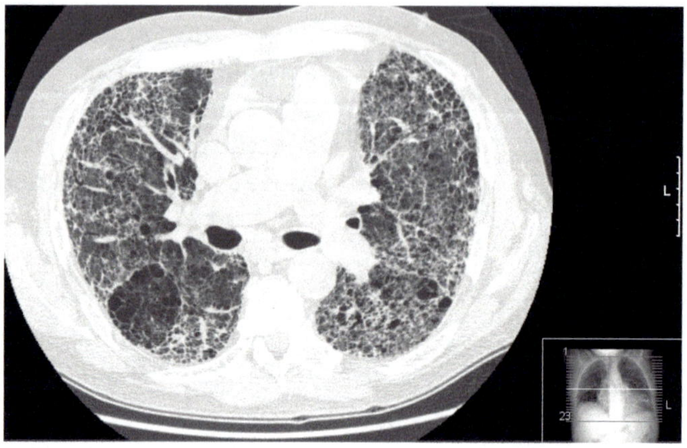

Figure 15.15. HRCT of lung showing extensive fibrosis possibly from usual interstitial pneumonitis. There is also a large bulla.

Source: https://upload.wikimedia.org/wikipedia/commons/8/81/Pulmon_fibrosis.PNG.

The GOLD helps clinicians by supplying standard approaches to diagnosing and managing COPD. In asthma management, the Global Initiative for Asthma (GINA) guidelines emphasize the importance of a stepwise approach to therapy based on symptom control and lung function metrics. Recent improvements in imaging technology have made it possible to monitor the progression of ARDS and pulmonary fibrosis more effectively. These structured approaches not only ensure accurate diagnosis but also assist in differentiating between various respiratory disorders, thereby optimizing management strategies for individuals (Bogun et al., 2017). Recognizing the symptoms and utilizing appropriate diagnostic tools are foundational to effective respiratory care, reducing the burden of these common and often debilitating disorders (Figure 15.15).

15.5. Respiratory Failure

Respiratory failure happens when the respiratory system cannot keep up with gas exchange, which results in major changes in the body's functions. There are two main types: Type I, which is mostly marked by hypoxemia without hypercapnia, and Type II, which has both hypoxemia and hypercapnia. Many different factors can lead to ARDS and pulmonary fibrosis, which are common causes of Type I ARDS. In contrast, Type II respiratory failure usually happens due to COPD, various systemic diseases or problems with the muscles used for breathing. Understanding the causes of respiratory failure is crucial, as it enables the selection of appropriate treatments to restore normal gas exchange and enhance the patient's overall well-being. In most cases, respiratory failure is managed through the use of advanced treatments, one of which is initiating ventilatory support. Non-invasive methods, such as Continuous Positive Airway Pressure (CPAP) and Bi-level Positive Airway Pressure (BiPAP), are frequently employed, particularly for patients exhibiting Type II respiratory failure due to COPD exacerbations. They help expand the lungs at the end of each breath, making breathing easier and supporting gas exchange. If the condition is severe, doctors may choose invasive mechanical ventilation to help the patient breathe properly and remove carbon dioxide. Clinicians should monitor for complications associated with long-term use of ventilatory support, such as ventilation-induced lung injury and weakening of the respiratory muscles, which may negatively impact the patient's overall recovery. Besides ventilation, the use of corticosteroids is crucial in treating the inflammation that often leads to respiratory failure. Corticosteroids control inflammation and can significantly decrease airway swelling in asthma and COPD, which helps these patients breathe better. As the understanding of corticosteroids and their diverse pharmacological effects evolves, the therapeutic approach must be tailored to the individual, balancing the benefits against potential adverse effects, such as osteoporosis and increased susceptibility to infections (Baloch et al., 2017). Additionally, ongoing research into emerging therapies and interventions aims to refine management strategies for respiratory failure, enhancing patient care and improving survival rates in increasingly complex clinical scenarios (Cagnone et al., 2018) (Figure 15.16).

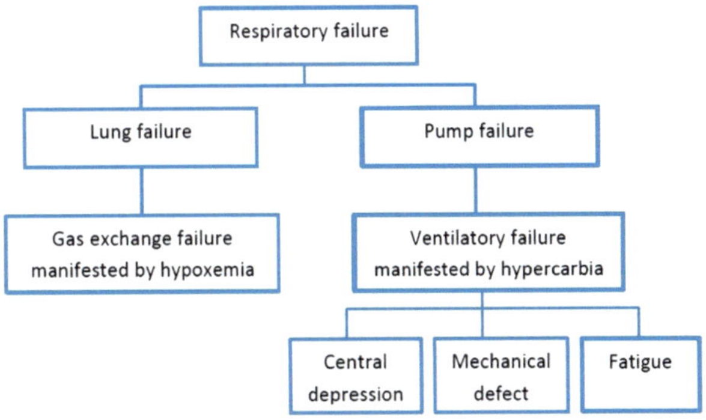

Figure 15.16. Respiratory failure.

Source: https://novapulmonary.com/wp-content/uploads/2020/03/Respiratory-Failure.jpg.

15.5.1. Definition and Classification of Respiratory Failure

Respiratory failure occurs when the respiratory system is unable to maintain adequate gas exchange in the body. A person with this disorder may experience hypoxemia, which is a condition characterized by low oxygen levels in the blood, or hypercapnia, which means too much carbon dioxide is retained in the body. Respiratory failure is typically classified into two types: Type I, which is hypoxemic respiratory failure, and Type II, known as hypercapnic respiratory failure. In Type I, problems such as ARDS and pneumonia are typical, and the lungs are unable to provide enough oxygen even though carbon dioxide levels are normal or close to normal. In Type II, the problem is insufficient ventilation, as seen in COPD and neuromuscular disorders, which leads to high carbon dioxide levels due to a reduced tidal volume or breathing rate. Respiratory failure affects more than just the process of gas exchange, as the correct classification helps determine the best way to manage the condition. When there is Type I respiratory failure, the main approach is to increase oxygen supply, which may involve extra oxygen or NIV. In Type II failure, the primary concern is managing carbon dioxide retention, and sometimes this necessitates the use of invasive mechanical ventilation. Understanding these classifications is crucial for enhancing patients' quality of life and overall well-being. It is also possible for patients to exhibit signs of both types, which makes it more challenging to diagnose and treat them. It is very important to use clinical signs, imaging, and biomarkers to assess and manage the condition accurately. New studies are shedding light on the understanding of respiratory failure and the underlying processes. For instance, BO, while not commonly classified under traditional respiratory failure, illustrates complexities in diagnostic criteria, affecting both obstructive and restrictive ventilatory patterns (King et al., 1989). Additionally, peptide patterns in BALF have shown promise in predicting outcomes in ALI and ARDS, demonstrating a relationship between inflammatory mediators and the severity of respiratory failure (Ben-David et al., 2011). As the reasons behind respiratory failure become better understood, the use of new diagnostic tools and biomarkers in clinical settings is crucial. This not only aids in classification but also informs targeted therapeutic strategies essential for improving patient care in the context of chronic respiratory disorders (Figure 15.17).

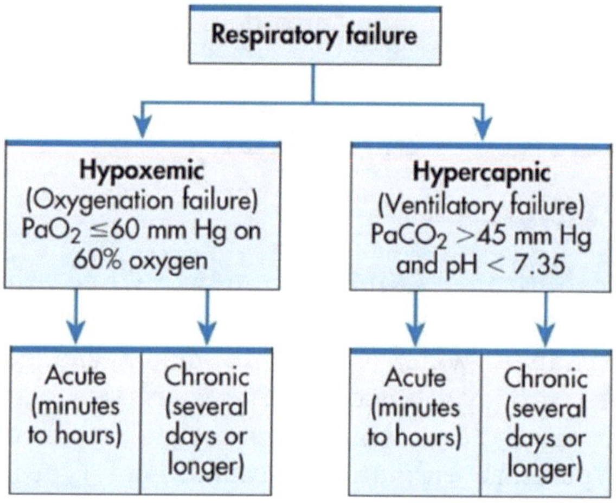

Figure 15.17. Classification of respiratory failure.

Source: https://image1.slideserve.com/3498844/classification-of-respiratory-failure-l.jpg.

15.5.2. Pathophysiology of Type I and Type II Respiratory Failure

Respiratory failure, which occurs when the lungs cannot meet the body's metabolic needs, presents in two main forms: Type I and Type II. Type I respiratory failure, which is hypoxemia without hypercapnia, usually happens due to problems with gas exchange at the alveolar-capillary membrane, including pulmonary edema, pneumonia, or ARDS. Under these conditions, the ventilation-perfusion (V/Q) mismatch results in inadequate oxygenation of the blood. As a result, organs do not receive enough oxygen, which can cause various organs to malfunction if not treated in a timely manner. The ability to assess pulmonary function through objective measures, such as ABGs, becomes crucial in distinguishing the type and severity of respiratory failure, guiding both diagnosis and subsequent management strategies (Cross et al., 2011). In contrast, Type II respiratory failure, also referred to as hypercapnic respiratory failure, is defined by an increase in carbon dioxide (CO_2) levels in the blood, accompanied often by hypoxemia. This kind of failure is usually because of ventilatory failure, when the body cannot get rid of CO_2 properly, often linked to COPD, asthma attacks, and neuromuscular problems. Decreased breathing, blockage of airways, or illnesses in the respiratory muscles can be part of the pathophysiology. In cases of severe hypercapnia, patients may experience confusion, lethargy, or potential coma, highlighting the importance of immediate and effective ventilatory support to restore normal CO_2 levels and improve gas exchange (Drasovean et al., 2023). Because there is much overlap between their symptoms, managing patients with both types of respiratory failure is often challenging. A combination of both types of respiratory failure can happen when someone has an acute worsening of a long-term lung disease or a very serious lung infection. Learning about the reasons for these failures supports treatment and increases the effectiveness of mechanical ventilation, which is important for managing both types. It is crucial to employ the correct ventilatory techniques, as each type of respiratory failure necessitates distinct settings to optimize oxygenation and ventilation. Clinicians must remain vigilant in monitoring their patient's conditions and adjusting therapies accordingly to prevent deterioration, underscoring the importance of a tailored approach to respiratory failure management (Cross et al., 2011) (Table 15.2).

Table 15.2. Types of Respiratory Failure

	Normal range	Respiratory failure			
		Type I (Hypoxaemic)	Type II (Hypercapnic)		
			Acute	Chronic	Acute on chronic
pH	7.35-7.45	Normal	< 7.35	Normal	< 7.35
PaO_2, mmHg	80-100	< 60	< 80	< 80	< 80
$PaCO_2$, mmHg	35-45	Normal	> 45	> 45	> 45
HCO_3,mM/L	22-28	Normal	Normal	> 28	> 28

Source: https://image.slideserve.com/960964/types-of-respiratory-failure1-l.jpg.

15.5.3. Clinical Implications and Management Strategies

To effectively manage respiratory illnesses, a customized approach should combine medical treatment with other complementary approaches. Bronchodilators and corticosteroids given by inhalation are key to easing symptoms and lowering the number of asthma or COPD attacks. Additionally, using PR can lead to a better quality of life for patients by enhancing their exercise capacity and respiratory function. The recent introduction of high-flow nasal therapy (HFNT) has expanded therapeutic options, especially in cases of acute respiratory failure. HFNT helps patients get more oxygen with less discomfort and better gas exchange. By promoting a multifaceted management strategy that includes patient education and lifestyle modifications, healthcare professionals can foster better adherence and ultimately improve outcomes in individuals suffering from these chronic diseases (Cortegiani et al., 2019). In addition, the effects of respiratory diseases can be seen both in the immediate care and in the long run, especially when patients have other conditions such as CVD or diabetes. COPD patients, for instance, frequently exhibit exacerbated responses to infections, as seen during the COVID-19 pandemic, making it essential to evaluate their risk profiles thoroughly (Awatade et al., 2023). If doctors monitor patients closely and detect early signs of an exacerbation, they can intervene promptly and prevent the disease from severely affecting the patient. Recent research shows that COPD patients are at a higher risk of being hospitalized during infections, which means doctors should create specific plans to monitor each patient. The goal is to help patients breathe more easily and support their overall health when they have other health issues. Proper ventilation remains crucial for treating severe lung conditions, including ARDS and respiratory failure. Knowing the principles of mechanical ventilation and the modes such as pressure-controlled and volume-controlled allows clinicians to tailor support for each patient. Selecting the most suitable adjunct therapies, such as sedation and neuromuscular blockade, is crucial for achieving effective ventilation and preventing complications. Regularly checking ABG results and lung function helps ensure the patient receives the correct ventilation. As advancements in technology prompt innovative approaches to ventilatory support, ensuring proficiency in these methods will be vital in enhancing recovery from serious respiratory events (Cortegiani et al., 2019). Every management plan should rely on the cooperation of a healthcare team to provide comprehensive care that meets patients' needs and is efficient with resources.

15.6. Interstitial Lung Disease (ILD)

ILD encompasses various disorders characterized by the presence of inflammatory cells and scarring in the lung tissue, which makes breathing and gas exchange more challenging. Because ILD can have many different causes and symptoms, it is essential to carefully classify them, which usually includes IPF, sarcoidosis, and ILDs related to connective tissue diseases. Inflammation and fibrosis are crucial steps in all forms of ILD, leading to lung damage and impairment. In radiology, these disorders usually show up as diffuse lung infiltrates, which can significantly reduce a patient's quality of life and how well they breathe. Because of the infections they are more likely to get, immunocompromised patients may experience more severe and confusing ILD symptoms.

It is essential to employ differential diagnosis in this group, as the treatment depends on distinguishing between infectious and non-infectious causes of lung infiltrates. An example is when graft-versus-host disease develops after hematopoietic stem cell transplantation, causing ILD due to an immune response, which makes the picture more confusing. It is essential to understand the connection between ILD and the immune system when developing treatments that support the lungs and manage the primary disease.

Doctors typically treat ILD by alleviating symptoms, slowing the progression of the disease, and managing any existing inflammation. In many cases where inflammation is a concern, conventional care often employs corticosteroids and immunosuppressive drugs. On the other hand, new therapies have emerged, such as antifibrotic agents, that target the fibrotic aspect of the disease. Clinicians should consider how the disease is affecting the patient and the patient's individual experience, as ILD can have various outcomes. As ongoing research continues to illuminate the complexities of ILD, a deeper understanding of its pathophysiology holds the promise of more effective interventions and improved patient care (Figure 15.18).

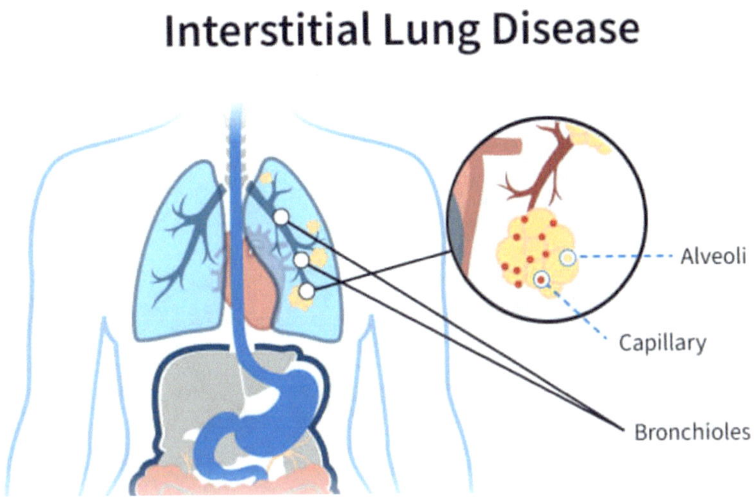

Figure 15.18. Interstitial lung disease.

15.6.1. Types of Interstitial Lung Diseases

ILDs comprise a heterogeneous group of pulmonary disorders, primarily characterized by inflammation and fibrosis of the lung interstitium. Such diseases typically result in impaired gas exchange and reduced lung function, which is often noticeable as dyspnea and cough. Of all ILDs, IPF is recognized for its severe outcomes and the progressive nature of its deterioration over time. IPF is characterized by a distinctive histopathological pattern known as usual interstitial pneumonia (UIP) and is especially prevalent in older adults. Sarcoidosis, which is an inflammatory condition that forms granulomas and ILDs linked to connective tissue diseases such as rheumatoid arthritis and systemic sclerosis, is another common ILD. Proper diagnosis and effective management require understanding the different types, as the treatment and outlook for each ILD can vary significantly. Genetic, environmental, and immune factors all work together to cause the pathophysiology of ILDs. Asbestos and silica are important factors in the development of asbestosis and silicosis, which are types of ILDs. It is also possible for certain medications to cause lung injury and clinicians must closely watch this. In ILDs, the inflammatory response typically involves numerous immune actions, including the attraction of inflammatory cells and the release of pro-fibrotic cytokines, which contribute to the formation of fibrotic tissue in the lungs. This causes the lungs to exchange gases less effectively, which is a significant reason for the main symptoms of these disorders. Because each ILD is address the distinct causes. Today, both symptom management and therapies that address the underlying causes of ILD are essential components of treatment. For example, IPF can be treated with antifibrotic drugs like nintedanib and pirfenidone which help slow the disease and improve how well the lungs function. Sometimes, sarcoidosis is treated with corticosteroids to reduce inflammation, primarily when the disease causes severe problems in the lungs or elsewhere in the body. If ILDs occur due to connective tissue disorders, it is essential to involve specialists from various fields to manage both the lung issues and the primary systemic condition. Additionally, emerging therapies, including immunomodulatory agents and biologics, offer new avenues for treatment, underscoring the need for ongoing research into the specific types of ILDs and their respective management protocols (Figure 15.19).

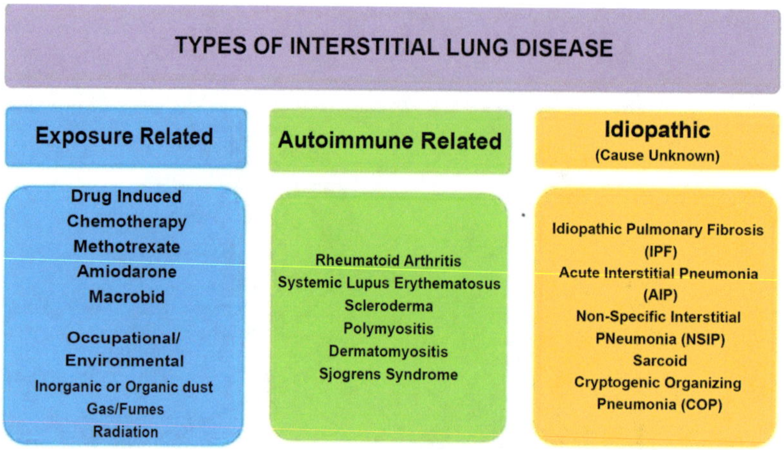

Figure 15.19. Interstitial lung diseases types.

Source: https://cdn-bejha.nitrocdn.com/kdUuIaPCsuCBPZpAHQVmXEokxbtoxcbd/assets/images/optimized/rev-598d290/respirehab.com/wp-content/uploads/2021/06/ILD-causes-interstitial-lung-disease-classification1.jpg.

15.6.2. Pathophysiological Changes in Lung Interstitium

The changes in the lung interstitium are essential for learning how respiratory disorders develop. The interstitium, which holds the lungs together, is made up of connective tissue and interstitial fluid that support the lung parenchyma. If someone has pulmonary fibrosis, this space between the air sacs is remodeled by collagen buildup and inflammation. Due to these changes, the interstitium becomes thicker, and this blocks the exchange of gases and reduces the lung's ability to expand. The stiffness in the lungs resulting from fibrosis can lead to restricted breathing patterns, a common occurrence in patients with ILDs. Therefore, it is essential to understand these changes in the body to develop treatments that can slow the progression of these disorders. The pathophysiology is further affected by the changes that occur in the small airways due to BO. The process causes the bronchiolar epithelium to thicken, resulting in excessive granulation tissue and tissue swelling between the air sacs. The fact that adjacent alveoli are involved indicates that interstitial changes and airway function are interconnected. BO can develop in various clinical scenarios, such as exposure to toxins and the presence of pre-existing systemic diseases. This may cause patients to show COPD-like symptoms, which makes it difficult to diagnose them. Due to these details, it is evident that understanding the relationship between the interstitium and airways is essential for a comprehensive understanding of respiratory diseases. Additionally, the effects of mechanical ventilation on lung tissue underscore the importance for clinicians to exercise caution when treating respiratory failure. Although mechanical ventilation is necessary to save lives, it may cause volutrauma and hyperoxia-related harm which can worsen the problems in the interstitium. Increased pressure inside the chest may cause changes in blood flow to the lungs, which can exacerbate interstitial edema and stiffen the lungs. When lung compliance decreases, the problems may worsen, making it more difficult to wean patients off ventilation. Balancing the therapeutic benefits of positive pressure ventilation (PPV) with the associated risks is crucial for optimal patient outcomes. Understanding the lung interstitium is important during mechanical ventilation, which points to the complexity of managing respiratory problems.

15.6.3. Clinical Presentation and Progression

The clinical presentation of common respiratory disorders often varies markedly among individuals, influenced by myriad factors, including age, sex, and underlying health conditions. Asthma and COPD patients typically report experiencing symptoms such as wheezing, difficulty breathing, and a persistent cough. Still, how severe and frequent the symptoms are may change depending on the environment, sticking to the prescribed plan, and any other health problems like obesity or anxiety. It appears that differences in sex and gender can significantly impact how respiratory conditions manifest and are experienced by patients. Some studies suggest that women with asthma may have a different set of symptoms and react differently to treatment because of the way hormones and social factors affect them. Most respiratory disorders tend to get worse in episodes, which can result in more health problems and, in some instances, death if not controlled. In asthma patients, acute exacerbations can occur due to viral infections or exposure to allergens, causing the airways to become overly sensitive and potentially requiring hospital care. Unlike other illnesses, COPD develops slowly, with lung function decreasing year by year, usually speeding up because of smoking or exposure to pollutants. Although there are differences, both conditions worsen over time, so regular checks and adjustments to treatment are necessary. Patients who have more than one diagnosis may exhibit a range of symptoms that make it difficult to treat and underscore the importance of treating them based on their individual needs. It is essential to understand how respiratory disorders manifest and progress to inform effective treatment and achieve better outcomes for patients. Clinicians need to consider both the physical and mental aspects that affect a patient, since anxiety and depression can make breathing problems worse and make it harder to manage the disease. Examples show that anxiety disorders are pervasive among those who have functional tic-like behaviors, highlighting how mental health and physical health can be closely connected. If healthcare providers consider both behavior and the environment, they can design more effective interventions. Taking this comprehensive approach helps precision medicine by addressing both the biology of respiratory diseases and the needs of each patient, which improves how care is delivered and makes patients happier.

15.7. Basics of Ventilatory Support

Ventilatory support is a cornerstone approach in managing various respiratory disorders, including COPD and ARDS. Being aware of the physiology behind ventilation helps choose and use the right support for patients. Mechanical ventilation is often used to help or replace breathing, making it easier for the patient to exchange gases. It is imperative when breathing on its own is not enough because of a disease or sudden event. Detailed guidelines are essential to help healthcare professionals determine when a patient requires ventilatory support, as each patient's needs are unique. The primary points in mechanical ventilation include settings, modes, and methods for monitoring the machine. Initially, the settings are typically adjusted to determine the tidal volume, respiratory rate, and oxygen level based on the patient's weight and medical needs. Literature points out that careful changes to these settings are necessary to ensure good oxygenation and to prevent VILI.

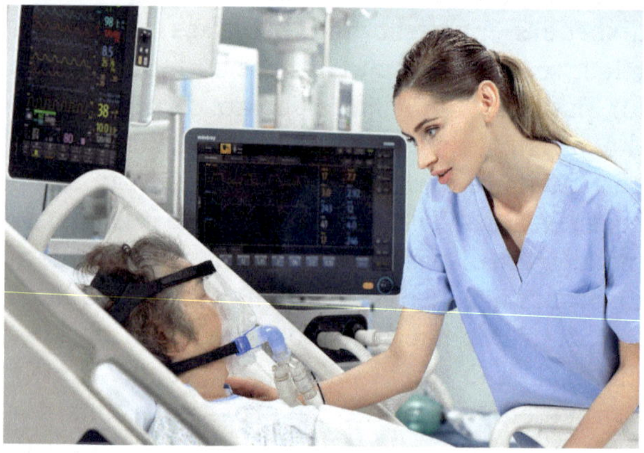

Figure 15.20. Clinical application of non-invasive ventilatory support in a patient with respiratory distress.

Source: https://scx2.b-cdn.net/gfx/news/hires/2020/ventilator.jpg.

The group's understanding enables healthcare providers to offer support tailored to each patient's specific needs. As the patient's condition evolves, the healthcare team must perform ongoing assessments to adjust ventilatory support effectively, incorporating findings from ABGs to guide therapeutic decisions and interventions (Drasovean et al., 2023). Incorporating both invasive and non-invasive modalities of ventilatory support can improve patient outcomes, particularly in cases of respiratory failure (Type I and II). The NIV is now recognized as an important method, as it helps patients feel more comfortable, reduces the risk of infection, and may prevent the need for endotracheal intubation. They mainly work by applying positive pressure to help tidal volume and oxygenation, without requiring invasive management of the airway. NIV can be helpful for many conditions, but it depends on how severe the patient's respiratory distress is and what health problem they have. Additionally, effective patient monitoring is crucial in ensuring that ventilatory support remains responsive to the dynamic nature of respiratory disorders, thereby facilitating the timely adjustment of treatment strategies (Cross et al., 2011) (Figure 15.20).

15.7.1. Overview of Ventilatory Support Methods

Various respiratory disorders are managed in critical care by using ventilatory support methods. They are generally grouped as invasive or non-invasive techniques. Mechanical ventilation is often given by inserting a tube through the mouth or nose into the trachea. It is often applied to patients who have severe trouble breathing, such as those with ARDS or when the airway is not adequately protected. Although invasive ventilation is effective, it can be risky, as it carries the risk of tracheal injury and infection. New studies suggest that selecting the right patients and procedures can reduce the risk of these complications. For example, weaning from mechanical ventilation can be monitored through different parameters, revealing essential insights about patient tolerance and recovery when using methods such as the T-tube or Expiratory Positive Airway Pressure (da Costa et al., 2009). NIV is used more often because it can help with respiratory failure without the need for intubation. NIV encompasses various modalities, including continuous positive airway pressure (CPAP) and BiPAP, which provide ventilatory support through a mask. This method has been effective in managing problems such as COPD, acute asthma attacks, and cardiogenic pulmonary edema. NIV brings more benefits than just avoiding intubation; it also provides patients with greater comfort and facilitates better collaboration between healthcare providers and patients. Moreover, NIV's flexibility makes it suitable for both acute and chronic respiratory failure in varied environments, ranging from ICUs to at-home management, significantly changing the landscape of respiratory support (Kumar et al., 2022). Several things are considered when deciding which ventilatory support method to use, such as the patient's condition, the reason for support, and their reaction to treatment.

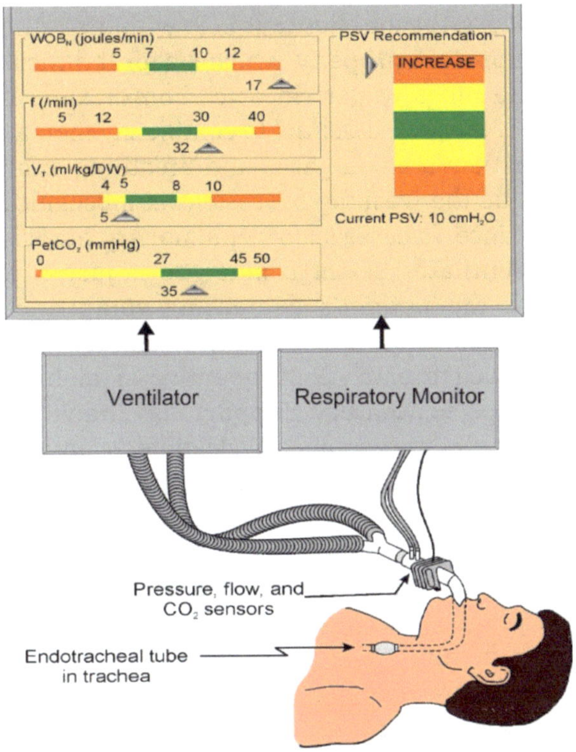

Figure 15.21. Open-loop pressure support ventilation advisory system.

Source: https://www.liebertpub.com/cms/10.4187/respcare.00656/asset/images/zrk0031154800001.jpg.

It is essential to establish optimal support to ensure oxygenation and ventilation, while minimizing the patient's effort required for breathing. For example, when weaning patients from machines, medical experts have examined Expiratory Positive Airway Pressure to determine its impact on breathing effort. In studies, evidence has indicated that while specific techniques, such as Expiratory Positive Airway Pressure, may increase the work of breathing, they do not necessarily induce significant cardiorespiratory changes compared to T-tube weaning methods (da Costa et al., 2009). Thus, understanding the nuances of each approach enables clinicians to implement care strategies that align with the unique needs of patients suffering from complex respiratory disorders, ultimately improving outcomes and recovery trajectories (Figure 15.21).

15.7.2. Indications for Mechanical Ventilation

The main reason for using mechanical ventilation on patients with respiratory disorders is severe failure of gas exchange. Many cases of COPD and ARDS result in respiratory failure, which may require the patient to be supported by a machine. Anyone who shows signs of hypoxemia and is not helped by extra oxygen or who has significant hypercapnia should be closely examined. It is imperative that respiratory rate supports gas exchange; if oral or non-invasive methods cannot keep oxygen levels steady or reduce carbon dioxide, the patient must be put on mechanical ventilation. This intervention not only aims to alleviate symptoms but also serves to prevent respiratory muscle fatigue and further compromise related to the underlying pathophysiology of the disorder, ensuring that the patient does not deteriorate further (Li et al., 2024). Assessing dyspnea is crucial in emergency situations to determine if mechanical ventilation is necessary. Since many people with acute dyspnea go to the emergency room, it is important to distinguish between cardiac and pulmonary issues quickly. Although standard methods have been used for this assessment, lung ultrasound is now a reliable tool in helping to determine if a person with dyspnea requires respiratory support. Non-invasive methods may provide temporary relief for some patients; however, in instances where respiratory failure is imminent or evident, immediate progression to mechanical ventilation is warranted (Santus et al., 2023). Because of this approach, patients get the proper care for their condition, which helps them recover better and reduces the chance of death. When deciding on mechanical ventilation, doctors also look at how the patient is likely to progress and what their outcome might be. Because asthma and pulmonary fibrosis worsen over time, doctors may need to monitor patients more closely and act promptly. Thoroughly checking ABGs and clinical signs helps healthcare providers choose the proper ventilatory support. Furthermore, understanding the multifactorial interplay between these conditions and their relationship with the lung microbiome, as suggested in recent literature, may influence therapeutic strategies (Li et al., 2024). Being an effective manager means spotting when intervention is necessary, anticipating issues that may arise, and providing the best care possible for each patient with a respiratory condition.

15.7.3. Complications and Considerations in Ventilatory Support

While ventilatory support is vital for dealing with respiratory failure and COPD or ARDS, it also has certain risks that must be considered. One significant complication is ventilator-associated pneumonia (VAP), which can develop in patients requiring prolonged mechanical ventilation. The usual cause of VAP is bacteria in the upper airways, which can move to the lungs because the body's defense mechanisms are weakened and invasive equipment is present. The threat of VAP emphasizes the importance of maintaining proper sedation, using clean procedures, and positioning patients to facilitate breathing and reduce the risk of aspiration. Additionally, prolonged use of mechanical ventilation can lead to VILI, a condition resulting from barotrauma or volutrauma caused by the high pressures and volumes applied to the lungs. The cumulative impact of these complications underscores the importance of meticulous monitoring and the implementation of evidence-based protocols in ventilatory management (Bogun et al., 2017). In addition to infections and lung injury, various changes in the body can occur during ventilatory support, making patient outcomes more challenging. Hypercapnia and acidosis may occur if the ventilation setup does not match the patient's specific condition and the way their lungs function. In many cases of obstructive disorders, the muscles that help with breathing may not work properly, which makes it difficult for the lungs to get rid of carbon dioxide. In light of this, it is essential to continually monitor the patient's blood gases and breathing effort to guide the weaning process from mechanical assistance. In cases such as pulmonary fibrosis, the ventilator settings must be adjusted to match the patient's decreasing compliance, which can affect the amount of air delivered with each breath. Consequently, an inability to adapt ventilatory support for individual pathologies may create a cycle of deterioration, underscoring the intricate relationship between ventilatory support and underlying lung pathophysiology (King et al., 1989). Long-term use of a ventilator can have important effects on a patient's psychological and physical health, which in turn affect their recovery and well-being. Many people on a ventilator for a long time often suffer from anxiety and depression, which can be made worse by being isolated and uncomfortable in the ICU. Sometimes, giving patients continuous sedation is important, but it may cause psychological issues that make it harder for them to recover. So, reducing sedation, having regular psychiatric reviews, and including family can create a better environment for the patient. Additionally, when patients are on mechanical ventilation, their muscles can weaken, a condition known as ventilator-induced diaphragm dysfunction, which can make it difficult for them to breathe independently. This multifaceted relationship between the physical and psychological aspects of ventilatory support underscores the need for a holistic approach, ensuring that both the physiological and emotional well-being of patients are prioritized throughout their care (Bogun et al., 2017).

SUMMARY

The way chronic COPD, asthma, ARDS, pulmonary fibrosis, and respiratory failure affect the lungs points out the need for careful and detailed understanding of lung function. Because each condition is different, it causes airflow problems, inflammation, and changes in the lung, so the treatment must be adjusted accordingly. The involvement of factors like environmental toxins and previous health problems makes it more challenging to control these disorders. This complexity is accentuated when considering the impact of concurrent respiratory threats like COVID-19, which poses heightened risks for individuals with COPD, as evidenced by recent studies indicating that COPD patients may experience worse outcomes from COVID-19 (Awatade et al., 2023). Additionally, having a good understanding of the changes in the body and diseases associated with these respiratory disorders helps doctors and public health officials. For example, understanding how airways become sensitive in asthma enables doctors to use bronchodilators and anti-inflammatory drugs effectively. In the same way, understanding the scarring in pulmonary fibrosis points to the need for early diagnosis and the chance for actions that may slow the progression of the disease. The intricate relationship between respiratory conditions and comorbidities underscores the need for ongoing research, enabling healthcare providers to develop comprehensive management plans that account for both immediate and long-term health implications for affected populations (Grobler et al., 2012). In the end, better understanding of pathophysiology will improve the way ventilatory support systems are used to treat respiratory failure. NIV is beneficial but should be adjusted to fit each person's specific condition. Because the field of respiratory health is constantly evolving, particularly with the emergence of new global health issues, it is crucial to make concerted efforts to support individuals with these conditions. In short, examining respiratory disorders in an integrated manner benefits healthcare and underscores the importance of ongoing research and public health efforts to address their issues and associated risks. It is essential to understand the causes of common respiratory disorders to manage and diagnose them well. Obstruction and inflammation of the airways are significant features of COPD and asthma. COPD is primarily caused by breathing in irritating gases or particles over years, leading to airflow problems. In contrast, asthma is usually caused by a combination of genetic and environmental factors. Conditions such as these involve excessive mucus, changes in the airways, and higher airway resistance, all of which lead to poor gas exchange. Spirometry and other tests allow doctors to assess lung function, which helps them tell the difference between obstructive and restrictive diseases and choose the proper treatment for each patient. ARDS and pulmonary fibrosis are significant conditions that make hospital treatment very challenging. ARDS develops rapidly and causes severe breathing problems because the alveolar-capillary membrane is damaged, leading to increased fluid in the lungs. Ventilatory support is necessary, mainly to prevent VILI. In another way, pulmonary fibrosis is a collection of ILDs that causes scarring in the lungs over time, which leads to reduced lung function. Recent studies have underscored the importance of assessing respiratory mechanics, emphasizing that traditional measurements of lung volume may not adequately reflect disease progression, particularly in ILD contexts, which highlights the need for non-invasive assessment techniques (Johnson et al., 2006). Moreover, respiratory failure, classified into Type I (hypoxemic) and Type II (hypercapnic) failure, further complicates the management of respiratory disorders. A Type I failure happens when there is not enough oxygen, and this is common in pneumonia and ARDS, whereas a Type II failure is marked by insufficient ventilation, which is usually seen in exacerbations of COPD. Effective ventilatory support strategies, including NIV modes and mechanical ventilation when required, play a pivotal role in stabilizing these patients (Drasovean et al., 2023).

CLOSER LOOK

BRONCHIOLITIS OBLITERANS

BO is a disease that results in obstruction of the smallest airways of the lungs (bronchioles) due to inflammation. Symptoms include a dry cough, shortness of breath, wheezing, and feeling tired. These symptoms typically worsen over several weeks to months. It is not related to cryptogenic organizing pneumonia, previously known as BO organizing pneumonia (Figure 15.22).

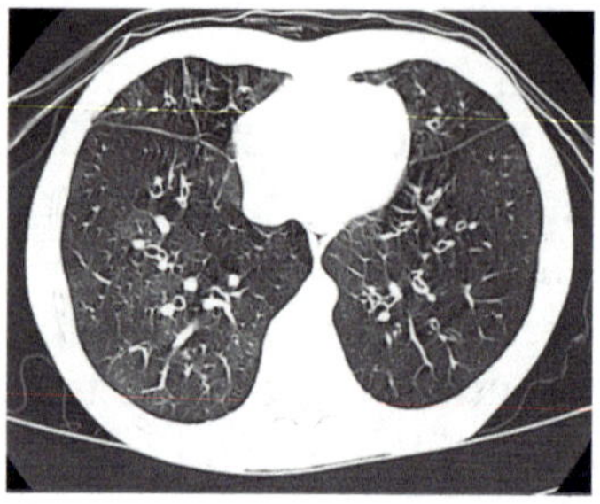

Figure 15.22. High-resolution computed tomography (HRCT) scan showing characteristic features of bronchiolitis obliterans (BO).

Source: https://upload.wikimedia.org/wikipedia/commons/thumb/a/ab/CTBO.png/800px-CTBO.png.

Causes include breathing in toxic fumes, respiratory infections, connective tissue disorder or complications following a bone marrow or heart-lung transplant. Symptoms may not occur until two to eight weeks following toxic exposure or infection. The underlying mechanism involves inflammation that results in scar tissue formation. Diagnosis is by CT scan, PFTs, or lung biopsy. A chest X-ray is often normal.

- **Signs and Symptoms:** BO results in worsening shortness of breath, wheezing, and a dry cough. The symptoms can start gradually, or severe symptoms can occur suddenly. These symptoms represent an obstructive pattern that is non-reversible with bronchodilator therapy, and need to be related to various lung insults. These insults include inhalation damage, post-transplant auto-immune injury, post-infectious disease, drug reactions, and several auto-immune diseases.
- **Cause:** BO has many possible causes, including collagen vascular disease, transplant rejection in organ transplant patients, viral infection (adenovirus, respiratory syncytial virus, influenza, HIV, cytomegalovirus), Stevens–Johnson syndrome, Pneumocystis pneumonia, drug reaction, aspiration, and complications of prematurity (bronchopulmonary dysplasia), and exposure to toxic fumes. Toxins believed to cause the condition are diacetyl, sulfur dioxide, nitrogen dioxide, ammonia, chlorine, thionyl chloride, methyl isocyanate, hydrogen fluoride, hydrogen bromide, hydrogen chloride, hydrogen sulfide, phosgene, polyamide-amine dyes, mustard gas, and ozone. It may also appear in people with IBD, systemic lupus erythematosus, juvenile idiopathic arthritis, rheumatoid arthritis, GERD, IgA nephropathy,

and ataxia telangiectasia. Aspirating activated charcoal can result in pneumonia. Eating large amounts of the vegetable *Sauropus androgynus,* which contains papaverine, is the reason. Additionally, the disorder may be idiopathic (without a known cause).

- **Mechanism:** The primary process is damage and inflammation to epithelial and sub-epithelial cells. The cells are no longer able to repair the tissue, and they especially cannot regenerate the outer layer, which results in too many cells forming and causing scarring. Many pathways of the disease have been identified, such as those involving fibrosis, lymphocytes, and antibodies. However, despite the different causes, the outcome is always injury and inflammation that lead to scarring in the lung tissue. The damaged tissue makes it more challenging to breathe out, and so air is not pushed out of the lungs. This is termed "air-trapping," which can be seen on medical imaging. Since there is permanent scarring, the disease usually stays the same or gets worse, and the cause can sometimes result in death.
- **Diagnosis:** BO is often diagnosed based on the symptoms of obstructive lung disease following lung injury. The definitive diagnosis is through biopsy, but due to the variable distribution of lesions, leading to falsely negative tests, and the invasive nature of this procedure, it is often not performed. Several tests are often needed to diagnose BO, including spirometry, diffusing capacity of the lung tests (DLCO), lung volume tests, chest X-rays, high-resolution CT (HRCT), and lung biopsy.
- **Prevention:** Stopping BO in people after lung transplant or HSCT is mainly done by using immunosuppression. The usual treatment after a lung transplant is to use a calcineurin inhibitor, a purine synthesis inhibitor, and a glucocorticoid. To determine if lung function is decreasing over time, people undergo a standard post-transplant lung function test. Most people following HSCT continue to use methotrexate and a calcineurin inhibitor to help prevent GVHD, which is a possible cause of BO.
- **Treatment:** The disease cannot be cured, but treatments can help stop it from getting worse. This may include the use of corticosteroids or immunosuppressive medication, which may affect the ability to receive a lung transplant if offered. If patients have difficulty breathing (hypoxemia), oxygen can be supplemented. Patients with chronic lung disease should get routine vaccinations to help avoid the complications of infections from pneumonia and influenza.

REFERENCES

1. Awatade, N., Wark, P., Chan, A., Mamun, S., Esa, N. M., Matsunaga, K., Rhee, C., Hansbro, P., & Sohal, S. (2023). The Complex Association between COPD and COVID-19. *Journal of Clinical Medicine, 12*(11), 3791. https://doi.org/10.3390/jcm12113791Azimi, S., Sahebnasagh, A., Sharifnia, H., & Najmeddin, F. (2020). Corticosteroids administration following COVID-19-induced acute respiratory distress syndrome: Is it harmful or life-saving? *4*, 43. https://www.semanticscholar.org/paper/28b34f8f4042566ae2508689305615347 30adf88 (accessed on 31st May 2025).

2. Baloch, N. U. A., Janahi, I. A., & Rehman, A. (2017). *Corticosteroids and Their Use in Respiratory Disorders.* https://core.ac.uk/download/322433793.pdf (accessed on 31st May 2025).

3. Bals, R., Becker, A. P., Danziger, G., Kamphorst, A., et al. (2022). Respiratory physiology of COVID-19 and influenza associated acute respiratory distress syndrome. J. Clin. Med. https://core.ac.uk/download/543579338.pdf (accessed on 31st May 2025).

4. Ben-David, A., Gamez-Pozo, A., Plymoth, A., Rose, A. S., Leroy, B., Schölkopf, B., De Torre, C., et al. (2011). Outcome prediction in pneumonia-induced ALI/ARDS by clinical features and peptide patterns of BALF determined by mass spectrometry. *PLoS ONE.* https://core.ac.uk/download/pdf/8623507.pdf (accessed on 31st May 2025).

5. Bogun, L., Brynza, M., Bychkova, O., Lysenko, T., et al. (2017). *Respiratory Failure & Cor Pulmonale.* https://core.ac.uk/download/144471261.pdf (accessed on 31st May 2025).

6. Cagnone, M., Chiarelli, L., Iadarola, P., Salvini, A., et al. (2018). The role of one- and two-dimensional electrophoretic techniques in proteomics of the lung. Electrophoresis – Life Sciences Practical Applications. https://core.ac.uk/download/322435800.pdf (accessed on 31st May 2025).

7. Calzetta, L., Cazzola, M., Matera, M. G., & Rogliani, P. (2020). *Pharmacological Management of COVID-19 Patients with ARDS (CARDS): A Narrative Review.* https://core.ac.uk/download/521224224.pdf (accessed on 31st May 2025).

8. Candemir, I. (2017). Advances in pulmonary rehabilitation for chronic obstructive pulmonary disease and associated conditions. *COPD – An Update in Pathogenesis and Clinical Management.* https://core.ac.uk/download/322433659.pdf (accessed on 31st May 2025).

9. Caudrillier, A., Coxon, A., Hochreiter-Hufford, A., McColl, A., Mulla, A., Rossi, A. G., Reis, A. C., et al. (2016). *Key Mechanisms Governing Resolution of Lung Inflammation.* https://core.ac.uk/download/322478305.pdf (accessed on 31st May 2025).

10. Cortegiani, A., Gregoretti, C., & Spoletini, G. (2019). Physiopathological rationale of using high-flow nasal therapy in the acute and chronic setting: A narrative review. Trends in Anesthesia and Critical Care. https://core.ac.uk/download/224993362.pdf (accessed on 31st May 2025).

11. Cross, M. (2011). *Occupational Respiratory Health Surveillance at Minara Resources, Murrin Murrin Mine Site.* https://core.ac.uk/download/41531903.pdf (accessed on 31st May 2025).

12. Da Costa, A. D., De Mello, R. M., & Vieira, S. R. R. (2009). Short-term effects of positive expiratory airway pressure in patients being weaned from mechanical ventilation. *Clinics.* https://core.ac.uk/download/pdf/8295365.pdf (accessed on 31st May 2025).

13. Drasovean, Y. (2023). *Breathe Easy: RT Student Resource for Mechanical Ventilation.* https://core.ac.uk/download/622362223.pdf (accessed on 31st May 2025).

14. Emiralioğlu, N., Karadoğan, D., Kızılırmak, D., Polat Yuluğ, E., et al. (2022). Turkish Thoracic Society Early Career Members Task Force Group's virtual congress notes: European Respiratory Society International Congress 2020. *Turk. Thorac. J.* https://core.ac.uk/download/553297700.pdf (accessed on 31st May 2025).

15. Falkenström, F., Granstrom, F., & Holmqvist, R. (2010). *Mechanical Ventilation*. https://core.ac.uk/download/pdf/35276663.pdf (accessed on 31st May 2025).

16. Ghahremani, M. H., Hajibabayee, M., Khajavi, M. R., Mandegari, M., et al. (2009). The role of glutathione-S-transferase polymorphisms on clinical outcome of ALI/ARDS patient treated with N-acetylcysteine. *Respir Med.* https://core.ac.uk/download/pdf/82646260.pdf (accessed on 31st May 2025).

17. Grobler, C., Maree, D. M., & Irusen, E. M. (2012). *Functional Evaluation in Respiratory Disorders.* https://core.ac.uk/download/322408718.pdf (accessed on 31st May 2025).

18. Humbert, M., Kovács, G., Hoeper, M. M., Badagliacca, R., Berger, R. M. F., Brida, M., Carlsen, J., et al. (2022). 2022 ESC/ERS guidelines for the diagnosis and treatment of pulmonary hypertension. *European Respiratory Journal, 61*, 2200879. https://doi.org/10.1183/13993003.00879-2022 (accessed on 31st May 2025).

19. Husebø, G. R. (2021). Systemic inflammatory markers as predictors of longitudinal outcomes in COPD: Results from the Bergen COPD Cohort Study. https://core.ac.uk/download/479093834.pdf (accessed on 31st May 2025).

20. King, T. E. (1989). *Bronchiolitis Obliterans*. https://core.ac.uk/download/323073306.pdf (accessed on 31st May 2025).

21. Kumar, S., Talwar, D., & Talwar, D. (2022). *Non-Invasive Ventilation in Acute Hypoxemic Respiratory Failure.* https://core.ac.uk/download/492703930.pdf (accessed on 31st May 2025).

22. Lee, J., Jang, J. Y., Park, S. M., & Yang, S. R. (2021). An update on the role of Nrf2 in respiratory disease: Molecular mechanisms and therapeutic approaches. *International Journal of Molecular Sciences, 22*. https://www.semanticscholar.org/paper/2e98939dae2b19a36cac0d9b67a1425ecd935ee2 (accessed on 31st May 2025).

23. Li, R., Li, J., & Zhou, X. (2024). Lung microbiome: New insights into the pathogenesis of respiratory diseases. *Signal Transduction and Targeted Therapy, 9*. https://doi.org/10.1038/s41392-023-01722-y (accessed on 31st May 2025).

24. Navarra, S., Congedo, M., & Pennisi, M. (2020). Indications for non-invasive ventilation in respiratory failure. *Reviews on Recent Clinical Trials*. https://www.semanticscholar.org/paper/8d0541bfd01234728d356ea9aae77be16fe91a26 (accessed on 31st May 2025).

25. Rudd, K. E., Johnson, S. C., Agesa, K. M., Shackelford, K. A., Tsoi, D., Kievlan, D., Colombara, D. V., et al. (2020). Global, regional, and national sepsis incidence and mortality, 1990–2017: Analysis for the Global Burden of Disease Study. *The Lancet, 395*, 200–211. https://doi.org/10.1016/s0140-6736(19)32989-7 (accessed on 31st May 2025).

26. Santus, P., Radovanovic, D., Saad, M., Zilianti, C., Coppola, S., Chiumello, D., & Pecchiari, M. (2023). Acute dyspnea in the emergency department: A clinical review. *Internal and Emergency Medicine, 18*, 1491–1507. https://doi.org/10.1007/s11739-023-03322-8 (accessed on 31st May 2025).

INDEX

C

D

E

F

P

R

S

T